PERINATAL
MEDICINE

Hugh E. Evans, M.D.

PROFESSOR OF PEDIATRICS, STATE UNIVERSITY OF NEW YORK,
DOWNSTATE MEDICAL CENTER; DIRECTOR, PEDIATRICS, JEWISH
HOSPITAL AND MEDICAL CENTER OF BROOKLYN, BROOKLYN, NEW YORK

Leonard Glass, M.D.

ASSOCIATE PROFESSOR OF PEDIATRICS, STATE UNIVERSITY
OF NEW YORK, DOWNSTATE MEDICAL CENTER; ASSOCIATE DIRECTOR,
PEDIATRICS, JEWISH HOSPITAL AND MEDICAL CENTER OF BROOKLYN,
BROOKLYN, NEW YORK

With illustrations by Ingram Chodorow

PERINATAL
MEDICINE

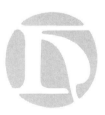

MEDICAL DEPARTMENT
HARPER AND ROW, PUBLISHERS
HAGERSTOWN, MARYLAND
NEW YORK, SAN FRANCISCO, LONDON

Library of Congress Cataloging in Publication Data
Evans, Hugh E   1934–
    Perinatal medicine.
    Includes bibliographies and index.
    1. Infants (Newborn)—Physiology. 2. Infants (Newborn)—Diseases. 3. Fetus—Diseases. 4. Pregnancy, Complications of. I. Glass, Leonard, 1933–   joint author. II. Title [DNLM: 1. Fetal diseases. 2. Infant, Newborn, Diseases. WS420 P445]
RJ254.E9   618.9′201   75–23391
ISBN 0–06–140791–7

Contents

Contributors

WALTER E. BERDON, M.D., F.A.C.R., F.A.A.P.

CHAPTER 24

Professor and Associate Director, Pediatric Radiology, Columbia University College of Physicians and Surgeons, Columbia-Presbyterian Medical Center, New York, New York

SANFORD N. COHEN, M.D.

CHAPTER 21

Professor and Chairman, Department of Pediatrics, Wayne State University School of Medicine; Pediatrician-in-Chief, Children's Hospital of Michigan, Detroit, Michigan

HUGH E. EVANS, M.D.

CHAPTERS 1, 2, 3, 4, 5, 6, 8, 9, 10, 11, 12, 13, 15, 16, 17, 18, 19, 20, 22

Professor of Pediatrics, State University of New York, Downstate Medical Center; Director, Pediatrics, Jewish Hospital and Medical Center of Brooklyn, Brooklyn, New York

DAVID L. FRANK, M.D.

CHAPTER 2

Staff Radiologist, Department of Radiology, John T. Mather Memorial Hospital, Port Jefferson, New York

JOSEPH H. GALICICH, M.D.

CHAPTER 23

Chief of Neurosurgery, Department of Surgery, Memorial Hospital; Associate Professor, Department of Surgery, Cornell University Medical College, New York, New York

SARASWATHY K. GANAPATHY, M.D.

CHAPTER 21

Assistant Professor of Pediatrics, New York University School of Medicine; Attending Neonatologist, Pediatrics, Bellevue Hospital, New York, New York; Director of Nurseries, Pediatrics, Booth Memorial Medical Center, Flushing, New York

WELTON M. GERSONY, M.D.

CHAPTERS 7, 22

Professor of Pediatrics and Director, Division of Pediatric Cardiology, College of Physicians and Surgeons of Columbia University, Babies Hospital, Columbia-Presbyterian Medical Center, New York, New York

MELVIN GERTNER, M.D.

CHAPTER 14

Assistant Professor, Pediatrics, Mount Sinai School of Medicine of the City University of New York, New York; Associate Director of Pediatrics, City Hospital Center at Elmhurst, Elmhurst, New York

LEONARD GLASS, M.D.

CHAPTERS 1, 2, 3, 4, 5, 6, 8, 9, 10, 11, 12, 13, 15, 16, 17, 18, 19, 20, 22

Associate Professor of Pediatrics, State University of New York, Downstate Medical Center; Associate Director, Pediatrics, Jewish Hospital and Medical Center of Brooklyn, Brooklyn, New York

S. FRANK REDO, M.D.

CHAPTER 23

Professor of Surgery, Cornell University Medical College; Attending Surgeon in Charge of Pediatric Surgery, The New York Hospital-Cornell Medical Center, New York, New York

CARL N. STEEG, M.D.

CHAPTERS 7, 22

Associate Professor of Clinical Pediatrics, College of Physicians and Surgeons of Columbia University; Director, Pediatric Cardiovascular Laboratory, Columbia-Presbyterian Medical Center, New York, New York

DAN J. TENNENHOUSE, M.D., J.D., F.C.L.M.

CHAPTER 25

Lecturer in Legal Medicine, Division of Ambulatory and Community Medicine, School of Medicine, University of California; Lecturer in Nursing Law, Department of Biodysfunction, School of Nursing, University of California, San Francisco; Adjunct Professor of Medical Law, School of Law, University of San Francisco, San Francisco; Assistant Professor of Medical Law, Hastings College of the Law, University of California; Associate Physician, Student Health Services, University of California Medical Center, San Francisco; Lecturer in Medical Law, University of California School of Law (Boalt Hall), Berkeley, California

Preface

The field of perinatal medicine has grown phenomenally in the past decade. Basic and clinical sciences have together enhanced diagnostic acumen and therapeutic efficacy in management of the fetus and the newborn infant. The results have led to a gratifying decrease in perinatal mortality and an increase in the number of neurologically intact survivors of severe perinatal illness. Progress is exemplified by such diagnostic procedures as amniocentesis, sonography, and fetal heart rate monitoring and such therapeutic developments as prevention of Rh isoimmunization, continuous distending airway pressure, and total parenteral alimentation.

PERINATAL MEDICINE brings together under one cover all aspects of fetal and neonatal medicine. Basic science and clinical information are presented, with stress on the latter. Each organ system and major disorder is introduced with embryologic and physiologic or biochemical background followed by differential diagnosis, methods of diagnostic evaluation, and current therapeutic modalities.

Many unresolved controversial areas are included here: problems of abortion, regionalization of care, cost factors, medicolegal and ethical concerns, fetal research, and interdisciplinary relationships. The efficacy and safety of certain therapeutic regimens, such as phototherapy, are still uncertain. PERINATAL MEDICINE presents controversial subjects as such, and varying opinions are discussed. Differences of opinion and interpretation, produced by the book's multiple authorship, are occasionally encountered in the text.

This volume is designed for both the student and the physician in practice. Extensive basic information in the areas of immunology, physiology, and biochemistry has been selected because of its relevance to clinical problems; this will provide more complete understanding of each problem for medical students, students in nursing and social work, and other professionals at all levels of training. The inclusion of practical information on each area of discussion will make this an exhaustive reference source for pediatric and obstetric house officers, pediatric practitioners, nurses, administrators, and public health authorities.

Of special interest is a section devoted to signs of illness in the newborn infant; a brief differential diagnosis emphasizes those conditions most frequently encountered and those which are amenable to therapy. A portion of the book discusses maternal disorders which may affect normal fetal development. Both normal and abnormal fetal growth and development are covered, together with the most recent methods of fetal diagnosis. The transition from fetal to neonatal life is considered.

The surgical chapter provides considerable information on operative technique and postoperative care. Other special sections deal with genetics, cardiology, pharmacology, radiology, and nursing. Devotion of an entire chapter to medicolegal problems is indicative of their growing importance. An extensive bibliography following each chapter will facilitate further reading.

It is hoped that this book will be helpful in dealing with emergency situations and day-to-day management of problems and in answering questions in detail about major disorders. For the sake of brevity, presentation of specific case material has been avoided.

H.E.E.
L.G.

Acknowledgments

The publication of this book would not have been possible without the support received by us over the past years.

We would like to pay special tribute to our wives, Ruth and Edith, and our children, without whose patience, loyalty, and understanding the book could not have been brought to fruition.

Recognition must be given to many of our mentors and colleagues who have guided us and who continue to be a source of inspiration. Among these are Mary Ellen Avery, Richard E. Behrman, Charles D. Cook, Robert E. Cooke, Edward C. Curnen, Jr., Richard L. Day, Horace L. Hodes, L. Stanley James, Eric J. Kahn, Vernon Knight, Doris Milman, William Nyhan, Jean Pakter, Sophie Pierog, Joseph B. Pincus, Morton Schiffer, William A. Silverman and Robert W. Winters.

Special acknowledgment must also be accorded Dr. Michael Levi who helped to initiate and lay the ground work for this book in its conceptual stages.

We express our gratitude to the Board of Trustees and the administration of the Jewish Hospital and Medical Center of Brooklyn, who have devoted considerable time and effort to the Department of Pediatrics and especially to the Neonatal Intensive Care Unit. Particularly helpful in this regard are Mrs. Sylvia Lowenstein, Mr. Max Koeppel, Mr. Martin Newman, Mr. Irving Baldinger, and Mr. Philip C. Abrams.

Preparation of the manuscript was greatly enhanced by the efforts of Mrs. Barbara Dabrowski, Miss Michele Gertner, Mrs. Susan Rinehart Weckesser, and Miss Marcia Kass.

H.E.E.
L.G.

PERINATAL

MEDICINE

1

Intensive Care

The most hazardous time in an infant's life is the perinatal period: the days immediately before and 28 days after birth. Rarely is the threat of death or irreversible central nervous system (CNS) damage as great. For those babies who survive, over seven decades of life may be anticipated.

Until the last decade of the nineteenth century, care of newborn infants was provided by midwives and other nonmedical personnel. At this time Budin recognized that incubator care was associated with improved survival of premature infants.

One of Budin's pupils, Martin Couney, introduced his ideas about premature infant care into the United States. From the early years of the twentieth century through the New York World's Fair of 1939–40, Couney exhibited premature infants in incubators at fairs and expositions throughout the United States. Although Couney was basically a showman, he employed well-qualified nurses and physicians to care for his patients.

His advances in incubator design and infant feeding enhanced the care of premature infants, and his influence on Dr. Julius Hess led, in 1922, to the establishment of a station for premature infants at Sarah Morris Hospital, the first of its kind in the United States. As Hess's program developed, an ambulance service was organized to transport premature infants born elsewhere in the city to his nursery. A specialized nursing service under Miss Evelyn Lundeen was established, as well as the first outpatient clinic for premature infants who had survived the neonatal period.

In the early 1930s most hospitals in the United States lacked special facilities for premature infants. In 1934 the Chicago City Health Department established a citywide plan for care of premature infants, and by 1940 a substantial decline in the premature infant mortality rate was noted.

In 1938 the New York City Department of Health initiated a citywide program directed toward improved hospital care of premature infants and in 1948 initiated a Premature Transport Service. Premature Centers were established throughout the city, and premature infants were transported to these centers in heated carriers under the care of specially trained nurses.

During the late 1930s and 1940s, many other municipal and statewide programs for premature infants were established throughout the United States. However, it was not until the late 1950s that the policy of active intervention in the care of the neonate, regardless of birth weight, became widespread. By the early 1960s assisted ventilation, umbilical arterial catheterization and the use of monitoring equipment had become general. By the mid- and late 1960s the effect of prenatal events on psychomotor development was recognized (5). Diagnostic techniques such as measurement of maternal urinary estriol levels, sonography, fetal electrocardiography and scalp blood sampling, which could evaluate fetal status, were developed. Amniocentesis was introduced as a diagnostic tool, and erythroblastosis fetalis was being treated by intrauterine transfusion. Techniques for evaluation and treatment of the sick newborn infant while en route from one hospital to another were developed. With this proliferation of knowledge and technology "neonatal intensive care units" developed rapidly in the late 1960s and early 1970s, and a new pediatric subspeciality, perinatal medicine, was established.

Many of the accomplishments in this discipline reflect application of knowledge and procedures originally used in other age groups. Advances in antibiotic therapy, anesthesiology, immunology, surgical techniques, blood bank procedures, biochemistry and physiology have all provided the keystones of contemporary practice in perinatal medicine.

REGIONALIZATION OF PERINATAL CARE

In the mid 1970s advanced technology and well-trained personnel led to improved perinatal survival and a decrease in impaired psychomotor development among high-risk neonates (1, 3, 6, 7, 9–12, 15–17, 20, 22). In order to gain maximum advantage for all newborn infants, the concept of regionalization of care for selected patients has been advocated. Under this system women with high-risk pregnancies are referred to designated centers with facilities for management of gestation, parturition and the newborn infant. Such concentration of effort has economic as well as medical advantages. Data from many areas of the United States and Canada with regionalized perinatal care show improved neonatal survival rates.

In cases in which unrecognized high-risk pregnancy results in the birth of a compromised infant, transport services are available to bring the patient rapidly and safely to the appropriate center. Regionalization may have certain disadvantages (7). It can be argued that a concentration of expertise at a limited number of centers weakens the quality of obstetric and neonatal care available at most hospitals. Since up to 50% of neonatal problems may follow a normal pregnancy, all hospitals with obstetric services must be able to diagnose and treat life-threatening conditions (e.g., neonatal asphyxia, hemorrhage and pneumothorax)

that may appear unexpectedly postpartum. Too, many general hospitals will be able to manage such relatively noncomplicated problems as neonatal jaundice, nondistressed large premature infants and many infections. Transport of infants to regional centers may be limited to the most seriously ill infants (such as those requiring assisted ventilation or major operative intervention).

Clearly, there is no universally appropriate formula for regionalization programs. Each area must balance the advantages of establishing these centers against the need for strong obstetric and pediatric services at numerous general hospitals.

Future social and political considerations may also have an effect on planning for regionalization. The acceptance of birth control methods, the legalization of abortion, population shifts and changes in economic conditions may all change the number of both total and high-risk pregnancies and neonatal complications in a particular region. Another consideration concerns future development of techniques that will facilitate identification of high-risk pregnancies and prevention of perinatal illness. If simplified, efficient techniques can be easily performed at most general hospitals, the need for regional centers may diminish.

In any event, maximum cooperation among members of the medical profession as well as between the profession and governmental health planning agencies is required for optimal delivery of perinatal care.

NEONATES REQUIRING SPECIAL CARE

Every newborn infant must be regarded as a potentially high-risk patient during the first 24 to 48 hours of life. Many, however, because of maternal history, adverse gestation or compromised clinical condition at birth are especially in peril.

The great majority of neonates are in no immediate distress and can be cared for in an admission or transitional care nursery immediately postpartum (4). Following careful observation for as long as 24 hours, most infants can be transferred to the normal full-term nursery. If problems arise,

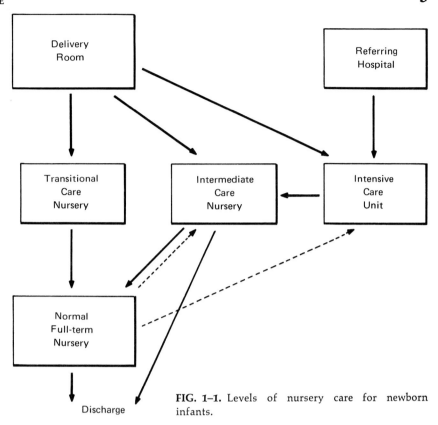

FIG. 1–1. Levels of nursery care for newborn infants.

transfer can be made to an intermediate or intensive care nursery, depending on the severity of the illness.

Those infants who demonstrate severe illness immediately postpartum require intensive medical care (Fig. 1–1). Although all hospitals with obstetric services should be able to provide emergency treatment to severely compromised infants immediately following birth, definitive care can be supplied only if facilities at the hospital of delivery are adequate. If the infant is seriously ill, he should be transferred to an intensive care unit (ICU) following stabilization of vital signs in the delivery suite. If this facility is absent at the hospital of birth, arrangements should be made for rapid transfer of the infant to a hospital with such a unit.

Among the problems that require intensive care are birth weight below 1500 g; respiratory insufficiency; major congenital anomalies; severe infections, e.g., sepsis or meningitis; preoperative and postoperative patients; hyperbilirubinemia requiring exchange transfusion; major metabolic disorders, such as hypocalcemia and hypoglycemia; and signs of major illness, e.g., apnea, convulsions, hemorrhage, cyanosis in the absence of a specific diagnosis.

Certain infants require treatment in intermediate care nurseries, which are available in most community hospitals. Asymptomatic premature infants, whose birth weights are greater than 1500 g, patients with hyperbilirubinemia requiring phototherapy, most infants of diabetic mothers and the majority of infants undergoing drug withdrawal are examples. Infants cared for in the ICU and whose clinical condition has improved may be transferred to the intermediate care nursery.

Infants with illnesses caused by highly communicable microorganisms, such as staphylococci, enteropathogenic *E. coli* and salmonellae, should be cared for in special

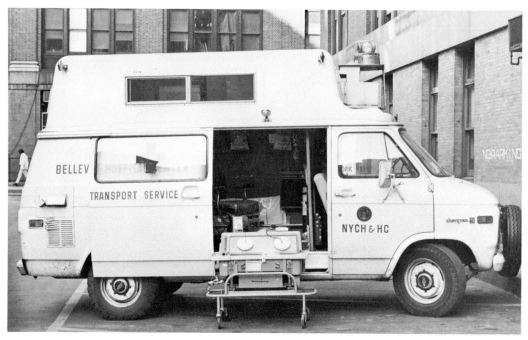

FIG. 1–2. New York City Health and Hospital Corporation infant transport ambulance. (Courtesy of Dr. A. Ferrara)

isolation areas manned by a nursing staff separate from that of the rest of the neonatal unit.

Each hospital must establish its own guidelines for the disposition of high-risk neonates, depending on the expertise of mediconursing staff and available facilities. If a hospital service attempts to exceed its capabilities in treating a sick neonate, a potentially avoidable death or serious neurologic damage may ensue.

Ultimately it is the individual physician who must decide the disposition of the infant, a conclusion that should be based on the medical history, physical examination and laboratory data. Even when detailed information is available, decisions on the disposition of such neonates are often among the most challenging in medicine.

REGIONAL TRANSPORT

Since the late 1960s, many sophisticated transport systems have been developed in the United States and Canada to facilitate the transfer of neonates requiring intensive care from the hospital of their birth to regional centers.

Whereas the Chicago and New York City premature infant transport systems were responsible for a significant decline in infant mortality rate, there were nevertheless limitations since active treatment could not be administerd during transit, and sick full-term infants were not being transported.

With the marked increase in interest during the 1960s in providing more-effective neonatal intensive care, reevaluation of methods of transporting sick babies to regional centers became necessary. In the ensuing years much effort and expense have gone into the design and construction of transport incubators, ambulances and aircraft capable of delivering sick infants to regional centers under optimum medical conditions. Also, medical and nursing personnel with experience in transporting these infants had been trained. However, by the early 1970s, there still remained much room for improvement (25).

Among the factors related to successful transfer of sick neonates from the hospital of birth to regional centers (26), the first is

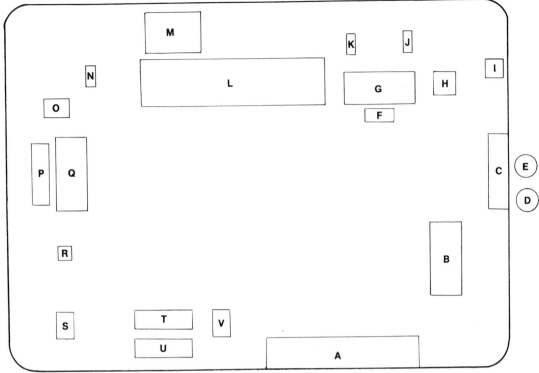

FIG. 1–3. Interior layout of New York City infant transport ambulance (not drawn to scale). Legend: (A) Entrance (side), (B) Incubator, (C) Air conditioner, (D) Oxygen tank, (E) Oxygen tank, (F) Suction apparatus, (G) Incubator, (H) Heater, (I) Controls for air conditioner, (J) Oxygen apparatus, (K) Oxygen apparatus, (L) Seating area, (M) Emergency exit window, (N) Oxygen apparatus, (O) Heart rate monitor, (P) Radiant heater, (Q) Pragle carrier,(R) Generator controls, (S) Circuit breaker controls, (T) Overhead lighting, (U) Counter space, (V) Heater. Contents of all cabinets are labeled.

maintenance of thermoneutrality during transit. For this purpose battery-powered transport incubators have been developed. Some transport vehicles are equipped with radiant heaters capable of maintaining a thermoneutral state for infants outside of incubators.

Maintenance of an intact airway and adequate oxygenation during transit are also vital. Assisted ventilation, either manually or with the aid of a respirator may be necessary for this purpose.

Intravenous administration of fluids and correction of acid-base disturbances through an umbilical arterial catheter may be of value during transit, especially if the trip lasts more than 30 minutes.

The design of transport ambulances varies (24), but all have similar features (Figs. 1–2 and 1–3). Most are equipped with radiant heaters and a stand up area for medical and nursing personnel to provide ready accessibility to the infant for diagnostic or therapeutic procedures. A source of oxygen, suction apparatus and equipment necessary for endotracheal intubation are universally available. In some ambulances, a respirator is present. A portion of the vehicle is set aside for the transport incubator. All carry a supply of emergency medications that may be necessary for treatment of the infant. Some ambulances have laboratory equipment for determining acid-base and oxygenation status, blood glucose and hematocrit. This may be of special value if long distances have to be traversed.

In sparsely populated areas where infants have to be transported more than 100 miles, both helicopter and fixed wing aircraft have

INFANT TRANSPORT SERVICE-MOTHER'S OBSTETRIC RECORD

NAME OF INFANT	SEX	RACE	RELIGION	BAPTIZED

☐ YES ☐ NO IF YES BY WHOM

ADDRESS	FLOOR OR APT.	BORO	ZIP CODE

HOME TELEPHONE NUMBER	RELATIVE OR NEIGHBOR'S NAME, ADDRESS AND TEL. NO:

PLACE OF INFANT'S BIRTH	DATE		WEIGHT AT BIRTH

TIME _____ ☐ AM ☐ PM

MATERNAL HISTORY

PRENATAL CARE ☐ YES ☐ NO   IF YES, SPECIFY WHERE   DATE STARTED

DATE LAST MENSTRUATION   DATE EXPECTED CONFINEMENT   FETAL AGE BY HISTORY _____ WEEKS.

SEROLOGY DATE   RESULT ☐ NEGATIVE ☐ POSITIVE   IF POSITIVE, SUMMARY OF TREATMENT

BLOOD TYPE, RH AND ANTIBODY TITRE

MOTHER'S HEALTH BEFORE AND DURING THIS PREGNANCY. HISTORY INCLUDING MEDICAL CONDITIONS, OPERATIONS AND INJURIES, DRUGS USED DURING PREGNANCY (GIVE DATES AND SPECIFICS)

DIABETES		
PYELONEPHRITIS		
TOXEMIA		
ADDICTION		
RUBELLA		
MEDICATION		
OTHER		

LABOR AND DELIVERY

DURATION 1ST STAGE HRS 2ND STAGE   POSITION OF FETUS AT DELIVERY   MEDICATIONS (INCLUDE DOSE AND TIME)

ANESTHESIA ☐ YES ☐ NO IF YES, SPECIFY _____

TYPE OF DELIVERY	PRECIPITATE	SPONTANEOUS	INDUCED (IF INDUCED, METHOD)	EPISIOTOMY ☐ YES ☐ NO

INSTRUMENTAL OR OPERATIVE PROCEDURES. (SPECIFY)

COMPLICATIONS OF THIS LABOR AND/OR DELIVERY, SPECIFY

NO. OF UMBILICAL ARTERIES	AMNIOTIC SAC RUPTURE DATE _____ TIME _____ ☐ AM ☐ PM	AMNIOTIC FLUID ☐ NORMAL	☐ POLYHYDRAMNIOS ☐ OLIGOHYDRAMNIOS ☐ MECONIUM STAINED ☐ PURULENT

PLACENTA DESCRIPTION

NAME OF ATTENDANT AT BIRTH	RESIDENT PHYSICIAN (IF OTHER SPECIFY)	TELEPHONE NUMBER
	PRIVATE PHYSICIAN	OFFICE TELEPHONE NUMBER

FAMILY HISTORY

NAME OF PARENTS OF BABY	AGE	RACE	OCCUPATION	MARITAL STATUS	HEALTH STATUS - (IF DECEASED CAUSE OF DEATH)
FATHER					
MOTHER'S MAIDEN NAME					

HISTORY OF PREVIOUS PREGNANCIES (List Chronologically) Total Number of Pregnancies:

YEAR	LIVE BIRTH OR FETAL DEATH	PREMATURE OR FULL TERM	AGE OR AGE AT DEATH	LIVING OR DEAD	ABNORMALITIES	PRESENT HEALTH CONDITION OR CAUSE OF DEATH

NAME OF SOCIAL SERVICE WORKER AT HOSPITAL OF BIRTH	CONTACT MADE ☐ YES ☐ NO

MOTHER'S SIGNATURE	WITNESSED BY

SIGNATURE AND TITLE OF HOSPITAL REPRESENTATIVE SUBMITTING THIS INFORMATION	TELEPHONE NUMBER . EXT.

21K (REV. 10/68) 10M-1121096 (69)

BUREAU OF MATERNITY SERVICES AND FAMILY PLANNING
DEPARTMENT OF HEALTH-THE CITY OF NEW YORK

been used with apparent success (23, 28, 30). Several problems have been encountered with this type of transport. Loss of heat may occur (because of cold outside environmental temperatures) if caution is not observed. Under certain circumstances, when free air is present in a body cavity (pneumothorax, pneumomediastinum or pneumoperitoneum), air transport may be hazardous because of exposure to low barometric pressures. With the use of helicopters, excessive noise and shaking are usually encountered. Helicopters are the vehicle of choice if the distance to be traversed is between 100 and 150 miles, while fixed wing aircraft are best used if the distance is more than 150 miles.

TRANSPORTING INFANTS

Whatever the means of transport, there are basic guidelines to assure arrival of the patient in the best possible condition.

The transfer of infants should be limited to those who are likely to benefit from care in the receiving center. Infants who are nonviable because of extreme prematurity or who have congenital anomalies incompatible with life should probably not be transported. In infants who are mildly or moderately compromised, the decision whether to transfer the infant to a special center will depend on the resources of the institution at which the birth occurred.

Personnel with expertise in transporting compromised infants should be in attendance both prior to and during the actual period of transfer. In certain cases, a nurse skilled in the care of these infants may be adequate. However, when active treatment of the infant is contemplated, the services of an experienced physician are required.

Immediately prior to transport, the clinical condition of the infant should be stabilized at the hospital of origin. A thermoneutral state should be established, the infant should be well oxygenated and stomach

contents removed to avoid possible vomiting and aspiration during the trip. The infant should be well secured in the ambulance in a lateral decubitus position. If esophageal atresia is present, the upper portion of the body should be elevated and the blind pouch suctioned frequently. With any other type of intestinal obstruction, an indwelling nasogastric tube should be in place and also suctioned frequently. Omphaloceles and myelomeningoceles should be covered with a moist, sterile dressing.

The obstetric (Fig. 1–4) and neonatal history (Fig. 1–5) including, if possible, a photocopy of the infant's and mother's hospital charts and x rays, should be sent to the receiving hospital. This should include all diagnostic tests performed and treatment already given. The name and telephone number of both the obstretrician and physician responsible for care of the infant at the hospital of birth should be included. If the infant requires special procedures at the receiving hospital, such as cardiac catheterization or emergency surgery, the team of physicians who will be performing the procedure should be notified ahead of time and should be awaiting the arrival of the infant at the center. A complete record of the actual transport of the infant must also be kept (Fig. 1–6).

Parental consent for both transfer and treatment at the receiving hospital should be obtained. It is essential that specimens of maternal and umbilical cord blood, properly labeled, accompany the infant.

In the days following admission of the infant to the receiving center, contact must be maintained between physicians at both the receiving and sending hospitals and the parents of the infant.

A regional transport service should be under the direction of a trained neonatologist. In many areas, such as New York City (27), the full-time services of one or more physicians are required to maintain efficient operations. With an ever-increasing experience, the new knowledge gained in transporting infants should facilitate their transfer to a regional center.

FIG. 1–4. New York City infant transport service—mother's obstetric record.

INFANT TRANSPORT SERVICE – NEWBORN RECORD

INFANT'S NAME	HOSPITAL	CONDITION AT BIRTH

MULTIPLE BIRTH

☐ YES ☐ NO   IF YES, SPECIFY_____

VITAMIN K (SPECIFY PREPARATION AND DOSE)	APGAR SCORE 1 MIN. _____ 5 MIN. _____	EYE PROPHYLAXIS: AGENT USED

RESUSCITATION REQUIRED

☐ YES ☐ NO   IF YES, SPECIFY METHOD_____

SECTION 1 TO BE COMPLETED BY NURSE

INFANT'S TEMPERATURE

INITIAL: DATE_____ TIME_____ ☐ RECTAL   ☐ AXILLARY

STOOLS AND VOIDING

FIRST STOOL: DATE_____ TIME:_____ FIRST VOIDING: DATE_____ TIME_____

LAST STOOL: DATE_____ TIME_____ LAST VOIDING: DATE_____ TIME_____

DESCRIPTION OF STOOLS:_____

FEEDINGS ☐ NIPPLE ☐ GAVAGE ☐ BREAST ☐ OTHER (SPECIFY _____	NAME OF FORMULA	VOLUME OFFERED.

ORAL FEEDING:

AGE AT TIME OF FIRST FEEDING_____ HOURS   LAST FEEDING: DATE_____ TIME_____ VOLUME TAKEN_____

SPECIAL TREATMENTS (E.G. RESUSCITATION, TRANSFUSION, SURGERY, INTRAVENOUS) (SPECIFY DATES)	MEDICATIONS (NAME, DOSAGE, INTERVAL, TIME OF LAST DOSE (SPECIFY DATES)

OXYGEN ADMINISTRATION

IN DELIVERY ROOM: TYPE OF INCUBATOR_____ RANGE OF CONCENTRATION_____ DURATION OF THERAPY: HRS__ MIN__

IN NURSERY   TYPE OF INCUBATOR_____ RANGE OF CONCENTRATION_____ DURATION OF THERAPY: HRS__ MIN__

REASONS FOR ADMINISTRATION OF OXYGEN:

LABORATORY TESTS AND X-RAYS (INCLUDE DATES AND RESULTS)

SUMMARY OF NURSING OBSERVATIONS (INCLUDE COLOR, FEEDING ABILITY, GENERAL BEHAVIOR, ANY ABNORMALITIES)	LAST WEIGHT	DATE

SIGNATURE AND TITLE OF PERSON SUBMITTING THIS INFORMATION	TELEPHONE	EXTENSION

SECTION 2 TO BE COMPLETED BY PHYSICIAN

PHYSICAL EXAMINATION AND MEDICAL SUMMARY OF NURSERY COURSE

SIGNATURE OF PHYSICIAN	TELEPHONE	EXTENSION
_____ M. D.		

21KA 10/68-10M-512088 (71)

BUREAU OF MATERNITY SERVICES AND FAMILY PLANNING
Department of Health—The City of New York

FIG. 1–5. New York City infant transport service—newborn infant's record.

RECORD OF INFANT'S TRANSPORT

INFANT'S NAME		BIRTH WEIGHT	DATE OF BIRTH

	FROM	TO		DATE	TIME	
TRANSPORTED						☐ AM ☐ PM

OBSERVATIONS AT HOSPITAL/HOME PRIOR TO TRANSFER

FORM FOR INFANT TRANSPORT SERVICE, OBSTETRIC RECORD AND NEWBORN RECORD COMPLETED. IF NO, GIVE REASON:

☐ YES ☐ NO

FOOT PRINTS RECEIVED

☐ YES ☐ NO   OXYGEN CONCENTRATION %

TEMPERATURE INFANT   °☐ RECTAL   °☐ AXILLA   INCUBATOR

5CC MOTHER'S CLOTTED BLOOD RECEIVED   IDENTIFICATION CHECKED WITH (NAME)

☐ YES ☐ NO

BABY SHOWN TO MOTHER   ☐ YES   ☐ NO   IF NO WHY?   FORM MNB 7 GIVEN TO (NAME)

CONDITION OF INFANT

OBSERVATIONS AND CARE OF INFANT DURING TRANSIT

OXYGEN ADMINISTERED AT _____ %

INCUBATOR TEMPERATURE _____ °

OBSERVATIONS AT RECEIVING HOSPITAL

CONDITION OF INFANT ON ARRIVAL   TIME OF ARRIVAL   ☐ AM ☐ PM

INFANT IDENTIFIED AND RECEIVED BY (NAME)

5CC MOTHER'S CLOTTED BLOOD LEFT WITH (NAME)

INFANT TRANSPORT SERVICE FORMS AND FOOTPRINTS LEFT WITH: (NAME)

TEMPERATURE INFANT   °☐ RECTAL   °☐ AXILLA   INCUBATOR   °   OXYGEN CONCENTRATION %

DURATION OF TRANSPORT

HOSP. OF BIRTH: DEPARTURE TIME: ___ AM PM TEMP. OF INCUBATOR: _____°   OXYGEN ADMINISTERED DURING TRANSPORT ☐ YES ☐ NO

PREMATURE CENTER: ARIVAL TIME: ___ AM PM TEMP. OF INCUBATOR: _____°   IF YES, CONCENTRATION _____ DURATION _____

SIGNATURE OF TRANSPORT NURSE (IF OTHER, SIGN NAME AND SPECIFY TITLE)

(21KB 10/68)-10M-1121096 (69)

**BUREAU OF MATERNITY SERVICES AND FAMILY PLANNING
DEPARTMENT OF HEALTH—THE CITY OF NEW YORK**

FIG. 1–6. New York City infant transport service—record of infant's transport.

ORGANIZATION OF A NEONATAL INTENSIVE CARE UNIT

Hospitals that accept the responsibility for providing intensive care to critically ill neonates must meet rigorous standards for the management of these infants. The set of standards for neonatal intensive care units (NICUs) recommended by the New York City Department of Health in 1973 is presented in Appendix 1.

A well-functioning NICU must have adequate space and modern equipment in good working order. Even more important is the continuous presence of a highly motivated and knowledgeable professional staff. The unit serves not only as a place for providing optimal medical care for the sick neonate, but as a center for teaching medical, nursing and ancillary personnel and as an area for clinical research. It must be capable of managing any type of medical or surgical problem at any given time.

ADMISSIONS TO THE UNIT

The unit should maintain a current set of written policies establishing guidelines for medical and nursing care. Because of rapidly growing knowledge in the area of perinatal medicine and the introduction of new techniques and equipment, these policies should be reviewed often and revised when necessary. Infants who require admission to the NICU are those needing constant medical and nursing care. Criteria for admission are discussed in the section Neonates Requiring Special Care.

The NICU (Fig. 1–7), as well as the newborn admissions unit should be located in close proximity to the delivery suite, preferably on the same floor, so that little time is lost in moving infants through corridors and on elevators following delivery.

Although 30 sq ft is usually adequate for each infant reared in an incubator, in the NICU as much as 80 sq ft per infant may be necessary to accommodate respirators, monitors, phototherapy units or other equipment and to provide sufficient room for professional staff.

In most instances the NICU is in physical proximity with the intermediate care nursery. The number of infants actually requiring intensive care at any one time varies, but an efficient unit should be able to manage six to ten critically ill neonates. The entire unit, including the intermediate care nursery, functions most efficiently when the bed capacity is 30 to 40. Smaller units tend to be economically inefficient; larger ones are difficult to manage, but under some circumstances (such as a statewide or province-wide regional unit) may be appropriate.

Traditionally, premature nurseries and NICUs have been subdivided into areas each capable of housing four to six incubators or bassinettes. In these rooms, electric outlets and sources of oxygen and suction have been located on the wall. To economize on space, offer more accessibility to the infant and introduce a greater flexibility, traditional walls have been eliminated and all sick infants have been grouped in one large room (33). The source of electric current, oxygen, suction and compressed air may be either a service module located on the ceiling or one located on the floor (Fig. 1–8).

The ambient air temperature of the unit must be maintained within the comfort zone for the staff (75°–78° F). Since wide fluctuations in air temperature affect incubator air temperature, room temperatures must be maintained at a relatively constant level. These room temperatures are also suited for larger infants being raised clothed and blanketed in bassinettes outside of the intensive care area.

EQUIPMENT, LIGHTING AND STORAGE SPACE

Superficially, the cost of properly equipping a NICU may seem large. However, in terms of the total and intact survival made possible by this equipment, the true cost is small.

In purchasing equipment, every attempt must be made to get the most value for the money being spent. However, any attempt to cut corners by purchasing equipment of questionable reliability should be avoided.

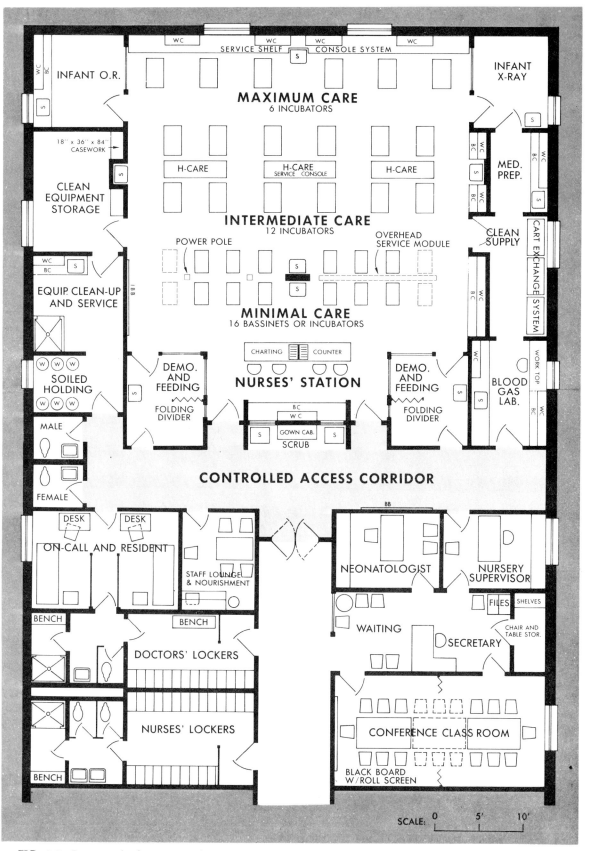

FIG. 1–7. Conceptual plan, neonatal intensive care unit. (Thogmartin BM, Tine MD: Design for Obstetric and Pediatric Facilities. Columbus, Ross Laboratories, 1972)

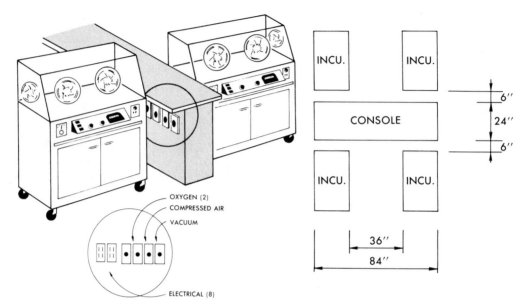

FIG. 1–8. Floor type of service console. (Thogmartin BM, Tine MD: Design for obstetric and pediatric facilities. Columbus, Ross Laboratories, 1972)

Incubators and Radiant Heaters

The primary item of equipment necessary for caring for small and compromised infants is the incubator. This serves a dual purpose: it regulates the thermal environment to which the infant is exposed and serves as a partial barrier to dust particles and airborne microorganisms. A major disadvantage is that it limits accessibility to the infant. It is now possible to raise small infants outside of incubators under radiant heaters in a thermoneutral environment (see Ch. 13, Thermoregulation). Accessibility of the infant to handling is increased under these circumstances, but the potential danger of airborne infection is also increased.

A sufficient number of incubators should be available, both to meet the immediate patient care demands and to allow for cleaning and repairs. Several incubators should be kept heated at all times in preparation for new admissions to the unit.

Battery-powered, portable transport incubators have enhanced the ability to safely transport infants from one area to another (delivery room to nursery, nursery to surg-

ical suite and so on) in a favorable thermal environment. Ideally there should be one warmed operative transport incubator in the delivery room and another in the nursery area at all times.

A radiant heater capable of maintaining the skin temperature of even the smallest premature infant at 36.5° C must be present in the treatment room. During prolonged procedures, such as exchange transfusions, umbilical vessel catheterizations and insertion of central venous catheters, use of this type of heater is mandatory.

Delivery of Supplementary Oxygen

Since the unit must contain a system for efficient delivery of oxygen, equipment that monitors environmental oxygen concentrations and the state of oxygenation of the infant is required. The source of oxygen should be a wall or ceiling outlet rather than a tank of compressed gas. Oxygen should be humidified and warmed before it is delivered to the infant. Although it is difficult to raise the oxygen concentration in the incubator above 70% and higher concentrations may be required at times, a special headbox designed for this purpose is commercially available.

The state of tissue oxygenation of the infant receiving supplementary oxygen is difficult to assess. Ambient oxygen concentrations of incubator air together with measurements of the partial pressure of oxygen in arterial blood (Pao_2) must be made at frequent intervals. A method of continuous Pao_2 measurement with an oxygen sensor built into the wall of the umbilical arterial catheter became commercially available in 1972, but in 1975 had not yet become widely used on a clinical basis. A noninvasive transcutaneous method of measuring tissue oxygenation is under evaluation in 1975.

Medical and nursing personnel must be experienced in the use of one or two types of mechanical ventilators (Fig. 1–9) as well as in administering constant distending airway pressure.

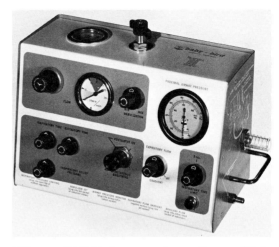

FIG. 1–9. BABYbird neonatal ventilator. (Bird Corporation, Mark 7, Palm Springs, Ca.)

Monitoring Devices

Precise continuous monitoring of vital functions in compromised infants has advanced markedly since the 1960s. Various instruments capable of monitoring respiratory rates, cardiac rates and rhythms and blood pressure have become available for clinical use. On occasion, so much hardware surrounds the sick infant that it is difficult to actually view the patient. This equipment has not decreased the nurse's responsibility of constantly attending the sick infant; rather, it has brought more burden since she must interpret not only the clinical reactions of the infant, but the output of the monitors as well. She must also be able to detect malfunction in these monitors.

Respiratory, or apnea, monitors have achieved a wide degree of popularity. One type of monitor, using impedance plethysmography, requires the attachment of two sensors to the chest wall. Another method, utilizing a special air mattress, has also been widely used.

Cardiac monitors (Fig. 1–10) are valuable in monitoring the heart rate; alarm systems attached to the cardiotachometer give warning when bradycardia occurs (this may be a prelude to an apneic attack). The electrocardiographic tracing may be viewed on the oscilloscope screen and arrhythmias detected. By use of telemetry, cardiac monitoring can be performed on even the smallest premature infants without wire attachments from the infant to the monitoring device.

Apparatus for measuring blood pressure both by direct and indirect methods should be present in the NICU.

It is advisable to have a portable electrocardiogram machine in addition to the cardiac monitor. The size of the electrodes should be appropriate for very small infants. A separate stethoscope should be kept for each infant.

A portable electroencephalograph (EEG) machine together with a skilled technician should be readily available for nursery use.

Both the widespread use of umbilical arterial catheters and the increasing popularity of total parenteral alimentation through a central venous catheter makes it imperative that several infusion pumps be available and in good working order at all times. At the slow rates of infusion required in small newborn infants, catheter blockage is minimized when these pumps are employed. Two basic types of pumps are available: 1) those using replaceable syringes, based on a turning screw type of mechanism and 2) rotary pumps, which apply a peristaltic-like pressure to the tubing at predetermined rates. It is desirable that the infu-

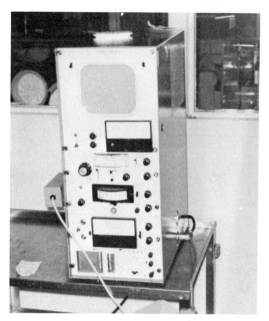

FIG. 1–10. IR-4 Cardiac and Respiratory Monitor. (Electronics for Medicine, White Plains, NY)

sion pump be able to run on a rechargeable battery, so that the infusion can be run continuously if the infant has to be transported.

Metric scales calibrated to the nearest 10 g are desirable for weighing the infant. A problem of heat loss will arise if small and sick infants have to be removed from the incubator to be weighed. Two alternatives are available: 1) having each scale placed under a radiant heater and 2) weighing the infant inside of the incubator using a cloth sling on a spring scale that is on top of the incubator hood. The latter method may be slightly less accurate, but it prevents chilling of the infant.

Various phototherapy units of about equal efficacy are commercially available. Wall-mounted units may save some floor space, but the mobility associated with portable units is then lost.

Closed waste disposal systems are of course a necessity in any nursery. Foot-controlled, covered containers for both trash and soiled linen should be present in each room.

An emergency cart must be fully stocked, with the following equipment in good work-

ing order: laryngoscopes with "premature" blades and functioning batteries and lights, nasotracheal and orotracheal tubes of various sizes; breathing bags capable of delivering a high concentration of oxygen, tape and silk thread necessary for fixing endotracheal tubes, various adapters for the tubes and drugs that are most likely to be used during resuscitative procedures and other emergencies, such as 7.5% sodium bicarbonate, 50% glucose, 10% calcium gluconate and 1:1000 epinephrine solutions, phenobarbital and digoxin.

The storage spaces of the unit must be stocked with necessary supplies, such as syringes, infusion sets, feeding tubes, sterile packs for catheterization, lumbar puncture and suprapubic bladder puncture. One nurse should be given the responsibility to inventory all supplies daily.

The general availability of prepared infant formula and disposable supplies obviates the need for a formula room and sterilization equipment. However, a gas sterilizer is still necessary for such reusable items as respiratory tubing and breathing bags.

An intercom system operating between the various areas of the nursery is useful, especially when emergencies arise.

In order to keep all equipment in good working order, a program of preventive maintenance is a necessity. This includes periodic checking of electric equipment for improper grounding and current leakage, since even a little current may cause serious injury or death in newborn infants, especially those with a low resistance pathway (umbilical catheter) to the heart (31, 34).

Adequate Illumination

Daylight fluorescent bulbs that provide 100 to 150 foot candles of light at the level of the incubator not only offer proper illumination, but may play a role in photooxidation of unconjugated bilirubin in the skin of nude jaundiced infants (32).

The walls should be painted a neutral color. Reflection from a wall painted yellow, green or blue may lead to a mistaken clinical diagnosis of jaundice or cyanosis.

Adequate storage space must be available in the immediate patient care area, so that all necessary supplies are immediately available.

Sinks with knee controls are necessary. Liquid antibacterial soaps for handwashing should be available in foot-controlled wall dispensers.

The degree of cleanliness of the air in the nursery probably affects the staff more than the infant in the incubator. Since dust and bacteria are to a great extent filtered out of the air entering the incubator, airborne infection is usually not a major problem in the nursery. However, bacteria emanating from the infants are transferred from the incubator to the room air. Although circulation and filtration of air probably reduces bacterial and dust levels, this appears to be of little clinical importance as long as the infants are cared for in incubators. The necessity for maintaining clean nursery air is of great importance if small infants are being cared for outside of incubators under radiant heaters.

Nursing stations should be so located that visual contact with all infants is provided at all times.

A treatment room for the performance of exchange transfusions, umbilical vessel catheterizations and other minor procedures should be adjacent to the patient care area. This room should have a radiant heater, monitoring devices, an available supply of oxygen, compressed air and suction devices and a scrub area.

A separate x-ray room within the confines of the unit is desirable but not absolutely necessary. Fine quality x rays can usually be taken with most portable machines with the infant remaining in the incubator. Good films more closely reflect the skill and dedication of the x-ray technician than the apparatus per se.

A small laboratory area within the confines of the unit is a necessity. At the least, this laboratory should be equipped to do routine hematologic examinations and urine analyses. A centrifuge for separating serum from whole blood should be present. Micromethods for determining blood sugar, total protein and total bilirubin should also be available. The apparatus for measuring Po_2, pH, Pco_2 and blood electrolytes should be located in a laboratory near the nursery area, if not within it. This must be operational on an around-the-clock, 7 days-a-week basis. It should be possible to do Gram stain examinations of body fluids within the nursery laboratory. However, a fully equipped bacteriology laboratory within the confines of the nursery area is not necessary (like the biochemistry laboratory, this should be within easy reach of the nursery).

A staff conference room plus a demonstration area (for teaching techniques to both staff and mothers of infants) are necessities. Adequate office space should be available for physicians, nurses, and social workers attached to the unit. A room with a bed should be provided so that a physician is physically on the premises 24 hours a day. An area should be set aside as a lounge for physicians and nursing staff.

PROFESSIONAL STAFF

The unit should be directed by a full-time pediatrician (37) with at least two years of formal training in neonatal medicine. He establishes all nursery policies, which should be recorded in a written manual. All members of the staff are ultimately responsible to this director. If the unit is large enough and there are sufficient clinical research and teaching responsibilities, additional full-time physicians should be assigned to the nurseries, as well as one or two fellows. At least two full-time house officers should be assigned to the unit (they can rotate night duties with the resident assigned to the normal full-term nursery).

The services of various medical specialists are required on a continuous basis. A pediatric surgeon must be available 24 hours a day, 7 days a week, as well as a pediatric cardiologist capable of performing cardiac catheterization and angiography. A radiologist knowledgeable in neonatal x-ray diagnosis must be on the staff. The ophthalmologist's role is discussed in the section Retrolental Fibroplasia, Chapter 3. In addition, consultants must be available in all of the medicosurgical subspecialities.

The physician who is in private practice may have patients in a unit that has a full-time director, and conflicts in the management of the patient have been known. Policies should be established making the practicing pediatrician part of the team, even though he is unable to be physically present in the nursery for more than a short period each day.

The nursing staff should consist of a supervisor and enough personnel to assure proper coverage, both in expertise and total numbers at all times. In the case of the sickest infants, skilled registered nurses should be in attendance; the ratio of nurses to patients should be 1:1 or 1:2. In recuperating or less seriously ill infants in the intermediate care nursery, the ratio of nursing personnel to infants should be no less than 1:4. One nurse should be responsible for the proper functioning of all intensive care equipment and for instructing the nursing staff with its use.

At least one full-time medical social worker is assigned to the unit and is responsible for facilitating communications with parents, physicians and nursing staff.

Ongoing Research and Education

The importance of education is reflected in daily medical rounds led by a senior pediatrician and attended by fellows, house officers, medical students and nursing personnel, as well as rounds by medical and nursing staff in the late afternoon and late evening to review pertinent new clinical, laboratory and x-ray findings of each infant.

Regularly scheduled clinical conferences, both intradepartmental and jointly with obstetricians, pathologists, anesthesiologists and radiologists are necessary. Special nursing and social service rounds should be conducted at least once a week.

Instruction and support of mothers of low birth weight and other compromised infants by mediconursing and social service

staff is necessary prior to discharge of the infants to their homes.

Research is another vital activity of the NICU. The great advances in neonatal medicine have been made possible because of controlled clinical trials that were carried out in these units. The NICU has many functions: it is a patient care area whose function is to enhance both total and intact survival of compromised infants; it is a place for educating students, medical and nursing staff; and it is a research area where advances in the care of sick newborn infants are to be made.

APPENDIX 1
NEW YORK CITY HEALTH DEPARTMENT STANDARDS FOR NEONATAL INTENSIVE CARE UNITS

1.00 GENERAL INFORMATION
1.10 *Definition*
The Neonatal Intensive Care Unit (NICU) shall be a physically distinct area staffed and equipped to provide for observation, preventive care or treatment of high risk newborns regardless of birth weight.
1.20 *Location*
The NICU may be located within an existing premature nursery, full-term nursery, or general intensive care facility, or it may exist as a freestanding, self-contained unit within a hospital.
1.30 *Accreditation*
The hospital in which the NICU is located shall be fully accredited by the Joint Commission on Accreditation of Hospitals, and furthermore shall have residency training programs in both Pediatrics, and Obstetrics and Gynecology, which are approved by the Council on Education of the American Medical Association, as well as by the American Board of Pediatrics and the American Board of Obstetrics and Gynecology, respectively.
1.40 *Types of Patients*
High risk newborns shall include infants born either at term or prematurely, who display severe asphyxia, acidosis, respiratory distress, metabolic disorders, seizures, infections, major congenital anomalies, and blood group incompatibilities requiring exchange transfusion, as well as neonates with cardiac disorders, surgical problems, diabetic or drug-addicted mothers, or other conditions requiring special care.
1.50 *Age Limitations*
Age limitations for admission to the NICU shall be determined by the medical director of that unit.

1.60 *Duration of Stay*
The duration of stay of patients in the NICU shall be limited only to the time the special services of the unit are required.

2.00 PERSONNEL
2.10 *Physicians*
2.11 Director: A full-time Board certified or eligible pediatrician, who has had special training or experience in newborn medicine, shall direct the unit. The director's total responsibility shall be to the institution's newborn service, and may include teaching, administrative and research activities customarily associated with such a position. The director shall supervise patient care, set policies and procedures, and, in collaboration with the Department of Nursing, maintain on-going teaching programs for both the medical and nursing staff.
2.12 House Staff: At least one pediatric house officer with a minimum of 6 months prior training in pediatrics shall be assigned exclusively to the newborn service, including the NICU, at all times. These residents shall have received training in resuscitative techniques, tracheal intubation, the utilization of assisted ventilation, the use of oxygen therapy, and the determination and treatment of acid-base and blood gas disorders. A senior house officer with more extensive experience in the care of newborns shall be on duty to supervise junior residents at all times.
2.130 Consultants: A diverse group of consultants is necessary in order to provide NICU patients with optimum care.
2.131 A Board eligible or certified surgeon with training and experience in pediatric surgery shall be a member of the active staff and available on call to the NICU.
2.132 A Board eligible or certified pediatric cardiologist as well as a team capable of performing cardiac catheterization and angiography within the hospital shall be available at all times.
2.133 A Board certified or eligible radiologist with training or experience in neonatal radiology shall be on the active staff of the hospital and available at all times.
2.134 Physicians with interest and training in newborn care in the following specialties shall be available for consultation: hematology, ophthalmology, neurology, neurosurgery, infectious disease, pulmonary physiology, pathology, anesthesiology, orthopedic surgery and oto-rhino laryngology.
2.20 *Nurses*
2.21 Staffing: A registered professional nurse with education and experience in neonatal intensive care shall be responsible for the nursing care in the unit on each tour of duty.
2.212 Registered professional nurses with orientation and experience in the care of sick neonate shall be assigned to the NICU in a ratio of at least one R.N. to every two infants.
2.213 The Table of Organization of the nursing staff and duty schedules shall reflect the maintenance of a stable core of nurses permanently assigned to the NICU, based on the recommended patient-to-nurse ratio of 2:1.
2.214 Additional nurses may be rotated through the NICU to enlarge the pool of available nurses experienced in the care of the sick neonates. These nurses may be drawn from other newborn and infant care areas, or from intensive care units, in the hospital.
2.22 In service Educational Program: A registered professional nurse with a background in teaching and clinical skills shall be responsible for, in collaboration with the medical director, planning and conducting an educational program in neonatal intensive care nursing.
2.30 *Social Worker*
2.31 The hospital shall have a Social Service Department headed by a full-time director qualified in the field of social work.
2.32 A professionally qualified social worker shall be assigned specifically to the unit with time allocation based on the size of the unit and the characteristics of the patient population.
2.40 *Clerical–Administrative Staff:* Clerical and secretarial assistance, and sufficient office space and equipment shall be assigned to the unit to assist the director in maintaining records, compiling statistics, corresponding, completing required governmental forms, referring discharged patients to followup facilities, etc.
2.50 *Inhalation Therapy:* An adequately staffed and equipped Department of Inhalation Therapy, directed by a qualified inhalational therapist, and operation on a 24-hour a day, 7 days per week basis, shall be maintained by the hospital in which the NICU is located.
2.60 *Supporting Personnel:* Sufficient ancillary nursing, housekeeping maintenance and messenger personnel shall be available to service the NICU on each tour of duty.

3.00 PHYSICAL FACILITIES
3.10 While the physical arrangement of individual intensive care units may vary considerably depending on circumstances, due consideration must be given important features such as the availability of sufficient floor space per patient, the environmental conditions in the nursery, the quality and intensity of illumination, the provision of adequate handwashing facilities, the inclusion of oxygen and compressed air outlets for each patient, and the availability of sufficient electrical outlets which are properly grounded and periodically inspected in order to minimize electrical hazards.
3.20 In general, the physical attributes of a NICU shall be consistent with the standards and

recommendations published by the American Academy of Pediatrics in "Hospital Care of the Newborn Infant," 5th Edition, 1971, pages 55–66, and pages 70–73.

4.00 LABORATORY FACILITIES

Adequacy of the diagnostic laboratories is a critical factor in the ability of any institution to render effective intensive care to newborns. The following represent minimal requirements:

4.10 *Intensive Care Supporting Laboratory*
This laboratory, which should be easily accessible to the intensive care unit, must make available on a 24-hour a day, 7 days a week basis, the following tests on an immediate basis; blood pH, Pco_2, Po_2, micro hematocrit, and examination of cerebral spinal fluid.

4.20 *Clinical Chemistry*
The following laboratory determinations must be available rapidly and performed by micro methods permitting analysis of capillary blood; serum Na, K, Cl, CO_2, calcium, magnesium, bilirubin, BUN, and blood glucose.

4.30 *Hematologic Services*
The facilities for obtaining, typing and cross-matching blood for transfusion, performing Coombs' test, and the availability of tests to detect disorders of blood coagulation including prothrombin time, PTT, fibrinogen, etc., shall be required.

4.40 *Clinical Microscopy*
The capacity to determine, at all times, CBC's, reticulocyte counts, platelet counts, red cell morphology and urinalysis is required.

4.50 *Microbiology*
Facilities for processing or holding bacteriologic, virologic and serologic materials shall be available in the institution at all times.

5.00 RADIOLOGY

5.10 The institution must contain the equipment and provide the staff for obtaining bedside x-rays in the NICU on a 24-hour basis, and for the performance of emergency contrast studies, angiography, or other specialized radiological procedures.

6.00 FOLLOW-UP

6.10 Medical and social service follow-up shall be available to patients discharged from the NICU in a regularly scheduled outpatient clinic supervised by the director of the NICU.

6.20 The patient's unit medical record shall be available for outpatient visits.

6.30 The duration of outpatient follow [up] shall be left to the discretion of the director of the NICU. Long-term observation of at least one year shall be encouraged.

7.00 RECORD KEEPING AND STATISTICS

7.10 Each Neonatal Intensive Care Unit shall maintain admission, health status, therapeutic and diagnostic records by birth weight and gestational age categories in such form as they may be submitted for review and comparison. Yearly statistics based on this data shall be prepared.

REFERENCES

REGIONALIZATION

1. Alden ER, Mandelkorn T, Woodrum DE, Wennberg RP, Parks CR, Hodson WA: Morbidity and mortality of infants weighing less than 1,000 grams in an intensive care nursery. Pediatrics 50:40, 1972

2. Committee on Fetus and Newborn, American Academy of Pediatrics. Standards and Recommendations for Hospital Care of Newborn Infants, 5th ed. Evanston, American Academy of Pediatrics, 1971

3. Carrier C, Doray B, Stern L, Usher R: Effect of neonatal intensive care on mortality rates in the province of Quebec, abstract. Pediatr Res 6:408, 1972

4. Desmond MM, Rudolph AJ, Phitaksphraiwan P: The transitional care nursery. Pediatr Clin North Am 13:651, 1966

5. Drage JS, Berendes H: Apgar scores and outcome of the newborn. Pediatr Clin North Am 13:635, 1966

6. Dweck HS, Saxon SA, Benton JW, Cassady G: Developmental assessment of the tiny premature infant, abstract. Pediatr Res, 6:408, 1972

7. Ellis WC, Bharara J, Snyder R: The regional newborn center—effect on neonatal mortality of referring hospitals (abstr). Pediatr Res 6:409, 1972

8. Erickson S: Infant I.C.U.s save lives—but too many units may add cost and hamper growth. Mod Hosp 115:80, 1970

9. Grassy RG, Barta RA, Zachman RD, Graven SN: Growth and development of low birth weight infants, abstract. Pediatr Res 7:402, 1973

10. Hunt JV, Tooley WH: Mental development in the first year for sick newly born infants, abstract. Clin Res 21:320, 1973

11. Indyk L, Cohen S: Newborn intensive care in the United States, east and west. Clin Pediatr 10:320, 1971

12. Kitchen WH, Campbell DG: Controlled trial of intensive care for very low birth weight infants. Pediatrics 48:411, 1971

13. Korones S: High Risk Newborn Infant: The Basis for Intensive Nursery Care. St. Louis, Mosby, 1972

14. Lucey JF: Why we should regionalize perinatal care. Pediatrics 52:488, 1973

15. Meyer BP, Harris TC, Daily WJR, Baum FK: Statewide reduction of neonatal mortality through effective regionalization of newborn intensive care, abstract. Pediatr Res 7:404, 1973

16. Murdock AI, Sutton M, Linsao L, Tilak K,

Reid M, Llewellyn MA, Swyer PR: Operational experience of a large urban neonatal referral unit. Can Med Assoc J 101:351, 1969

17. Rawlings G, Reynolds EOR, Stewart A, Strang LB: Changing prognosis for infants of very low birth weight. Lancet 1:516, 1971

18. Schlesinger ER: Neonatal intensive care: planning for services and outcomes following care. J Pediatr 82:916, 1973

19. Silverman W: Intensive care of the low birth weight and other at-risk infants. Clin Obstet Gynecol 13:87, 1970

20. Stahlman MT: What evidence exists that intensive care has changed the incidence of intact survival. In: Problems of Neonatal Intensive Care Units, Report of the Fifty-Ninth Ross Conference on Pediatric Research. Edited by JF Lucey. Columbus, Ross Laboratories, 1969

21. Swyer PR: The regional organisation of special care for the neonate. Pediatr Clin North Am 17:761, 1970

22. Teberg AJ, Wu P, Hodgman JE: Developmental and neurologic outcome of infants with birth weight under 1500 grams, abstract. Clin Res 21:322, 1973

REGIONAL TRANSPORT

23. Arp LJ, Dillon RE, Tom Long M, Boatwright CL: An emergency air–ground transport system for newborn infants with respiratory distress syndrome. Med Ann DC 38:261, 1969

24. Baker GL: Design and operation of a van for the transport of sick infants. Am J Dis Child 118:743, 1969

25. Chance GW, O'Brien MJ, Swyer PR: Transportation of sick neonates, 1972: an unsatisfactory aspect of medical care. Can Med Assoc J 3:847, 1973

26. Cunningham MD, Smith FR: Stabilization and transport of severely ill infants. Pediatr Clin North Am 20:359, 1973

27. Ferrara A, Cohen SN: NYC infant transport system (ITS): a program of regionalized care in an urban setting (abstr). Pediatr Res 7:401, 1973

28. Jung J: Neonatal ICU reaches out via air-lift. Hosp Pract 7:115, 1972

29. Segal S (ed): Manual for the Transport of High-risk Newborn Infants. Can Pediatr Soc, 1972

30. Shepard KS: Air transportation of high risk infants utilizing a flying intensive care nursery. J Pediatr 77:148, 1970

ADMISSIONS TO THE UNIT

31. Chernick V, Raber M: Electrical hazards in the newborn nursery. J Pediatr 77:143, 1970

32. Giunta F, Ruth J: Effect of environmental illumination in prevention of hyperbilirubinemia of prematurity. Pediatrics 44:162, 1969

33. Gluck L: Design of a perinatal center. Pediatr Clin North Am 17:777, 1970

34. Lubin D: Stringent grounding control, last-minute checks, needed for electrical safety. Mod Hosp 113:88, 1969

35. Segal S, Pirie G: Equipment and personnel for neonatal special care. Pediatr Clin North Am 17:798, 1970

36. Thogmartin BM, Tine MD: Design for obstetric and pediatric facilities. Columbus, Ross Laboratories, 1972

37. Usher R: Role of the neonatologist. Pediatr Clin North Am 17:199, 1970

2

High-Risk Pregnancy and Fetal Monitoring

HIGH-RISK PREGNANCY

Numerous obstetric factors, singly or in combinations, may be directly related to an increased risk of perinatal morbidity and mortality. Among these are the following:

Demographic and socioeconomic
   Maternal age less than 15 or greater than 40 years
   Low socioeconomic status
   Illegitimacy
   Low educational level
   Poor dietary intake
   Use of addictive drugs
Past obstetric history
   Primiparity or grand multiparity
   Premature delivery
   Abortion
   Perinatal death
   Major congenital malformations
   Blood group incompatibility
   Cesarean section
   Uterine abnormality
Medical and obstetric disorders
   Diabetes mellitus
   Hypertension and cardiovascular disease
   Infectious disease
   Metabolic and endocrinologic disorders
   Hematologic disease
   Preeclampsia

Multiple pregnancy
Placenta previa
Premature rupture of membranes
Intrapartum complications
   Fetal hypoxia
   Abruptio placentae
   Amnionitis
   Administration of depressant drugs to mother

In order to obtain the best possible result from a high-risk pregnancy, the obstetrician must first identify the patient at risk and then combine careful observations with appropriate diagnostic tests.

FACTORS ASSOCIATED WITH HIGH-RISK PREGNANCY

Demographic and Socioeconomic Factors

Pregnancies occurring at the extremes of reproductive age (less than 15 and greater than 40 years) are associated with the highest perinatal risk. A first pregnancy in a woman older than 35 is also associated with increased risk. Among the very young, the high incidence of illegitimacy is another factor leading to poor reproductive performance. There is greater perinatal morbidity and mortality among nonwhites than whites, primarily due to differences in socioeconomic status (see section Prematurity, Ch. 4).

The section Ultrasound (p 26ff) was prepared by David L. Frank.

Adverse socioeconomic factors, such as low income, public assistance, low educational level and poor housing, are associated with poor pregnancy outcome. Others, such as lack of motivation to seek prenatal care, inadequate diet during pregnancy and use of addictive drugs can also be considered sociomedical factors.

Obstetric History

Obstetric history has a direct bearing on the present pregnancy (see Ch. 17, History, Physical and Neurologic Examinations). Fetal risk is increased in primiparous and grand multiparous women. If there has been a previous history of premature delivery, abortion, perinatal death, excessively large infant (over 9 lb), major congenital malformation, blood group incompatibility, cesarean section, uterine abnormality or incompetent cervix, fetal well-being may be jeopardized.

Medical and Obstetric Disorders

Many medical and obstetric disorders have a deleterious effect on the fetus. From the medical point of view, diabetes mellitus, hypertension and infectious diseases are the most commonly encountered. The latter category includes venereal diseases, viral and protozoal infections, pyelonephritis and amnionitis. Metabolic, endocrinologic, hematologic and cardiac disorders may also affect the fetus.

Preeclampsia, multiple pregnancy, placenta previa and premature rupture of membranes are the major obstetric factors leading to increased risk.

Intrapartum Period

Complications during the intrapartum period may be superimposed on a high-risk pregnancy or may appear in one that has previously been uncomplicated. These are usually related to fetal anoxia, but may also be associated with hemorrhage, infection or administration of depressant drugs to the mother.

Most of the factors associated with high-risk pregnancy, are discussed throughout the text. A few, such as hypertension and multiple pregnancy, are discussed in this chapter.

PREECLAMPSIA AND HYPERTENSION

Elevated maternal blood pressure (an increase in systolic pressure of 30 mm Hg, in diastolic pressure of 15 mm Hg, or an initial reading of 140/90 mm Hg when normal pressure is not known), occurring either prior to or superimposed on a pregnancy, is hazardous to both mother and fetus. Proteinuria and generalized edema may occur either as isolated findings or in conjunction with the hypertension.

Preeclampsia refers to all three signs occurring together after the 20th week of gestation. The disorder may occur in various degrees of severity. The criteria for the less-severe form of the disorder are generalized edema without pulmonary involvement or anasarca, urinary protein loss of less than 5 g/24 hours and mild to moderate elevations of blood pressure. In severe preeclampsia, blood pressure elevations of 60/30 mm Hg above normal (or 170/100 mm Hg) are observed, together with proteinuria of over 5 g/24 hours, anasarca and pulmonary edema. Visual and central nervous system (CNS) abnormalities may be observed. If a convulsion supervenes, the disorder is classified as eclampsia.

If a patient has preexisting renal or hypertensive vascular disease, the condition is known as superimposed preeclampsia or eclampsia.

Etiology and Pathophysiology

The exact etiology of preeclampsia is uncertain, but certain predisposing factors exist, among which are teenage and multiple pregnancy, diabetes mellitus, hydatidiform mole and first pregnancy. It occurs three times more frequently among blacks than among whites, and there is an eight-fold increase in twin pregnancies.

Uterine ischemia is characteristic and is the factor most closely related to increased perinatal morbidity and mortality. Salt and water retention and various endocrinologic disturbances may also be present.

Clinical Aspects

Preeclamptic patients should be treated with bedrest, restriction of sodium intake and sedation. If the blood pressure rises above 150/100 mm Hg, proteinuria is greater than 1 g/24 hours, edema is progressive, urinary output is decreased or CNS symptoms appear, hospitalization is required.

Hydrochlorothiazide may be administered as both an antihypertensive agent and diuretic. Magnesium sulfate, administered intravenously or intramuscularly during the intrapartum period, effectively decreases neuromuscular irritability and prevents the appearance of preeclampsia.

Fetal monitoring is vital in patients with preeclampsia since the fetal mortality rate is as high as 20%. If the condition is progressive in spite of optimal medical therapy, delivery should be expedited, even in the presence of fetal immaturity.

MULTIPLE PREGNANCY

The human, like most other mammalian species having a gestational period of more than 150 days, usually produces one offspring with each pregnancy. The presence of two fetuses greatly increases the likelihood of maternal morbidity and perinatal morbidity and mortality. (Fetal and neonatal loss is about three to four times greater in twin than in singleton pregnancies.) The rare occurrence of triplets, quadruplets and quintuplets is associated with a progressive increase in perinatal loss.

Because of increased risk associated with multiple pregnancy, early knowledge of the presence of two or more fetuses is advantageous. When multiple births are anticipated, plans must be made for delivery at a facility capable of providing intensive care.

Twins may be either monozygotic (originating from a single fertilized ovum that has split in two at some time following fertilization) or dizygotic (originating from two separate ova that have been fertilized simul-

taneously). Although monozygotic twins are genetically identical, dizygotic twins are no more alike than siblings who happened to be conceived at the same time.

Incidence

The incidence of monozygotic twinning appears to be constant throughout the world and is independent of racial or ethnic background. It is a chance occurrence and not familial. Dizygotic twinning, on the other hand, occurs most frequently among the black population and least commonly among Asiatics. The incidence of twinning is about 1:93 births in the white population and about 1:73 in the nonwhite (over 90% black) population of the United States. The incidence of twinning is only about 1:155 among the Japanese.

Monozygotic Twins

Monozygotic (Fig. 2–1) twinning occurs following the splitting of a single blastocyst at some time prior to the tenth day after fertilization of the ovum; its etiology remains unknown. If splitting occurs before the third day after fertilization, each twin has its own amnion and chorion (25% to 30% of monozygotic twins). If it occurs between the third and eighth days, there are two amnions but one chorion (70% to 75% of monozygotic twins). Splitting after the eighth day (about 1% of the time) results in monochorionic, monoamniotic twins, who have a very poor prognosis. The umbilical cords of these twins become twisted around one another, leading to a very high incidence of fetal death. Splitting after the tenth day results in either conjoined twins or monsters.

Hazards

The hazards of multiple pregnancy are related to both the suboptimal intrauterine conditions and increased hazards of the intrapartum period. They are as follows: intrauterine growth retardation (occurring in monochorionic and dichorionic twins);

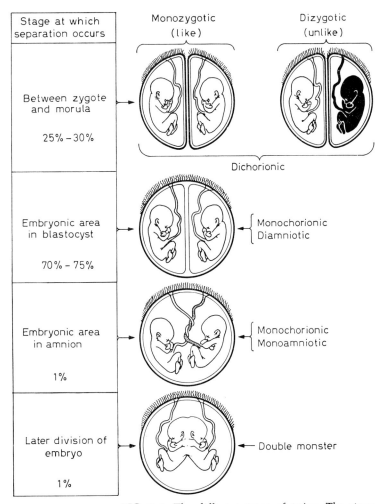

FIG. 2–1. The different types of twins. The stage of development at which separation occurs determines the variety of monozygotic twin. Dichorionic twins may be either monozygotic or dizygotic in origin. Monozygotic dichorionic twins form during the first to the third day of ovulation age when the embryo consists of only a few cells. Diamniotic monochorionic twins form before the eighth day, and monoamniotic monochorionic twins probably before the tenth day. Implantation occurs about the sixth to seventh day. After day 13 the germ disc shows the appearance of a single axial arrangement and can no longer divide into equal parts. Then only conjoined twins or monsters could form. (Morison JE: Foetal and Neonatal Pathology, 3rd ed. New York, Appleton-Century-Crofts, 1970)

increased perinatal mortality (incidence greater in monochorionic twins); intertwin transfusion syndrome (occurring in monochorionic twins); congenital malformations (incidence greater in monochorionic twins); hypoglycemia (occurring in the smaller of either monochorionic or dichorionic twins); decreased IQ (occurring in the smaller of either monochorionic or dichorionic twins); and increased intrapartum asphyxia (occurring in monochorionic and dichorionic twins, more often in the second born twin).

Intrauterine Growth Retardation. Both intrauterine growth retardation and premature delivery are associated with multiple pregnancy; the larger the number of fetuses present, the greater the degree of both prematurity and intrauterine growth retardation.

In his thorough study of 365 twin pregnancies, Gruenwald (8) was able to detect a decreased rate of intrauterine growth beginning early in the third trimester. This continued lag in weight gain continued through the last trimester; a mean peak weight of about 2700 g was reached at 39 weeks.

Singletons remaining in utero continue to grow through the 42nd week. The peak time of delivery for twins is about 38 weeks (11), compared to 40 weeks for singletons (Fig. 2–2). This relatively slow weight gain occurs in spite of the fact that the size of the placenta in relation to fetal size is greater in twins than in singletons up to 36 weeks of gestation. This latter phenomenon may represent a compensatory mechanism for decreased efficiency of placental exchange that occurs with multiple pregnancies.

Single Chorion. Gruenwald (8) has demonstrated the importance of intrauterine environment on the development of twin fetuses. The presence of a single chorionic

cavity appears to be associated with increased mortality when compared to dichorionic twinning. In the latter circumstance, both monozygotic and dizygotic varieties are affected in a similar manner with respect to morbidity and mortality. The relatively late splitting of the blastocyst that leads to monochorionic twinning may predispose to twins of unequal size. The placental vascular anastomoses that almost universally occur in these twins (6) may lead to the intertwin transfusion syndrome, in which the donor twin may become severely anemic while the recipient twin is polycythemic. The recipient twin is usually larger than the donor twin. In many cases, these anastomoses lead to the intrauterine death of a fetus, usually the donor twin. Congenital malformations also appear to occur more frequently in monochorionic than in dichorionic twins, regardless of zygosity. In Gruenwald's series (8) the perinatal mortality rate was 7.1% among monochorionic twins, 4.6% among the same sex dichorionic twins and 3.6% among opposite sex dichorionic twins. Significant differences in size (occurring most frequently among monochorionic twins) have been related to

FIG. 2–2. Intrauterine growth curves of dichorionic and monochorionic twins with Lubchenco's intrauterine growth curves for single born infants. (Naeye R et al, Pediatrics 37:409, 1966)

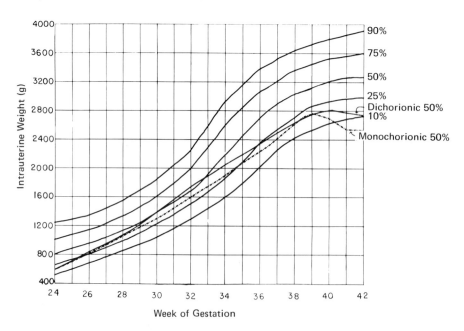

increased neonatal morbidity and long-term sequelae. Reisner et al (12) have shown that if there is a 25% or more discrepancy in birth weight, the smaller twin is likely to develop hypoglycemia. It has been shown that the IQ of the larger twin of similar sex is likely to be higher than that of the smaller (7, 10). Whether this is related to intrauterine malnutrition or neonatal hypoglycemia in the smaller twin can only be speculated.

Pregnancies with more than two fetuses present may be due to either fertilization of more than one ovum, the splitting of a blastocyst following fertilization or any combination of the two. The rising morbidity and mortality rates accompanying increased "litter" size is associated with both increasing fetal growth retardation and increased risk of premature delivery. With the use of hormonal therapy to treat sterility in women who are unable to ovulate, there has been a marked increase in the frequency of pregnancies in which three or more fetuses have been conceived.

Intrapartum Period

The intrapartum period is particularly hazardous, and perinatal loss is excessively high. The twin perinatal loss according to Guttmacher and Kohl (9) is four times that of the singleton, with mortality of the first born being 118:1000 and the second 148:1000. However, there is disagreement concerning increased risk of perinatal mortality in the second twin. Some factors predisposing to increased perinatal morbidity and mortality are premature delivery, intrauterine growth retardation, intrauterine anoxia (especially in the case of the second twin) and intrapartum bleeding. The latter may occur because of a high incidence of velamentous insertion of the umbilical cord in twins and, in monozygous twins, of the second twin bleeding through the cut end of the placental segment of the first twin's cord.

If multiple pregnancy is not suspected, there may be delay in delivery of the second twin, with an increased possibility of traumatic delivery, hypoxia and hemorrhage.

Preparation for Multiple Births

Because of increased neonatal morbidity and mortality, preparation for care of the infants should be made if multiple pregnancy has been diagnosed antenatally, and a pediatrician should be present in the delivery room. Admission to an intermediate or intensive care nursery is often necessary.

Vascular Anastomoses and Intertwin Transfusions

Examination of the placentas, both grossly and microscopically, is important and should be performed routinely. The macroscopic presence of vascular anastomoses and the microscopic absence of chorionic tissue between the two amniotic cavities confirms the diagnosis of monochorionic twinning. Vascular anastomoses between dichorionic placentas is almost unheard of in humans. Determination of zygosity by placental examination in similar sex dichorionic twins is not possible. At any rate, this determination is of little clinical importance in the neonatal period and may be made later if necessary by blood grouping techniques.

A difference in hemoglobin concentration of more than 5 g/100 ml in monochorionic twins in whom placental blood vessel anastomoses may have been present (provided that one infant is polycythemic) confirms the diagnosis of the intertwin transfusion syndrome. If the venous hematocrit exceeds 60% to 65%, or hemoglobin concentration 20 g/100 ml, the viscosity of the blood may be increased, and the plethoric infant may show signs of cardiac hypertrophy, polyuria, hypertension, sluggishness, irritability and respiratory distress. The treatment usually consists of a partial exchange transfusion with plasma (described in the section Polycythemia, Ch. 8). In the case of the anemic twin (hemoglobin concentration less than 15 g/100 ml or hematocrit less than 45%), a judicious transfusion of packed red blood cells should be given. If the twins are monochorionic (and therefore monozygotic), the blood removed from the recipient twin may be retransfused into the donor twin.

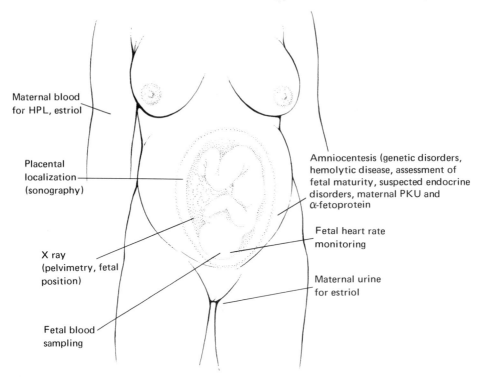

Maternal blood
for HPL, estriol

Placental
localization
(sonography)

X ray
(pelvimetry, fetal
position)

Fetal blood
sampling

Amniocentesis (genetic disorders,
hemolytic disease, assessment of
fetal maturity, suspected endocrine
disorders, maternal PKU and
α-fetoprotein

Fetal heart rate
monitoring

Maternal urine
for estriol

FIG. 2–3. Major diagnostic techniques used to assess fetal well-being.

Long-Term Prognosis

After the neonatal period, unequal growth may continue, especially if one twin has had severe intrauterine growth retardation. This may be accompanied by a decreased level of intelligence.

The management of multiple pregnancies, both in the antenatal and neonatal period presents a great challenge, and only through the utmost diligence can the very high perinatal morbidity and mortality rate be lowered.

DIAGNOSTIC TESTS

Numerous diagnostic techniques developed during the 1960s and 1970s enable the obstetrician to assess fetal development and well-being prior to the onset of labor. Used either alone or in combination, these proce-

dures are valuable in management of the high-risk pregnancy (Fig. 2–3).

In this section we will consider ultrasonic techniques, measurements of placental lactogen and estrogen concentrations in maternal body fluids and amniocentesis in diagnosis of fetal disorders.

ULTRASOUND*

In recent years, the use of ultrasound in medical diagnosis has undergone rapid development and become widespread throughout the world. It is a noninvasive technique that produces no discomfort, is apparently safe for mother and fetus and can be repeated as often as necessary.

The principles of medical ultrasound owe much to the use of sonar in the navy to detect the presence of enemy submarines. Initially, ultrasound was used primarily for therapeutic purposes. Its diagnostic application to obstetrics and gynecology was first described by Donald et al in 1958 (16).

* The section Ultrasound was prepared by David L. Frank.

Physical Principles

Ultrasound refers to mechanical energy with a frequency greater than audible sound (over 20,000 cycles per second). At these high frequencies (in the megahertz range), the wave length is of the same order as visible light, so that ultrasound exhibits similar properties of refraction and diffraction. In other respects, however, ultrasound displays the same characteristics as audible sound.

The main functioning element of an ultrasound machine is a transducer that houses a crystalline ceramic, such as barium titanate or lead zirconate titanate, having an asymmetric structure with one or more polar axes. Such crystals exhibit the piezoelectric effect. In this phenomenon, the shape of the crystal changes when an electric field is applied. Thus when an alternating current is used, the crystal alternately expands and contracts, producing mechanical waves of rarefaction and compression. In this way electric energy is converted into sound energy. When sound is reflected back to the transducer, the crystal acts in reverse to convert mechanical energy into electric potential (which can be measured by appropriate electronic devices) on the surface of the crystal. Thus the crystalline transducer serves as both transmitter and receiver.

The ultrasonic beam is composed of both longitudinal waves and transverse, or shear, waves. In longitudinal waves the particles of the medium oscillate in the direction of propagation, and in transverse waves particle motion is perpendicular to the direction of propagation. In gasses and liquids, only the longitudinal waves occur; in solids, both types of motion can take place. With the exception of bone, the tissues of the body behave as fluids, and therefore the main form of propagation in the human body is that of longitudinal wave motion.

The sonographic signal may be displayed on an oscilloscope in one of a number of forms. One-dimensional information is supplied by A mode, or amplitude modulation in which echoes are represented as spikes on a line. The intensity of the echo determines the amplitude of the spike, and the distance between interfaces is represented by the distance between the spikes. In B mode, or brightness modulation, each echo is represented by a dot, the brightness of the dot varying with the intensity of the echo. In B scanning the moving transducer picks up echoes from various points in the body, and a computer within the scanner arranges the dots on the screen according to their exact anatomic location to depict a two-dimensional cross section of the body. In M mode, or motion mode, the transducer remains fixed, but the anatomic part being examined moves. An electronic sweep causes the echo pattern to move across the face of the oscilloscope. This is used chiefly in cardiac work. The Doppler apparatus, which utilizes a slightly different principle, is also used in clinical sonography (14).

Diagnostic ultrasound has proven to be safe for both mother and fetus. No clinical evidence of harmful effects has ever been shown, and the few laboratory experiments in which damage could be produced used power levels far above those used in diagnostic pulsed ultrasound.

Hellman et al (20), in a follow-up of 3297 patients who had ultrasound examinations, found an incidence of fetal abnormalities no higher than that in the general population, even though many of these patients had been examined because of abnormal pregnancies.

Equipment and Technique

B scanning is the method in clinical use at our institution. The image on the oscilloscope screen can be photographed for a permanent record by a Polaroid camera.

Patients are examined with the bladder full. This displaces the gas-filled bowel, which reflects sound, out of the pelvis and provides a transsonic window through which the pelvic organs can be visualized. This is especially important in the early stages of pregnancy when the pelvic organs are relatively small, but for simple measurement of the fetal head in the last trimester it may not be necessary. The patient's abdomen is liberally coated with mineral oil to

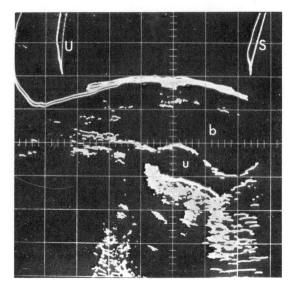

FIG. 2–4. Normal nonpregnant uterus. Longitudinal cross section, L + 1. Top of picture is anterior. As in all longitudinal sonograms in this text, cephalad is at left, caudad at right. The patient has a full bladder, b, to provide a transsonic window. Small u, uterus; large U (at left), Umbilicus; S, symphysis pubis.

improve contact and eliminate sound-reflecting air pockets between the transducer and the skin.

The transducer is then moved manually back and forth across the abdomen, first in the longitudinal direction and then in the transverse. The mechanical carriage of the scanner advances the transducer from one place to the next, so that the entire abdomen is covered. When an area of interest is localized, Polaroid films are taken. By convention, longitudinal scans are marked L, with the location of the plane of section designated in centimeters to the left or right of the umbilicus. Thus L+3 is 3 cm to the right of the umbilicus; L−4 is 4 cm to the left of the umbilicus, and so on. Transverse scans are marked in centimeters above or below the umbilicus, T+3 being 3 cm above the umbilicus, T−5 5 cm below. The probe is sometimes angled to bring it perpendicular with tissue planes. Occasionally an oblique scan is helpful in the delineation of multiple pregnancy or fetal presentation.

The examination usually takes from fifteen minutes to half an hour. Ordinarily the patient is quite comfortable except for bladder distension, although occasionally the supine hypotensive syndrome may interfere with the procedure.

Clinical Applications

The Normal Nonpregnant Patient. The normal nongravid uterus (Fig. 2–4) appears as an elongated oval-shaped structure, 4 to 8 cm long, behind the distended bladder. It may be slightly displaced from the midline. A retroverted uterus is more difficult to demonstrate than one that is anteverted. The normal non-gravid uterus is echo free even during menstruation. Normal ovaries ordinarily cannot be visualized.

Normal Pregnancy. The pregnant uterus is ideally suited for the use of ultrasound as it is filled with both amniotic fluid and solid intrauterine structures, providing interfaces of highly contrasting acoustic impedance. Also, the radiation hazards of x-ray and isotope methods are avoided.

The diagnosis of pregnancy can be made by demonstration of the gestational sac (Fig. 2–5), which appears as a ringlike structure within the uterine cavity as early as the fourth week of gestation and is consistently found from the fifth through the tenth week. As the uterus enlarges, the gestational sac grows proportionately. Contrary to traditional teachings that the early growth of the uterus is spheroidal, it has been shown that the increase in length of the uterus in the first half of pregnancy exceeds its growth in the anteroposterior diameter.

The gestational sac disappears between the 10th and 12th week. However, the placenta can be visualized at this time. The fetal head appears as a well-defined round structure between the 11th and 13th weeks (19).

Although the gestational sac and the fetal head are both ringlike structures, they can be differentiated by four criteria:

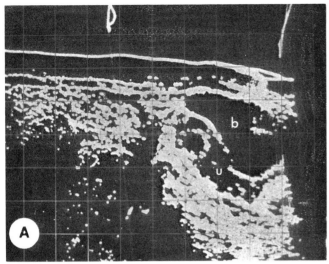
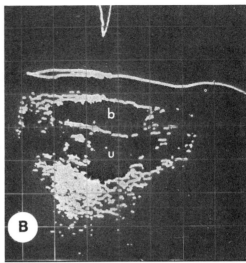

FIG. 2–5. Early pregnancy, 7 weeks (b, bladder; u, uterus). **A.** longitudinal cross section, L — 2. Circle within uterus represents gestational sac. A few echoes within bladder were not constant and are artifacts. Marker at left is for umbilicus; marker at right is for symphysis pubis. **B.** transverse cross section, T — 5. Marker is for midline.

1. The uterus is larger at the time of appearance of the fetal head than in the early stage of pregnancy when the gestational sac is present.
2. The fetal head (Fig. 2–6) has a smooth round or oval-shaped contour, whereas the gestational sac has an irregular contour produced by the chorionic villi.
3. The fetal head is visible even at the lower sensitivity settings, whereas increased sensitivity is often necessary to bring out the gestational sac.

4. The sac is fixed in position, whereas the head may move during the examination.

Fetal Presentation and Lie. The presentation and lie of the fetus can easily be determined by localization of their relative positions. The body, which is not as sharply defined as the head, is round or oval shaped in its transverse cross section and elongated in its longitudinal section. Often, internal organs can be detected within the fetal trunk. If doubt exists as to whether a rounded contour represents the head or the trunk, this can be resolved by scanning the same area in the perpendicular plane.

In breech presentation (Fig. 2–7) the fetal mortality rate is four-and-a-half times higher than that in vertex presentation. Hence it is important that the condition be recognized so that it can be properly managed. Sonography provides a reliable method of diagnosis.

Fetal Size and Gestational Age. It has been demonstrated that fetal head measurements correlate well with gestational age. Direct x-

FIG. 2–6. Fetal head, 9.6 cm, 39 weeks.

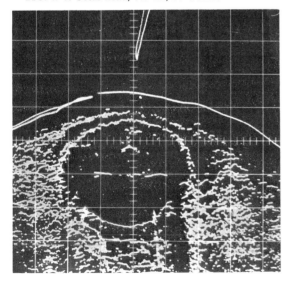

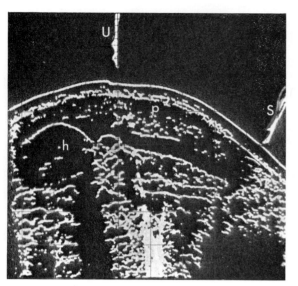

FIG. 2–7. Breech presentation. Longitudinal cross section, L + 7. Marker, U (at left) for umbilicus; S, symphysis pubis; h, fetal head; p, placenta.

ray cephalometry has been used, but it cannot be employed during the early stages of pregnancy since the fetal skeleton can rarely be seen before the 16th week of gestation. Even after this period x-ray cephalometry has not been reliable. Prediction of fetal maturity by radiologic detection of ossification centers is also of limited value. Measurement of head size by sonography is, however, extremely predictive of gestational age (Fig. 2–8).

In the case of elective cesarean section cephalometry, along with measurement of amniotic fluid phospholipids (see section Respiratory Distress Syndrome, Ch. 6) should be used to assess fetal maturity in order to prevent delivery of a premature infant. Thompson et al (23) found that when the biparietal diameter of the fetal head was over 8.5 cm, there was a 91% chance of the birth weight being greater than 2500 g. If it was more than 9 cm, the probability of a 2500 g birth weight was 97%. Lee et al (22), in their series of 63 patients, found that when the biparietal diameter exceeded 8.7 cm, every infant weighed over 2500 g.

Early diagnosis of impaired intrauterine growth (see section Intrauterine Growth Retardation, Ch. 4) is important since there is an eight-fold increase in perinatal mortality in this group when compared to normally grown infants of similar gestational age. To distinguish this group of fetuses from those with normal intrauterine growth in whom the maternal menstrual history is incorrect, it is essential that serial determinations be performed (15). Candidates for serial sonography would include

1. Patients with a history of previous fetal deaths associated with placental insufficiency.
2. Patients with systemic diseases such as hypertension or renal disease in which impaired fetal growth may occur.

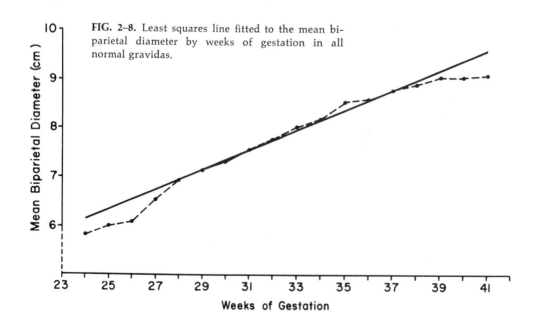

FIG. 2–8. Least squares line fitted to the mean biparietal diameter by weeks of gestation in all normal gravidas.

3. Patients in whom the uterus is small for the chronologic gestational age.

The fetal head (biparietal diameter) normally grows at the rate of about 1.8 mm per week, with some leveling off in the last few weeks of pregnancy. A significant deceleration of head growth may be a major factor in electing to deliver the infant early. It has been observed that fetal death secondary to placental insufficiency occurs most commonly about four weeks after growth failure is detected.

The technique of ultrasound cephalometry takes time to master and may not yield reliable results in the hands of the beginner (18). It is important to demonstrate the midline echo, which is believed to represent the medial aspect of each cerebral hemisphere. As this indicates the true longitudinal diameter of the fetal head, the biparietal diameter is perpendicular to it. The most common difficulty is encountered with a fetus in the direct occiput anterior or occiput posterior position so that the ultrasonic beam, entering the anterior aspect of the body, cannot pass through the biparietal diameter. Often a satisfactory scan can be obtained by oblique scans, by turning the patient on her side or by repeating the examination a few

days later. Other sources of error include exaggerated biparietal bosses, limited definition in the B-scan apparatus and incompleteness of the skull ellipse.

Charts and graphs have been constructed for the estimation of gestational age by measurements of fetal head size. During the first ten weeks of pregnancy, gestational age can be determined by the size of the gestational sac. Exact estimation of fetal weight by cephalometry is of limited value.

Multiple Pregnancy. An unusually large uterus may be indicative of multiple pregnancy (Fig. 2–9), excessive amniotic fluid (hydramnios), a large fetus or a tumor mass. Sonographic examination will usually establish the correct diagnosis. The entire uterus should be scanned in both planes so that a second fetal head will not be missed. In the case of twins, both heads can be shown on one picture by an oblique scan. This is more difficult however, when more than two fetuses are present.

Fetal Death in Utero. After the 12th week of gestation, fetal death is associated with changes in acoustic impedance that can be detected within 48 hours (13). Caused by seepage of amniotic fluid into fetal soft tissues, these changes result in new tissue-fluid interspaces. This produces a coarsened or brush-stroke appearance of the fetal outline. This phenomenon may also be encountered in diabetic pregnancies or in isoimmunized fetuses.

Twelve to 48 hours after fetal death, an increase in coarseness of body parts is seen, the skull collapses, and the normal, round well-defined contour is lost. Apparent overriding of bones is noted. There are increased echoes within the calvaria, and the normal midline echo cannot be identified.

The thorax also shows signs of collapse with fragmentation and overriding of its walls. Often a double line "echo," believed to represent the motionless mediastinum, can be demonstrated within the thorax.

In a series of 113 patients, Gottesfeld was able to detect fetal death with 98% accuracy (17).

FIG. 2–9. Twin pregnancy. Longitudinal cross section, L + 3. Two fetal heads, h, are shown. Placenta, p, in anterior.

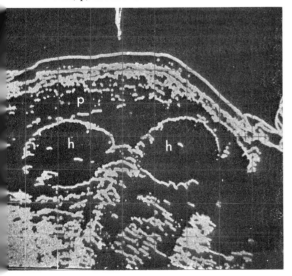

Evaluation of Fetal Heart and Circulation

Doppler Technique. The Doppler effect is based on the principle that sound or radio waves are reflected back to the transmitting source at an altered frequency when they strike a moving object. This property of detecting and describing motion has been utilized in the human body in blood flow studies, the detection of fetal life and the observation of fetal heart motion.

The difference in frequency between the emitted energy and the reflected energy can be demonstrated in a variety of ways. It can be converted into audible sound, delineated on an oscilloscope or recorded on paper or magnetic tape. As the audible sound is simply an electronic representation of alteration in wave motion, it is not identical with the sound heard through the stethoscope. Nevertheless, a number of distinct ultrasound patterns have been detected in the pregnant uterus. These correspond to: 1) the fetal heart, 2) major fetal blood vessels, 3) the umbilical cord, 4) the placenta, 5) movement of fetal extremities and 6) the maternal circulation.

At 20 weeks of gestation, the fetal pulse can be counted and recorded 17% of the time by this method. The inability to detect cardiac motion is a presumptive sign of fetal death. A misdiagnosis of fetal death has been reported, however, in the presence of hydramnios (13).

The Doppler apparatus can be used for intermittent observation of the fetal pulse or for continuous monitoring of the fetal heart during labor, as in cases of premature labor, prolapse of the cord, abruptio placentae and placenta previa or to monitor the second twin.

The Doppler technique has been used in placental localization, but it does not approach the accuracy or precision of the B scan.

M Mode Pulsed Ultrasound

When an electronic pulse hits an echo-producing structure moving in the direction of the ultrasound beam, i.e., changing in its distance from the surface, it will be reflected on the oscilloscope by an alteration of the position of the echo on the base line. If a time sweep is added to the horizontal axis of the oscilloscope, a time-motion display, or M mode, can be produced. This gives information as to the depth of a structure from the surface, the relative velocity of motion and cardiac rate and rhythm.

The region of the fetal heart can be first localized by B scanning, and the heart then studied by M mode. By this method, a fetal pulsation curve has been recorded as early as the ninth week of gestation. Although cardiac echoes are difficult to obtain in early and middle pregnancy and have little value except to demonstrate that the fetus is alive, a good echocardiogram can be obtained in the late stages of pregnancy or during labor.

Ectopic and Abdominal Pregnancy. Ectopic and abdominal pregnancy can be diagnosed by sonography. In the latter condition, the fetal head can be demonstrated outside of the uterus. The extrauterine placenta may be difficult to depict because of insufficient amniotic fluid, multiple adhesions and overlying bowel loops.

Fetal Anomalies. Anencephaly is a rare condition often associated with hydramnios. On sonography a normal skull cannot be demonstrated by longitudinal and transverse scanning, although a shapeless collection of echoes may be found. One must be careful not to confuse this condition with a normal fetal head lying low in the pelvis where it is difficult to scan. The diagnosis can be confirmed by x ray.

Hydrocephalus can be diagnosed by seeing an extremely large fetal head or a fetal head that is disproportionately large when compared with a cross section of the fetal body.

Placental Localization. Placental localization is important in patients with antepartum hemorrhage in whom placenta previa must be ruled out and in those patients requiring

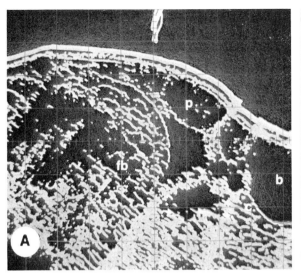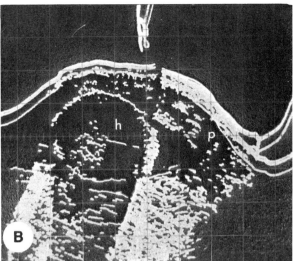

FIG. 2–10. Anterior total placenta previa. A. Longitudinal cross section, L + 3. Area of cervical os, c, is just behind bladder, b; p, placenta extends over os and onto posterior wall of uterus; fb, fetal body. B. Longitudinal cross section, T − 4; p, placenta; h, fetal head.

amniocentesis. Ultrasound provides a safe, reliable method of evaluation that causes no discomfort. In studies in which placental localization was confirmed at cesarean section or by manual exploration of the uterus during the third stage of labor, accuracy of 95% or better has been attained.

On the sonogram the placenta is represented by a semilunar speckled area demarcated by the inner wall of the uterus on the maternal side and an interrupted white line representing the chorionic plate on the fetal side. The chorionic plate can be best demonstrated when there is amniotic fluid separating the placenta and fetus. In a posterior placenta, the speckled effect is not always seen because of the attenuating effect on the fetus, although where the energy traverses only amniotic fluid in its path to the placenta, the internal echoes of the placenta are often seen. In general, a posterior placenta is more difficult to demonstrate than an anterior one (Figs. 2–10 and 2–11), and it is usually necessary to increase the sensitivity. It is very important for the patient to have a full bladder, as this provides better delineation of the lowermost margin of the placenta, the cervix and lower uterine segment and shows to what extent the placenta covers the internal os. As the relationship of the lower border of the placenta to the internal os can be determined, ultrasound is more precise in this respect than methods in which placental location can only be related to the symphysis pubis.

A placenta previa is best shown when there is a breech presentation or transverse lie. In such cases the chorionic plate is in contact with free amniotic fluid, creating a well-defined interface. The most-difficult cases are those of posterior placenta previa with vertex presentation, as in this situation the fetal head obscures the adjacent chorionic plate. Gentle manipulation of the fetus or a change in the patient's position may introduce amniotic fluid between the fetus and placenta.

In cases of isoimmunization, diabetes and syphilis, the placenta is found to be larger, thicker and less transonic than usual.

Kobayashi et al (21) have shown that in abruptio placentae the placenta is extremely thick, with clear spaces representing hematomas between the placenta and uterine wall.

Miscellaneous Conditions. Sonography has been of value in the diagnosis of hydatidiform moles, hydramnios and certain pelvic tumors associated with pregnancy.

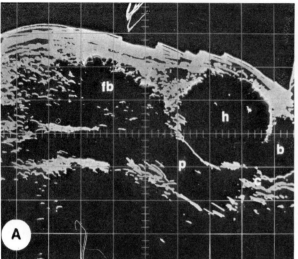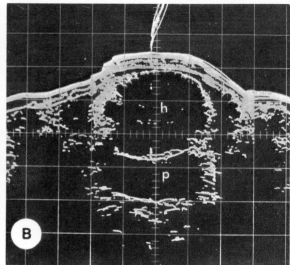

FIG. 2–11. Posterior partial placenta previa (h, fetal head; fb, fetal body). **A.** Longitudinal cross section, L + 1. Cervical os, c, is directly behind bladder, b. Note how placenta, p, extends to internal os. **B.** Longitudinal cross section, T − 8. Placenta directly behind fetal head.

ESTRIOL MEASUREMENTS

Measurement of maternal urinary estriol excretion is widely used in assessing fetal well-being during the third trimester (Table 2–1). Placental estrogens (primarily estriol) are produced in increasing amounts during the second half of pregnancy. Estriol synthesis requires a precursor (16 α-hydroxy-dehydroepiandrosterone), produced by the fetal zone of the fetal adrenal cortex. Urinary estriol levels therefore reflect both fetal adrenocortical and placental function, and abnormally low values usually indicate failure of the fetoplacental unit.

Following synthesis by the placenta, estriol is transferred to the fetal circulation, converted to a glucuronide in the fetal liver and excreted by the kidney into amniotic fluid. Estriol is then transferred to the maternal circulation and excreted via maternal urine. Although estriol concentrations in both amniotic fluid and plasma are low (measurable in nanograms/ml), the 24-hour urinary estriol excretion normally increases from 2 to 6 mg at 20 weeks to 12 to 40 mg at term.

Clinical Aspects

Measurements of urinary estriol secretion are valuable in assessing fetal status in such conditions as maternal diabetes mellitus, toxemia, hypertension, suspected intrauterine growth retardation and postmaturity (24, 27). In hemolytic disease secondary to Rh incompatibility, urinary estriol excretion may be normal even though the fetus is in jeopardy, and measurement of amniotic fluid estriol levels may be more useful.

Single measurements of urinary estriol excretion are usually of little value because of normal early variations. Sequential changes in estriol excretion over several weeks are more informative. If, for example, intrauterine growth retardation with placental insufficiency is suspected at 34 weeks, the absence of normally increased daily excretion as term approaches would support the diagnosis. On the other hand, if estriol excretion has been normal at 41 weeks but begins to decline thereafter, placental failure secondary to postmaturity may be suspected.

At term, a 24-hour estriol excretion of 2 mg or less is usually indicative of fetal death. In the range of 2 to 4 mg, the fetus may be severely compromised and unable to survive vaginal delivery. Values of 4 to 12 mg are considered borderline; in diabetes

TABLE 2–1. Normal Estriol Values

	Weeks of Gestation				
	32	34	36	38	40
Urine (mg/24 hours) (10th and 90th percentiles) (24)	8–23	9–27	10–32	11–35	12–40
Amniotic fluid (ng/ml) (95% confidence limits) (28)			2–10	4–12	5–18
Plasma (ng/ml) (mean) (29)	7.5	8	9	10	12.5

mellitus, excretion of less than 7 to 9 mg/24 hours is often associated with a poor prognosis, and delivery by cesarean section may be required.

In maternal hypertension or severe toxemia, poor renal function may lead to decreased urinary estriol excretion, even though the fetus is not jeopardized (25). Measurements of plasma estriol concentrations may point to a more-specific clinical picture.

With an anencephalic fetus, estriol production is severely impaired because the fetal adrenal cortex is nonfunctional. Similarly, maternal use of corticosteroids may impair estriol synthesis through suppression of adrenocortical function. Adrenal hypoplasia is also associated with decreased maternal estriol excretion.

While estriol measurements are of proven value, they must be used in conjunction with a variety of other tests, such as sonography, lecithin–sphingomyelin (L–S) ratio and monitoring of fetal heart rate in order to obtain as complete an assessment as possible about the fetal condition.

HUMAN PLACENTAL LACTOGEN

One placental protein of clinical significance in evaluating fetal status is human placental lactogen (HPL). It consists of a single polypeptide chain having a molecular weight of 20,000 and an amino acid sequence and immunologic reactivity comparable to pituitary growth hormone. This protein is also known as chorionic growth hormone, prolactin (CGP), purified placental protein (PPP) and human chorionic somatomammotropin (HCS). Human placental lactogen is synthesized and stored in the syntrophoblast cells of the placenta, which secrete the protein into the intervillous space and maternal blood pool. Little HPL reaches the fetus and none can be measured in either fetal or maternal urine. It has several known metabolic effects including induction of lipolysis, elevation of free fatty acids, inhibition of glucose uptake and enhancement of gluconeogenesis, thereby sparing glucose and protein and acting as a diabetogenic agent.

Human placental lactogen can be measured in small volumes (0.2 ml) of maternal serum accurately and rapidly using a radioimmunoassay technique; hence, mass screening is feasible. The serum concentration, which reflects placental mass, is detectable after the fourth or fifth week and increases progressively over the first two trimesters to a mean of about 7.7 μg/ml. This value persists from 35 weeks to term. In general, a rising HPL level is reassuring in pregnancies complicated by bleeding and cramping. Conversely, a declining level is associated with spontaneous abortion. In hypertension and toxemia the concentration of HPL per gram of placental tissue is lower than normal, and hence serum levels are generally low. Fetal death is often predictable in these pregnancies and is associated with decreased HPL values. Likewise, low levels of HPL are associated with intrauterine growth retardation. Human placental lactogen levels are not consistently altered in postmaturity, maternal diabetes or Rh sensitivity, nor are they clearly correlated with fetal heart rate or five-minute Apgar score. In sickle cell crisis and anemia HPL levels may be elevated. Low serum concentrations have been associated with fetal hypoxia and death, but the extent of this correlation is unclear. False positive results have also been observed (32).

Because of the close correlation between abnormally low levels and fetal distress and the ease with which the test can be performed, HPL determinations are of great potential importance in monitoring high-risk pregnancies.

AMNIOCENTESIS

Examination of amniotic fluid obtained by amniocentesis plays an important role in evaluation of the clinical condition of the fetus. Indications for diagnostic amniocentesis are as follows:

Early diagnosis of genetic disorders

Management of fetal hemolytic disease secondary to Rh isoimmunization

Measurement of surface-active phospholipids for assessment of fetal lung maturity

Management of suspected fetal endocrine disorders, e.g., hypothyroidism or hyperthyroidism, congenital adrenal hyperplasia

Management of fetuses of phenylketonuric mothers

Antenatal diagnosis of neural tube defects (α-fetoprotein)

Its major application has been in early diagnosis of genetic and biochemical disorders, management of the fetus with hemolytic disease secondary to Rh sensitization and assessment of fetal lung maturity. It has also been used successfully in a variety of other situations.

The technique is relatively simple (Fig. 2–12). After the placenta is localized by sonography, a No. 20 needle is inserted into the amniotic cavity under sterile conditions and approximately 15 ml of amniotic fluid is aspirated. Although the procedure is associated with minimal morbidity, such complications as bleeding, abortion, amniotic fluid leak, infection and even sudden fetal death have been observed (36). Therefore, the potential benefits of the procedure must clearly outweigh the risks.

Genetic Disorders

The use of amniocentesis for diagnosis of genetic disorders is discussed in detail in Chapter 14, Genetic Disorders. In this situation, amniocentesis is performed late in the first or early in the second trimester for determination of karyotype and for biochemical and enzymatic analysis. Knowledge gained from this procedure has a direct

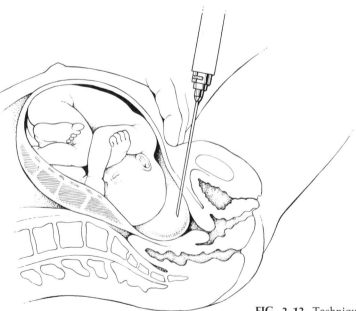

FIG. 2–12. Technique of diagnostic amniocentesis.

bearing on further management of the pregnancy.

Rh Incompatibility

Examination of amniotic fluid for bilirubin and related pigments in sensitized fetuses is discussed in the section Rh Incompatibility, Chapter 8. When amniotic fluid is removed for this purpose, the determination of amniotic fluid estriol concentrations may give further information concerning fetal well-being.

Phospholipid Measurements

The most-frequent reason for performing amniocentesis is assessment of fetal lung maturity by the L–S ratio or bubble stability test. This is discussed in detail in the section Respiratory Distress Syndrome, Chapter 6.

Other Determinations

Assessment of amniotic fluid volume may be of diagnostic value to the obstetrician. Excessive fluid (hydramnios) may portend a high intestinal obstruction, while decreased volume may reflect a genitourinary anomaly.

Amniotic fluid osmolarity decreases with advancing gestational age. A sudden increase in osmolarity may be an indication of fetal distress.

Measurement of amniotic fluid creatinine concentration (which normally increases after the 34th week) is another means of assessing fetal maturity. This is of limited diagnostic importance because of wide overlap of values.

Amino acids and various protein components of amniotic fluid have been measured, but have limited diagnostic value. In some instances, however, they may play a significant role in management of the pregnancy. For example, knowledge of the amniotic fluid phenylalanine concentration is important in managing the fetus of a phenylketonuric woman.

Elevated levels of amniotic fluid α-fetoprotein have been observed as early as the second trimester in the presence of severe neural tube defects, such as anencephaly and myelomeningocele. The practical use of this test is mainly among women whose previous pregnancies have terminated with infants having neural tube defects and in whom the chance for a second affected infant is 1 in 20 and for a third 1 in 10. Sonographic confirmation should, however, be performed in all suspicious cases.

Amniocentesis is of potential importance in the antenatal diagnosis of certain endocrine disorders. Elevated amniotic fluid concentrations of 17-ketosteroids and pregnanetriol have been observed in the presence of congenital adrenal hyperplasia (34). These determinations are indicated if a previous pregnancy has terminated in a child with this disorder.

Thyroid function studies on amniotic fluid are of potential importance in the presence of maternal hyperthyroidism or familial history of hypothyroidism.

Amniocentesis plays a major role as a diagnostic tool in perinatal medicine. It is likely that the number of useful diagnostic tests will greatly increase in the future.

AMNIOSCOPY

With the use of an amnioscope that can be inserted through the cervical canal, the color of the amniotic fluid can be observed in the presence of intact membranes. Meconium staining of the amniotic fluid, usually secondary to fetal hypoxia, is an ominous sign associated with increased perinatal morbidity and mortality.

When detected, membranes should be ruptured and fetal scalp blood pH determined. If acidosis (pH below 7.20) is present, immediate delivery of the infant is indicated.

REFERENCES

HIGH-RISK PREGNANCY

1. Nesbitt REL Jr, Aubry RH: High-risk obstetrics. II. Value of semiobjective grading system in identifying the vulnerable group. Am J Obstet Gynecol 103:972, 1969

2. Osofsky HJ (ed): High Risk Pregnancy with Emphasis upon Maternal and Fetal Well-Being. Clin Obstet Gynec, Vol 16, 1973

3. Shapiro S, Schlesinger ER, Nesbitt REL Jr: Infant, Perinatal, Maternal and Childhood Mortality in the United States. Cambridge, Harvard Univ Press, 1968

PREECLAMPSIA AND HYPERTENSION

4. De Alvarez RR: Hypertensive disorders in pregnancy. Clin Obstet Gynecol 16:47, 1973

5. Hendricks CH, Brenner WE: Toxemia of pregnancy: relationship between fetal weight, fetal survival, and the maternal state. Am J Obstet Gynecol 109:225, 1971

MULTIPLE PREGNANCY

6. Aherne W, Strong SJ, Corney G: The structure of the placenta in the twin transfusion syndrome. Biol Neonat 12:121, 1968

7. Babson SG, Phillips DS: Growth and development of twins dissimilar in size at birth. N Engl J Med 289:937, 1973

8. Gruenwald P: Environmental influences on twins apparent at birth. Biol Neonate 15:79, 1970

9. Guttmacher A, Kohl SG: The fetus of multiple gestations. Obstet Gynecol 12:528, 1958

10. Kaelber CT, Pugh TF: Influence of intrauterine relations on the intelligence of twins. N Engl J Med 280:1030, 1969

11. Naeye RL, Benirschke K, Hagstrom JWC, Marcus CC: Intrauterine growth of twins as estimated from liveborn birth-weight data. Pediatrics 37:409, 1966

12. Reisner SH, Forbes AE, Cornblath M: The smaller of twins and hypoglycaemia. Lancet 1:524, 1965

ULTRASOUND

13. Brown RE: Detection of intra-uterine death. Am J Obstet Gynecol 102:965, 1968

14. Brown RE: Doppler ultrasound in obstetrics. JAMA 218:1395, 1971

15. Campbell S, Dewhurst CJ: Diagnosis of the small-for-dates fetus by serial ultrasonic cephalometry. Lancet 2:1002, 1971

16. Donald I, MacVicar J, Brown TG: Investigation of abdominal masses by pulsed ultrasound. Lancet 1:1118, 1958

17. Gottesfeld KR: The ultrasonic diagnosis of intrauterine fetal death. Am J Obstet Gynecol 108:623, 1970

18. Hellman LM, Kobayashi M, Fillisti L, Lavenhar M, Cromb E: Sources of error in sonographic fetal mensuration and estimation of growth. Am J Obstet Gynecol 99:662, 1967

19. Hellman LM, Kobayashi M, Fillisti L, Lavenhar M, Cromb E: Growth and development of the human fetus prior to the twentieth week of gestation. Am J Obstet Gynecol 103:789, 1969

20. Hellman L, Duffus GM, Donald I, Sunden B: Safety of diagnostic ultrasound in obstetrics. Lancet 1:1133, 1970

21. Kobayashi M, Hellman LM, Fillisti L: Placenta localization by ultra sound. J Obstet Gynecol 106: 279, 1970

22. Lee BO, Major FJ, Wingold AB: Ultrasonic determination of fetal maturity at repeat Caesarean section. Obstet Gynecol 38:295, 1971

23. Thompson HE, Holmes JH, Gottesfeld KR, Taylor ES: Fetal development as determined by ultrasonic pulse echo techniques. Am J Obstet Gynecol 92:44, 1965

ESTRIOL

24. Beischer NA, Brown JB, Smith MA, Townsend L: Studies in prolonged pregnancy. II. Clinical results and urinary estriol excretion in prolonged pregnancy. Am J Obstet Gynecol 103:485, 1969

25. Galbraith RS, Low JA, Boston RW: Maternal urinary estriol excretion in patients with chronic fetal insufficiency. Am J Obstet Gynecol 106:352, 1970

26. Lundy LE, Wu CH, Lee SG: Estrogen assessments in the high risk pregnancy. Clin Obstet Gynecol 16:279, 1974

27. Ostergard DR, Kushinsky S: Urinary estriol as indicator of fetal well being. Obstet Gynecol 38:74, 1971

28. Sciarra JJ, Tagatz JE, Notation AD: Estriol and estetrol in amniotic fluid. Am J Obstet Gynecol 118:626, 1974

29. Tulchinsky D, Hobel CJ, Yeager E, Marshall JR: Plasma estrone, estradiol, estriol, progesterone and 17-hydroxyprogesterone in human pregnancy. I. Normal pregnancy. Am J Obstet Gynecol 112:1095, 1972

PLACENTAL LACTOGEN

30. England P, Larrimer D, Fergusson JC, Moffatt AM, Kelly AM: Human placental lactogen: the watchdog of fetal distress. Lancet 1:5, 1974

31. Saxena BN, Emerson K Jr, Selenkow HA: Serum placental lactogen (HPL) levels as an index of placental function. N Engl J Med 281:225, 1969

32. Spellacy WN: Human placental lactogen in high risk pregnancy. Clin Obstet Gynecol 16:298, 1973

AMNIOCENTESIS AND AMNIOSCOPY

33. Cassady G: Amniocentesis. Clin Perinatol 1:87, 1974

34. Jeffcoate TNA, Fliegner JRH, Russell SH, Davis, JC, Wade AP: Diagnosis of the adreno-

genital syndrome before birth. Lancet 2:553, 1965

35. Rajan R: Amniotic fluid assays in high-risk pregnancy. Clin Obstet Gynecol 16:313, 1973

36. Robinson A, Bowes W, Droeyemueller W, Pack M, Goodman S, Skikes R, Greenshur A: Intrauterine diagnosis: potential complications. Am J Obstet Gynecol 116:937, 1973

3
Oxygenation

OXYGENATION OF THE FETUS AND NEWBORN INFANT

Both fetus and newborn infant depend on a constant and adequate supply of oxygen for the continuation of normal metabolic processes and proper growth. Deviations from this standard may result in permanent damage both to the CNS and to other vital organs.

During fetal life, inadequate oxygenation is a continuous danger, and a primary goal of fetal medicine is the prevention of its occurrence. Overoxygenation, on the other hand, is a virtual impossibility.

Inadequate oxygenation postpartum may lead to diffuse tissue damage, as it does in the fetus. Overcorrection of this deficiency by excessive administration of oxygen may, however, lead to permanent retinal and pulmonary damage. An understanding of oxygen transport and utilization during the perinatal period is therefore vital for those physicians involved in the care of the fetus and neonate.

OXYGEN TRANSPORT

Although small quantities of oxygen are physically dissolved in plasma (the amount dissolved being directly proportional to the partial pressure of oxygen with which it is in equilibrium), oxygen transport depends primarily on the erythrocyte—and specifically on hemoglobin. This molecule, which contains iron, globin and a heme moiety, serves to chemically bind oxygen, transport it and release it at the cellular level, where it is taken up by the mitochondria. Between 40

and 70 times as much oxygen is carried by hemoglobin as by plasma (Fig. 3–1).

Each gram of hemoglobin, whether fetal or adult, maximally combines with 1.34 ml of oxygen at $38°$ C. The oxygen capacity of blood is the maximum amount of oxygen that can be bound at a given hemoglobin concentration. Thus at a hemoglobin concentration of 15 g/100 ml, the oxygen capacity is 20.1 ml. Oxygen saturation represents the actual percentage of oxygen bound to hemoglobin in relationship to the oxygen capacity. Oxygen content represents the total amount of oxygen in a given sample of blood and is the sum total of oxygen bound to hemoglobin and dissolved in plasma.

The oxygen tension or partial pressure of oxygen (Po_2) is measured in mm Hg and represents a driving force (analogous to voltage in electric terminology) and measures the ability of oxygen to escape from one phase to another (such as from air to hemoglobin or from hemoglobin to cells).

The partial pressure of oxygen bound to hemoglobin in arterial blood is the Pao_2. The relationship of Pao_2 to oxygen saturation of hemoglobin can be described by a sigmoid-shaped oxyhemoglobin dissociation curve that is derived by 1) equilibrating hemoglobin solutions with oxygen under various partial pressures in closed tonometers at constant temperature, pH and Pco_2 (all of which affect the affinity of hemoglobin for oxygen) and 2) measuring the saturation of hemoglobin at different partial pressures. At relatively low partial pressures hemoglobin becomes rapidly saturated with oxygen. The slope of the curve begins to flatten out at a Pao_2 of 70 or 80

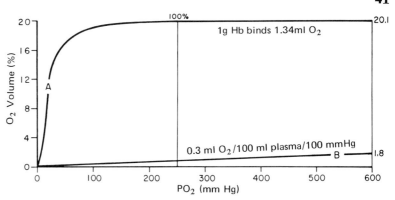

FIG. 3–1. The dissociation curve of hemoglobin (15 g/100 ml) at pH 7.40 and temperature 38° C (curve A) compared with the amount of oxygen dissolved in plasma (curve B) for P_{O_2} going from 0 to 600 mm Hg. (Duc: Pediatrics 48:469, 1971)

mm Hg, with the percentage of oxygen saturation being in the low 90s at this level. With increments in Pa_{O_2}, saturation of hemoglobin with oxygen increases little, and hemoglobin becomes fully saturated at a Pa_{O_2} of about 250 mm Hg.

FETAL OXYGENATION

Optimal oxygenation, along with normal acid-base balance, primarily depends on adequate gaseous exchange across intact placental membranes. To remain viable the fetus must be able to remove oxygen from the maternal circulation and return carbon dioxide in exchange for it.

The exchange of gases across the placenta occurs because of differences of both P_{O_2} and P_{CO_2} between maternal and fetal circulations. Oxygen diffuses poorly across the placenta, which has about 1/50th the capacity of the lung. There is a stepwise decrement of P_{O_2} from the maternal uterine artery (90 mm Hg) to the intervillous space (40 mm Hg) to umbilical vein (25–30 mm Hg) to umbilical artery (10–15 mm Hg). The difference in P_{O_2} between maternal arterial and intervillous blood probably represents shunting of partially desaturated blood from uterine musculature into the intervillous spaces. The low fetal Pa_{O_2} may also reflect the high oxygen consumption of the placenta (in the fetal lamb, one-third of the oxygen uptake from maternal blood is utilized by the placenta).

Fetal oxygen consumption is the driving force for maintaining a difference in oxygen tension between maternal blood in the intervillous spaces and fetal blood in the villous capillaries. Owing to the inefficiency of this oxygen transport system, the fetus must maintain normal aerobic metabolism at a Pa_{O_2} of about one-third that of maternal blood. That the fetus is able to do this is beyond dispute; however, the reasons are unclear. The fetus may have a richer tissue bed capillary supply, diffusion of oxygen into tissues may be more efficient or utilization of oxygen may be decreased. Other relevant factors might include the relatively large cardiac output of the fetus and the high oxygen capacity of fetal blood, which is secondary to a high hemoglobin concentration. Perhaps high fetal hemoglobin concentration is a response (like that of mountain climbers) to a low degree of oxygenation.

Because of the characteristics of the oxyhemoglobin dissociation curve, maternal arterial oxygen saturation remains relatively high even in the presence of hypoventilation. At the relatively low P_{O_2} of maternal blood in the intervillous spaces, oxygen is dissociated from maternal hemoglobin with comparative ease.

Several factors (Fig. 3–2) favor the uptake of oxygen by fetal blood, including the nature of the oxyhemoglobin dissociation curve of fetal hemoglobin, which is "to the

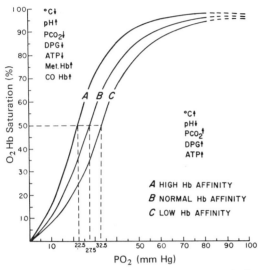

FIG. 3–2. Factors influencing the position of the oxyhemoglobin-dissociation curve (P_{50}). Curve B was obtained in a normal adult at 38° C, pH 7.40, P_{CO_2} 35.0 mm Hg. Curves A and C illustrate the effect on P_{50} of variations in temperature (°C), pH, P_{CO_2}, 2,3-diphosphoglycerate (DPG), adenosine triphosphate (ATP), methemoglobin (Met Hb), carboxyhemoglobin (COHB). Factors in the left upper portion of the diagram lead to a "left shift" of the dissociation curve, while those in the right lower portion lead to a "right shift." (Duc G: Pediatrics 48:469, 1971)

left" of adult hemoglobin (the lower the gestational age, the more pronounced the shift to the left). This means that fetal hemoglobin has a greater affinity for oxygen than has adult hemoglobin, and at the same P_{O_2} (all other conditions being equal) fetal hemoglobin has a higher oxygen saturation than has adult hemoglobin. In order to measure the position of an oxyhemoglobin dissociation curve, the P_{O_2} at which 50% of the hemoglobin is saturated is chosen as a reference point. This P_{O_2} is known as the P_{50}. A low P_{50} represents a high affinity of hemoglobin for oxygen, as is the case with fetal hemoglobin, and a relatively high P_{50} —as seen in adult hemoglobin—represents the opposite. The P_{50} for fetal hemoglobin is about 20 mm Hg, whereas that of adult hemoglobin is about 27 or 28 mm Hg (Fig. 3–3). In general the P_{50} increases with advancing postconceptional age (or shifts to the right) (12, 13).

The molecular basis for this important difference in oxyhemoglobin dissociation curves between fetal and adult hemoglobin appears to be due to an organic polyphosphate: 2,3-diphosphoglycerate in erythrocytes (14). Other phosphates are present within the erythrocyte, but 2,3-diphosphoglycerate is the most important, and its concentration averages about 5 mmol/ml of red blood cells (RBCs). It is bound to the β chain found in adult, but not in fetal, hemoglobin. This molecule forms a complex with reduced or deoxygenated hemoglobin, thereby inhibiting the binding of oxygen and facilitating the release of oxygen from the erythrocyte.

The concentration of 2,3-diphosphoglycerate does not vary between fetal and adult erythrocytes, the physiologic difference being that binding to hemoglobin is far greater in adult than in fetal cells.

There are instances, however, where maternal blood has a greater affinity for oxygen than has fetal blood. Parer (15) has shown that mothers who are homozygous for hemoglobin Ranier (whose dissociation curve is to the left of fetal hemoglobin) have normal reproductive histories and are able to provide adequate oxygenation of their fetuses. Other factors are involved in addition to differences in affinity for oxygen between fetal and adult hemoglobin that are responsible for transplacental transfer of oxygen.

The effect of pH on the affinity of oxygen for hemoglobin (Bohr effect) plays a role in oxygen transfer from maternal to fetal blood. As blood pH decreases, the affinity of hemoglobin for oxygen is decreased, and the dissociation curve shifts to the right. Conversely, with a rising pH the curve shifts to the left. When carbon dioxide passes from the fetal to maternal side of the placenta, the pH of the fetal blood rises, increasing its affinity for oxygen. Carbon dioxide entering the intervillous blood on the maternal side lowers the pH, thus decreasing its affinity for oxygen and making it available for transplacental diffusion.

At parturition, the mechanics of labor

may interfere with maternofetal gaseous exchange, especially if placental dysfunction is present.

There is evidence that administration of supplementary oxygen during labor may improve fetal oxygenation (11). A slight increase in the oxygen that is physically dissolved in maternal plasma may lead to a small increment in the Po_2 of poorly saturated fetal hemoglobin (on the steep portion of the oxyhemoglobin dissociation curve).

ASSESSMENT OF FETAL OXYGENATION

For many years, transabdominal auscultation of the fetal heart during labor was the only available clinical assessment of the adequacy of fetal oxygenation. Cardiac rates below 120 and above 160 beats per minute were considered indicative of fetal distress. However, this technique was found to be limited since the subtle changes in rate and rhythm that reflect inadequate oxygenation could not be detected. Biophysical and biochemical tests were thus developed, permitting the determination of fetal oxygenation prior to delivery. Certain changes in the fetal heart rate and an abnormally low fetal blood pH are two indicators of fetal hypoxia that warn the obstetrician that the fetus is in jeopardy.

FETAL HEART RATE MONITORING

The most widely used method of assessing the adequacy of fetal oxygenation during labor in the mid-1970s is direct monitoring of the fetal heart rate (FHR) (9, 17). The normal FHR is 120 to 160 beats per minute; sustained decreases or increases (for more than ten minutes) are called bradycardia and tachycardia. Although these may be indicative of fetal hypoxia, the most useful early indicator of fetal asphyxia is the relationship of transient decreases of cardiac rate (decelerations) to uterine contractions (Fig. 3–4).

In the presence of normal fetal oxygena-

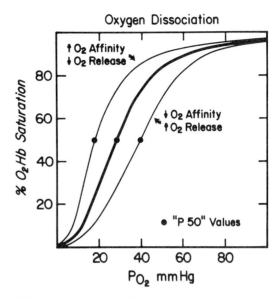

FIG. 3–3. The oxygen dissociation curve of normal adult blood (center curve). The P_{50} is approximately 27 mm Hg. As the curve shifts to the right, the oxygen affinity of hemoglobin decreases and more oxygen is released at a given oxygen tension. With a shift to the left, the opposite effects are observed. (Oski FA, Delivoria-Papadopoulos M: Pediatrics 48:853, 1971)

tion, the onset of uterine contractions is associated with a transient decrease in FHR. As contractions subside, the FHR returns to baseline values. This physiologic phenomenon is thought to be mediated through a vagal reflex when pressure is applied to the fetal head by the contracting uterus.

Late deceleration of FHR, however, is a pathologic finding associated with uteroplacental insufficiency and indicative of inadequate fetal oxygenation. Here, the decline in FHR begins late in relation to the onset of uterine contraction, with a return to normal well after the contraction has ended. Late decelerations occur when uterine contractions further impair oxygen transport to a fetus who is already either marginally or poorly oxygenated because of uteroplacental dysfunction. Both early and late deceleration patterns have a fairly uniform shape.

A third pattern frequently encountered, especially late in labor, is that of variable

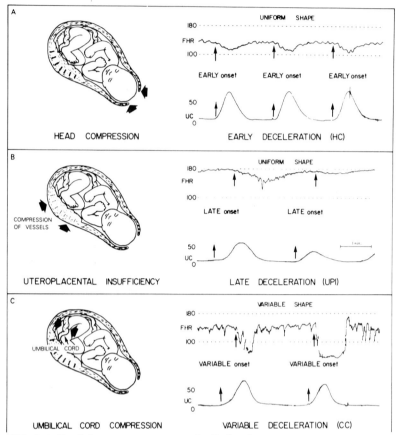

FIG. 3–4. Fetal heart rate patterns. **A.** Early deceleration caused by compression of the fetal head; **B.** Late deceleration caused by uteroplacental insufficiency; **C.** Variable deceleration caused by umbilical cord compression. (Hon EH: Clin Perinatol 1:149, 1974)

deceleration. Here, FHR deceleration may begin at any time relative to the onset of uterine contraction. This pattern is associated with compression of the umbilical cord and is usually not associated with fetal asphyxia. However, when a decelerated FHR lasts for more than one minute, fetal distress is likely.

Oxytocin Stress Test

The oxytocin stress test is designed to determine placental reserve prior to the onset of labor. After a baseline recording of FHR and uterine activity, oxytocin is administered intravenously at the rate of 0.5 mU per minute. The rate of infusion is increased by 0.5

mU every 15 minutes until the patient has three firm uterine contractions. If at least two uniform late decelerations are observed, the test is considered positive (indicating decreased placental reserve).

Clinical Considerations

Direct fetal monitoring can be instituted after membranes have ruptured and there is 1 cm of cervical dilatation. A stainless steel electrode is applied directly to the fetal head, and a catheter, attached to a strain gauge in order to measure intrauterine pressure during contractions, is inserted into the uterine cavity through the cervix. Using a 2-channel recorder, a permanent record of both FHR and intrauterine pressures can be obtained (Fig. 3–5).

The FHR can also be monitored by means of an external electrode attached to the mother's abdomen. Because of the high de-

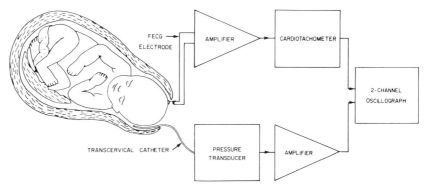

FIG. 3–5. Direct technique for intrapartal fetal monitoring. (Hon EH. Clin Perinatol 1:149, 1974)

gree of interference with the signal, this technique is most useful prior to the onset of cervical dilatation.

When FHR patterns indicative of fetal distress are observed, several measures can be promptly undertaken. Changing the position of the mother, especially if she is supine, may relieve pressure on the umbilical cord. Decreasing the dosage of oxytocic drugs (if they are being administered) may lessen the strength of uterine contractions and enhance uterine blood flow. Administration of oxygen to the mother may be of value. Analysis of fetal blood samples for pH may aid assessment of fetal oxygenation.

If there is no improvement in FHR patterns after about 30 minutes of therapy, delivery should be accomplished in the most expeditious manner.

Fetal heart rate monitoring has gained wide acceptance in evaluation of fetal well-being during labor in both high-risk and normal pregnancies. Although evidence exists that its use is associated with decreased perinatal mortality (16), studies are in progress (in the mid-1970s) more fully to explore its usefulness.

FETAL BLOOD SAMPLING

When fetal oxygenation is inadequate, lactic acid and carbon dioxide accumulate, with a resultant acidosis. Measurements of pH on small blood samples obtained from the presenting part during labor therefore reflect the state of fetal oxygenation (10), correlat-

ing well with both FHR and Apgar score (3). The Po_2 and Pco_2, which may change from moment to moment, are not reliable indicators of the state of fetal oxygenation.

The technique involved is relatively straightforward. The sacrum is elevated and the perineum cleansed, and under aseptic conditions, a Teflon endoscope is guided through the cervix and held firmly against the presenting part to prevent leakage of amniotic fluid.

After the exposed skin is dried, a drop of silicone is applied to enhance blood droplet formation, and a small skin incision is made by a blade attached to a rod. The blood sample is collected in long, heparinized capillary tubes, and a determination of the pH is immediately made. After the blood is collected, the wound is dried with a cotton swab and observed for at least one contraction to ensure that hemostasis has been achieved. Although this procedure is usually well tolerated by the fetus, adverse side-effects (bleeding and infection) have been described.

Indications

Fetal blood sampling during labor is helpful when the FHR is abnormal, when meconium has been passed by a fetus in a vertex presentation (this phenomenon may be normal with a breech delivery) and when there is previous evidence of fetal distress, e.g., low maternal urinary estriol excretion.

Interpretation of Results

If the blood pH is over 7.25, there is little risk of fetal asphyxia. If the pH is between 7.20 and 7.25, the fetus may be in jeopardy, and the determination should be repeated immediately. If the pH is less than 7.20, it is likely that the fetus is in jeopardy.

There are instances when a relatively high pH is observed, yet the fetus is depressed at birth (false normals); on other occasions a low pH is found, but the fetus appears well oxygenated at birth (false abnormals). Bowe et al (2) found either false normals or abnormals in 18% of their cases.

The most common cause of false normals is maternal oversedation. Other contributing causes are fetal infections, major congenital anomalies and asphyxial episodes occurring after the blood sample was taken.

False abnormals are usually a reflection of maternal acidosis, occurring after a long and arduous labor.

NEONATAL PERIOD

Following delivery, a smooth transition from placental to pulmonary respiration must occur in order to maintain adequate tissue oxygenation. An inability to carry out this transition leads to neonatal morbidity, possible neurologic sequelae and, often, neonatal mortality. Factors associated with neonatal hypoxia are incomplete lung development, increased pulmonary vascular resistance, right-to-left shunting of blood, alveolar hypoventilation, ventilation perfusion inequality, shock, cardiac failure and high fetal hemoglobin concentration.

Several conditions must be met for adequate neonatal oxygenation to occur. The lung must be capable of providing for normal gaseous exchange. Developmental immaturity, leading to respiratory distress syndrome (RDS) is the most important cause of abnormal neonatal oxygenation. In the premature infant, incomplete anatomic development of the lung results in a relatively small surface area for gaseous exchange. There is also an increase in the relative volume of anatomic dead space (con-

ducting airways) in this group. Although 25% of the tidal volume is dead space in full term infants, this rises to about 40% in premature infants and to as much as 70% in infants with RDS. All of these factors interfere with optimal oxygenation.

Aspiration pneumonia, pneumothorax and hypoplastic lungs are other conditions that may interfere with normal gaseous exchange in the lung.

Once the lungs have expanded and are supporting respiration, certain circulatory adjustments occur that are necessary for the continuation of normal oxygenation. When the lung expands, pulmonary vascular resistance falls, permitting a marked increase in blood flow to the lung. With poor oxygenation, pulmonary vascular resistance is increased, and blood flow to the lung is impaired. This leads to the establishment of a vicious cycle of increasing pulmonary vascular resistance, decreased oxygenation and worsening hypoxia. Hypoxia itself then causes a further decrease in pulmonary perfusion (4).

With normal oxygenation, the ductus arteriosus closes. In the presence of hypoxia, it remains open, and because of increased pulmonary vascular resistance, a right-to-left shunting of blood occurs, further perpetuating the hypoxia.

Certain congenital cardiac anomalies (see Ch. 7, Cardiovascular Disorders) associated with right-to-left shunting of blood may lead to decreased oxygen saturation of hemoglobin and subsequent tissue hypoxia.

Hypoventilation, usually secondary to CNS depression, can also be responsible for decreased gaseous exchange, leading to both inadequate oxygen uptake and carbon dioxide retention.

A decreased concentration of hemoglobin, even in the presence of normal pulmonary and cardiovascular function, may lead to tissue hypoxia. Although each erythrocyte may transport a normal volume of oxygen under these circumstances, the total quantity of oxygen being delivered to the tissues may be inadequate to support normal oxidative metabolism.

In the presence of shock (which may accompany RDS or follow severe perinatal asphyxia), both the total quantity of hemoglobin and the amount of oxygen carried by each erythrocyte may be sufficient, yet tissue hypoxia may still be present because of inadequate blood flow and consequent decreased uptake of oxygen by the cells. A similar picture may occur in congestive heart failure.

The high affinity of fetal hemoglobin for oxygen may be yet another factor promoting tissue hypoxia, especially among infants of low gestational age with RDS. The relatively high percentage of fetal hemoglobin present in the erythrocytes of these premature infants and their inability to regenerate 2,3-diphosphoglycerate appear to be factors preventing the release of adequate amounts of oxygen into cells even at a very low Po_2. The falling blood pH secondary to worsening hypoxia, may cause a shift of the dissociation curve to the right, temporarily enhancing oxygen release to the tissues, but this phenomenon is short-lived, and unless oxygenation is improved, tissue hypoxia will continue to worsen.

CLINICAL MANAGEMENT

High-risk infants require both thorough clinical evaluation and laboratory investigations in order to avoid both hypoxia and hyperoxia.

Careful observation of the infant is of primary importance. Cyanosis, labored or rapid respiration, retractions, flaring of the alae nasi, respiratory depression and pallor are important physical signs associated with hypoxia. It should be noted that about 3 g of unsaturated hemoglobin/100 ml of blood are necessary before cyanosis becomes clinically apparent. Therefore, some infants may be hypoxic, yet cyanosis is inapparent.

LABORATORY DIAGNOSIS

Some basic laboratory tests are necessary to evaluate the state of oxygenation. Knowledge of the hemoglobin concentration (or hematocrit) is important in assessing the oxygen capacity. In the presence of acute hemorrhage, the hemoglobin concentration may be initially high in the presence of a low blood volume. It must also be remembered that a hemoglobin or hematocrit determination performed on peripheral blood yields a higher value than that of venous or arterial blood, especially when there is poor perfusion of the extremities.

Measurements of Pao_2 are vital in assessing the state of oxygenation of the infant. At present this is best carried out on small quantities of blood removed from the abdominal aorta via an indwelling umbilical arterial catheter. Although these Po_2s may be slightly lower than those of arterial blood perfusing the brain (because of right-to-left shunting of blood across a patent ductus arteriosus), the values obtained are usually satisfactory in evaluating the state of oxygenation. An alternate satisfactory means of assessing Pao_2 is analysis of blood sampled by temporal, brachial or radial artery puncture. Determinations of the Po_2 on arterialized capillary blood should generally be avoided, if possible, since they may be low when compared to arterial blood. However, in the hands of some investigators, there is good correlation between arterial and arterialized capillary Po_2 at tensions below 55 to 60 mm Hg (7).

An indwelling oxygen sensor built into the wall of umbilical arterial catheters is now commercially available for continuous monitoring of Po_2 (8). Since discrepancies have been observed between readings obtained by this method and comparative laboratory blood gas measurements, further modifications must be made in this system before it can be utilized to give a completely accurate picture of the state of oxygenation of the infant.

A method of continuously monitoring Pao_2 by a transcutaneous surface electrode is undergoing clinical evaluation in 1975. This noninvasive method has the advantage of avoiding umbilical arterial catheterization and frequent removal of blood samples for biochemical analysis (9a).

The purpose of frequent Pao_2 measurements is to maintain an optimal level of oxygenation. Since hypoxia may develop below a Pao_2 of 40 to 50 mm Hg, and hyperoxic retinopathy at a Pao_2 of more than 100 mm Hg, it is recommended that aortic

Pao$_2$ be maintained in the range of 60 to 80 mm Hg (see section Retrolental Fibroplasia).

Measurements of oxygen saturation alone are inadequate to evaluate the status of oxygenation, especially at a Pao$_2$ greater than 70 to 80 mm Hg (where the oxyhemoglobin saturation curve begins to flatten out) and where large changes in Pao$_2$ are associated with very small changes in oxygen saturation. However, a determination of both Pao$_2$ and oxygen saturation on the same blood sample may be of value in assessing the affinity of the infant's hemoglobin for oxygen.

The change in Pao$_2$ following administration of supplementary oxygen may be of diagnostic value. If decreased oxygenation is caused by a right-to-left shunt, the administration of oxygen will have little effect on the Pao$_2$. However, if hypoventilation is the primary cause of inadequate oxygenation, an increase in alveolar oxygen concentration will improve oxygenation. In conditions such as RDS, in which poor oxygenation leads to pulmonary vascular constriction, the administration of oxygen appears to play a role in lowering the pulmonary vascular resistance, thereby improving the state of oxygenation.

Measurements of the blood pH and Pco$_2$ are necessary in evaluating oxygenation status. A metabolic acidosis in an infant with RDS is usually a reflection of poor oxygenation; carbon dioxide retention is usually indicative of either a ventilation-perfusion imbalance or hypoventilation.

Direct arterial blood pressure determinations via an indwelling umbilical arterial catheter are valuable, especially in asphyxiated infants or those with RDS who may be hypotensive. Even though hemoglobin concentration and Pao$_2$ are normal in these infants, tissue oxygenation may suffer because of decreased tissue perfusion.

THERAPEUTIC CONSIDERATIONS

The treatment of hypoxia in the newborn infant must be directed toward providing adequate tissue oxygenation without incurring the risk of either retinal or pulmonary oxygen toxicity. Although the former is due to an elevated PaO$_2$, the latter appears to be the result of direct exposure of lung tissue to high concentrations of oxygen.

When the PaO$_2$ cannot be maintained between 60 to 80 mm Hg by increasing the oxygen concentration in inspired air, assisted ventilation is indicated (see section Assisted Ventilation, Ch. 6). If the hemoglobin concentration is low (below 15 g/100 ml), a transfusion of whole blood should be given. Treatment of hypotension with either whole blood or plasma may be beneficial.

Another semiexperimental approach to the treatment of the hypoxic infant with RDS is exchange transfusion with fresh adult blood. The shift of the infant's oxyhemoglobin dissociation curve to the right is associated with improved oxygenation, and in the experience of Delivoria-Papadopoulos et al (5), with decreased morbidity and mortality.

Prompt diagnosis and treatment of fetal and neonatal hypoxia are necessary for intact survival. The introduction of new and improved techniques in these areas is the primary goal of physicians practicing perinatal medicine.

PERINATAL ASPHYXIA AND RESUSCITATION

Perinatal asphyxia refers to suboptimal oxygenation of the fetus just prior to delivery and of the newborn infant in the hours and days just following birth. A partial rather than complete lack of oxygenation leads to the most frequently seen clinical picture (27). One long-standing, minimal oxygenating defect associated with chronic placental insufficiency and decreased rates of fetal growth is discussed in the section Intrauterine Growth Retardation, Chapter 4.

Asphyxia is a leading cause of fetal and neonatal death and neonatal morbidity. Among survivors of moderate or severe asphyxia, there is an increased incidence of brain damage and developmental retardation. Early recognition of asphyxia in both the fetus and newborn infant is therefore of great importance to both obstetrician and pediatrician since it should lead to prompt therapeutic intervention.

Prior to delivery the obstetrician must be able to identify those situations associated with a high incidence of intrauterine hypoxia and to use all diagnostic methods available to him, e.g., urinary estriol determinations, fetal heart rate monitoring and scalp blood sampling, to confirm his diagnosis. If the fetus is compromised, every effort must be made to deliver a viable infant.

Lines of communication must be kept open between obstetrician and pediatrician so that the latter is present in the delivery room when a presumptively asphyxiated fetus is being delivered. The pediatrician should be well trained in resuscitation of the newborn infant. Since a substantial number of asphyxiated infants are born without any forewarning, obstetricians as well as anesthesiologists must also be trained in neonatal resuscitative methods.

PATHOPHYSIOLOGY OF PERINATAL ASPHYXIA

During the intrapartum period and prior to the onset of breathing, there is normally an interruption of transplacental gaseous exchange secondary to both placental separation and compression of the umbilical cord. Arterial blood pH and Po_2 fall; Pco_2 rises. This mild hypoxia and hypercarbia probably stimulates the respiratory center, and normal breathing patterns are quickly established. With the onset of spontaneous respirations, pH, Po_2 and Pco_2 rapidly return to normal levels. If the fetus has been asphyxiated prior to the onset of labor, establishment of spontaneous respirations may be delayed or impossible. In the latter situation prompt resuscitation becomes a lifesaving procedure.

Experimental Studies

Most of the knowledge concerning the pathophysiology of perinatal asphyxia and the rational approach to its treatment have been gained through the study of animal models. It has been known for about 300 years that newborn animals are better able than adults of the same species to withstand oxygen deprivation. This ability decreases with advancing postnatal age.

In the complete absence of transplacental transfer, the oxygen content of fetal blood decreases rapidly and is exhausted within one-and-a-half to two minutes. The ability of the fetus to remain alive in the presence of a decreased oxygen supply depends, therefore, on anaerobic metabolism. There is evidence that the major source of energy substrate for this process is cardiac glycogen, with the accumulation of lactic acid as a breakdown product (25). The ability to withstand perinatal asphyxia therefore depends to a large extent on the preexisting concentration of cardiac glycogen. (In human fetuses, unlike those of other species, cardiac glycogen concentrations reach their highest levels at term.) The rate of decline of cardiac glycogen during asphyxia decreases with the lowering of the environmental temperature. In certain species, hypothermia is associated with a beneficial effect on asphyxiated neonates. This may be secondary to the slowing of cardiac rather than brain metabolism. However, hypothermia has never been demonstrated to be of benefit in the treatment of the asphyxiated human newborn infant.

Because of its phylogenetic closeness to the human newborn infant, the newborn monkey has, in recent years, been investigated to gain a further understanding of human perinatal asphyxia. Acute total asphyxia produces primarily brain stem lesions in those animals, while partial asphyxia results in cerebral cortical swelling and necrosis (as is usually seen in severely asphyxiated human infants). Hence most human asphyxia is accepted as being partial rather than complete (27).

With complete asphyxia (Fig. 3–6), the animals breathe for several minutes. There is an initial elevation and then a fall in systemic blood pressure. Hypotonia, vasoconstriction and possibly a convulsion ensue. Respirations then cease for 30 to 60 sec-

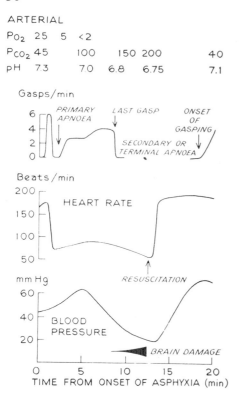

ARTERIAL

P_{O_2}	25	5	<2		
P_{CO_2}	45	100	150 200	40
pH	7.3	7.0	6.8 6.75	7.1

FIG. 3–6. Physiologic changes in rhesus monkeys during asphyxia and on resuscitation by positive pressure ventilation. Brain damage was assessed by histologic examination some weeks or months later. (Dawes GS. Foetal and Neonatal Physiology. Chicago, Year Book Med Pub, 1968)

onds. This is the period of primary apnea. Following this, there are gasping respirations at the rate of six per minute. This gasping soon weakens and slows. After the last gasp, the period of secondary apnea begins. The time to the last gasp depends on both species and arterial pH at the time of delivery. At a very low blood pH (under 6.8) there may be no gasping at all. During the period of primary apnea, and in the absence of respiratory depressant drugs, physical stimulation is sufficient to elicit gasping. An increase in intratracheal pressure during this period usually elicits a rhythmic respiratory effort. If gasping is present when resuscitation is instituted, readmission of air into the lungs is usually sufficient for recovery unless the gasps are very feeble and systemic arterial blood pressure is low. During the period of secondary

apnea, artificial ventilation or rapid correction of low blood pH (acidemia) by infusion of alkali, or both, are the only means by which gasping can be reinstituted. (The alkali appears to exert its beneficial effect by maintaining the intracellular pH necessary for the glycolytic process to proceed.) The first sign of recovery in this situation is cardiac acceleration accompanied by an increase in systemic arterial pressure. If the period of secondary apnea is prolonged, the rise in blood pressure is slow. In the newborn monkey who has entered a period of secondary apnea each delay of one minute before artificial ventilation is begun is associated with additional delays of two minutes before gasping begins again and four minutes before a rhythmic breathing pattern is reestablished. Following the end of the period of primary apnea, the time interval to the last gasp is about eight minutes in newborn monkeys. What this time period is for human newborn infants is not known.

The reason why a neonate can withstand apnea to a greater degree than the adult is not completely understood. A possible explanation may be that energy requirements of the neonatal brain are decreased.

Role of Barbiturates

The use of barbiturates as an adjunct in the treatment of neonatal asphyxia has been studied in several animal species (22). The pretreatment of these mothers prior to delivery with a short-acting barbiturate, e.g., pentobarbital, seems to prolong the time to the last gasp and affords some protection against CNS damage. However, there have been no reported studies showing that asphyxiated human newborn infants benefit from administration of barbiturates to the mother.

CLINICAL CONSIDERATIONS

Physical Setup of the Delivery Room

The delivery room must be properly equipped for neonatal resuscitation. An area must be set aside for procedures to be performed under thermoneutral conditions.

This can be provided by use of an overhead radiant heater. The equipment necessary for resuscitation consists of a laryngoscope with a pencil handle and premature blade, suction tube, an available source of oxygen plastic airways and Cole endotracheal tubes of various sizes with stilettes. An Ambu bag and a premature face mask must also be available. A wall clock with a second hand should be in full view.

Immediate Postnatal Period

Upon delivery the head should be held down while the umbilical cord is clamped and cut. The infant should then be placed supine under a radiant heater and quickly dried. The head should be kept below the level of the thorax while the nose, mouth and oropharynx are suctioned. During this time the nurse or physician should monitor the heartbeat and indicate the rate by tapping a finger. If the infant is extremely depressed with absent respirations, distant and slow heartbeat and poor muscle tone and reflex irritability, resuscitative measures must be immediately undertaken with endotracheal intubation since these findings indicate severe intrauterine asphyxia. In less-severe cases in which respiratory efforts are not present, but the heartbeat and reflex irritability are good, physical stimulation, such as lightly slapping the soles of the feet, may initiate a respiratory effort. This latter situation probably resembles the period of primary apnea seen in experimental animals, while the severely asphyxiated infant with poor cardiac function, muscle tone and reflex irritability is similar to the animal with secondary apnea.

At 60 seconds after delivery, the infant's clinical condition must be carefully evaluated. This is summarized in the one-minute Apgar score (20), which usually reflects the severity of fetal asphyxia (Table 3–1). However, depressant drugs and anesthesia given to the mother may produce low Apgar scores in the absence of asphyxia. Other conditions that may lead to a depressed infant are fetomaternal infection, congenital pneumonia, severe anomalies of the CNS and acute hemorrhage. A full knowledge of the maternal history, with special reference to maternal medication, is imperative.

Apgar Score

The Apgar score should be assigned by someone other than the individual who delivered the infant since complete objectivity on the part of this person may not be possible.

The Apgar score is based on evaluation of heart rate, respiratory effort, color, muscle tone and reflex irritability. A numerical score of zero to two is assigned to each of these factors. Absence of heartbeat and respiratory effort, generalized cyanosis or pallor, absence of muscle tone and reflex irritability are each given a score of zero. A heart rate below 100 per minute, slow or irregular respirations, blue extremities with a pink body, and slight muscle tone and response to a light slap on the heel with a weak cry or grimace are each given a score of one. A heart rate greater than 100 per minute, good respiratory effort, pink color, good muscle tone and cry are each given a score of two. Infants scoring seven to ten at one minute are clinically well and require no further resuscitation.

Those infants scoring four to six are usu-

TABLE 3–1. Apgar Scoring Chart

Sign	0	1	2
Heart rate	Absent	Below 100	Over 100
Respiratory effort	Absent	Slow, irregular	Good, crying
Muscle tone	Flaccid	Some flexion of extremities	Active motion
Reflex irritability	No response	Cry	Vigorous cry
Color	Blue, pale	Body, pink; extremities, blue	Completely pink

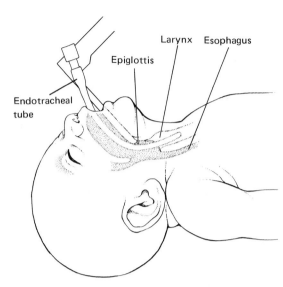

Larynx Esophagus

Epiglottis

Endotracheal
tube

FIG. 3–7. Endotracheal intubation in the newborn infant.

ally mildly to moderately depressed (often associated with maternal anesthesia and analgesia). Oxygen may be administered by bag and mask. A plastic oropharyngeal airway may be inserted to facilitate this procedure. In the vast majority of these infants, oxygen reaching the stretch receptors in the respiratory bronchioles will be adequate to stimulate spontaneous respirations (23). Infants who do not breathe spontaneously following these maneuvers require endotracheal intubation and assisted ventilation (Fig. 3–7).

In those severely asphyxiated infants having one-minute scores of zero to three who have not yet been intubated, the following procedure must be carried out immediately:

1. Place infant under radiant heater
2. Clear upper airway
3. Remove meconium (if present) from trachea by suction under direct visualization
4. Insert endotracheal tube and begin mouth-to-tube ventilation
5. If heart rate remains < 70 beats/minute, begin cardiac massage
6. If infant is still unresponsive at five minutes, inject sodium bicarbonate, 3 mEq/

kg, through umbilical catheter. With poor clinical response, repeat up to 2 mEq of sodium bicarbonate
7. If clinical condition is still poor, inject 0.5 ml of 1:1000 epinephrine through umbilical catheter, followed by a slow infusion of 1 to 2 ml of 50% glucose solution

The Apgar score is again determined at two and at five minutes. The one-minute Apgar score serves several purposes. Its immediate value is as a guide to the method of resuscitation that must be performed. It is also a prognostic indicator of neonatal mortality, with the latter being inversely proportional to the one-minute Apgar score. Correlation between this score and neurologic abnormalities at one year of age were reported in the National Institutes of Health Collaborative Study of Cerebral Palsy (26). With scores of zero to three, there was a 3.6% incidence of abnormality; scores of four to six were related to a 2.8% incidence and of seven or higher, a 1.6% incidence. In the same study, it was noted that the five-minute score serves as a better prognosticator for neurologic damage at age one year. Infants with five-minute scores of three or less had a 7.4% incidence of deficit, with scores of four to six, a 5.3% incidence, and with scores of seven or over, a 1.6% incidence. It was also found that infants with the lowest birth weights within their five-minute score categories had the worst prognosis.

Endotracheal Intubation

Once the decision to intubate the infant has been made, the procedure must be executed promptly. The infant is held in the supine position with the head slightly extended. If the physician is right-handed, the laryngoscope handle is grasped with the left hand while the right hand steadies the infant's head and holds it in line with the body.

The blade is inserted into the right corner of the mouth, advanced for about 2 cm between tongue and palate and then swung toward the midline with further advance. The epiglottis is visualized, and the tip of the blade is advanced gently into the space between the epiglottis and base of the tongue. The blade is elevated slightly, and the vocal cords and glottis are visualized. Visualization of the larynx may be enhanced by using the little finger of the left hand to compress the hyoid bone.

The endotracheal tube is inserted into the right corner of the mouth and then passed down the side of the laryngoscope blade so that the tip of the tube is approximately 2 cm below the level of the cords. If meconium, blood or mucus is present, the endotracheal tube is slowly withdrawn while gentle suction is applied. This is repeated until as much of the obstructing material as possible is removed. Assisted ventilation must not be attempted until the airway has been cleared!

Assisted Ventilation

Direct mouth-to-tube breathing is probably the safest and most efficient way of inflating the infant's lungs. If supplementary oxygen is required, a tube leading from an oxygen source may be led directly into the operator's mouth. The mouth-to-tube breathing should be carried out at the rate of about one per second until there is evidence of spontaneous, rhythmic respiration. Full expansion of the lungs with each assisted respiration is necessary, and the chest should be allowed to completely deflate during the expiratory phase.

In some infants with moderate asphyxia, gasping may occur very shortly after the initiation of mouth-to-tube ventilation. In the more severely asphyxiated infants, the first gasp usually occurs within 3 to 8 minutes, but assisted ventilation of up to 30 minutes may be necessary. If the heart rate is less than 70 per minute and has not risen promptly after the first three or four ventilations, external cardiac massage with the thumb pressed over the sternum at the rate of 2 per second may improve cardiovascular integrity by raising the systemic blood pressure and delivering gluclose and oxygen to the compromised brain. If artificial ventilation and cardiac massage are performed

simultaneously, the development of pneumothorax or pneumomediastinum becomes a real possibility. These two maneuvers should therefore be performed alternately.

Infusion of Alkali

Infusion of alkali plays an important role in the resuscitation of the severely asphyxiated newborn infant. Alkali solution is injected into the infant by means of a catheter inserted into one of the umbilical blood vessels. Although the vein is usually quite easy to catheterize, several potential dangers exist when this route is used. A large volume of alkali solution may cause liver necrosis if the tip of the catheter is in one of the branches of the hepatic vein. Introduction of a catheter into the umbilical vein is also associated with a relatively high incidence of infection. The umbilical artery may be relatively easy to catheterize in the asphyxiated neonate because of the relaxation of its muscular layer. One advantage of using this vessel is that the alkali delivered into the abdominal aorta is quickly diluted and dissipated. A potential disadvantage is that if the tip of the catheter cannot be visualized radiographically following its placement, a hypertonic solution may be introduced near the branching of the renal or mesenteric arteries from the aorta, with the attendant risk of arterial thrombosis.

The alkali solution to be infused may be prepared by mixing a 7.5% solution of sodium bicarbonate with an equal volume of 5% or 10% glucose solution, the latter providing an energy source for cardiac and cerebral metabolism. It is suggested that approximately 3 mEq/kg of sodium bicarbonate be infused over a 2 to 5-minute period (each ml of this solution contains approximately 0.5 mEq of sodium bicarbonate). The blood pH and P_{CO_2} should be determined several minutes after the infusion is completed. If there is a poor biochemical and clinical response, up to 4 ml of this solution may be infused after 10 to 15 minutes. The umbilical catheter should be left in place so that the infusion of glucose solution can be continued.

Other Measures

If in spite of the above therapy the infant remains unresponsive, 1 ml of 1:1000 epinephrine solution is diluted in 10 ml of a 10% glucose solution, and 0.5 ml of this solution is infused through the umbilical catheter. If there is still no clinical response 1 to 2 ml of a 50% glucose solution may be infused slowly through the catheter.

If there is no response at all to any of these measures after 30 minutes, the prognosis must be considered grave.

The use of analeptic drugs, such as nikethamide (Coramine), in the delivery room is to be condemned since they play no role in the resuscitation of severely asphyxiated infants. Those less severely asphyxiated infants who do respond to these drugs would have probably responded to physical stimuli alone.

Narcotic antagonists should only be used if there is either a high degree of suspicion or actual knowledge that the infant's depressed state is secondary to narcotics administered to the mother.

NURSERY CARE

All infants who have been asphyxiated should be transferred to the neonatal intensive care unit. If not already in place, an umbilical arterial catheter should be inserted for both blood sampling and monitoring arterial blood pressure. Any sign of seizure activity that may have been produced by cerebral anoxia should be managed in the manner described in the section Neonatal Convulsions, Chapter 9.

If anemia due to acute blood loss is present, it should be treated with a transfusion of whole blood. Suspected infection should be treated with appropriate antimicrobial therapy, and metabolic abnormalities, such as hypoglycemia and hypocalcemia, should be treated as indicated.

The long-term outlook for brain damage is greater in infants requiring resuscitation at birth than in normal infants. However, prompt establishment of aerobic metabolism, restoration of normal circulation and normalization of the internal environment may minimize this possibility.

UMBILICAL BLOOD VESSEL CATHETERIZATION

The three umbilical blood vessels (two arteries and a vein) offer unique sites for blood sampling, administration of parenteral fluids, exchange transfusion, monitoring of blood pressure and administration of contrast material for certain diagnostic radiologic procedures.

Although umbilical venous catheters were first used for exchange transfusions in 1947, it was not until the mid-1960s that both arterial and venous catheters were widely employed in neonatal intensive care units. Marked improvements in patient care were associated with this development. However, it soon became evident that serious complications were occasionally observed with the use of both arterial and venous catheters, and hence the benefits derived from their use should outweigh potential risks in any particular case.

INDICATIONS

Exchange Transfusion

Exchange transfusion is an absolute indication for catheterization of umbilical vessels. The umbilical vein may be used for both withdrawing and injecting blood. When this method is used, a polyvinyl feeding tube with side holes is preferred, with the tip of the catheter in the inferior vena cava. (With an end-holed arterial catheter, there is a risk of sucking up the blood vessel wall into the tube during the removal of blood).

Both vessels may be used concurrently for exchange transfusion, or the umbilical artery alone may be used in those infants with indwelling arterial catheters previously inserted.

Delivery Room

Infusion of alkali through umbilical vessel catheters in the delivery room is an integral part of resuscitation of the asphyxiated newborn infant. This is discussed in the section Perinatal Asphyxia and Resuscitation.

INDWELLING CATHETERS

The use of indwelling umbilical arterial catheters has become a routine part of neonatal intensive care. With this type of catheter in place, blood can be easily withdrawn from the infant for biochemical analysis, IV fluids and medications can be infused and arterial blood pressure directly measured.

The umbilical vein is ordinarily unsatisfactory for blood gas and pH determinations. The Po_2 is much lower than that of arterial blood, the Pco_2 is about 5 mm Hg higher and the pH 0.02 to 0.03 units lower. However, if a venous catheter can be passed through a patent foramen ovale in to the left atrium, blood samples obtained from this site will be similar to those obtained from the aorta.

Umbilical vessels should not be used routinely for the sole purpose of administering IV fluids since peripheral veins offer a safer route with fewer complications.

The umbilical vessels can be used, under some circumstances, for cardiac catheterization and for injection of contrast media for angiography.

Umbilical Artery

The technique for catheterizing the umbilical artery can be mastered readily. However, gentle handling of the involved tissues and strict sterile technique are absolute requirements. Preferably one group of physicians will be responsible for the performance of all umbilical arterial catheterizations since the incidence of complications seems to decrease when the procedure is performed by highly experienced personnel.

Catheterizations should be performed in a treatment area separate from the patient care area of the nursery. They should be carried out as surgical procedures, with the operators properly gowned and masked. Since they are performed outside of the incubator, thermoneutral conditions should

prevail, using an overhead radiant heater as the source of additional heat. Oxygen should be available, preferably via a plastic head box. A functioning laryngoscope and an endotracheal tube should also be available.

The catheter best suited for this procedure is the Argyle Umbilical Arterial Catheter. The No. 3½ French is generally indicated for infants weighing less than 1500 g, while the No. 5 is preferable for those over this weight. The characteristics that make the use of this catheter advisable for arterial catheterization are its softly rounded end hole, radiopacity and relatively small dead space.

When performing the procedure, the infant should be lightly bound to the treatment table. After careful preparation of the abdominal skin, the umbilical cord is cut, leaving a stump of 1.0 to 1.5 cm. The two arteries should be identified; since they are usually constricted, the one to be used is gently dilated before the catheter is inserted. This is done by placing the tip of a fine, curved eye forceps into the lumen of the vessel, releasing it and repeating the maneuver several times.

Before inserting the catheter, the dead space of the system may be decreased by cutting off the last 8 or 9 cm of the catheter and inserting a blunt needle attached to a three-way stopcock into the cut end. The catheter is then gently advanced. Obstruction may be encountered either slightly below the abdominal wall or at the entrance of the internal iliac artery. If very gentle pressure does not overcome the obstruction, 0.1 to 0.2 ml of 2% lidocaine (without epinephrine) is injected to attempt to release the spasm. If resistance persists in spite of this, catheterization of the other artery should be attempted.

The tip of the catheter should be in a position away from major arterial branches, e.g., renal arteries and celiac axis (Fig. 3–8). The most frequently used location is just above the aortic bifurcation (about 2 cm past the point where blood is first obtained); an alternate site for the tip is about 1 cm above the diaphragm.

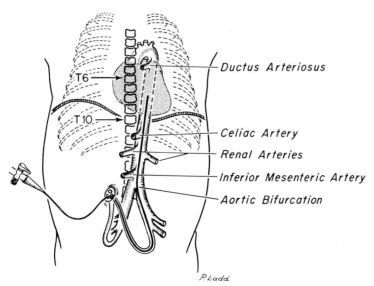

P Ladd

FIG. 3–8. Position of umbilical artery catheter. Major artery-aortic junctions are noted. (Weaver RL, Ahlgren EW. Am J Dis Child 122:499, 1971. Copyright American Medical Association)

Various formulas have been devised for the length of catheter that is to be inserted into the vessel (32). This distance can be ascertained by referring to Table 3–2. These measurements are just approximations, and posteroanterior and lateral x rays of the abdomen must be taken to assess accurately the location of the catheter (28).

The catheter should be held in place by a purse-string suture around the cord stump, and a sterile dressing with topical antibiotic ointment applied. The dressing should be changed daily, the area being inspected for evidence of infection.

There is no evidence to suggest that the use of prophylactic systemic antibiotics or even topical antibiotics applied to the umbilicus decreases the incidence of infection with indwelling umbilical arterial catheters (30).

Successful catheterization of the umbilical artery can usually be accomplished through the third day of life. Although the average duration of arterial catheterization is about two days, the catheter can often be left in place for up to one week if necessary.

When a blood sample is being withdrawn, the infant should be at rest, and the ambient oxygen concentration should be kept constant for at least 5 to 10 minutes.

Kitterman et al (33) suggest that when

TABLE 3–2. Mean Length of Umbilical Catheter Required to Reach Various Anatomic Points

Anatomic Points	No. of Observations	Total or Crown-heel Length (%)	Shoulder-umbilicus Length (%)
Umbilical vein			
V1 The diaphragm	43	17.6	60.0
V2 The left atrium	35	21.4	74.3
Umbilical artery			
A1 Bifurcation of aorta	26	16.5	55.8
A2 The diaphragm	26	31.3	106.4
A3 Aortic valves	24	47.5	159.9

(Modified from Dunn PM: Arch Dis Child 41:69, 1966)

withdrawing blood, three times the dead space of the catheter system (0.4 ml when blood is taken through the stopcock) be removed before the necessary sample is drawn into a herparinized syringe. The original volume of blood should then be reinjected through the catheter, along with a volume of fluid equal to the size of the specimen.

Removal of the catheter must be carried out by the physician with great care under sterile conditions comparable to those that were required when the catheter was inserted. During the removal procedure, a purse-string suture should be placed around the stump of the cord and tightened as soon as the catheter has been removed.

Umbilical Venous Catheterization

The procedure for insertion of an umbilical venous catheter is comparable to that for inserting an arterial catheter. A catheter with side holes, such as a polyvinyl feeding tube, is preferable to an open-ended arterial catheter. Insertion of a venous catheter is usually less difficult than that of an arterial catheter. Certain points, however, must be carefully followed during this procedure.

Although the umbilical vein does not have to be dilated, it must be free of clots before the catheter (which should be fluid filled) is inserted. The tip of the catheter should be advanced so that it passes through the ductus venosus into the inferior vena cava; it should not be allowed to remain in the portal vein or in any of its branches. The location of the tip of the catheter can be determined by posteroanterior and lateral x rays of the abdomen.

With both arterial and venous catheters, any impediment either in the flow of an infusion or in the ability to withdraw blood may be associated with formation of a clot within the lumen of the catheter. If this occurs, the catheter should be removed and a new one inserted. The blocked catheter should never be flushed since a dislodged thrombus may enter the infant's circulation.

Heparin has been added to the infusate and used as a flushing solution in an attempt to enhance catheter patency, but it appears to be ineffective for this purpose and has been shown to have an adverse effect on the infant's blood coagulability (36). However, 0.1% heparin may be used to fill the catheter initially when it is inserted.

COMPLICATIONS

Complications of umbilical vessel catheterization may be divided into acute and long term. Hemorrhage may occur through accidental perforation of the vessel wall. Blanching of a lower extremity may occasionally be seen with umbilical artery catheterization and is probably due to vascular spasm. When this occurs, the catheter should be removed and replaced in the other artery. Thrombosis and infection are major sequelae of deep vessel catheterization. Wigger et al (40) found at postmortem examination that 12.5% of all infants with umbilical catheters had vascular thromboses. Stasis and direct trauma to the vessel walls were considered major factors in the pathogenesis of this finding. Larroche (35) found a 33% incidence of thrombosis associated with umbilical venous catheterization. With umbilical arterial catheterization (in infants who came to autopsy), he found a 25% rate of thrombosis if the catheter was in place for less than 12 hours, 53% if the duration was 24 hours and 61% at 48 hours.

Neal et al (37) hand injected contrast material through the catheter as the tip was being withdrawn through the umbilical artery. They were able to demonstrate thrombus formation in 18 out of 21 cases.

Embolization, leading to gangrene of toes or even an entire lower extremity has been reported following arterial catheterization (38).

The experimental use of a radiopaque silicone rubber umbilical arterial catheter has resulted in a marked decrease in thrombus formation. Further evaluation is necessary, however, prior to widespread clinical use of this catheter (30a).

Infection, in the form of umbilical cellulitis, sepsis or multiple abscesses, is more often a problem with venous than with arterial catheterization (29). Bacterial colonization of umbilical arterial catheters is very common (34), with a 60% to 70% recovery rate for staphylococci, pseudomonas and other organisms. This is not reduced by the application of topical antibiotics. In only a small proportion of cases is there evidence of associated clinical infection.

Perforation of the large bowel has been reported following exchange transfusion during which umbilical venous catheterization has been performed (31). This may be secondary to disturbances of blood flow caused by the catheter located in the portal circulation.

Saline-filled indwelling catheters offer little resistance to passage of an electric current. Since extremely small currents are potentially capable of inducing ventricular fibrillation, all electric equipment must be adequately grounded.

Although umbilical blood vessel catheterization has greatly enhanced the care of sick newborn infants, the use of indwelling catheters should be limited to those instances where potential benefits outweigh the risk of complications.

RETROLENTAL FIBROPLASIA

Retrolental fibroplasia (RLF) exemplifies a very important therapeutic dilemma involving the use of oxygen facing physicians caring for newborn infants. The use of a quantity of oxygen insufficient to meet the needs of a hypoxic newborn infant usually leads to a perpetuation of the problem, with subsequent death of the infant or neurologic sequelae. The use of an excessive amount prevents damage to the CNS but, in the case of an infant of low gestational age, may lead also to total or partial blindness secondary to RLF (42, 47).

Although oxygen is one of the most widely used "drugs" in the neonatal nursery, the threshold of Pao_2 at which RLF may occur has not been precisely established, nor has its maximum safe dosage. A system for measuring Pao_2 on a continuous basis is available, but its clinical use has been limited. Biochemical measurements of Pao_2, which may be done only once every few hours, may lead to inadvertent hyperoxia over a period of time long enough for RLF to develop. Frequent examinations of the optic fundi of premature infants receiving supplementary oxygen may be of limited value in detecting the early vasoconstrictive phase of RLF (44).

Despite all the knowledge gained about RLF, it is still sporadically encountered among premature infants receiving supplementary oxygen therapy.

HISTORY

Retrolental fibroplasia was not recognized as a clinical entity prior to 1942. In that year, Terry (51) recognized that blindness occurred in certain premature infants. However, neither he nor other observers recognized the relationship between RLF and hyperoxia. In the decade between 1940 and 1950 the incidence of blindness secondary to RLF rose precipitously. By the end of the decade, RLF had become the major cause of blindness in children in the United States. Numerous etiologies other than oxygen toxicity were investigated, and the mystery remained unsolved. It was most commonly observed in the best-equipped premature nurseries, which had modern incubators capable of delivering high concentrations of oxygen. Its incidence was relatively rare where premature centers did not exist and oxygen was used sparingly.

In 1954 hyperoxia was definitely confirmed as the cause of RLF. Marked restrictions were then placed on the use of oxygen, and there was a subsequent decrease in the incidence of RLF. Oxygen concentrations greater than 40% were virtually never used. However, many hypoxic infants requiring higher concentrations remained underoxygenated, with an apparent increase in the mortality rate of low birth weight infants with RDS and a probable increase in the incidence of neurologic sequelae among survivors (43). By the mid-1960s, when the monitoring of Pao_2 became available to clinicians, concentrations of over 40% could be administered with a decreased risk of hyperoxia. In spite of this, sporadic cases of RLF continued to be seen. The development in the early 1970s of an oxygen sensor capable of continuous monitoring of Pao₂ may decrease the possibility of inadvertent overoxygenation and thus further decrease the incidence of RLF.

EMBRYOLOGY

For a fuller understanding of the pathogenesis and prevention of RLF, an appreciation of the process of vascularization of the retina and the effect of overoxygenation on developing retinal blood vessels is necessary.

Up to the third month of fetal life, the retina does not have its own blood supply but is apparently dependent on neighboring choroidal capillaries. With subsequent thickening of the retina, an additional blood supply is required. At this time, branches of the hyeloid artery begin to grow into the nerve fiber layer of the retina, advancing laterally toward the ora serrata. The temporal arteries form earlier than the nasal vessels and are longer at all stages of development (they have a longer distance to traverse to the ora serrata since the optic disc is located medially). By the eighth month of gestation, the vessels have reached the ora serrata, and the retina is considered fully vascularized.

Infants born prior to the eighth month of gestation must complete retinal vascularization following birth. During this period (as is amply demonstrated in experimental newborn animals) the retinal vessels are susceptible to the toxic effects of hyperoxia. Once vascularization has been completed, hyperoxia does not damage retinal vessels.

PATHOPHYSIOLOGY

The initial effect of increased oxygen tension on immature retinal vessels is vasoconstriction. Ashton et al (42) noted that newborn animals with immature retinal vasculature who were exposed to oxygen concentrations about 35% showed a marked constriction of arteries and arterioles, followed by a contraction of the entire capillary bed. Then the main arteries and veins constricted, leaving an avascular retina. These changes started within minutes after exposure to the oxygen, began peripherally and spread posteriorly. This initial process could be reversed by removing the animals from oxygen and placing them back in room air. After exposure to oxygen for three or more days, the process became irreversible.

This immediate vasoconstriction on exposure to high oxygen concentrations is noted in the retinal vessels of premature infants but not in the vasculature of any other organ. The mechanism responsible for this unique effect on retinal blood vessels has never been elucidated.

Following removal from an oxygen-enriched environment, the premature infant with preretrolental fibroplasia (constriction of retinal vessels) may show no further sequelae. On the other hand, within three to ten weeks, signs of the active stage, followed by cicatricial changes may occur. If vasoconstriction persists for more than 15 or 20 minutes after removal of the infant into room air, permanent changes of RLF are likely.

Following the period of latency, the first recognizable lesion of RLF can be found in the nerve fiber layer of the retina. Endothelial and mesenchymal cells proliferate, forming nodules, and whorls of capillaries are seen.

As the active disease progresses, hemorrhages may appear, and capillary tufts may sprout into the vitreous through the internal limiting membrane. Retinal detachment can occur following transudate in the retina and organization of intravitreal hemorrhages. The active stage may regress with spontaneous resolution or procede to the cicatricial stage. The duration of the active stage varies. It may be very rapid or may linger for weeks. It does not, however, continue after the sixth month of life. Owens (46) found that 44% of infants with active RLF had no permanent sequelae.

TABLE 3–3. Active Stages of Retrolental
Fibroplasia

Stage	Conditions
Preretrolental Fibroplasia	Marked constriction of vessels
Stage 1	Dilatation of tortuosity of retinal vessels
Stage 2	The retinal stage; stage 1 plus vascularization and some peripheral retinal clouding
Stage 3	The stage of early proliferation; stage 2 plus retinal detachment in the periphery of the fundus
Stage 4	The stage of moderate proliferation; hemispheric or circumferential retinal detachment
Stage 5	The stage of advance proliferation; complete retinal detachment

(Modified from Patz A: Survey Ophthalmol 14:1,
1969)

Active Stages

A classification of the active stages of RLF
proposed by Reese et al (50) in 1953 was
modified by Patz (49) in 1969. Table 3–3
gives this classification.

Cicatricial Stages

After the acute stage subsides, a wide variety of ocular changes can be seen in those
infants in whom the process does not completely resolve. These changes range from
small retinal scars with minor visual disability to the formation of a mass of fibrous
tissue filling the entire space behind the lens
and causing total blindness.

Table 3–4 is Patz's modification of the
grading of the cicatricial phase of RLF.

CLINICAL CONSIDERATIONS

The incidence of RLF is generally correlated
with both low birth weight and magnitude
of the peak level of Pao_2, although this entity has been observed in full-term infants
and in infants receiving minimal supplemental oxygen.

Aranda et al (41) found the highest incidence of RLF among infants weighing less
than 1500 g. Among their patients, vasoconstriction was never noted if umbilical
arterial Po_2 remained less than 100 mm Hg.
Although vasoconstriction was noted between Pao_2 levels of 100 to 200 mm Hg,
the active stage of the disease was noted
only in cases where peak Pao_2 was greater
than 200 mm Hg. It has also been observed
that the risk of RLF is increased following
blood transfusion (41a). A possible explanation of this finding is the shift in oxygen-hemoglobin affinity caused by transfusing
the neonate with adult erythrocytes, thus increasing the availability of oxygen to retinal
vessels and tissues.

Patz (48) has also found that examination
of the fundi of premature infants receiving
supplementary oxygen is of some value in
the prevention of RDS. Cantolino et al (44),
however, have found the evaluation of retinal vasoconstriction in these infants to be
extremely difficult. This may be at least partially due to a velum, or membrane, that
exists as a normal structure at certain stages
of embryonic development.

At the present time, biochemical measurement of Pao_2 at frequent intervals offers
the best means of averting hyperoxia and

TABLE 3–4. Cicatricial Stages of Retrolental
Fibroplasia

Grade	Condition
Grade 1	Minor changes; small mass of opaque tissue in periphery of the fundus without visible retinal detachment
Grade 2	Disc distortion; larger mass of opaque tissue in periphery of the fundus with some localized retinal detachment
Grade 3	Retinal fold; larger mass of opaque tissue in periphery incorporating a retinal fold that extends to the disc
Grade 4	Incomplete retrolental mass; retrolental tissue covering part of the pupillary area
Grade 5	Complete retrolental mass; retrolental tissue covering entire pupillary area

(Modified from Patz A: Survey Ophthalmol 14:1,
1969)

subsequent RLF. A well-functioning, atraumatic arterial oxygen sensor would replace this method, which requires frequent blood sampling.

SPECIFIC RECOMMENDATIONS

Because of limitations in following Pao_2s in infants receiving supplementary oxygen, the Committee on the Fetus and Newborn of the American Academy of Pediatrics has formulated the following set of guidelines regulating the administration of oxygen (45):

1. A normal newborn infant has an oxygen tension in arterial blood of 60 to 100 mmHg. It is recommended that, when newborn infants breathe oxygen-enriched mixtures, the oxygen tension of arterial blood be kept close to this normal range.
2. Inspired oxygen may be needed in relatively high concentrations to maintain the arterial oxygen tension in the normal range.
3. If blood gas measurements are not available, a mature infant who is not apneic but has generalized cyanosis may be given oxygen in a concentration just high enough to abolish the cyanosis. However, the infant born before 34 weeks gestation or weighing less than 2,000 gm (4 lb., 7 oz.) who requires an inspired oxygen concentration greater than 40% for more than brief periods should be treated, where feasible, in a hospital at which the inspired oxygen concentration can be regulated on the basis of blood gas measurements.*
4. The ideal sampling sites for arterial oxygen tension studies are the radial or temporal arteries. In most circumstances, however, in hospitals where well established experience has reduced the technical hazards, a sample from the descending aorta through an indwelling umbilical arterial catheter is satisfactory.
5. Equipment for the regulation of oxygen concentration (as provided by some incubators

* The Committee recognizes that, at the present time, this represents an optimal standard of care; and, it may well be impossible to arrange for such transfer because of lack of facilities and transport problems. The Committee hopes that, by making this recommendation, all concerned in the delivery of health care to the newborn infant will work toward making this standard a reality.

and respirators) and devices for mixing oxygen and room air may not function properly; therefore, it is essential that, when an infant is placed in an oxygen-enriched environment, the concentration of oxygen be measured with an oxygen analyzer at least every 2 hours. The performance of the oxygen analyzer must be checked daily by calibration with room air and 100% oxygen.
6. Mixtures of oxygen and room air may be delivered to an infant by endotracheal tubes, masks, funnels, hoods, or incubators. Regardless of the method used, the mixture should be warmed and humidified.
7. The condition of infants requiring oxygen may improve rapidly. Under these circumstances, the inspired oxygen concentration should be lowered carefully in decrements that maintain the oxygen tension of arterial blood in the normal range.
8. It should be appreciated that oxygen is toxic to organs other than the retina, e.g., lungs, which may be damaged even if the foregoing criteria are adhered to. To avoid prolonged hyperoxic exposure of the lungs, if very high ambient concentrations of oxygen are required to maintain a normal arterial oxygen tension, a reasonable compromise may be to lower the oxygen concentration progressively after the first 1 or 2 days, even though this may result in a somewhat lower arterial oxygen tension than normal.
9. A person experienced in recognizing retrolental fibroplasia (retinopathy of prematurity) should examine the eyes of all infants born at less than 36 weeks gestation or weighing less than 2,000 gms (4 lb., 7 oz.) who have received oxygen therapy. This examination should be made at discharge from the nursery and again at 3 to 6 months of age. If there are no fundal abnormalities on discharge from the hospital, no further eye examination is necessary.

It is apparent that any premature infant requiring oxygen therapy should be managed in a fully equipped neonatal center. Prompt transfer to such a center should be mandatory if proper facilities for monitoring Pao_2 are not available at the hospital of birth. In addition to the great risk of blindness when hyperoxia has gone unrecognized, there is also a great likelihood of litigation against the physician whose patient has developed RLF. Large judgments against such physicians have been common in recent years. It cannot be overemphasized that physicians must not only pay meticulous attention to the type of oxygen therapy that they prescribe for premature infants, but to the keeping of careful records as well.

REFERENCES

OXYGENATION OF THE FETUS AND NEWBORN INFANT

1. Bartels D: Prenatal Respiration. New York, American Elsevier, 1970
2. Bowe ET, Beard RW, Finster M, Poppers PJ, Adamsons K, James LS: Reliability of fetal blood sampling. Am J Obstet Gynecol 107:279, 1970
3. Caldeyro-Barcia R, Casacuberta C, Bustos R, Giussi G, Gulin L, Escarcena L, Mendez Bauer C: Correlation of intrapartum changes in fetal heart rate with fetal blood oxygen and acid-base state. In: Diagnosis and Treatment of Fetal Disorders. Edited by K Adamsons. New York, Springer-Verlag, 1967, p 205
4. Chu J, Clements JA, Cotton E, Klaus MH, Sweet AY, Thomas MA, Tooley WH: Preliminary report: the pulmonary hypoperfusion syndrome. Pediatrics 35:733, 1965
5. Delivoria-Papadopoulos M, Morrow G, Oski FA: Exchange transfusion in the newborn infant with fresh and "old" blood: The role of storage on 2,3,-diphosphoglycerate, hemoglobin oxygen affinity and oxygen release. J Pediatr 79:898, 1971
6. Duc G: Assessment of hypoxia in the newborn. Pediatrics 48:469, 1971
7. Glasgow JF, Flynn DM, Swyer PR: A comparison of descending aortic and "arterialized" capillary blood in the sick newborn. Can Med Assoc J 106:660, 1972
8. Harris TR, Nugent M: Continuous arterial oxygen tension monitoring in the newborn infant. J Pediatr 82:929, 1973
9. Hon EH: Biophysical intrapartal fetal monitoring. Clin Perinatol 1:149, 1974
9a. Huch R, Huch A. Lübbers DW: Transcutaneous measurements of blood PO_2 (tcPO_2): Method and applications in perinatal medicine. J Perinat Med 1:183, 1973
10. James LS: Fetal blood sampling. Clin Perinatol 1:141, 1974
11. Khazin AF, Hon EH, Hehre FW: Effects of maternal hyperoxia on fetus. I. Oxygen tension. Am J Obstet Gynecol 109:628, 1974
12. Novy MJ, Frigoletto FD, Easterday CL, Umansky I, Nelson NM: Changes in cord blood oxygen affinity after intrauterine transfusions for erythroblastosis. N Engl J Med 285:589, 1971
13. Orzalesi MM, Hay WW: The regulation of oxygen affinity of fetal blood. I. In vitro experiments and results in normal infants. Pediatrics 48:857, 1971
14. Oski FA: The unique fetal red cell and its function. Pediatrics 51:494, 1973
15. Parer JT: Reversed relationship of oxygen affinity in maternal and fetal blood. Am J Obstet Gynecol 108:323, 1970
16. Paul RH, Hon EH: Clinical fetal monitoring. V. Effect on perinatal outcome. Am J Obstet Gynecol 118:529, 1974
17. Shifrin BS: Fetal heart rate monitoring during labor. JAMA 222:96, 1972
18. Stern L: The use and misuse of oxygen in the newborn infant. Pediatr Clin North Am 20:447, 1973

PERINATAL ASPHYXIA AND RESUSCITATION

19. Adamsons K, Myers RE: Perinatal asphyxia: Causes, detection and neurologic sequelae. Pediatr Clin North Am 20:465, 1973
20. Apgar V: The newborn (APGAR) scoring system: reflections and advice. Pediatr Clin North Am 13:645, 1966
21. Behrman RE, James LS, Klaus M, Nelson N, Oliver T: Treatment of the asphyxiated newborn infant. J Pediatr 74:981, 1969
22. Brown AW, Montalvo JM: Barbiturates and asphyxia. Pediatr Clin North Am 17:851, 1970
23. Cross KW: Resuscitation of the asphyxiated infant. Br M Bull 22:73, 1966
24. Dawes G: Birth asphyxia, resuscitation and brain damage. In Foetal and Neonatal Physiology, A Comparative Study of the Changes at Birth. Chicago, Year Book Med Pub, 1968, p 141
25. Dawes GS, Mott JC, Shelley HJ: The importance of cardiac glycogen for the maintenance of life in foetal lambs and newborn animals during anoxia. J Physiol (Lond) 146:516, 1959
26. Drage JS, Berendes H: Apgar scores and outcome of the newborn. Pediatr Clin North Am 13:635, 1966
27. Myers RE: Two patterns of perinatal brain damage and their conditions of occurrence. Am J Obstet Gynecol 112:246, 1972

UMBILICAL BLOOD VESSEL CATHETERIZATION

28. Baker DH, Berdon WE, James LS: Proper localization of umbilical arterial and venous catheters by lateral roentgenograms. Pediatrics 43:34, 1969
29. Balagtas RC, Bell CE, Edwards LD, Levin S: Risk of local and systemic infections associated with umbilical vein catheterization: a prospective study in 86 newborn patients. Pediatrics 48:359, 1971
30. Bhatt DR, Hodgman JE, Tatter D: Evaluation of prophylactic antibiotics during umbilical catheterization in newborns. Clin Res 18:217, 1970

30a. Boros SJ, Thompson TR, Reynolds JW, Jarvis CW, Williams HJ: Reduced thrombus formation with silicone rubber (silastic) umbilical artery catheters (abstr). Pediatr Res, 9:363, 1975

31. Corkery JJ, Dubowitz V, Lister J, Moosa A: Colonic perforation after exchange transfusion. Br Med J 4:345, 1968

32. Dunn PM: Localization of the umbilical catheter by postmortem measurements. Arch Dis Child 41:69, 1966

33. Kitterman JA, Phibbs RH, Tooley WH: Catheterization of umbilical vessels in newborn infants. Pediatr Clin North Am 17:895, 1970

34. Krauss AN, Albert RF, Kannan MM: Contamination of umbilical catheters in the newborn infant. J Pediatr 77:965, 1970

35. Larroche JC: Umbilical catheterization: Its complications. Biol Neonate 16:101, 1970

36. Merenstein G, Blackmon L: Heparin and umbilical arterial catheters (abst). Clin Res 20:282, 1972

37. Neal WA, Reynolds JW, Jarvis CW, Williams HJ: Umbilical artery catheterization: demonstration of arterial thrombosis by aortography. Pediatrics 50:6, 1972

38. Schenker MD: Gangrene of the extremities of a newborn premature infant. Clin Pediatr 12:285, 1973

39. Symansky MR, Fox HA: Umbilical vessel catheterization: indications, management, and evaluation of the technique. J Pediatr 80:820, 1972

40. Wigger HJ, Bransilver BR, Blanc WA: Thromboses due to catheterization in infants and children. J Pediatr 76:1, 1970

RETROLENTAL FIBROPLASIA

41. Aranda JV, Saheb N, Stern L, Avery ME: Arterial oxygen tension and retinal vasoconstriction in newborn infants. Am J Dis Child 122:189, 1971

41a. Aranda JV, Clark TE, Maniello R, Outerbridge EW. Blood transfusion (BT): Possible potentiating risk factor in retrolental fibroplasma (RLF) (abstr). Pediatr Res 9:362, 1975

42. Ashton N, Ward B, Serpell G: Effect of oxygen on developing retinal vessels with particular reference to the problem of retrolental fibroplasia. Br J Ophthalmol 38:397, 1954

43. Avery ME, Oppenheimer EH: Recent increase in mortality from hyaline membrane disease. J Pediatr 57:553, 1960

44. Cantolino SJ, O'Grady GE, Herrera JA, Israel C, Justice J, Flynn JT: Ophthalmoscopic monitoring of oxygen therapy in premature infants. Am J Ophthalmol 72:32, 1971

45. Committee on Fetus and Newborn, American Academy of Pediatrics: Standards and Recommendations for Hospital Care of Newborn Infants, 5th ed. Evanston, American Academy of Pediatrics, 1971

46. Owens WC: Spontaneous regression in retrolental fibroplasia. Trans Am Ophthalmol Soc 51:555, 1953

47. Patz A: Oxygen studies in retrolental fibroplasia. Am J Ophthalmol 36:1511, 1953

48. Patz A: New role of ophthalmologist in prevention of retrolental fibroplasia. Arch Ophthalmol 78:565, 1967

49. Patz A: Retrolental fibroplasia. Survey Ophthalmol 14:1, 1969

50. Reese AB, King M, Owens EC: Classification of retrolental fibroplasia. Am J Ophthalmol 36:1333, 1953

51. Terry TL: Extreme prematurity and fibroplastic overgrowth of persistent vascular sheath behind each crystalline lens. I. Preliminary Report. Am J Ophthalmol 25:203, 1942

4

Prematurity, Postmaturity and Intrauterine Growth Retardation

PREMATURITY

Those infants born prior to the completion of 37 weeks of gestation are premature. The major problems associated with premature delivery are related to physiologic immaturity rather than the infant's birth weight. The vast majority of neonatal deaths occur in this group of infants, primarily during the first 24 to 48 hours of life (Fig. 4–1). In addition, a disproportionately high incidence of psychomotor retardation has been noted among survivors of premature delivery (2, 4, 8–11, 15). One of the major goals of perinatal medicine is to reduce the prevalence of prematurity and increase "high-quality" survival among those in whom prevention has not been possible.

The exact number of premature infants born annually in the United States is not known. During the mid-1960s approximately 300,000 infants weighing less than 2500 g (the definition of prematurity recommended by the World Health Assembly in 1948) were born each year. However, this number presumably includes many infants of a gestational age greater than 37 weeks and disregards many infants weighing more than 2500 g who were premature by gestation age.

The prevalence of prematurity varies among different ethnic groups and is strongly influenced by socioeconomic factors. Prior to the advent of liberalized abortion laws in the early 1970s, about 7% of white and 14% of nonwhite newborn infants weighed less than 2500 g. In the Netherlands, Denmark and India the prevalence has been 3.5%, 4.6% and 34.7%, respectively.

ETIOLOGY

The factors responsible for prematurity are incompletely understood but probably include poor maternal socioeconomic status, intrauterine infection, drug abuse, multiple births, intrauterine contraceptive device in gravid uterus, second trimester induced abortion and maternal diabetes mellitus, as well as etiologies of obscure origin. Poor socioeconomic status is an extremely important antecedent (1). Poor maternal health, increased frequency of infections, anemia, fatigue, poor sanitation, drug abuse, inadequate prenatal medical care, poor housing and education may all contribute to the outcome.

The possibility that intrauterine infection plays an important role in the etiology of prematurity was discussed by Naeye et al (12), who found that this was the major factor related to premature delivery in a group of heroin-addicted gravidas.

Maternal height, weight and cardiac output all influence birth weight; however, low maternal weight, short stature and decreased cardiac output may be related primarily to decreased rates of intrauterine growth rather than to a shortened gestational period.

Multiple births prior to the 37th week are a known cause of both prematurity and intrauterine growth retardation. The greater the number of fetuses present, the earlier in gestation is the pregnancy likely to terminate.

Another infrequently encountered cause of prematurity is the presence of an intra-uterine contraceptive device in a gravid uterus.

Prior to legalized abortion, an unusually high number of live-born infants weighing between 500 and 1000 g were encountered at Harlem Hospital. The number of these infants, whose mortality rate was about 98%, was significantly reduced when legal abortions became widely available. It is likely that illegal second trimester abortions caused the birth of many of these nonviable premature infants (7).

FIG. 4–1. Neonatal classification and mortality risk (per 100 live births) by birth weight and gestational age. (Lubchenco LO et al: J Pediatr 81:814, 1972)

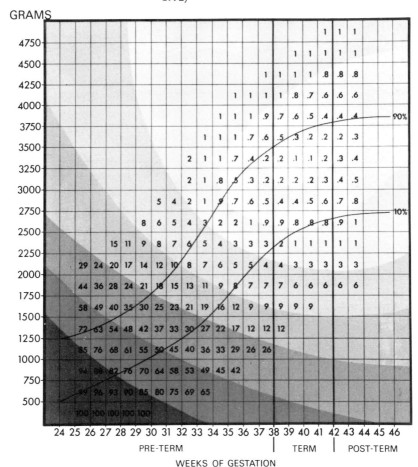

Interpolated data based on mathematical fit from original data
University of Colorado Medical Center newborns, 7/1/58 – 7/1/69

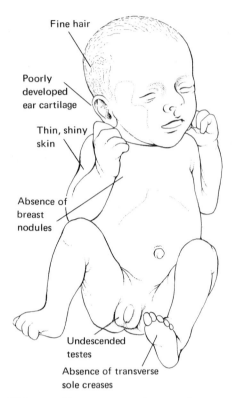

Fine hair

Poorly
developed
ear cartilage

Thin, shiny
skin

Absence of
breast
nodules

Undescended
testes

Absence of transverse
sole creases

FIG. 4–2. Characteristics of a typical premature infant of 32 weeks' gestation weighing 1500 g.

Low birth weight associated with maternal cigarette smoking is usually due to intrauterine growth retardation rather than to a shortened period of gestation.

Maternal diabetes mellitus is frequently associated with premature delivery. These infants are usually large for gestational age, but in spite of their relatively high birth weight, they encounter all the problems of prematurity.

In the majority of cases, however, premature delivery occurs spontaneously, and no specific cause can be identified.

The physical and neurologic characteristics of the premature infant (Fig. 4–2) are discussed in the section on physical examination of the newborn infant, Chapter 17.

The physiologic immaturity of these infants places them at high risk for both mortality and neurologic impairment. Characteristics of premature infants include low body weight (except in infants of diabetic mothers), decreased ability to secrete pul-

monary surfactant, poor muscle tone, decreased ability to suck and swallow, low gastric capacity, poor fat and vitamin D absorption, decreased hepatic and renal function, hypocalcemia, decreased glucose tolerance, immunologic defects and poor temperature control. As these problems are discussed throughout the book, they will be outlined only briefly here.

The major factor limiting survival of premature infants is functional immaturity of the lung. The inability to synthesize pulmonary surfactant in adequate quantities to sustain extrauterine respirations leads to the development of the respiratory distress syndrome (RDS), which is a leading cause of death among premature infants. For those with RDS who do survive, inadequate cerebral oxygenation may lead to psychomotor retardation.

Because of physiologic immaturity of the central nervous system (CNS), coordination between efficient sucking and swallowing is usually absent until the 33rd or 34th week of gestation. Therefore the premature infant must be fed either by intermittent gavage or by indwelling nasogastric tube. A low gastric capacity makes it virtually impossible to provide the premature infant with his full caloric requirements by the oral route during the early days of life. Fat absorption is decreased in the premature infant; his formula must therefore contain vegetable oils, which are more easily absorbed than animal fats. Poor gastrointestinal (GI) absorption of vitamin D may lead to rickets in the premature infant if adequate supplements are not provided.

Hepatic function is often suboptimal in premature infants. Their inability to conjugate bilirubin may lead to hyperbilirubinemia. The use of certain drugs, such as chloramphenicol, whose metabolism and excretion require good hepatic function, should be avoided in premature infants.

The nephrons of premature infants are usually incompletely developed. This limits their ability to excrete both concentrated and dilute urine. Clearance of urea, chloride, potassium and phosphorus is diminished, and acid-base homeostasis is impaired.

Hypocalcemia may occur in premature infants because of physiologic immaturity of the parathyroid glands; decreased glucose tolerance is secondary to decreased secretion of insulin by pancreatic islet cells.

Predisposition to infection, so commonly seen in these infants, reflects various immunologic deficiencies and such nonspecific handicaps as poor suck and gag reflexes. Breaks in their delicate skin may be portals of entry of infectious agents.

Temperature regulation is a major problem among premature infants. Difficulties in both production and conservation of heat will lead to hypothermia if the physician does not intervene by placing the infant in an incubator or under a radiant heater.

It is evident that the premature infant, with his poorly developed homeostatic mechanisms, requires a great deal of medical and nursing attention if he is to survive the neonatal period neurologically intact.

PREVENTION AND TREATMENT

One of the major goals of both the obstetrician and pediatrician is a decrease in the frequency of premature deliveries. Although this can be accomplished to a large extent by improved antenatal obstetric care, family planning and improvement in socioeconomic status, there will nevertheless continue to be a significant number of premature deliveries in the United States.*

Intensive perinatal care in the mid-1970s is directed primarily towards improving the chances for intact survival of infants born prematurely. Fetal heart rate monitoring and sonography have assumed major importance. Measurements of amniotic fluid surfactant content can identify a fetus who is likely to develop RDS if delivery is imminent. It is now possible to enhance fetal surfactant synthesis prior to delivery by administering corticosteroids to mothers of fetuses at risk. If the premature infant does develop RDS, therapeutic regimens, such as continuous positive airway pressure, may play a major role in intact survival of the infant.

Methods of IV alimentation are available that can provide the premature infant with

* See Appendix A, Addendum 1.

both the total calories and protein, which cannot be adequately administered by the oral route.

Treatment of hyperbilirubinemia, infection and acid-base and electrolyte imbalance have all contributed to improved survival of these infants.

It is increasingly clear that meticulous medical and nursing care of premature infants have led to a significant increase in intact survival in this group (5, 6, 13). This is true even among those of very low birth weight in whom neurologic sequelae had been encountered with great frequency. Hopefully the number of premature deliveries will further decline and the future will see advances in the management of infants born following a shortened gestational period.

POSTMATURITY

Any pregnancy that is terminated after 43 completed weeks of pregnancy may be considered postterm or postmature. Zwerdling (19) found the incidence of postmaturity to be 7.3% in a longitudinal study of almost 10,000 pregnancies in Oakland, California, and 5.4% in a retrospective study of approximately 300,000 birth certificates in New York City.

Postterm delivery is of clinical importance because prolonged gestation is associated with a twofold increase in the perinatal mortality rate, serious neonatal morbidity and an increased mortality rate during the first two to three years of life (Table 4–1).

TABLE 4–1. Death Rates for First Two Years of Life for Post-term and Term Infants, New York City, 1957–1959

Age at Death (months)	Deaths Per 1000 Live Births	
	43+ wk	37–42 wk
Neonatal	11.2†	5.9†
1–11	5.3*	4.3*
12–23	1.7|	0.9†

Difference between 43+ and 37 to 42 weeks significant at P<1% (†) and P<5%(*).
(From Zwerdling: Pediatrics 40:202, 1967)

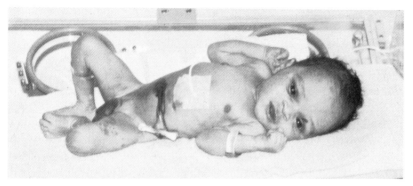

FIG. 4–3. Postmaturity with dysmaturity. Infant was born at 43+ weeks' gestation. Birth weight was 3200 g, head circumference 35 cm and length 52 cm; there were clinical characteristics of dysmaturity. (Andrews BF, Lorchirachoonfsul V, Shott RJ: Pediatr Clin North Am 17:185, 1970)

The basic pathophysiologic problem associated with postmaturity is that placental function begins to decline as the pregnancy extends past 40 weeks. In most instances, the fetuses continues to gain weight until the 42nd week. However, the further beyond term that the pregnancy progresses, the greater the likelihood that the fetus will be adversely affected.

CLINICAL FEATURES

An impaired gaseous exchange and inadequate transfer of nutrients to the fetus across a malfunctioning placenta leads to typical clinical problems.

Deceleration of fetal growth may be followed by actual weight loss when fat reserves are mobilized to provide an energy substrate. Depletion of subcutaneous fat stores may cause the fetus to appear extremely thin. If weight loss is severe and the postmature fetus weighs less than 2500 g, there is a sevenfold increase in perinatal mortality.

The postmature fetus (Fig. 4–3) has long nails and abundant scalp hair. There is a decrease in the amount of vernix caseosa; following delivery, the infant usually has an alert appearance. Certain enzyme systems, such as those responsible for the conjugation of bilirubin, are well developed, and physiologic jaundice is extremely rare. The skin may appear pale, with a desquamated, parchmentlike epithelium.

As placental function worsens, decreasing transport of oxygen to the fetus leads to tissue hypoxia. Of special importance is the effect of lack of oxygen on the brain. Relaxation of the anal sphincter causes passage of meconium in utero. The asphyxiated fetus begins to gasp, and meconium is aspirated into his lungs.

The ultimate outcome of the pregnancy depends on the duration and degree of cerebral hypoxia. The management of distressed postmature infants is discussed in the sections Perinatal Asphyxia and Meconium Aspiration, Chapters 3 and 6.

The increased morbidity and mortality secondary to prolonged gestation are potentially preventable. When a pregnancy has advanced past the 40th week, the gravida must be followed closely by the obstetrician. Evaluation of maternal estriol or placental lactogen levels may identify the jeopardized postterm fetus. In this way, delivery of a neurologically intact infant may be facilitated.

INTRAUTERINE GROWTH RETARDATION

Decreased rates of intrauterine growth are attributed to various causes. The range of severity is related to both the duration and magnitude of the underlying etiology.

Although many observers had recognized that certain small newborn infants appeared unusually mature and vigorous for their body size, it was not until the early 1960s that intrauterine growth retardation was clearly differentiated from a shortened gestational period (prematurity) as a cause of low birth weight (36, 62). It soon became clear that about one-third of all infants who had previously been identified as premature (birth weight of less than 2500 g) had retarded intrauterine growth.

ETIOLOGY

Intrauterine growth retardation may occur as a result of an inherent defect of the fetus, placental dysfunction, maternal factors or a combination of these. Some of the major etiologic factors in intrauterine growth retardation are shown on the accompanying list.

Intrauterine infection (39, 46): rubella, toxoplasmosis, cytomegalovirus, h. simplex and syphilis.

Chromosomal abnormalities (54): mongolism, trisomy D, trisomy E, cri-du-chat syndrome, Turner's syndrome, Fanconi's anemia, and Bloom's syndrome (chromosomal breakage).

Conditions not associated with chromosomal abnormalities (67): Cornelia de Lange syndrome, osteogenesis imperfecta, dyschondroplasia and various types of dwarfism.

Multiple births (44)

Maternal use of drugs: tobacco (52), narcotics (49, 68) and antimetabolites, e.g., methotrexate.

Fetal malnutrition (20, 25, 47, 51, 57): maternal factors (maternal malnutrition); maternoplacental factors (preeclampsia, hypertension (45); placental factors (placental failure secondary to postmaturity, placental hemangiomas, vascular anomalies of the placenta, abnormal insertion of the umbilical cord, single umbilical artery); and unknown reasons.

These infants have higher perinatal morbidity and mortality rates than normally grown infants of comparable gestational age (35, 42, 43). During the immediate neonatal period special problems arise in clinical management (such as hypoglycemia, increased risk of infection and difficulties in maintaining normal body temperature). From a point of view of long-term growth and development, many will never attain normal body size, and a substantial number will have some degree of neurologic impairment (24, 29, 32, 55, 63).

Some causes of intrauterine growth retardation may be preventable. A successful vaccine for the prevention of rubella has offered the promise of eliminating this etiology, but in spite of widespread immunization and the reliance on "herd immunity" to prevent epidemics, rubella's appearance in pregnant women has not been completely eliminated. Improvement in maternal nutrition and further knowledge of the etiology of toxemia of pregnancy, leading to both improved treatment and prevention, may eliminate these causes of fetal growth failure.

Obstetricians should be able to recognize significantly retarded fetal growth. Affected fetuses must be carefully monitored both by physical and biochemical means, so that delivery of a viable fetus can be accomplished (when possible) before irreversible damage or death has occurred.

During the neonatal period, the ability to recognize the infant with intrauterine growth retardation is important in providing for optimal clinical management. If the cause is not obvious, diagnostic tests must be performed to establish an etiology. After discharge from the nursery, the infant must be carefully followed in order to detect retarded physical growth and psychomotor development.

INTRAUTERINE INFECTION

Congenital infections, such as rubella, cytomegalovirus, toxoplasmosis, h. simplex and congenital syphilis may be associated with retarded intrauterine growth. During the rubella epidemic of 1964, large numbers of infants with intrauterine infection were small for their gestational age. This finding led to studies that went far to elucidate the mechanisms of growth retardation in intra-uterine infection.

A villous placentitis accompanies the viremic phase of maternal rubella and is associated with damage to the placental vasculature. The virus then enters the fetus and invades fetal cells. Metabolic activity of the cells is impaired without their actually being destroyed. The incidence of chromosomal breakage is high, and cells divide poorly. This is consistent with the observations of Naeye and Blanc (46), who have found a markedly decreased cell number in many organs in fatal cases. Brain weights were generally low, and there was a decreased number of cells. Both hearts and livers were large in proportion to body size, but these were small and contained subnormal numbers of cells when compared to the infants' gestational ages. The thymus was generally small, with a minimal amount of lymphoid tissue present.

Infants who survive congenital rubella usually continue to secrete the virus from various sites for one to two years after birth, and they continue to grow at a very slow rate.

Although rubella has served as the prototype for the study of intrauterine infections, there is evidence that the manifestations of this group of infections are similar, regardless of the causative organism. The earlier in the gestational period that infection occurs, the greater the teratogenic and developmental risk to the fetus. The organs most affected are those undergoing development at the time of infection.

With the exception of congenital syphilis, the treatment of infections causing intrauterine growth retardation is either nonexistent or ineffectual. Thus, prevention of these diseases is the only means by which their devastating effects on the fetus may be controlled. The program of mass immunization against rubella is an example of this.

Any febrile illness in a pregnant woman, especially if accompanied by rash and lymphadenopathy, raises the suspicion of an illness that may adversely affect the fetus. This is of particular importance when the infection occurs during the first half of pregnancy. Virologic and serologic studies are indicated, and if infection with rubella is confirmed, the opportunity for a therapeutic abortion should be presented to the mother. Gamma-globulin administration has not been documented to be of value but may be utilized when abortion is not possible.

While intrauterine growth retardation secondary to rubella and syphilis are now largely preventable diseases, investigations directed towards prevention of fetal infection by other relatively common organisms, e.g., *Toxoplasma*, cytomegalovirus or h. simplex, must continue.

FETAL MALNUTRITION

It is postulated that the leading cause of intrauterine growth retardation is poor fetal nutrition (60). The nutritional status of the fetus depends on maternal blood perfusing the placenta, composition of the maternal blood (e.g., hemoglobin level and concentrations of various nutrients) and the ability to transfer nutrients and oxygen across the placenta to the fetus.

Fetal growth occurs in three phases. The first period, in which organ growth depends solely on cellular division (hyperplasia), is associated with an increase in the amount of deoxyribonucleic acid (DNA) within the organ; the second is the period when cells are both dividing and increasing in size (hypertrophy), and this phase is associated with an increase in both DNA and ribonucleic acid (RNA) within the organ; in the third period organ growth occurs primarily by an increase in the size of cells. Inadequate fetal nutrition during any period may impair growth; however, when it occurs at a time when growth is primarily secondary to cell division, there may be a permanent impairment of growth potential (66).

Pathophysiologic Factors

The effect of intrauterine malnutrition on fetal growth depends on both the duration and severity of the insult. With severe maternal malnutrition, interference with fetal growth may begin early in pregnancy and lead to impairment of linear growth, weight gain, and brain growth (as measured by head circumference). Maternal chronic renal disease or hypertension may interfere with fetal growth during the second trimester and have a similar effect. If growth continues normally until the middle or late third trimester (as with pre-eclampsia), weight gain will be impaired more than linear growth or head circumference. If malnutrition begins near, at or postterm, the fetus usually has a normal length and head circumference but a decreased body weight secondary to starvation of relatively short duration.

Intrauterine malnutrition has a differential effect on organ growth both in the human and in newborn animals. The brain, which is the most vital organ, suffers the least both in terms of diminished size and total cell number. Other vital organs, such as heart, lung and kidney, suffer to a lesser extent than do the liver, spleen, pancreas and adrenals. There is a concurrent decrease both in size and cell number of the placenta (37, 38).

A postnatal growth spurt may accompany efficient nutritional intake. However, affected infants will often not attain the same growth potential as infants having normal birth weight for their gestational age. When fetal malnutrition is compounded by poor diet following birth, growth potential is further impaired.

The risk of intrauterine death from asphyxia during the intrapartum period is about ten times higher in infants who are fetally malnourished than in infants who are normally grown for corresponding gestational age.

Maternal Malnutrition. Excellent experimental evidence in several subhuman species indicates that inadequate maternal nutrition can retard fetal growth (27, 64, 65) and have a permanent effect on body size. There is now a mounting body of evidence that maternal malnutrition can adversely affect human fetal growth. The severe malnutrition that affected the populations of Rotterdam (58) and Leningrad (21) during World War II was apparently responsible for a significant decrease in birth weights. It is probable that suboptimal

nutritional status (but above the level of starvation) may also be responsible for diminished birth weight. It is now well established that an abnormally low weight gain during pregnancy is associated with a slow rate of fetal weight gain. In the United States, Great Britain and many developing countries, low maternal socioeconomic status is associated with decreased birth weight. Controlled studies are now in progress to determine whether improved maternal nutrition during pregnancy can have a beneficial effect on fetal weight gain.

Vascular Disorders. Microvascular changes associated with toxemia of pregnancy, maternal hypertension, chronic renal disease and diabetes mellitus may be responsible for a decrease in blood flow to the uterus and placenta. This is usually associated with a decrease in placental mass. Localized or gross infarcts may occasionally be seen, but this is not common. Gruenwald (35) has found that microscopic placental lesions, especially the presence of avascular terminal villi, are more common than gross defects. Very often only a small placenta with neither microscopic nor macroscopic defects is seen. Here, the problem appears to be preplacental. When the placenta is unusually small, there is a decreased area for diffusion of both gases and nutrients, and a decreased amount of hormone-producing tissue.

Other placental factors associated with decreased fetal growth are abnormal insertion of the umbilical cord, hemangiomas of the placenta and cord and vascular anomalies of the placenta. Single umbilical arteries are associated with both an increased incidence of congenital anomalies and a low birth weight.

Since placental reserves decline toward the end of pregnancy, the relationship of placental insufficiency to fetal malnutrition becomes more pronounced as term approaches.

MULTIPLE PREGNANCY

Multiple pregnancies are a well-recognized cause of intrauterine growth retardation.

Since the human uterine cavity and placenta are intended by nature to support only one fetus, the presence of two or more fetuses usually leads to impaired fetal growth. The normal intrauterine growth curve for twins is about the same as that for singleton fetuses until about the 34th week of gestation, at which time it begins to fall below the singleton curve. As the number of fetuses increases, the intrauterine growth curve begins to deviate from the normal singleton curve at a progressively earlier gestational age.

In certain instances, there is a gross discrepancy between the sizes of twins. While one may be of relatively normal size for gestational age, the other may be severely undergrown. This phenomenon is usually due to an unequal placental mass supplying each twin but may be secondary to the intertwin transfusion syndrome.

GENETIC OR INTRINSIC FACTORS

Chromosomal and Nonchromosomal Disorders

Intrinsic factors may cause intrauterine growth retardation. All common chromosomal aberrations are associated with decreased intrauterine growth. In Down's syndrome, there is a small decrease in the intrauterine growth rate. Growth retardation is more pronounced in the fetus with D trisomy, and extremely severe in the E trisomy syndrome.

Seventy percent of infants with the cri-du-chat syndrome are below the tenth percentile for gestational age, and about one-third of infants with Turner's syndrome weigh less than 2500 g.

Intrauterine growth retardation is also present in fetuses with Fanconi's anemia and Bloom's syndrome, two conditions associated with chromosomal breakage.

There is also a group of infants who show retarded intrauterine growth with congenital disorders in which no chromosomal aberrations have yet been detected. This group includes the Cornelia de Lange syndrome, osteogenesis imperfecta, dyschondroplasia, Russell-Silver dwarfs, primordial dwarfs of Conradi and the bird-headed dwarfs of Virchow.

The high incidence of serious congenital malformations in infants who are small for gestational age is striking. The basis for these defects may be either a chromosomal abnormality not yet detected or intrauterine infection.

MATERNAL DRUGS

Drugs used during pregnancy for medicinal or nonmedicinal purposes may be associated with intrauterine growth retardation.

Antimetabolites, such as methotrexate, are teratogenic and seriously impair fetal growth. Their use during pregnancy should be limited to life-saving situations.

The use of tobacco during pregnancy is related to both impaired fetal growth and an increased risk of fetal death. There is evidence, however, that if cigarette smoking is discontinued prior to the fourth month of pregnancy, a decreased risk of intrauterine growth retardation results. The adverse effect of smoking on fetal growth is directly related to the total number of cigarettes smoked during the pregnancy. The constrictive effect of nicotine on the placental vasculature is probably the basis for impaired fetal growth.

The use of heroin during pregnancy is also associated with both true prematurity and impaired fetal growth. The basis for these findings is unknown.

SICKLE CELL TRAIT

Brown et al (26) found a decrease in the birth weights of infants of mothers with sickle cell trait that was significant when compared to a normal population of similar gestational age. This may be related to deprivation of oxygen for the developing fetus.

DIAGNOSIS

A diagnosis of intrauterine growth retardation can be made when the birth weight is found to be below the tenth percentile for

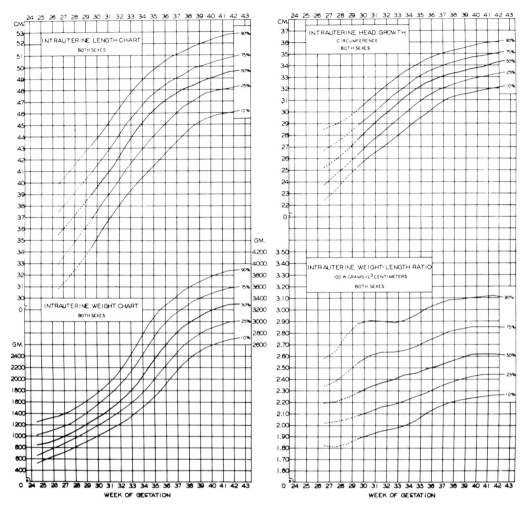

FIG. 4–4. Intrauterine growth—weight, length, head circumference and weight-length ratio. (Lubchenco et al: Pediatrics 37:403, 1966)

gestational age; when it is below the third percentile, the degree of growth retardation may be considered severe.

Several standards (Fig. 4–4, Table 4–2) available for the assessment of fetal growth have been compiled by investigators who surveyed large numbers of singleton live-born infants delivered over a wide range of gestational ages (22, 33, 34, 40, 59–61, 67).

An accurate gestational age must be established to assess fetal growth. One way of doing this is by questioning the mother regarding the date of her last regular menstrual period. However, a history of irregular menses or post-conceptional bleeding may cloud the issue. The determination of gestational age prior to the termination of pregnancy, either through physical exami-nation, sonography or biochemical examina-tion of the amniotic fluid is inexact.

Physical and Placental Examination

The physical and neurologic characteristics of the infant may be helpful in assignment of gestational age. However, many pitfalls exist, and this approach too, may be inexact. For example, the breast nodules may be relatively small in an infant of advanced gestational age with moderate or severe intrauterine growth retardation. This is due to diminished estriol production and secre-tion by a failing fetoplacental unit. Develop-

TABLE 4–2. Birth weight in relation to gestational age

Weeks from last menstrual period	Standard deviation from mean					Percentiles						
	−2	−1	Mean	+1	+2	5	10	25	50	75	90	95
28	430	750	1050	1400	1750	500	620	850	1080			
29	500	870	1200	1570	1910	620	790	1000	1200			
30	630	1000	1380	1750	2120	760	920	1150	1350			
31	760	1190	1580	1940	2330	900	1080	1300	1540			
32	920	1340	1750	2150	2560	1080	1240	1500	1750			
33	1100	1520	1950	2370	2800	1280	1420	1700	1980			
34	1290	1720	2170	2610	3040	1500	1620	1920	2240			
35	1500	1940	2390	2840	3270	1740	1840	2150	2450			
36	1720	2150	2610	3080	3490	1970	2060	2380	2650			
37	1940	2370	2830	3300	3700	2200	2280	2600	2850	3200	3480	3700
38	2150	2560	3050	3480	3900	2400	2500	2780	3030	3330	3610	3820
39	2310	2750	3210	3630	4070	2510	2630	2920	3170	3450	3730	3940
40	2400	2830	3280	3720	4170	2580	2720	3000	3260	3570	3850	4060
41	2450	2890	3350	3800	4260	2630	2780	3050	3320	3650	3970	4170
42	2480	2930	3400	3860	4340	2660	2840	3100	3370	3700	4030	4230
43	2450	2930	3410	3900	4400	2650	2830	3100	3400	3750	4060	4280
44+	2430	2930	3420	3940	4460	2590	2820	3100	3420	3750	4080	4300

(Gruenwald: Am J Obstet Gynecol 94:1112, 1966)

ment of sole creases may normally be less advanced in black than in white infants. A completely reliable neurologic examination cannot be performed until about 48 hours after delivery. In the first hours of life, evaluation of muscle tone and recoil ability of the upper and lower extremities and the sucking ability of the infant may be of value in establishing an approximate gestational age. However, in the presence of hypoxia or heavy maternal sedation, muscle tone and suck may be diminished. On the other hand, muscle tone may be increased if the infant is undergoing heroin withdrawal.

The placenta should be thoroughly examined, and its size and the presence of malformations or infarcts noted. In multiple pregnancies (especially in the case of discordant twins), special attention should be paid to the placenta(s). Both routine and phase microscopy may be useful in determining some of the histologic placental abnormalities associated with intrauterine growth failure. The number of umbilical arteries should be counted.

Infants with chromosomal abnormalities usually have a characteristic appearance, particularly Down's syndrome. The presence of "rocker bottom feet" and a characteristic facial profile suggest trisomy E. Many syndromes not associated with chromosomal defects, e.g., renal anomalies with "Potter's facies," dyschondroplasia, Cornelia de Lange syndrome, will also present with a unique appearance.

Intrauterine infection may be accompanied by microcephaly, jaundice, hepatosplenomegaly and a rash. Infants with congenital rubella may have obvious cardiac and eye involvement, and hydrocephalus may be present in toxoplasmosis.

Dubowitz et al (30) have devised a grading system that combines physical and neurologic examination in assignment of gestational age; this has proven reasonably reliable and is widely used (see Ch. 17, History, Physical, and Neurological Examinations).

The electroencephalogram (EEG) may be accurate in determining gestational age within a two-week period. Measurement of nerve conduction times, when available, may be an even more accurate method (53). The appearance of the distal femoral and proximal tibial epiphyses at 36 to 38 weeks of gestation is a useful radiologic finding in assessing gestational age.

Laboratory and Radiologic Assays

Since chronic intrauterine infections may have similar presenting symptoms, proper use of the laboratory and x-ray examination may be of great value in establishing a correct diagnosis. The rubella virus may be grown from a throat, urine or other culture. Positive serologic tests for toxoplasmosis, syphilis and rubella may indicate a fetal infection or may be a reflection of transplacentally transmitted maternal antibodies. However, specific fluorescent antibody tests for toxoplasmosis and syphilis may be of value in establishing a specific diagnosis. Elevation of cord blood levels of IgA and IgM may either reflect an antibody response to intrauterine infection or a nonspecific antigenic stimulus and therefore are not necessarily diagnostic of intrauterine infection. Serologic determinations in the first weeks of life may be a more-specific finding in fetomaternal infection. The identification of inclusion bodies in cells of urinary sediment may be diagnostic of cytomegalovirus; however, these cells are also found in infants who have no clinical evidence of infection.

In both congenital cytomegalovirus and toxoplasmosis, x rays of the skull may reveal cerebral calcifications. In congenital rubella, the long bones may have a typical "moth-eaten" appearance, while in congenital syphilis, osteochondritis may be apparent.

Since encephalitis may accompany nonbacterial intrauterine infection, a lumbar puncture must be considered when this diagnosis is entertained.

The diagnosis of intrauterine infection as a cause of fetal growth retardation is of practical value since there is effective antimicrobial therapy for congenital syphilis, and experimental agents are available for the treatment of h. simplex and toxoplasmosis. If a diagnosis of rubella is made, strict isolation procedures must be followed since the infant will continue to shed virus for a prolonged period of time.

Absence of Specific Etiology. If no specific etiology can be determined, it is likely that the cause is fetal malnutrition. The skin of these infants is often thin and dry, with poor development of subcutaneous tissue. The head will often appear large in propor-

tion to the remainder of the body and will give the impression of hydrocephalus. These infants may appear unusually vigorous and alert for their small body size. Respiratory distress syndrome is not common, and when pulmonary signs occur, the diagnosis of intrauterine pneumonia, meconium aspiration, pneumothorax and pneumomediastinum should be considered. Some of these infants may be depressed because of intrauterine asphyxia.

If the intrauterine growth retardation was due to maternal preeclampsia, lethargy, respiratory depression and sluggish or absent reflexes may be due to magnesium sulfate that has been administered to the mother. In this case, the serum magnesium concentration must be measured.

Fetal malnutrition is associated with a high incidence of hypoglycemia (see section Carbohydrate Metabolism, Ch. 12) due primarily to depletion of liver glycogen stores prior to delivery. Other factors are increased utilization of glucose by a brain that is relatively large in relation to the rest of the body and a decreased ability to secrete epinephrine when blood concentrations of glucose are low. The clinical manifestations of hypoglycemia are lethargy, tremulousness, poor suck, apneic episodes and occasionally convulsions. In many instances, hypoglycemia may occur in the absence of specific signs. Both frequent measurements of blood glucose concentrations with treatment of hypoglycemia when it is found and early feedings appear to play an important role in the prevention of brain damage that may follow untreated hypoglycemia.

Many of these infants may have very high hemoglobin concentrations and hematocrit levels because of chronic intrauterine hypoxia. Since polycythemia may be harmful to the newborn infant, measurements of either the hemoglobin concentration or hematocrit should not be overlooked (see section Polycythemia, Ch. 8).

Metabolic Acidosis. Acid-base measurements on the blood of malnourished infants may reveal a metabolic acidosis shortly after delivery secondary to chronic hypoxemia. Since pulmonary function is usually adequate in these infants, effective postnatal oxygenation can be established fairly rapidly, with a favorable adjustment of the infant's acid-base status occurring within a short period of time. Hyperventilation with decreased levels of Pco_2 (compensatory respiratory alkalosis) may sometimes be noted. Alkali therapy should be given with caution to these infants, and only after measurements of acid-base status, to avoid overcorrection and possible hypocalcemic tetany.

Leukocytes isolated from umbilical cord blood of infants with fetal malnutrition have shown decreased activity of two energy-generating enzymes, pyruvic kinase and adenylic kinase (42). Since these enzymes may also be deficient in the leukocytes of the mothers as well, a prenatal assay may point to the possibility of fetal malnutrition.

There is evidence that infants who have suffered from intrauterine malnutrition have increased metabolic requirements following delivery when compared to infants of comparable gestational age whose intrauterine growth has been normal. Since these infants have poor glycogen and fat stores to draw upon in the critical first days of life, adequate calories must be supplied shortly after birth to meet their requirements. In order to decrease caloric expenditure, resting oxygen consumption must be minimized. This may be accomplished by maintaining a thermoneutral environment until the infant is receiving an optimal caloric intake (56).

PROGNOSIS

Both the short-term and long-term outcome for infants who are small for gestational age depends both on the etiology of the fetal growth failure and its severity. In infants who have had intrauterine infection, CNS involvement often portends retarded psychomotor development provided the infant survives the neonatal period.

Infants with genetic causes for intrauterine growth failure usually have a poor prognosis for a normal life. The ultimate outcome for infants whose intrauterine growth

has been retarded because of maternal use of narcotics or tobacco is not known.

This group of infants generally have a less stormy neonatal course than normally grown premature infants of comparable birth weight. However, there is an increased incidence of morbidity and mortality when compared to normally grown infants of comparable gestational age. These infants tend to take feedings well, and their rate of weight gain is usually relatively rapid. The ultimate outcome for these infants following discharge from the nursery, however, is not completely clear. Many never achieve "normal" weight and height, and there is some evidence that their head circumferences remain abnormally small (24, 31).

While some investigators have shown no difference in IQ levels between infants with intrauterine growth retardation and normal infants of comparable gestational ages (23, 48), others have found an increase in the incidence of "minimal brain damage" in this group of infants (32).

Further prospective studies must be performed in order to more fully evaluate the ultimate prognosis for infants who are small for gestational age. These studies must take into account not only the varied etiology of intrauterine growth retardation, but the effect of postnatal influences as well.

REFERENCES

PREMATURITY

1. Drillien CM: The social and economic factors affecting the incidence of premature birth. I. Premature births without complications of pregnancy. J Obstet Gynaecol Br Commonw 64:161, 1957

2. Drillien CM: Growth and development in a group of children of very low birth weight. Arch Dis Child 33:10, 1958

3. Drillien CM: The Growth and Development of the Prematurely Born Infant. Baltimore, Williams & Wilkins, 1964

4. Drillien CM: The incidence of mental and physical handicaps in school age children of very low birthweight. Pediatrics 39:238, 1967

5. Dweck HS, Saxon HS, Benton JW, Cassady G: Early development of the tiny premature infant. Am J Dis Child 126:28, 1973

6. Fitzhardinge PM, Ramsay M: The improving outlook for the small prematurely born infant. Dev Med Child Neurol 15:447, 1973

7. Glass L, Evans HE, Swartz DP, Rajegowda BK, Leblanc W: Effects of legalized abortion on neonatal mortality and obstetrical morbidity at Harlem Hospital Center. Amer J Publ Health 64:717, 1974

8. Janus-Kakulska A, Lis S: Developmental peculiarities of prematurely born children with birthweight below 1250 grams. Dev Med Child Neurol 8:285, 1966

9. Katz CM, Taylor PM: Incidence of low birth weight in children with severe mental retardation. Am J Dis Child 114:80, 1967

10. Lubchenco LO, Delivoria-Papadopoulos M, Butterfield LJ, French JH, Metcalf D, Hix IE, Danick J, Dodds J, Downs M, Freeland E: Long-term follow-up studies of prematurely born infants. I. Relationship of handicaps to nursery routines. J Pediatr 80:501, 1972

11. Lubchenco L, Delivoria-Papadopoulos M, Searls D: Long-term follow-up studies of prematurely born infants: II. Influence of birth weight and gestational age on sequelae. J Pediatr 80:509, 1972

12. Naeye RL, Blanc W, Leblanc W, Khatamee MA: Fetal complications of maternal heroin addiction: abnormal growth, infections, and episodes of stress. J Pediatr 83: 1055, 1973

13. Rawlings G, Reynolds EOR, Stewart A, Strang LB: Changing prognosis for infants of very low birth weight. Lancet 1:516, 1971

14. Silverman WA: Dunham's Premature Infants, 3rd ed. New York, Harper & Row, 1964

15. Wright FH, Blough RR, Chamberlin A, Ernest T, Halstead WC, Meier P, Moore RY, Naunton RF, Newell FW: A controlled follow-up study of small prematures born from 1952 through 1956. Am J Dis Child 124:506, 1972

POSTMATURITY

16. Evans TN, Koeff ST, Morely GW: Fetal effects of prolonged pregnancy. Am J Obstet Gynecol 85:701, 1963

17. Lucas WE, Anetil AO, Callagan DA: The problem of post-term pregnancy. Am J Obstet Gynecol 91:241, 1965

18. McClure-Browne JC: Postmaturity. Am J Obstet Gynecol 85:573, 1963

19. Zwerdling MA: Factors pertaining to prolonged pregnancy and its outcome. Pediatrics 40:202, 1967

INTRAUTERINE GROWTH RETARDATION

20. Ademowore AS, Courey NG, Kime JS: Relationships of maternal nutrition and weight gain to newborn birthweight. Obstet Gynecol 39:460, 1972

21. Antonov AN: Children born during the siege of Leningrad in 1942. J Pediatr 30:250, 1947

22. Babson SG, Behrman RE, Lessel R: Fetal growth. Liveborn birthweights for gestational age of white middle class infants. Pediatrics 45:937, 1970

23. Babson SG, Kangas J: Preschool intelligence of undersized term infants. Am J Dis Child 117:553, 1969

24. Beargie RA, James VL, Greene JW: Growth and development of small-for-date newborns. Pediatr Clin North Am 17:159, 1970

25. Birch HG: Functional effects of fetal malnutrition. Hosp Pract 6:134, 1971

26. Brown S, Merkow A, Wiener M, Khajezadeh J: Low birth weight in babies born to mothers with sickle cell trait. JAMA 221:1404, 1972

27. Chase HP, Dabiere CS, Welch NN, O'Brien D: Intrauterine undernutrition and brain development. Pediatrics 47:491, 1971

28. Clifford SH: Postmaturity—with placental dysfunction: clinical syndrome and pathologic findings. J Pediatr 44:1, 1954

29. Drillien CM: The small-for-date infant: etiology and prognosis. Pediatr Clin North Am 17:9, 1970

30. Dubowitz LMS, Dubowitz V, Goldberg C: Clinical assessment of gestational age in the newborn infant. J Pediatr 77:1, 1970

31. Fitzhardinge PM, Steven EM: The small-for-date infant. I. Late growth patterns. Pediatrics 49:671, 1972

32. Fitzhardinge PM, Steven EM: The small-for-date infant. II Neurological and intellectual sequelae. Pediatrics 50:50, 1972

33. Ghosh, S, Bhargava SK, Madhavan S, Taskar AD, Bhargava V, Nigam SK: Intra-uterine growth of north Indian babies. Pediatrics 47:826, 1971

35. Gruenwald P: Chronic fetal distress and placental insufficiency. Biol Neonate 5:215, 1963

34. Gruenwald P: Growth of the human fetus. 1. Normal growth and its variation. Am J Obstet Gynecol 94:1112, 1966

36. Gruenwald P, Dawkins M, Hepner R: Panel discussion: chronic deprivation of the fetus. Sinai Hosp J 11:51, 1963

37. Gruenwald P, Minh HN: Evaluation of body and organ weights in prenatal pathology. I. Normal standards derived from autopsies. Am J Clin Path 34:247, 1960

38. Gruenwald P, Minh HN: Evaluation of body and organ weights in perinatal pathology. Am J Obstet Gynecol 82:312, 1961

39. Hughes WT: Infections and intrauterine growth retardation. Pediatr Clin North Am 17:119, 1970

40. Lubchenco LO, Hansman C, Boyd E: Intrauterine growth in length and head circumference as estimated from live births at gestational ages from 26 to 42 weeks. Pediatrics 37:403, 1966

41. Lubchenco LO, Searls DT, Brazie JV: Neonatal mortality rate: relationship to birth weight and gestational age. J Pediatr 81:814, 1972

42. Metcoff J, Yoshida T, Morales M, Rosado A, Urrusti J, Sosa A, Yoshida P, Frenk S, Velasco L, Ward A, Al-Ubaidi Y: Biomolecular studies in fetal malnutrition in maternal leukocytes. Pediatrics 47:180, 1971

43. Miller HC: Fetal growth and neonatal mortality. Pediatrics 49:392, 1972

44. Naeye RL: The fetal and neonatal development of twins. Pediatrics 33:546, 1964

45. Naeye RL: Abnormalities in infants of mothers with toxemia of pregnancy. Am J Obstet Gynecol 95:276, 1966

46. Naeye RL, Blanc W: Pathogenesis of congenital rubella. JAMA 194:1277, 1965

47. Naeye RL, Blanc W, Paul C: Effects of maternal nutrition on the human fetus. Pediatrics 52:494, 1973

48. Neligan GA: The clinical effect of being "light for dates." Proc R Soc Med 60:881, 1967

49. Rajegowda BK, Glass L, Evans HE, Masó G, Swartz DP, Leblanc W: Methadone withdrawal in newborn infants. J Pediatr 81:532, 1972

50. Reisman LE: Chromosome abnormalities and intrauterine growth retardation. Pediatr Clin North Am 17:101, 1970

51. Rush D, Davis H, Susser M: Antecedents of low birthweight in Harlem, New York City. Int J Epidemiol 1:393, 1972

52. Rush D, Kass EH: Maternal smoking: reassessment of association with perinatal mortality. Am J Epidemiol 96:183, 1972

53. Schulte FJ, Michaelis R, Linke I, Nolte R: Motor nerve conduction velocity in term, pereterm, and small-for-date newborn infants. Pediatrics 42:17, 1968

54. Shanklin DR: The influence of placental lesions on the newborn infant. Pediatr Clin North Am 17:25, 1970

55. Sinclair JC, Coldiron JS: Low birth weight and postnatal physical development. Dev Med Child Neurol 11:314, 1969

56. Sinclair JC: Heat production and thermoregulation in the small-for-date infant. Pediatr Clin North Am 17:147, 1970

57. Singer JE, Westphal M, Nisewander K: Relationship of weight gain idurng pregnancy to birth weight and infant growth and development in the first year of life. Report from collaborative study of cerebral palsy. Obstet Gynecol 3:417, 1968

58. Smith CA: Effect of wartime starvation in Holland upon pregnancy and its product. Am J Obstet Gynecol 53:599, 1947

59. Tanner JM: Standards for birth weight or intrauterine growth. Pediatrics 46:1, 1970

60. Usher R, McLean F: Intrauterine growth of liveborn caucasian infants at sea level: Standards obtained from measurements in 7 dimensions of infants born between 25 and 44 weeks of gestation. J Pediatr 74:901, 1969

61. Van den Berg BJ, Yerushalmy J: The relationship of the rates of intrauterine growth of infants of low birth weight to mortality, morbidity and congenital anomalies. J Pediatr 69:531, 1966.

62. Warkany J, Monroe BB, Sutherland BS: Intrauterine growth retardation. Am J Dis Child 102:249, 1961

63. Wedgwood M, Holt KS: Longitudinal study of dental and physical development of 2-to-3 year old children who were underweight at birth. Biol Neonate 12:214, 1968

64. Winick M, Noble A: Quantitative changes in DNA, RNA and protein during prenatal and postnatal growth in the rat. Dev Biol 12:451, 1965

65. Winick M, Noble A: Cellular response in rats during malnutrition at various ages. J Nutr 89:300, 1966

66. Winick M: Cellular growth in intrauterne malnutrition. Pediatr Clin North Am 17:69, 1970

67. Yerushalmy J: The classification of newborn infants by birth weight and gestational age. J Pediatr 71:164, 1967

68. Zelson C, Lee SJ, Casalino M: Neonatal narcotic addiction: comparative effects of maternal intake of heroin and methadone. N Engl J Med 289:1216, 1973

5

Skin
Disorders

The skin is the one organ of the newborn infant that is completely visible to the eye and is therefore a source of considerable information concerning the infant's clinical condition.

FETAL DEVELOPMENT

Fetal skin consists of a single layer of cells until about the sixth week of gestation. At this time it doubles its thickness to form an inner stratum germinativum and an outer periderm. Eccrine sweat glands arise from an epidermal downgrowth at this stage of development, and by the third or fourth month the stratum intermedium, which will be the prickle cell layer, arises from the stratum germinativum. Hair follicles begin to form at about three months, and sebaceous glands differentiate primarily from the epithelial portion of these follicles. They develop as an outpouching from the upper one-third of the follicles. Their marked activity seems to be governed by maternal androgen secretion. Apocrine glands develop somewhat later, originating from and emptying into the hair follicles.

Melanocytes migrate from the neural crest to the basal layer of the skin at the fifth to sixth month of fetal life. At term the amount of melanin is limited, but it increases over the first few weeks of postnatal life. Certain areas, such as the scrotum, areola and linea alba may appear much more pigmented because of a response to maternal and placental hormones that enter the fetal circulation.

The dermis, mesodermal in origin and metabolically active, contains ground substance, fibrous elements, elastin, nerves, blood vessels and lymphatics. Collagen comprises more than 90% of the dermis at term. After 20 to 22 weeks of gestation the concentration of collagen nitrogen increases markedly, indicating increased deposition of collagen after this time. The attachment of the dermis to epidermis does not become secure until a few weeks after birth (even in full-term infants), thus predisposing the newborn infant to blistering.

At 13 to 14 weeks the water content of the skin is 92%, and at 20 to 22 weeks it is about 90%. At term the skin is about 83% water. As water content of the skin decreases, there is a concomitant increase in both total and colloid nitrogen content.

During the early stages of gestation (12 to 16 weeks) transfer of water may occur across the fetal skin, a function that is lost as term approaches (3). The ability of relatively immature skin to act as a permeable membrane is vivid in premature infants up to 35 weeks of gestation. Nachman and Esterly (8) demonstrated local cutaneous blanching in these premature infants following the topical application of a 10% phenylephrine solution. Some evidence also indicates that the skin of a full-term infant can absorb drugs. Curley et al (4) showed a significant increase in the blood levels of hexachlorophene (HCP) in 50 newborn infants following several baths using this agent.

Vascularization of the skin begins early in fetal development. Three networks of anastomosing arteries supply the skin, the most superficial of which is the subepidermal (or papillary) plexus. The deepest is at the junction of dermis and subcutaneous tissue. These arterial networks anastomose freely, not only with themselves, but with the five networks of veins present in the skin. The necessity for all of these anastomoses is undoubtedly related to the skin's thermoregulatory role.

The blood supply to the skin varies widely (flowrates are from 0.1 to 150 ml/100 g tissue per minute). Vasomotor tone (and therefore blood supply to the skin) is largely under the control of the sympathetic and parasympathetic nervous systems and probably of the hypothalamus as well.

Innervation of the skin also begins early in gestation, cutaneous nerves appearing to overlap in their areas of innervation. Special sense organs are found in the skin at birth, although maturation of Meissner's tactile organs occurs postnatally.

Sympathetic nerves supply arterioles and erector pili muscles, norepinephrine serving as the chemical mediator. Eccrine gland function, on the other hand, is mediated by acetylcholine.

NEONATAL PERIOD (see Ch. 17, History, Physical and Neurologic Examinations)

At birth the nails are well formed, even in premature infants. Sweat glands are also present in both term and premature infants but are generally less physiologically active in the latter group. The full-term infant usually sweats poorly, if at all, during the first one to two days of life. When sweating begins, it appears first on the forehead, later on the palms. Infants of heroin-addicted mothers have a greater propensity to sweat both spontaneously and after stimulation with various pharmacologic agents (2).

In full-term infants the pH of the skin is nearly neutral for the first two days postpartum (the pH of vernix is about 7.4), and in premature infants, slightly lower. The pH steadily declines so that by the end of the first month it is about 5.5. (Bacterial colonization of the skin is discussed in Ch. 19, Bacterial Infection.)

Care of the skin is an important part of neonatal nursing care, especially in the very thin, poorly keratinized and easily traumatized skin of the premature infant.

Postpartum washing of the skin with HCP has been advocated as a means of decreasing staphylococcal colonization and hence decreasing the likelihood of skin infection. During the 1960s when staphylococcal skin disease was a serious problem, this was an effective means of preventing nursery epidemics of staphylococcal origin. However, the number of major nursery epidemics caused by staphylococci declined sharply after that period. The realization that HCP may be absorbed through the skin and have a damaging effect on the CNS has caused application of this agent to fall into relative disfavor. Routine HCP washes were discontinued at Harlem Hospital in 1966, despite which a low rate of staphylococcal colonization of the skin has been noted, together with a low incidence of staphylococcal skin disease. Many other centers, however, have reported a recrudescence of staphylococcal infection following cessation of bathing infants with HCP (see section Staphylococcal Disease of the Newborn Infant, Ch. 19).

Breaks in the skin, especially in premature infants, e.g., after infiltration of an IV infusion, or denudation of skin following removal of tape, may serve as a portal of entry for potentially pathogenic bacteria. An antibiotic ointment that is effective against both gram-positive and gram-negative bacteria, such as a combination of neomycin, polymxin and bacitracin, should be applied to traumatized neonatal skin. Potentially pathogenic skin bacteria can be introduced into the hip joint by femoral puncture, with a subsequent septic arthritis (1); therefore, this procedure must be approached with caution.

NONPATHOLOGIC CONDITIONS

Erythema Toxicum

Erythema toxicum is a very common eruption, appearing primarily on the face, trunk and buttocks, but it may occur at any site. Its incidence increases with gestational age and is rarely seen in infants of less than 30 weeks. It generally occurs early in the first week of life, usually after the first 24 to 48 hours. It is occasionally seen as late as the 14th day.

Erythematous papules or splotches are seen, and often there are small whitish or pale yellow pustules that are subcorneal and perifollicular. The erythematous areas blanch on pressure. These pustules contain an eosinophilic exudate and are bacteriologically sterile. The etiology is not known, but the presence of eosinophils may indicate that this benign condition represents a local allergy to a component of amniotic fluid.

The principal importance of erythema toxicum is that it may be confused, by inexperienced observers, with staphylococcal pustules. Usually the distinction can be made on a clinical basis since the pustules in erythema toxicum are very small, and the erythema and papules look like flea bites. In doubtful cases the exudate should be stained with Gram's and Wright's stains. The absence of bacteria and polymorphonuclear neutrophiles (PMNs) helps to establish the diagnosis. The rash usually disappears within a few days, and no therapy is necessary.

Milia

About 40% of full-term infants have numerous pearly white or yellowish papules located on the cheeks, forehead, nose and occasionally elsewhere (Fig. 5–1). They are small epidermal cysts that contain keratinous material. The lesions exfoliate spontaneously during the first few weeks of life. Their persistence beyond this point is rare and may be associated with one of several unusual syndromes.

Miliaria

Miliaria crystallina are superficial, noninflammatory, clear vesicles that may appear on the face, scalp, forehead and intertriginous areas as early as the first day after birth. They are due to postnatal retention of sweat secondary to obstruction of eccrine gland ducts; high environmental humidity

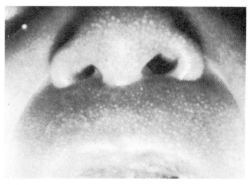

FIG. 5–1. Hyperplastic sebaceous glands in the nasolabial region of a full-term infant. A solitary epidermal inclusion cyst (milium) is on the right cheek. (Hodgman JE et al: Pediatr Clin North Am 18:713, 1971)

may prolong the presence of the rash (Fig. 5–2).

Miliaria rubra is also due to sweat retention but is accompanied by erythema and usually occurs after the first week of life. The sweat retention is intradermal.

Epstein's Pearls

Epstein's pearls are located on the palate or —occasionally—on the alveolar ridges. They are comparable histologically to milia.

Mongolian Spots

Another commonly encountered benign lesion is Mongolian spots. They occur in over 90% of Negroes, Orientals and American Indians and are also found in 1% to 5% of Caucasian infants. Usually found in the lumbosacral area they may occasionally be located elsewhere. They have irregular borders, may be single or multiple, vary widely in size and are slate blue or gray. On biopsy, spindle-shaped melanocytes are seen: these may represent cells that have not completely migrated from the neural crest to the epidermis. The lesions usually fade within the first year or two but occasionally persist for an indefinite period.

Harlequin Color Change

When the infant is placed on his side, there may be a deep erythema of the dependent

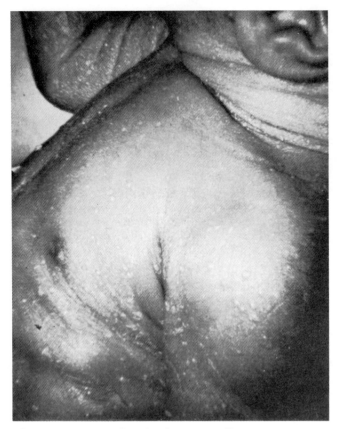

FIG. 5–2. Diffuse vesicles of miliaria crystallina in an immature full-term infant cared for in an incubator. At 24 hours of age, the infant developed a fever and vesicular eruption. (Hodgman JE et al: Pediatr Clin North Am 18:713, 1971)

portion and pallor of the superior half of the body. The phenomonon is more common in the premature than in the full-term infant. It is usually transient, lasting from 30 seconds to 20 minutes. Episodes may be single or multiple and are rarely seen after the third week of life. This is a completely benign condition unassociated with any known disease.

Cutis Marmorata

Exposure of an infant to a low environmental temperature ay lead to a marble-like vascular pattern on the skin. On rewarming, the configuration disappears. This phenomonon may be seen in normal infants and is common in neonates with Down's syndrome, trisomy E or the Cornelia de Lange syndrome.

POTENTIALLY PATHOLOGIC CONDITIONS

Skin Dimples and Tags

Skin dimples may appear over various bony prominences and are usually of no diagnostic significance. They are occasionally seen in the rubella syndrome and in several rare chromosomal abnormalities.

Skin tags are minor unilateral or bilateral developmental abnormalities. They are usually on the face, close to the mandible or hyoid arch. They are often seen in infants with severe anomalies of the ears and face.

ABNORMAL CONDITIONS

Skin Infections

Skin infections are discussed in Ch. 19, Bacterial Infection.

Petechiae

Petechiae are small areas of bleeding into the skin; in contrast to macules and erythema, they do not blanch with pressure. Ordinarily after a normal vaginal delivery a few petechiae may be observed on the face and in the conjunctivae, and after a breech delivery on the buttocks and in the perineal area. Large numbers of them, especially on the trunk and lower extremities, raise the question of thrombocytopenia, which may accompany intrauterine infection or disseminated intravascular coagulation, or they may exist as an isolated problem. Their number and distribution do not differentiate the etiologic basis for the lesion.

Acne

Neonatal acne is rare, but it may occasionally be seen on the face (usually in male infants). Papules, pustules and comedones are present, just as in adolescent acne. Treatment is conservative, and the rash usually disappears within several months.

Subcutaneous Fat Necrosis

Subcutaneous fat necrosis is a well-demarcated lesion, usually seen in large infants following a difficult delivery. The characteristic firm, moveable nodules range in diameter from 1 or 2 mm to 10 cm. They are usually colorless and nontender, but occasionally a mild inflammatory reaction may be noted. The lesions most often appear late in the first week or early in the second week of life, are most common over pressure points and are frequently seen over the cheeks following a forceps delivery. They also appear over the shoulders, back, thighs and buttocks.

The etiology is imperfectly understood but is most likely due to local tissue ischemia. On microscopic examination, fat crystals and a chronic inflammatory infiltrate with giant cells can be seen.

The lesions usually disappear slowly, often taking a few months to completely re-solve. The nodules may calcify, and elevations of serum calcium may be noted.

If overlooked in the nursery, they may cause diagnostic confusion on follow-up visits with lesions due to trauma, tumors or infection.

Sclerema

Sclerema neonatorum is a serious entity characterized by a "woody" hardening of the subcutaneous tissue that makes it impossible to pinch or lift the skin. It affects the entire body with the exception of palms, soles and genitalia, usually beginning on the thighs and back. It is generally seen only in infants who have serious systemic illness, most often infection, and occurs more often in premature than in full-term infants. Although it was fairly common several years ago, we have encountered this entity only once in the past decade among premature infants. Since all low-birth-weight infants are now raised under thermoneutral conditions during the first week of life, it is probable that subthermoneutral environmental temperatures superimposed on a serious systemic illness play a role in the etiology of this disorder.

The basic underlying defect is not known. Microscopic examination shows neither fat necrosis nor an inflammatory reaction; however, some thickening of the trabeculae of the subcutaneous fat is noted.

Treatment is supportive, with principal therapy directed towards the underlying illness. There is no evidence that treatment with corticosteroids increases survival.

Traumatic Lesions

Traumatic lesions of the skin are occasionally noted at birth. Blisters in various stages of healing (often only areas of denuded skin are seen) are occasionally encountered on the upper extremities of full-term infants. These are thought to be secondary to intrauterine sucking.

Traumatic injury to the vertex in vaginal delivery is called caput succedaneum. The hemorrhage and edema noted here usually subside fairly rapidly.

Punched-out ulcerated lesions, especially of the scalp, are seen occasionally (Fig. 5–3). With pressure necrosis secondary to the process of vaginal delivery, the skin may appear normal at birth, but shortly thereafter become erythematous and swollen. There is subsequent breakdown of the skin, with draining ulcerated lesions that heal slowly. An occasional infant is seen at birth with one or more punched-out ulcers of the scalp. Whether this is caused by intrauterine pressure necrosis or has some other etiology is not known. This type of lesion heals by scarring. Defects of the scalp are also noted in the trisomy D syndrome.

Transplacental Passage of Drug or Antibody

Skin eruptions in the newborn infant have been reported secondary to transplacental passage of drugs ingested by the mother and of abnormal maternal antibody. Hodgman et al (5) report a generalized desquamating eruption in an infant whose mother had ingested bromide, and in whom the serum bromide level was elevated.

Infants of mothers with systemic lupus erythematosus (LE) can develop dermatologic manifestations of discord lupus during the first month of life, together with a positive LE preparation. These lesions, which have an erythematous periphery and pale center, tend to fade after several months, often leaving atrophic scars. With permanent regression of skin lesions in the infant, the LE preparation becomes negative.

Icthyosis

Icthyosis describes a variety of congenital disorders of keratinization (with several modes of inheritance) that may be present at birth. The most common type is ichthyosis vulgaris, which may appear at birth or shortly thereafter. It varies in severity from mild scaling and dryness to severe fissuring, with the lesion resembling fish scales (Fig. 5–4). This form of ichthyosis is transmitted by an autosomal dominant gene; it may

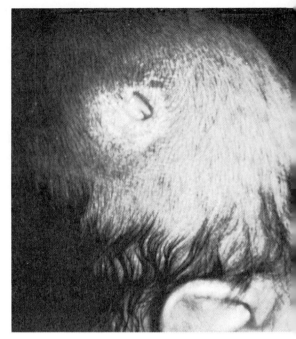

FIG. 5–3. Punched-out ulcer in the parietal region secondary to pressure necrosis. (Hodgman JE et al: Pediatr Clin North Am 18:713, 1971)

either regress spontaneously or progress into later life.

The "collodian" baby (Fig. 5–5) (lamellar exfoliation of the newborn) is covered either partially or completely at birth by a restrictive membrane that resembles dried collodian. Many of these infants are of low birth-weight. Shedding begins after a day or two but may not be complete for several weeks or months. The skin underlying this membrane often appears edematous. This entity may represent the neonatal form of X-linked ichthyosis or nonbullous congenital ichthyosiform erythroderma, which has an autosomal recessive mode of inheritance. In the former condition, the collodian membrane may not be present at birth. There may be only hyperkeratosis (or even no findings) in the neonatal period. The thick yellowish scales that evolve do not affect the palms, soles and flexures of the extremities. There are usually no systemic manifestations. Since there is an X-linked mode of inheritance, this condition is limited to males.

The latter condition (nonbullous congenital ichthyosiform erythroderma) may present with only mild scaling and hyperkeratosis. This usually leads to denudation of skin and secondary infection. Corticosteroids may be of some value.

Incontinentia Pigmenti

Incontinentia pigmenti is a developmental anomaly of the skin that eventually affects other organ systems, such as the eyes, teeth, bone and the CNS. The cutaneous manifestations, which may begin in utero, undergo three phases. At first there is a papulovesicular eruption, which is often linear in configuration. The presence of eosinophils in the vesicular fluid may cause some confusion with erythema toxicum. Warty nodules then appear and are eventually replaced by pigmented whorls. The whole process may occur in utero, so that at birth only the pigmented whorls may be seen. This syndrome is familial and seen almost universally in females. It is felt that the responsible gene is an X-linked dominant that usually causes intrauterine death in male fetuses.

Epidermolysis Bullosa

Epidermolysis bullosa is a group of disorders manifested by vesicle and bulla formation. It may first appear either in utero or during the neonatal period, often secondary to mild trauma to the skin (Fig. 5–6).

The most common and least dangerous of this group is epidermolysis bullosa simplex,

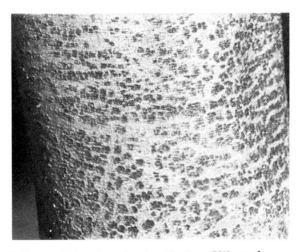

FIG. 5–4. Icthyosis vulgaris. (Korting GW et al: Diseases of the Skin in Children and Adolescents. Philadelphia, Saunders, 1969)

which is transmitted through an autosomal dominant gene. Vesicle formation may begin in utero, with denuded areas of skin appearing at birth, or shortly after delivery. These vesicles are most often located over points of friction, such as the heels, soles of feet and knuckles, but they may occur anywhere over the body. They heal without scarring since the defect is located within basal layer of the epidermis. However, secondary infection in the denuded areas may pose a problem in care of the infant. Nails and mucous membranes are not involved in this form of the disease. By adolescence the tendency to form vesicles has usually diminished markedly and may disappear altogether in adult life.

FIG. 5–5. Collodian baby. (Hodgman JE et al: Pediatr Clin North Am 18:713, 1971)

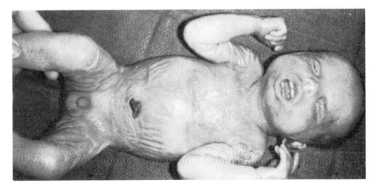

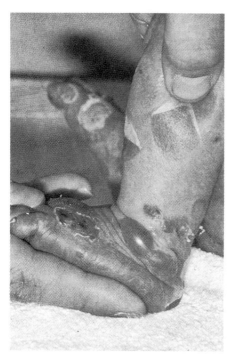

FIG. 5–6. Epidermolysis bullosa hereditaria with positive Nikolski sign. (Korting GW et al: Diseases of the Skin in Children and Adolescents. Philadelphia, Saunders, 1969)

The dystrophic types of epidermolysis bullosa are much less common than the simple type. The autosomal dominant variant of the dystrophic type is relatively not serious. The vesicles and bullae may first appear at any time from intrauterine life to early infancy. The hands, feet, knees and elbows are commonly affected, as are the nails, which may show a clawlike deformity. There is occasionally mild involvement of the mucous membranes. Since the basic defect is located in the upper cutis, the healing phase is associated with scarring. The autosomal form of dystrophic epidermolysis bullosa is not associated with an increased mortality rate.

The recessive type of dystrophic epidermolysis bullosa is extremely serious although rare. As in the dominant type, the basic defect is in the connective tissue just below the epidermis. Large hemorrhagic bullae may be present at birth. The hands and feet usually show severe involvement, and in healing, extreme scarring and deformity occur, with fusion of digits, resorption of

bone and loss of nails. The mucous membranes of the eye and mouth may also be involved, as well as dental enamel. Nodules (or milia) may appear at the sites of scarring. Anemia often complicates this disorder. Secondary infection can pose a major problem and often leads to death in infancy. In those who do survive into adult life, the severity of the disorder may decrease during adolescence. Treatment is aimed mainly at preventing both trauma and the formation of new bullae. Corticosteroids are of little value.

The extremely rare letalis form of this disorder has an autosomal recessive mode of inheritance. It is seen immediately after birth. Large sheets of epidermis desquamate over the entire body after minimal trauma, with nails and mucous membranes usually being involved. The denuded areas, which ulcerate easily and become secondarily infected, heal very slowly. Those lesions that do heal leave no scars since the defect appears to be between the upper layer of dermis and the basement membrane of the epidermis. Although corticosteroids may be of some value, death usually occurs in early infancy.

Urticaria Pigmentosa

Urticaria pigmentosa may appear in the neonatal period. This disorder is due to an abnormal accumulation of nests of histamine-secreting mast cells in the dermis. Local trauma to the skin causes release of histamine with subsequent formation of urticarial wheals and bullae, which may be localized or widespread. Deposition of pigment characterizes the healing phase of this lesion; this, however, does not usually become widespread until after six months of age. Despite these lesions, systemic health of the infant is usually good.

Nevi

Nevi, either vascular or pigmented, are local skin malformations that probably do not fit into the category of tumors.

The most common type of vascular nevus seen in the newborn infant is the salmon

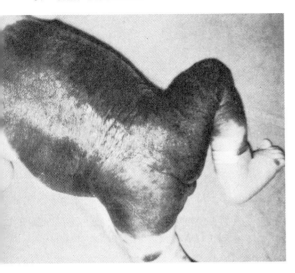

FIG. 5–7. Giant pigmented nevus. (Hodgman JE et al: Pediatr Clin North Am 18:713, 1971)

patch, or nevus simplex, which is most often located on the nape of the neck but is also seen over the eyelids, lips, nasolabial folds and forehead. Most of these regress spontaneously.

The port wine stain (nevus flammeus) is red or purple and is most commonly found on the face. It is made up of newly formed, but mature, capillaries that do not proliferate after birth. These flat and sharply demarcated lesions represent major cosmetic defects. Port wine nevi rarely regress spontaneously.

If a port wine stain follows the distribution of the trigeminal nerve, the diagnosis of Sturge-Weber syndrome may be considered. This is associated with intracranial hemangiomas, whose calcification may lead to a convulsive disorder.

Pigmented nevi are nests of melanin-containing nervus cells of neuroectodermal origin that are related to melanocytes and lie within the dermis. Nearly all pigmented nevi seen in the neonatal period are benign.

The giant nevus (Fig. 5–7) is always present at birth. It often follows the area of distribution of an article of clothing (bathing trunk, coat sleeve). This deeply pigmented lesion, which may be hairy and verrucous, often presents a serious cosmetic problem. It may also undergo malignant degeneration

in later life. Therefore, removal of this nevus, whenever possible, is generally indicated. However, the large area involved in many of these often makes complete removal impossible.

Hemangiomas

Several varieties of hemangiomas may be seen in the neonatal period. The capillary hemangioma, or strawberry mark, is an extremely common finding in the neonatal period. For some reason, these are rarely, if ever, seen on the day of birth but usually appear during the first week of life. They seem to be more common in premature than in full-term infants and are seen more often in females than in males. They are usually small (about the size of a pinhead) when first seen, but they grow progressively larger. The lesion is most often solitary, appearing primarily on the face. Lesions are elevated, well demarcated, blanch on pressure and resemble the outside of a strawberry; most of them grow fairly rapidly during the first half year of life and by the second year begin to regress. By age five, about 50% disappear, and by age seven, about 70%.

Since these tumors are all benign and most regress spontaneously, no specific therapy is necessary unless they interfere with vital function, e.g., impinge on the orbit. Parental reassurance is necessary during the period of rapid growth of these lesions. When therapy is required, surgical incision, solid carbon dioxide applications or short intensive courses of corticosteroid therapy may be of value.

Cavernous hemangiomas (Fig. 5–8) are more deeply located in the dermis and are made up of mature interconnected venules and vascular sinuses. In contrast with strawberry hemangiomas, they are always present at birth. They have a spongy feeling, are easily compressible and give a bluish tint to the skin. These hemangiomas do not have the same rapid growth pattern as the capillary variety; they grow in proportion to the rest of the body. They do not involute spontaneously, and occasionally reconstructive surgery is required. Both capillary and venous elements may exist together in a combined hemangioma.

A complication of widespread hemangiomatosis is sequestration of platelets and thrombocytopenia (Kasabach-Merritt syndrome). Bleeding and anemia may be severe, and splenomegaly may occasionally be noted. Platelet survival is decreased, and a variety of coagulation disorders are observed.

This syndrome is a life-threatening entity, requiring fresh blood and platelet transfusions. Removal of the lesions by surgery or radiotherapy is required following treatment of the coagulation disorder.

Lymphangiomas

Lymphangiomas, which are much less common than hemangiomas, affect not only the skin but the deeper structures as well.

Phlebectasia

Congenital phlebectasia is a rare condition in which networks of superficially dilated veins are present at birth, usually on an extremity. These may regress spontaneously, or venous ligation may occasionally be required during childhood.

Café-au-lait Spots

Café-au-lait spots are tannish macules that may be the only manifestation of neurofibromatosis in the neonatal period. About 20% occur as an isolated finding. More than five or six of these macules on the body of a newborn infant should raise the suspicion of this diagnosis.

The disorder occurs in 1:3000 live births and is inherited as an autosomal dominant trait. Although other abnormalities are seen in later life, only the skin lesion is observed during the neonatal period.

White Spots

About 90% of newborn infants who will develop tuberous sclerosis have white macules

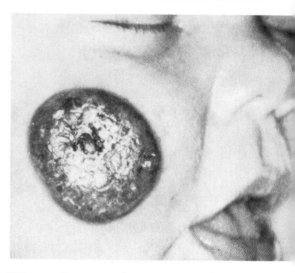

FIG. 5–8. Cavernous hemangioma with central necrosis. (Solomon LM, Esterly NB: Neonatal Dermatology. Philadelphia, Saunders, 1973)

that may be present anywhere over the body. These lesions may be demonstrated by use of the Wood's lamp.

REFERENCES

1. Asnes RS, Arendar GS: Septic arthritis of the hip: a complication of femoral venipuncture. Pediatrics 38:837, 1966

2. Behrendt H, Green M.: Nature of the sweating deficit of prematurely born neonates; observations on babies with the heroin withdrawal syndrome. N Engl J Med 286:1376, 1972

3. Brown AK, Scoggin WA: Studies of bilirubin and water transfer across umbilical cord and fetal skin. Am Pediatr Soc Inc and Soc Pediatr Res; Program and Abstract, p 264, 1971

4. Curley A, Hawk RE, Kimbrough RD, Nathenson G, Finberg L: Dermal absorption of hexachlorophene in infants. Lancet 2:296, 1971

5. Hodgman JE, Freedman RI, Levan NE: Neonatal dermatology. Pediatr Clin North Am 18:713, 1971

6. Jacobs AH (ed): Symposium on Pediatric Dermatology (Pediatr Clin North Am 18:3). Philadelphia, Saunders, 1971

7. Korting GW: Diseases of the Skin in Children and Adolescents. Philadelphia, Saunders, 1969

8. Nachman RL, Esterly NB: Increased skin permeability in preterm infants. J Pediatr 79:628, 1971

9. Solomon LM, Esterly NB: Neonatal Dermatology. Philadelphia, Saunders, 1973

6

Pulmonary Function and Disorders

DEVELOPMENT AND ADAPTATION

IN UTERO MATURATION

The in utero process of pulmonary maturation prepares the lung to replace the placenta as the organ of gas exchange postpartum. The fetal lung has no known physiologic function except for its small contribution to the production of amniotic fluid.

The epithelial-lined bronchial tree is derived from gut endoderm outpouching from the primordial gastrointestinal (GI) tract (Fig. 6–1). Beginning at the 24th day of gestation, this is known as the glandular phase. Branching, which is asymmetric and dichotomous, begins during the 6th week and continues through the 16th week (canalicular phase), with peripheral growth progressing at a greater rate than proximal growth. Between the 10th and 14th weeks, 65% to 75% of branchings occur.

Bronchial epithelium, which develops as early as the tenth week, consists of a superficial layer of columnar cells and a deeper layer of irregularly appearing cells resting on a well-defined basement membrane. The newly formed bronchial branches are lined with epithelial cells whose height progressively diminishes until cuboidal epithelium is reached in the bronchioles.

By the 16th week respiratory bronchioles begin to differentiate by branching of the terminal bronchioles, which at first are lined continuously with cuboidal epithelial cells. The proliferation of vascular tissue around the respiratory bronchioles is associated with a progressive loss of continuity of this cuboidal epithelial lining—a hallmark of the canalicular phase.

Cilia are found as early as the 10th week, and mucous glands begin to appear by the 12th week. Goblet cells, appearing in the trachea and large bronchi at 13 weeks, proliferate gradually during the next 20 weeks, at which time they appear in the same segments as the mucous glands.

Recognizable tracheal cartilage is seen at 7 weeks, its peripheral growth and development continuing until the 24th week. The principal connective tissue of fetal lung is collagen, which is first seen at 18 to 20 weeks' gestation in the septa that provide the framework for the lobes. This material gives support to the air passages and blood.

Smooth muscle development is limited during fetal life; only during the last weeks of gestation is a small amount noted in perialveolar tissue.

Lymph channels are noted by the 20th week of gestation and are fully mature by term.

Airway canalization begins by the 20th week. The growing bronchial tree extends into an area containing mesenchyme, from which is derived connective tissue, septa and blood vessels. As development proceeds, air spaces become more complex, con-

89

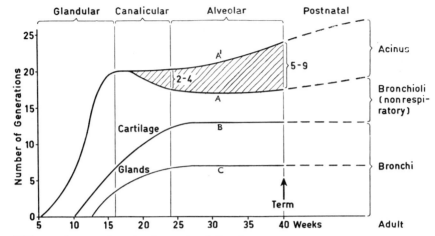

FIG. 6–1. Intrauterine development of the bronchial tree. A, Number of bronchial generations; A¹, Respiratory bronchioles and alveolar ducts; B, Extension of cartilage along the bronchial tree; C, Extension of mucous glands. (Bucher U, Reid L: Thorax 16:207, 1961)

nective tissue thins out and capillaries begin to pouch into the walls of the alveoli.

At about the 24th week alveolar capillary complexes are sufficiently developed to permit a minimal diffusion of oxygen and carbon dioxide.

At about 26 to 30 weeks' gestation, two types of cells are observed lining the air spaces. Type I cells are small, have attenuated cytoplasm and cover most of the alveolar surface. Type II cells—larger, cuboidal and with distinct lamellae and osmiophilic granules—are the source of pulmonary surfactant (8), which protects alveoli from total collapse at the end of expiration. It is at about this time that the fetal lung becomes capable of supporting life in an extrauterine environment.

Lung maturation is in many ways under hormonal control, with both corticosteroids (10) and thyroid hormone (11) playing a role in the maturation of processes leading to the synthesis of pulmonary surfactant. Corticosteroids are especially important in the choline incorporation (see section Respiratory Distress Syndrome) pathway of lecithin synthesis. This action appears to be mediated through the specific corticosteroid receptor sites of fetal lung necessary for the initiation of surfactant synthesis (3). Corti-

costeroid receptor sites are also found in other fetal cells (6, 7); hence intrauterine administration of corticosteroids may affect multiple organs in addition to the lungs.

LUNG DEVELOPMENT AND RESPIRATION

A considerable portion of lung growth occurs postnatally. The more premature the infant is at birth, the less well developed his lung. Following delivery, there is a postpartum increase both in the number of bronchiolar divisions and in the total number of alveoli. Whereas roughly 24 million are present at birth, 300 million have developed by four to eight years. Alveolar diameter increases from 50μ at term to 120μ at two months to 150 to 200μ in older children. Although the number of alveoli between birth and adulthood increases about 10-fold, the surface area for gas exchange increases about 20-fold.

Fetal respiratory movements can be observed indirectly through the gravid abdominal wall in about one-third of pregnancies near term. These movements, which are probably present in all fetuses during the second half of pregnancy, can be recorded with an ultrasound A scan (4). There is preliminary evidence that hypoxia and hypoglycemia depress fetal respirations and that use of this noninvasive diagnostic method may aid in the evaluation of fetal well-being (5).

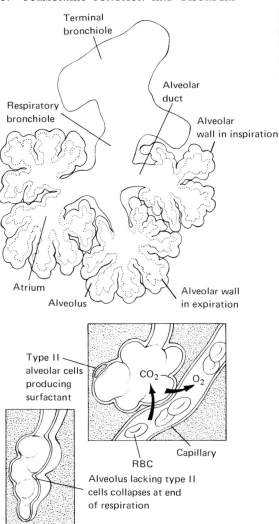

Terminal bronchiole

Alveolar duct

Respiratory bronchiole

Alveolar wall in inspiration

Atrium

Alveolus

Alveolar wall in expiration

Type II alveolar cells producing surfactant

CO_2 O_2

RBC

Capillary

Alveolus lacking type II cells collapses at end of respiration

FIG. 6–2. Following delivery, gaseous exchange occurs between expanded alveoli and the pulmonary capillary bed. In the absence of pulmonary surfactant, alveoli collapse at the end of expiration, and gaseous exchange is impaired.

As the infant passes through the birth canal during a normal vaginal delivery, its thorax is compressed and fluid is forced from the upper portion of the lung and removed from the nose and mouth. After delivery of the chest, there is recoil of the thorax and a small amount of air enters the chest. A rapid change in pulmonary blood flow occurs and (under normal circumstances), the lungs are then perfused by virtually the entire blood volume rather than the 10% or less present during fetal life. The remainder of the lung fluid is absorbed, and the infant is able to take his first postnatal breath (Fig. 6–2).

The mechanisms responsible for initiation of the first breath have not been completely defined. The hypoxemia, acidosis and hypercarbia that occur during parturition, mediated through carotid and aortic chemoreceptors, undoubtedly play a major role. These metabolic changes reflect decreased maternal blood flow to the placenta, placental separation and umbilical cord compression during the intrapartum period. However, severe asphyxia, acidosis and administration of depressant drugs to the mother interfere with the initiation of respiration. Certain physical factors occurring at birth also play an important role in the initiation of respiration. Hypothermia is a major stimulus, its effect being mediated by facial sensory receptors. Tactile stimuli produce gasping but do not induce a sustained respiratory effort.

TABLE 6–1. Normal Pulmonary Function in a 3 kg
Full-Term Infant*

Function	Normal Values
Respiration	30–50/minute
Tidal volume	20–25 ml
Physiologic dead space	6–8 ml
Total lung volume	160 ml
Crying vital capacity	120 ml
Inspiratory capacity	80 ml
Function residual capacity	80 ml

Occlusion of the umbilical cord leads to a transient elevation of blood pressure, which may also be a respiratory stimulus.

With the first breath a very high negative intrapleural pressure (often as high as 70 cm of water) is required to overcome the surface tension opposing the opening of air spaces. About 50 to 80 ml of air enter the lung with the first breath, 20 to 30 ml of which establish the functional residual capacity. Normal values of pulmonary function for term infants are shown in Table 6–1.

Evidence indicates that the placenta continues as the primary organ of respiration for the first five breaths (9), with the lungs taking over after this time. With inflation of the lungs pulmonary vascular resistance decreases. Left atrial pressure begins to rise and soon exceeds that of the right atrium, causing closure of the foramen ovale. Ligation of the umbilical blood vessels leads to increased pressure and resistance in the systemic circulation. When systemic exceeds pulmonary pressure, blood begins to flow in a left-to-right direction across the ductus arteriosus. Closure of the ductus normally occurs 8 to 24 hours postpartum, probably as a result of increased oxygenation. In hypoxia, closure of the ductus may be delayed and a high pulmonary pressure may persist, secondary to pulmonary arteriolar constriction.

STABILIZATION

During the first 30 minutes following delivery (first reactive phase), respirations are usually irregular and shallow, and flaring, grunting and chest retractions may be pres-ent. After this interval there is usually a period of sleep, during which respirations are rapid and shallow. At about three to six hours of age a second reactive phase occurs, marked by an irregular respiratory effort. Following this phase, respirations normally stabilize at a rate of 30 to 50 per minute. These respiratory rates, which are considerably higher than those found in older children and adults, may be secondary to an active Hering-Breuer reflex, which is mediated through vagal pathways.

RESPIRATORY DISTRESS SYNDROME

The respiratory distress syndrome (RDS) is an acute disorder of newborn infants, especially those of less than 38 weeks' gestation. Clinical manifestations, which usually appear shortly after birth, include retraction of the chest wall, expiratory grunt and cyanosis in room air. The clinical course usually lasts from three to five days, ending in recovery of the infant or death. Occasionally, chronic lung disease with a course protracted over several months is encountered following recovery.

There is a predilection of RDS for males, and a tendency to recur in families has been described. Together with prematurity, RDS is associated with maternal diabetes mellitus, cesarean section and third trimester bleeding (24, 29).

The mortality rate from this disorder has been estimated to be between 30% and 60%, resulting in about 25,000 neonatal deaths annually in the United States. Diagnostic and therapeutic modalities introduced in the early 1970s have substantially reduced this number. It is by far the most important life-threatening illness that the physician caring for newborn infants encounters, and a major proportion of the effort of neonatal intensive care units is directed towards the treatment of this disorder.

ETIOLOGY

The etiology of RDS remained an enigma for many years. Various factors, including aspiration of amniotic fluid, asphyxia, congestive heart failure, decreased blood volume, shock, pulmonary hypoperfusion, disturbed autonomic regulation and a fibrinolytic enzyme defect were all proposed as underlying causes of RDS (15, 26, 30, 32, 35). Although all of these problems have been encountered at one time or another in infants with RDS, none were ever definitely proven to be a causative factor.

The weight of evidence now points to a deficiency of pulmonary surfactant, a surface-active phospholipid (primarily comprised of dipalmitoyl lecithin) that maintains alveolar stability and prevents their collapse at the end of expiration, as the probable cause of RDS.

Pulmonary Surfactant

The association between lack of a surface-active material and the atelectasis observed in infants dying with RDS was made by Avery and Mead in 1959 (12). They noted that lung extracts of premature infants who die of RDS have a much higher surface tension than those of full-term infants who die of other causes. Extensive studies by many investigators over the next decade, culminating in the findings of Gluck et al (22, 23), have elucidated some of the mechanisms involved in the production of pulmonary surfactant by the fetus and newborn infant. These findings have been correlated with the clinical manifestations of RDS and have led to the development of tests for its antenatal diagnosis.

Pulmonary surfactant is necessary for prevention of alveolar collapse at the end of expiration. Since an alveolus can be compared to a spherical bubble, its surface tension tends to increase with a decreasing radius (end expiration) according to La Place's law (P = 2T/R, where P is the pressure of the gas within the alveolus, T the surface tension in dynes and R is its radius). Surfactant, which decreases surface tension in the wall of the alveolus at the end of expiration, is the factor responsible for the residual air that is normally present in lungs at the end of expiration.

Surfactant is produced by osmiophilic granules found within the cytoplasm of type II alveolar lining cells. It is synthesized primarily through the phosphocholine (cytidyl) transferase pathway (pathway I), which is responsible for more than 95% of surfactant production. Synthesis of surfactant through this pathway begins early in pregnancy but does not become fully developed until the 35th to 37th week of gestation. At this time, a marked elevation in the lecithin concentration of amniotic fluid is observed, reflecting maturation of pathway I.

A secondary mechanism, the methyltransferase pathway (pathway II), accounts for less than 5% of surfactant production. It begins to function at the 20th to 22nd week of gestation in human fetuses and is inhibited by such stresses as acidosis and hypoxia, both prenatally and postnatally.

Gestational and Postnatal Episodes

The ability of a newborn infant to successfully accommodate an air-breathing environment (and to avoid developing RDS) therefore depends on the continued synthesis of surfactant by alveolar lining cells. In fetuses less than 35 to 37 weeks' gestation, in whom surfactant production is limited, various prenatal stresses can further predispose to the development of RDS, including familial (history of previous siblings with RDS); gestational (prematurity, diabetes mellitus); intrapartum (hypoxia, acidosis, maternal hemorrhage or hypotension, cesarean section and early clamping of umbilical cord); and postnatal (hypoxia, acidosis and chilling). On the other hand, IU infection (31), prolonged rupture of fetal membranes (37) and maternal use of heroin (19) appear to protect against its development. However, Jones et al (25a), in a retrospective analysis of over 16,000 birth records, found no association of antenatal hemorrhage with increased frequency of RDS, nor was prolonged rupture of the fetal membranes associated with a decreased occurrence of this disorder.

Events occurring during the intrapartum

period may also relate to the development and severity of RDS. Cesarean section is associated with an increased incidence of RDS (35). This is probably related to certain underlying indications for the operation, such as maternal hemorrhage or fetal hypoxia. However, inadvertent hypotension caused by maternal anesthesia may also play a role. Early clamping of the umbilical cord resulting in a decreased blood volume may intensify the illness in affected infants. Chilling of the infant following delivery appears to be a factor in the pathogenesis of RDS. This may be secondary to the pulmonary vascular constriction and resultant acidosis and decreased oxygenation that occurs following exposure to low environmental temperatures.

Once the infant is thrust by birth into an air-breathing environment, surfactant must be rapidly replenished or the signs of RDS will soon develop. In its absence or when production is decreased, alveoli collapse at the end of expiration, so that with each breath the infant must reexpand an atelectatic lung. Lung compliance is markedly reduced under these circumstances, and an extremely high work effort is necessary to maintain respirations. In the more severe forms of the illness, a vicious cycle that may lead to the demise of the infant develops.

Progressive atelectasis ensues if the infant's ability to expand alveoli with each breath begins to fail. With the development of atelectasis, portions of lung are perfused by blood but ventilated either inadequately or not at all. This leads to decreased oxygenation, asphyxia and metabolic acidosis. Hypoxia and acidosis further perpetuate the problem by causing pulmonary vasoconstriction, diminishing the amount of blood available to perfuse ventilated alveoli. A right-to-left shunting of blood across a patent ductus arteriosus accompanies the decreased pulmonary blood flow.

With progressive hypoventilation and marked inequalities in ventilation and perfusion in the atelectatic lung, hypoxia and acidosis worsen. Retention of carbon dioxide leads to a respiratory acidosis; this may be a factor in increased cerebral venous blood flow and in the pathogenesis of the intraventricular hemorrhage seen in RDS.

After several hours, a membrane composed of the components of the infant's serum (including fibrin, immune globulins, albumin, α-2 macroglobulins and α-1 antitrypsin) plus debris from alveolar lining cells begins to line terminal bronchioles, alveoli and alveolar ducts. Because of the staining properties on histologic examination, they are called hyaline membranes (and hence the name hyaline membrane disease, which had been used synonymously with RDS for many years). These membranes further interfere with gaseous exchange. If the infant survives, the membranes are reabsorbed after several days. When death occurs within the first few hours of life, the membranes are usually not observed on postmortem examination.

If the infant remains alive for three or four days, surfactant synthesis usually accelerates, and the clinical picture and pulmonary function begin to improve.

CLINICAL MANIFESTATIONS

The infant most likely to develop RDS usually has a gestational age of 28 to 37 weeks. Its occurrence is uncommon in infants born during the second trimester or near term. The lower the gestational age, the more severe the disease.

Signs usually are observed shortly after birth and include tachypnea, chest retractions, expiratory grunt, flaring of alae nasi, cyanosis in room air, apneic episodes, "see-saw" respirations, diminished breath sounds, hypotension, peripheral edema, hypothermia, systolic murmur and diminished GI motility. With close observation tachypnea and chest retraction may be noted in the delivery room. Grunting appears shortly thereafter, and flaring of the alae nasi may occur. Signs may progress to include cyanosis in room air and apneic episodes (often an ominous prognostic sign). A see-saw respiratory pattern may be observed, with the abdomen protruding during inspiration. Breath sounds are usually diminished bilaterally. Inspiratory rales are rarely heard and may be indicative of a pneumonic process. However, auscultation may not be helpful in establishing a diagnosis. A systolic murmur usually secondary to a patent ductus arteriosus (a nonspecific finding in newborn infants that is frequently associated with hypoxemia) may sometimes be detected on cardiac auscultation.

The expiratory grunt that accompanies RDS is actually a modified Valsalva maneuver (expiration against a partially closed glottis) (25). It is thought to be a compensatory mechanism to combat alveolar collapse occurring at the end of expiration. This disappears following endotracheal intubation.

The heart rate is usually normal except for terminal bradycardia. Hypotension is common and may be associated with a decreased blood volume. Peripheral circulation is poor, with a pallid, dusky appearance being common. Peripheral edema, which may be found in any premature infant, is usually more pronounced in infants with RDS. Hypothermia may also be noted, especially in those hypoxic infants whose heat-producing capabilities have been impaired. Hyperbilirubinemia is a common finding with an increased risk of kernicterus among those who are most immature, hypoproteinemic, hypoxic and acidotic. Decreased urinary output is secondary to the shocklike state and hypotension. Diminished peristalsis leads to paralytic ileus.

Intraventricular hemorrhage is a frequently associated finding, usually leading to death of the infant within the first 48 hours. The precipitating factor here may be disseminated intravascular coagulation or venous stasis within the CNS, or both.

The clinical course of the illness is variable. Often, a mild variety (type II RDS) is seen (34), and transient signs may disappear within the first 24 hours of life. This type of RDS may be at least partially secondary to inadvertent chilling of the infant. More typically, the acute course of RDS runs from three to five days, with most deaths occurring within the first two days. Occasionally, in severe RDS, especially with respiratory failure and dependence on a respirator, the course may be markedly protracted and associated with chronic lung disease (bronchopulmonary dysplasia). Another possibility is that the infant may recover from RDS only to die at five to ten days of age of another complication of prematurity, such as generalized infection.

DIFFERENTIAL DIAGNOSIS

Although a typical syndrome is described for RDS, other neonatal disorders can easily be confused with it.

Rapid respirations may be noted in transient tachypnea of the newborn. This disorder is of uncertain etiology, but it may be related to a decreased rate of reabsorption of lung fluid. Retractions and grunting are absent, but mild cyanosis is occasionally seen. The chest x ray may show evidence of small pleural effusions or interstitial edema.

Tachypnea is a primary finding in the neonatal narcotic withdrawal syndrome. Here, all infants are pink in room air, blood acid-base studies usually show a primary respiratory alkalosis, and chest x rays are normal.

Intrauterine aspiration of amniotic fluid (often mixed with meconium) may occur in the presence of fetal hypoxemia. This condition is discussed in the section Meconium Aspiration.

Congenital pneumonia, which may be accompanied by generalized infection, is suggested by a history of prolonged rupture of membranes, prolonged labor and amnionitis and is associated with respiratory distress after delivery. This syndrome is often associated with fetal or early neonatal death. The clinical picture may be almost identical to that seen in RDS; often the history and chest x ray (usually showing diffuse infiltration with hilar accentuation) aids in making the correct diagnosis. Rales are usually present on auscultation; fever is generally absent (as in RDS, hypothermia is a more common finding).

Pneumothorax and pneumomediastinum may also mimic (or accompany) RDS. A chest x ray confirms the diagnosis.

Lobar atelectasis may develop after four

or more symptom-free hours of life. Localized dullness, diminished breath sounds,
heart and mediastinum shifted toward the
side of dullness, together with a chest x ray
showing a large homogenous area of radiopacity with compensatory emphysema on
the opposite side establish the diagnosis.

Diaphragmatic hernia often presents as
severe respiratory distress, typically with a
scaphoid abdomen, bulging thorax with
bowel sounds heard in the chest and dullness to percussion posteriorly; it is an acute
surgical emergency. X rays are confirmatory, and supportive therapy must be
started immediately while preparations for
the earliest possible operation are made. In
mild cases the diagnosis may be confusing
until the x rays are available.

Esophageal atresia with tracheoesophageal fistula may also present with early dyspnea, but the vomiting of copious frothy
mucus and the inability to pass a catheter
(and contrast material) into the stomach is
diagnostic.

Bleeding into the liver and adrenal gland
may also produce a clinical syndrome similar to RDS. Falling hematocrit along with a
shocklike picture and, on occasion, a palpable abdominal mass may suggest the diagnosis.

Symptomatic congenital cardiac disease
very often presents with respiratory symptoms and may sometimes be confused with
RDS. This is discussed in Chapter 7, Cardiovascular Disorders.

ANTENATAL DIAGNOSIS

Since the insufficient production of surfactant is related to the development of RDS,
tests based on the examination of amniotic
fluid can predict the likelihood of RDS appearing postnatally (Table 6–2).

Lung secretions contribute to the formation of amniotic fluid, and the phospholipid
and protein compositions of both fluids are
similar. Therefore, the measurement of surface-active phospholipids in amniotic fluid
is one means of measuring the production
of phospholipids by the fetal lung.

TABLE 6–2. Antenatal Diagnosis of RDS

L–S Ratio*	Bubble Stability (Shake) Test	Risk of RDS
<1.0	Negative	Almost 100%; severe
1.0–1.49	Negative	Usually present; moderately severe
1.5–1.99	Intermediate	May be present or absent; usually mild if present
>2.0	Positive	Nil

*These correlations are true in the vast majority of cases; however, exceptions have been noted.

Lecithin-Sphingomyelin Ratio

Gluck et al (20) have devised a relatively
simple method of using thin-layer chromatography to measure the ratio of lecithin
to sphingomyelin (L–S ratio) (Fig. 6–3).
Until the 30th week of gestation sphingomyelin is the predominant phospholipid in
amniotic fluid, and the L–S ratio is usually
about 1.0 or less. At about this time lecithin
production begins to increase slowly; at
about the 35th week of gestation there is a
sharp increase in lecithin synthesis, whereas
the concentration of sphingomyelin declines. During the last weeks of pregnancy
the L–S ratio is usually 2.0 or more. An L–S
ratio of less than 1.0 is almost always predictive of very severe RDS following delivery. A ratio of 1.0 to 1.49 denotes a
somewhat more advanced state of pulmonary maturity and is usually associated with
a less severe form of RDS. Ratios of 1.50 to
1.99 are borderline and may or may not be
associated with RDS, whereas ratios of 2.0
or more, which indicate pulmonary maturity, are almost always associated with the
absence of RDS. Determinations may be repeated approximately every two weeks if
the initial L–S ratio is low.

Because of methodologic differences, variations in interpretation of the L–S ratio may
be observed in individual centers. Therefore,
each laboratory performing the test must
establish its own criteria for the antenatal
determination of pulmonary maturity.

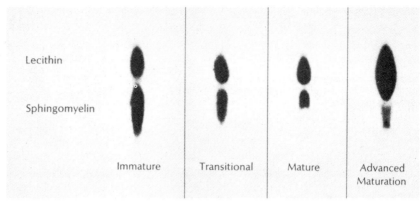

FIG. 6–3. Thin-layer chromatogram of amniotic fluid phospholipids shows changing relationship of lecithin to sphingomyelin as pulmonary maturation nears. The L–S ratios of specimens above were (left to right) 0.7, 1.8, 3.2, 8.4; a ratio of 2.0 signifies fetal maturity. (Gluck L: Hosp Pract 5:45, 1971)

Bubble Stability Test

Clements et al (16) have developed a rapid screening test for surfactant in amniotic fluid that depends on the ability of pulmonary surfactant to generate stable foam in a test tube in the presence of ethanol. The absence of stable bubbles in all tubes, correlating with a marked deficiency of surface-active material, is usually associated with the development of RDS and clear-cut bubble stability is almost always associated with the absence of RDS. An intermediate test is associated with RDS in about one-half of the cases.

This screening test is of value since it can be performed rapidly at the bedside using simple materials.

Amniotic Fluid Cortisol Levels

Fencl and Tulchinsky (17a) have shown that concentrations of amniotic fluid cortisol rise sharply after the 34th week of gestation. In their experience, concentrations of greater than 60 ng/ml are usually associated with L–S ratios of more than 2.0, while concentration of less than 40 ng/ml are associated with L–S ratios of less than 1.5.

The usefulness of this measurement in assessing fetal lung maturity requires further investigation.

POSTNATAL DIAGNOSIS

In addition to the physical findings, a wide range of tests are useful in substantiating the diagnosis, in aiding in the therapeutic approach and, to some degree, in establishing a prognosis. These tests include

1. Biochemical
   Decreased Pao_2, even when supplementary O_2 is administered
   Metabolic and respiratory acidosis
   Hypoproteinemia
   Decreased serum α1-antitrypsin
   Low L–S ratio and decreased PDME in tracheal fluid
   Hyperkalemia
2. Radiologic
   "Ground glass" appearance and air bronchogram effect on chest x ray
3. Pulmonary function
   Decreased lung compliance
   Decreased total lung volume
   Decreased functional residual capacity
   Increased dead space
   Ventilation perfusion inequality

Radiologic

The chest x ray is of great importance in establishing the diagnosis of RDS. The pulmonary parenchyma assumes a typical "ground glass" appearance, which is a manifestation of diffuse atelectasis. The air bronchogram effect that is characteristic of these x rays represents air passages silhouetted against poorly aerated lungs. In the mild, or type II RDS, the chest x ray may appear normal.

Other Diagnostic Tests

Measurements of phosphatidyl dimethyl-ethanolamine (PDME) in tracheal aspirate may be of value in the diagnosis of RDS. Wu et al (36) have found that this compound (a precursor of lecithin synthesized in the methylation pathway) is absent in infants with RDS and that its reappearance in tracheal aspirates coincides with clinical improvement of the infant.

Evans et al (17) found that *serum trypsin inhibitor levels* are significantly decreased in cord bloods of infants who developed RDS and that survival is associated with a rise in these levels.

Low *serum protein concentrations* have also been correlated with RDS. About one-half of low-birth-weight infants with cord blood serum protein concentrations of less than 4.6 g/100 ml develop RDS (14). The basis for this finding is unknown, and likewise the role of the hypoproteinemia in the pathogenesis of RDS is uncertain.

Since marked changes in *acid-base status* may occur with RDS, frequent determination of pH and Pco_2 should be made. Since both a metabolic and respiratory acidosis occur in RDS, knowledge of the Pco_2 as well as of the blood pH is vital. For these determinations, either arterial or arterialized capillary blood may be used.

Measurements of *arterial oxygen tension* (Pao_2) are important since hypoxemia in room air is one of the major manifestations of RDS, and supplementary administration of oxygen is always necessary. Since hypoxemia may lead to neurologic impairment and hyperoxemia to retrolental fibroplasia and pulmonary damage, frequent determinations are necessary. These should be performed on arterial blood, which is usually obtained via an indwelling umbilical arterial catheter, although samples may also be obtained by direct puncture of the temporal, radial or brachial arteries. Use of arterialized capillary blood is often unreliable. However, Glasgow et al (18) have found that at a

Pao_2 below 60 mm Hg, there is good correlation between arterialized capillary and arterial blood, and under some circumstances, the former method of blood sampling may be used. The development of a noninvasive transcutaneous method of measuring Pao_2 may eliminate the need for frequent blood sampling.

Measurements of *systemic arterial blood pressure* by an indwelling umbilical arterial catheter in infants with RDS has also been recommended. This not only detects the systemic arterial hypotension that is often present in RDS but also monitors the patency of the catheter lumen.

If any question exists about the presence of infection, a diagnostic evaluation for sepsis should be performed.

Since disseminated intravascular coagulation (DIC) may occur in infants with RDS, measurements of blood coagulation factors may be useful in the prevention of full-blown manifestations of this disorder.

Other routine determinations, such as measurements of hematocrit, blood glucose, serum electrolytes, calcium and phosphate, urinalyses and frequent determinations of the infant's weight, should not be overlooked.

PREVENTION AND TREATMENT

Respiratory distress syndrome is predominantly observed among premature infants. Hence, factors reducing the frequency of prematurity will necessarily cause a decreased prevalence of RDS. Improved socio-economic conditions, nutrition, prenatal medical care and reduced numbers of pregnancies in high-risk groups all contribute to a diminished number of premature deliveries and therefore to a reduced incidence of RDS.

Even when premature labor occurs, RDS may be prevented by administration of corticosteroids to the mother. These agents promote surfactant maturation in lambs and have been evaluated in humans by Liggins and Howie (27). In a prospective, controlled study, premature labor was temporarily halted by IV administration of ethyl alcohol, and betamethasone was administered to mothers on a random basis. Among those at 32 weeks' or less gestation, the prevalence of RDS was significantly reduced.

Baden et al (13) administered corticosteroids to infants who had already developed signs of RDS and no demonstrable change in the course of the illness occurred.

Further studies are underway (in 1975) to evaluate corticosteroids in the prevention and treatment of RDS and to explore their possible effects on the growth and development of other fetal organs.

Since there is no specific treatment for RDS, therapy is basically supportive and aimed at maintaining homeostasis in the affected infant until pulmonary function begins to improve spontaneously. Therapy includes:

1. Maintenance of Pao_2 at 60–80 mm Hg
   Distending airway pressure if Pao_2 < 60 mm Hg at F_Io_2 of 60%
   Mechanical ventilation if infant is apneic or distending airway pressure is unsuccessful
2. Maintenance of thermoneutral state
3. Administration of IV fluids
4. Correction of acid-base and electrolyte disturbances
5. Meticulous nursing care in neonatal intensive care unit

Oxygenation and Thermoneutrality

Maintaining normal oxygenation of the infant is the most important aspect of the therapeutic regimen. In mild or moderate cases, this can often be accomplished by increasing the inspired oxygen concentration (F_Io_2). Artificial ventilation has played a role in improving survival rates among these infants. The introduction of constant distending airway pressure has led to both improved oxygenation and a significant increase in survival rates of infants with moderate and severe RDS (see section Assisted Ventilation).

Infants with RDS must be reared in a thermoneutral environment (preferably in servocontrolled incubators or under radiant heaters with abdominal skin temperatures maintained at 36.5° C) to minimize the resting metabolic rate. Subthermoneutral environmental temperatures may be associated with acidosis, decreased Pao_2, impairment of the methyl transferase pathway of surfactant synthesis and increased mortality rates.

Infusions and Intensive Care

The use of IV infusions to maintain hydration, electrolyte and acid-base balance, as well as a source of calories, is imperative in the treatment of RDS (see Ch. 10, Renal Function and Fluid and Electrolyte Balance).

Proper management of an infant with RDS is possible only in a competently staffed intensive care unit. A well-trained physician must be available 24 hours a day. In severe cases the infant may require the undivided attention of a nurse on a round the clock basis. Only with meticulous attention to detail can both total and intact survival of infants with RDS be improved.

PATHOLOGIC FACTORS

On inspection, the lungs of infants who have succumbed to RDS appear heavy and airless and sink in water. Microscopically (Fig. 6–4) the air spaces lined with a hyaline-like eosinophilic membrane are most prominent in the dilated alveolar ducts and terminal bronchioles, and the most peripheral air spaces are collapsed. In infants who have lived for less than six hours, hyaline membranes are usually not present. They are likewise absent among survivors who succumb after five or more days to another disease. By this time, the membranes have usually been resorbed.

Alpha-1-antitrypsin, an antiproteolytic enzyme has been shown by fluorescent methods to be sequestered by the hyaline membrane (28). This may have a pathophysiologic role in the slow resorption of the membrane.

Lymphangiectasis is an important morphologic finding in RDS and is associated with increased pulmonary water content and capillary distension. Pulmonary arteriolar constriction may be evident, with thickening of the muscularis a prominent finding.

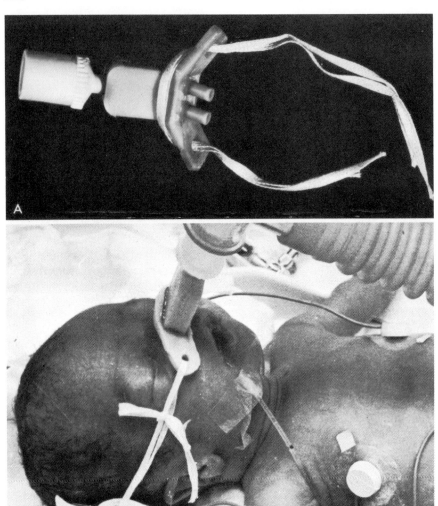

FIG. 6–4. Nasal continuous positive airway pressure (CPAP). **A.** Silastic device for administration of nasal CPAP; **B.** Nasal CPAP unit in place on infant. (Klaus MH, Fanaroff AA: Care of the High-Risk Neonate. Philadelphia, Saunders, 1973)

Other postmortem pulmonary findings in RDS are pneumothorax, pneumopericardium and hemorrhage.

Intraventricular hemorrhage is frequently a concomitant finding (see section Intracranial Bleeding, Ch. 9).

FOLLOW-UP OF INFANTS WITH RDS

High concentrations of oxygen and mechanical ventilation will in certain instances lead to bronchopulmonary dysplasia with some long-term impairment of pulmonary function. Prior to the concept of neonatal intensive care, a majority of the survivors of RDS manifested long-term neurologic impairment. A mounting body of evidence now indicates that with meticulous attention to detail in the treatment of RDS, survival is usually accompanied by an intact CNS (33).

PROLONGED RESPIRATORY DISTRESS

WILSON-MIKITY SYNDROME

The syndrome described by Wilson and Mikity in 1960 is a disorder limited to infants of very low birth weight and gestational age (39, 42). Most of the affected infants do not have the typical clinical signs of RDS and usually receive little or no supplementary oxygen therapy.

The signs of chest retractions, mild cyanosis, tachypnea and occasional apneic episodes usually do not occur until late in the first week of life, although they have been described as early as the first day.

Although usually mild at first, signs become progressively more severe, lasting for several weeks and requiring increasing amounts of supplementary oxygen in order to maintain normal tissue oxygenation. The mortality rate during this period varies from 25% to 50%. Signs gradually subside among survivors, and resolution is usually complete by the end of the first year. Ausculation of the lungs usually reveals rales, wheezing or harsh breath sounds.

During the early stages of the illness, x-ray examination of the chest usually reveals bilateral coarse streaky infiltrates and widely distributed small cystic areas. These areas tend to enlarge and, at the bases, coalesce, resulting in hyperexpanded lower lobes and flattening of the diaphragms.

Except for measurements of blood gases, laboratory testing is usually of no particular aid in clinical management. A decreased Pao_2 and elevated Pco_2 are frequently encountered in this disorder (40).

The lungs at necropsy have a "hobnailed" appearance, with areas of uneven aeration. Some portions appear overaerated; fibrosis and inflammatory cells have been noted (Fig. 6–5).

Except for oxygen in treating the cyanosis, therapy is symptomatic and supportive.

BRONCHOPULMONARY DYSPLASIA

It has been known for many years that oxygen is toxic to the human lung. In 1967 Northway et al (41) found that very high concentrations of oxygen administered by respirator to infants with RDS for a prolonged period of time could result in a form of bronchopulmonary disease that had not been previously described.

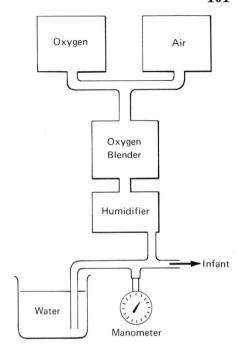

FIG. 6–5. Continuous positive airway pressure. The level of water is adjusted to obtain the desired positive pressure.

Acute, subacute and chronic changes, involving alveoli, mucous membranes and blood vessels were recognized, with those infants receiving therapy for over 150 hours usually developing the chronic form of the illness.

In its early stages, pulmonary oxygen toxicity cannot be clinically differentiated from severe RDS, both having a typical "ground glass" appearance on x ray. In infants who die during this phase, an acute exudative reaction may accompany the typical pathologic findings of RDS (38).

By the end of the first week of life, infants with pulmonary oxygen toxicity require supplementary oxygen to remain acyanotic. Radiologically, the lungs remain opacified. Infants dying during this phase show hyaline membranes still present. Bronchiolar necrosis and squamous metaplasia have also been noted.

The radiologic picture gradually changes, so that areas of lucency alternate with areas of irregular density (honeycomb lesions). Proliferative lesions, mucosal metaplasia and areas of emphysema and atelectasis are seen in infants who die during the second and third week of life. In infants who survive for a longer time, interstitial fibrosis, emphysema and cystic bronchiectasis may occur. Deaths during the late neonatal period are often accompanied by a patent ductus arteriosus, cor pulmonale and congestive heart failure.

Since new pulmonary tissue is being regenerated during the course of this disease, it is often reversible, and many infants recover with little or no loss of lung function. Every effort must therefore be made to provide optimal medical and nursing care for these infants during the weeks or months they must remain in the nursery.

PRIMARY APNEA OF PREMATURITY

Episodes of apnea are frequently observed in premature infants who are free of RDS, intracranial bleeding, systemic infection and other serious disorders. While the exact etiology of primary apnea is unknown, cessation of breathing for time intervals as short as 15 seconds may lead to bradycardia, hypoxemia and subsequent neurologic impairment.

Studies performed in the early 1970s (42a, 42b) have demonstrated that oral administration of theophylline, 1.5 to 4.0 mg/kg every 6 hours leads to a significant decrease in the number of apneic episodes. The mechanism of action of this drug on the respiratory center is not known.

PULMONARY HEMORRHAGE

Pulmonary hemorrhage, which is most commonly observed among low-birth-weight infants, almost always occurs in already distressed neonates. It has been observed in 9% to 28% of autopsies performed on newborn infants and is often encountered in postmortem examinations of stillborn fetuses (44–46).

Hemoptysis, the presenting sign of pulmonary hemorrhage, is usually observed early in the first week of life in infants with such underlying disorders as sepsis, pneumonia, RDS, perinatal asphyxia, bronchopulmonary dysplasia, aspiration of gastric fluid, hemolytic disease, coagulation defects, cold injury and severe congenital anomalies.

The acute bleeding episode is almost always preceded by respiratory collapse and bradycardia. In most cases, the fluid appearing in the trachea, throat and mouth is a sanguinous transudate rather than frank blood. Cole et al (43) have demonstrated that this fluid is a plasma filtrate containing a small proportion of whole blood.

Studies carried out during the early 1970s have suggested that left ventricular failure secondary to asphyxia and acidosis is the major mechanism responsible for pulmonary hemorrhage (43). Rapid blood transfusion and congenital heart disease may also predispose to left ventricular failure. With an increase in left atrial and pulmonary capillary pressure (secondary to the left ventricular failure), transudation of edema fluid into the interstitial tissues of the lung may cause destruction of lung tissue, with subsequent bleeding.

Decreased colloid osmotic pressure in pulmonary capillaries, secondary to hypoproteinemia, may play a role in the net filtration of fluid into pulmonary interstitial tissues.

Mechanical ventilation and oxygen therapy may also contribute to tissue breakdown and pulmonary bleeding, but these are probably not the initiating factors in pulmonary hemorrhage.

Coagulation disorders, such as disseminated intravascular coagulation, probably also play a secondary rather than primary role in the pathogenesis of pulmonary hemorrhage.

There is no specific treatment for pulmonary hemorrhage. When resuscitative measures (particularly, assisted ventilation through an endotracheal tube) are carried out, there is often a temporary improvement in cardiac and respiratory function, but therapy is usually ineffective and the overall mortality extremely high.

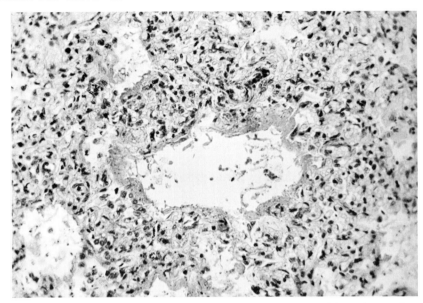

FIG. 6–6. Microscopic section of lung from infant with fetal RDS. Hyaline-like membranes can be seen lining collapsed alveoli. (Courtesy of Dr. Weiner Leblanc)

MECONIUM ASPIRATION

Fetal aspiration of meconium mixed with amniotic fluid is a relatively common occurrence associated with significant perinatal morbidity and mortality. Passage of meconium by the fetus in utero is usually secondary to asphyxia in vertex presentations (Fig. 6–6), but it may occur normally in breech presentations (47). Although it is often associated with prenatal aspiration into the lungs, many of the infants are born —and remain—asymptomatic.

Placental insufficiency, prolapse of the umbilical cord, abruptio placentae, placenta previa and maternal hypotension may lead to inadequate fetal oxygenation, causing not only cerebral hypoxia but relaxation of the anal sphincter and passage of meconium as well. The hypoxic fetus may begin to gasp and cause meconium to be aspirated into the tracheobronchial tree.

The earliest sign of this disorder may be passage of meconium-containing amniotic fluid following rupture of the fetal membranes. It may also be detected by amnioscopy, which may be performed if there is evidence of fetal distress.

When passage of meconium has been detected either as a single finding or in conjunction with other signs of distress, fetal monitoring should be instituted and the infant delivered in the most expeditious manner.

At birth the infant may appear depressed, a one-minute Apgar score of less than 4 is common, and respirations may either be absent or markedly labored. Meconium staining of the skin, umbilical cord and nails may be present, together with desquamation of skin and loss of subcutaneous tissue.

Immediately after delivery, direct visualization of the vocal cords by laryngoscopy and removal of meconium present in the trachea by aspiration are indicated. This must be done before attempts at performing positive pressure ventilation in depressed infants (see section Perinatal Asphyxia and Resuscitation, Ch. 3). If ventilation is attempted first, the meconium may be forced distally into the tracheobronchial tree. The stomach should also be aspirated to remove any meconium that has been swallowed.

CLINICAL MANIFESTATIONS

After spontaneous respirations have been established, transfer of the infant to the neonatal intensive care unit is mandatory. The severity of illness varies from a very mild aspiration pneumonia and transient depression to severe pulmonary disease with massive aspiration and a CNS so badly damaged that establishing spontaneous respirations is impossible.

Both posteroanterior and lateral x rays of the chest must be taken immediately. Diffuse areas of infiltration, often interspersed with areas of hyperaeration, may be present. The diaphragms may appear depressed and the posteroanterior diameter of the chest enlarged because of entrapment of air (48).

Pneumomediastinum

Pneumomediastinum, either alone or in combination with pneumothorax may be present. Bronchioles obstructed with plugs of meconium may allow air to enter but not leave alveoli (ball-valve effect), causing alveolar overdistension and rupture, with passage of air along vascular sheathes into the mediastinum. Although pneumomediastinum is usually asymptomatic and does not require operative intervention, pneumothorax may be symptomatic and may require removal of the air from the pleural space.

SUPPORTIVE MANAGEMENT

Warmth, adequate oxygenation, maintenance of normal acid-base balance and adequate administration of fluid and calories must be provided. Although meconium pneumonitis is basically chemical in nature, meconium is an excellent culture medium, and systemic treatment with antibiotics is usually indicated. Corticosteroids have not been shown to be advantageous in treating this disorder.

Clinical and radiologic signs usually disappear within a few days, but they may persist for weeks, with extremely slow radiologic resolution; in the latter case physical therapy (percussion and postural drainage), along with bronchodilators, may be indicated.

Central nervous system damage associated with this syndrome may lead to long-term psychomotor disability. Survivors must be carefully monitored following discharge from the nursery because of the high incidence of neurologic sequelae.

Postmortem examination of infants who succumb to this disorder reveals firm and congested lungs with areas of emphysema and atelectasis. The tracheobronchial tree contains meconium and other debris, and areas of hemorrhage may be present. The brain may be edematous, with venous congestion and areas of petechial (and less commonly) gross hemorrhage.

ASSISTED VENTILATION

The use of artificial ventilation in the treatment of respiratory failure dates back to biblical times. It was not until the poliomyelitis epidemics of the 20th century, however, that mechanical ventilators were successful. Mechanical ventilation of newborn infants with respiratory failure, which was introduced on a wide scale during the mid-1960s, enhanced the possibilities of successful treatment. The discovery by Gregory et al (55) that continuous distending airway pressure significantly improved oxygenation of noncompliant lungs (as occurs in RDS) has led to even further refinements in the treatment of RDS in the 1970s.

Respiratory failure is reflected biochemically by worsening hypoxemia (even when supplementary oxygen is administered), carbon dioxide retention and acidosis. Clinical signs include cyanosis, irregular respirations, apneic episodes, cardiovascular collapse and respiratory arrest.

The two most common causes of respiratory failure in the neonate are RDS and intrauterine asphyxia, but other causes include CNS bleeding, systemic infection, hypoglycemia, hypomagnesemia, depressant drugs, surgical conditions (diaphragmatic hernia or tension pneumothorax), neonatal tetany and chronic lung disease (Wilson-Mikity syndrome or bronchopulmonary dysplasia).

The type of assisted ventilation used depends on several factors: the nature of the disorder, clinical and biochemical manifestations and the facility of the medical staff in the use of various types of equipment.

CONTINUOUS DISTENDING AIRWAY PRESSURE

The use of constant distending airway pressure in the neonate is primarily limited to the treatment of RDS, where alveolar collapse occurs at the end of each respiratory cycle. This increase in pressure may be used in conjunction with a mechanical respirator or administered to an infant who is breathing spontaneously.

In an uncontrolled study, Gregory et al (55) administered continuous positive airway pressure to 20 infants with RDS who were breathing spontaneously. Indications for therapy were the inability to maintain a Pao_2 of at least 50 mm Hg at an F_{IO_2} of 100% or repeated episodes of apnea, bradycardia and cyanosis at an F_{IO_2} of 70% to 100%. An endotracheal tube was used in 18 infants and a pressurized head chamber in 2. The Pao_2 rose in all infants, and there were 16 survivors.

Other studies were performed over the ensuing years utilizing face masks, head chambers, nasal prongs and constant negative external pressure applied below the neck (49, 50, 54, 56, 57, 59). They all demonstrated that distending airway pressure improves oxygenation and in many cases eliminates the need for mechanical ventilation with a respirator.

CLINICAL CONSIDERATIONS

We have successfully used the method of Kattwinkel et al (57) in treating infants with RDS whose Pao_2 is less than 60 mm Hg at an F_{IO_2} of 60%. A Silastic nasal piece with prongs that extend about 1 cm proximal to the nares is sealed with hydrocortisone cream to prevent gas leakage and mucosal ulcerations.

The nasal piece is secured to the infant's face (Fig. 6–7) so that it will not be dis-

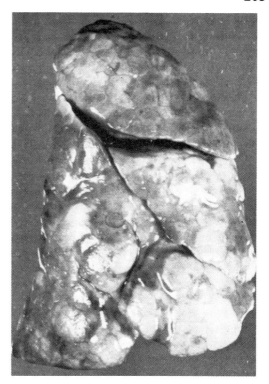

FIG. 6–7. Inflated right lung of an infant (birth weight 750 g) who died at age 145 days of Wilson-Mikity syndrome. Many discrete hyperexpanded areas may be observed. (Swyer PR, Delivoria-Papadopoulos M, Levison H, Reilly BJ, Balis JU: Pediatrics 36:374, 1965)

lodged by spontaneous movements and is connected to the apparatus (Fig. 6–8). The initial positive pressure of 6 cm H_2O may be raised as high as 12 cm H_2O (if necessary) before blowoff of air through the mouth occurs. The initial F_{IO_2} should be comparable to the level prior to initiating therapy. Usually there is a significant improvement in oxygenation. However, hyperoxia (with the attendant risk of retrolental fibroplasia) may occur. Since in a few cases, an adequate Pao_2 (60 to 90 mm Hg) may not be attained, blood gas measurements should be made about 15 minutes after therapy is initiated.

If the Pao_2 rises above 90 mm Hg, the F_{IO_2} should be gradually lowered until an F_{IO_2} of 40% is reached; at this time, positive pressure is reduced 2 cm H_2O at a time until the infant is able to maintain a normal

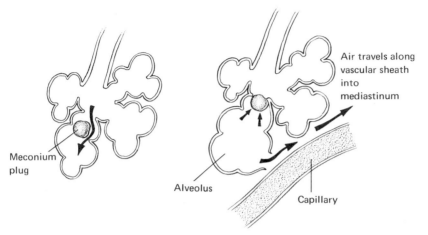

Air travels along vascular sheath into mediastinum

Meconium plug

Alveolus

Capillary

FIG. 6–8. Pathogenesis of pneumomediastinum in meconium aspiration syndrome. Plugs of meconium act as ball-valves, allowing air to enter but not leave alveoli. Overexpanded alveoli rupture, and free air travels along vascular sheaths into the mediastinum.

Pa_{O_2} without continuous positive airway pressure. If the Pa_{O_2} remains below 60 mm Hg, positive pressure rather than the $F_{I_{O_2}}$ is increased. Increasing positive airway pressure instead of $F_{I_{O_2}}$ to maintain a normal Pa_{O_2} lessens the danger of pulmonary oxygen toxicity.

Insertion of an orogastric tube provides a means of preventing gastric distension and providing calories by the enteric route, if the infant's clinical condition permits.

Although respiratory acidosis (carbon dioxide retention) is usually alleviated when ventilation is improved, hypercapnea may nonetheless persist. In this case, the Pa_{CO_2} may be lowered by intermittent use of bag and mask.

If respiratory failure persists in infants with RDS treated with distending airway pressure, the use of a mechanical respirator is indicated.

MECHANICAL VENTILATORS

Therapy with mechanical respirators is indicated for all infants with respiratory failure secondary to conditions other than RDS. In the latter disorder, it is indicated only if the infant is not breathing spontaneously or if initial treatment with constant distending airway pressure has failed. When mechanical ventilation is used in infants with RDS, distending airway pressure is usually maintained at the end of expiration in order to prevent alveolar collapse. In infants with severe antenatal asphyxia in whom spontaneous respirations were never established, use of mechanical ventilators is usually not associated with long-term survival because of associated severe CNS damage. Similarly, premature infants whose respiratory failure is secondary to intraventricular or pulmonary hemorrhage usually do not survive despite mechanical ventilation.

On the other hand, mechanical ventilators in forms of respiratory failure due to paralysis of respiratory musculature (such as tetanus neonatorum or hypermagnesemia) are usually associated with a favorable outcome.

Respirators

Both positive and negative pressure respirators have been used successfully in mechanical ventilation of newborn infants (52). Since there is no apparent advantage in the use of any one particular type of respirator, it is desirable that medical and nursing staff use the type with which they have gained expertise. However, mechanical problems make the use of negative pressure respirators in infants weighing less than 1500 g extremely difficult, and their use is not advised in this group.

Respirators designed for the newborn infant must be able to deliver small tidal volumes at rapid rates. The pressure must vary over a wide range since increased pressures, as high as 35 to 40 cm H_2O, may be necessary to expand the atelectatic lungs of infants with RDS. Inspiratory flowrates should be adjustable, as well as the inspiration to expiration ratio. A method of warming and humidifying the gas mixture must be available.

Most of the respirators in common use are intermittent positive pressure devices. Both the Bennett PR-2* and BABYbird† are relatively inexpensive and have been widely used in the treatment of respiratory failure in the neonate. Both are pressure cycled; this refers to the fact that a preset inspiratory pressure rather than the desired tidal volume is selected. Inspiration ceases when this pressure is reached. The inspiratory to expiratory time ratio can be adjusted on both of these instruments. Both of these respirators are designed to deliver either 40% or 100% oxygen, but they can be modified to deliver intermediate concentrations.

The Bourns Pediatric Respirator Model LS104-150‡ ventilator is specifically designed for the newborn infant and is volume cycled. The desired tidal volume, concentration of oxygen and respiratory rate can be preset, and it is sensitive in the "assist" as well as the "control" mode. The major problem that has limited its widespread use is its high cost.

The Air-Shields Negative Pressure Respirator§ is a double-chambered, time-cycled incubator. Its advantage is that infants can be ventilated without endotracheal intubation; however, small infants weighing under 1500 g cannot be adequately ventilated with this respirator (58).

MEDICAL AND NURSING ASPECTS

Since the success of mechanical ventilation depends more on meticulous technique than on the type of ventilator used, the nursery staff must be well trained in methods of in-

* Puritan-Bennett, 15 Worth St, South Hackensack, NJ
† Bird Corp., Mark 7, Palm Springs, CA
‡ Bourns, Inc, Life Systems, 6135 Magnolia Ave, Riverside, CA
§ Air-Shields, Inc, Hatboro, PA

tubation and principles of intensive medical care applicable to infants who are being ventilated. A nurse must be assigned full time to each infant being treated with a respirator and, with the medical staff, must be able to recognize complications that frequently arise.

TRACHEAL INTUBATION

With positive pressure ventilation, either nasotracheal or orotracheal intubation is necessary. Both types of tubes have certain advantages and disadvantages. An orotracheal tube is easier to pass, but it is also dislodged more easily. It is usually necessary to change the tube every two or three days.

The diameter of the tube should be as large as possible for the particular infant. In the smallest infants, an internal diameter of 2.5 mm should be used, with progressively larger sizes for infants of higher birth weights. When using a nasotracheal tube, its length (anterior nares to carina) should be about 21% of the infants crown to heel length (51) (Fig. 6–9).

Intubation should be performed as rapidly as possible, with the infant well oxygenated prior to the procedure. If intubation is unsuccessful and hypoxia ensues, the patient should be reoxygenated by bag and mask before another attempt is made. Before the tube is fixed, both lungs should be carefully examined to ascertain that breath sounds are equal. It is relatively easy to pass a tube into a main stem bronchus, thus preventing aeration of one lung. It is vital that the tube be securely fixed so that dislodgment is not possible. Following intubation, posteroanterior and lateral x rays of the chest are necessary to ascertain that the tip of the tube is in the proper location (just above the carina).

Medical Management

Close monitoring of the infant is essential with any mode of assisted ventilation. A thermoneutral environment must be maintained, preferably with the use of a radiant heater (to provide easy accessibility to the

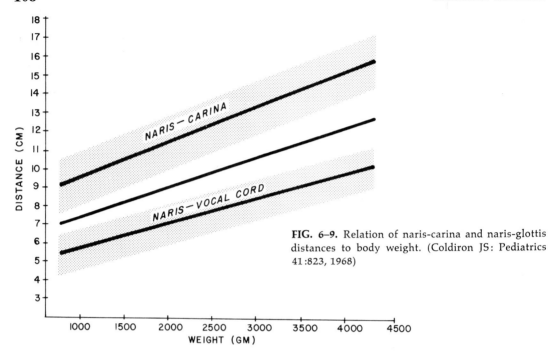

FIG. 6–9. Relation of naris-carina and naris-glottis distances to body weight. (Coldiron JS: Pediatrics 41:823, 1968)

infant). Fluid and caloric demands must be met, and normal acid-base and oxygenation status maintained. An indwelling umbilical arterial catheter must be inserted for blood sampling, measurement of blood pressure and infusion of fluids.

The gas mixture administered must be warmed and humidified and the tracheal tube suctioned hourly to prevent inspissation of secretions. Dailey and Cave-Smith (53) suggest using physiotherapy (percussion and vibration) in infants who are undergoing prolonged mechanical ventilation. They also suggest using nebulized isoproterenol if wheezes are heard on auscultation. Secretions should be cultured, and if there is any sign of superimposed infection, appropriate antibiotic therapy should be instituted. Frequent portable chest x rays should be taken since both atelectasis and pneumothorax may be complications of mechanical ventilation.

Weaning the infant from the respirator should be attempted as soon as it is feasible. Prolonged tracheal intubation may be associated with both squamous metaplasia and pulmonary fibrosis. The former is probably due to irritating qualities of the tube,

whereas the latter is probably secondary to oxygen toxicity. Following removal of the tube, the infant must still be monitored very carefully, with frequent suctioning, and adequate oxygenation must be maintained. Intravenous fluids should be continued in the period immediately following extubation in order to prevent aspiration of formula.

When all details of good medical care have been adhered to, the long-term intact survival of infants who have received assisted ventilation is good (58).

REFERENCES

1. Avery ME, Fletcher BD: The Lung and Its Disorders in the Newborn Infant. Philadelphia, Saunders, 1974
2. Symposium on Respiratory Disorders in the Newborn. Pediatric Clinics of North America. Philadelphia, Saunders, May 1973

DEVELOPMENT AND ADAPTATION

3. Ballard PL, Ballard RA: Cytoplasmic receptor for glucocorticoids in lungs of the human fetus and neonate. J Clin Invest 53:477, 1974
4. Boddy F, Robinson JS: External method for detection of fetal breathing in utero. Lancet 2:1231, 1971

5. Dawes GS: Breathing before birth in animals and man. N Engl J Med 290:557, 1974

6. Doell RG, Kretchmer N: Intestinal invertase: Precocious development of activity after injection of hydrocortisone. Science 143:42, 1963

7. Jacquot R: Some hormonally controlled events of liver differentiation in the perinatal period. In: Hormones in Development, 1st ed. Edited by M Hamburgh, EJW Barrington. New York, Appleton-Century-Crofts, 1971

8. Klaus M, Rein OK, Tooley WH, Piel C, Clements JA: Alveolar epithelial cell mitochondria as a source of the surface active lung lining. Science 137:750, 1962

9. Marquis L, Ackerman BD: Placental respiration in the immediate neonatal period. Am J Obstet Gynecol 117:358, 1973

10. Motoyama EK, Orzalesi MM, Kikkawa Y, Kaibara M, Wu B, Zigas CJ, Cook CD: Effect of cortisol on the maturation of fetal rabbit lungs. Pediatrics 48:547, 1971

11. Redding RA, Douglas WHJ, Stein M: Thyroid hormone influence upon lung surfactant metabolism. Science 175:994, 1972

RESPIRATORY DISTRESS SYNDROME

12. Avery ME, Mead J: Surface properties in relation to atelectasis and hyaline membrane disease. Am J Dis Child 97:517, 1959

13. Baden M, Bauer CR, Colle E, Klein G, Taeusch HW, Stern L: A controlled trial of hydrocortisone therapy in infants with respiratory distress syndrome. Pediatrics 50:526, 1972

14. Bland RD: Cord-blood total protein level as a screening aid for the idiopathic respiratory distress syndrome. N Engl J Med 287:9, 1972

15. Chu J, Clements JA, Cotton E, Klaus MH, Sweet AY, Thomas MA, Tooley WH: Preliminary report: the pulmonary hypoperfusion syndrome. Pediatrics 35:733, 1965

16. Clements JA, Platzker AC, Tierney DF, Hobel CJ, Creasy RK, Margolis AJ, Thibeault DW, Oh W: Assessment of the risk of the respiratory distress syndrome by a rapid new test for surfactant in amniotic fluid. N Engl J Med 286:1077, 1972

17. Evans HE, Keller S, Mandl I: Serum trypsin inhibitory capacity and idiopathic respiratory distress syndrome. J Pediatr 81:588, 1972

17a. Fencl MdeM, Tulchinsky D: Total cortisol in amniotic fluid and fetal lung maturation. N Engl J Med 292:133, 1975

18. Glasgow JF, Flynn DM, Swyer PR: A comparison of descending aortic and "arterialized" capillary blood in sick newborn. Can Med Assoc J 106:660, 1972

19. Glass L, Rajegowda Bk, Evans HE: Absence of respiratory distress syndrome in premature infants of heroin addicted mothers. Lancet 2:685, 1971

20. Gluck L: Pulmonary surfactant and neonatal respiratory distress. Hosp Prac 5:45, 1971

21. Gluck L, Kulovich MV, Borer RC, Brenner PH, Anderson CG, Spellacy WN: Diagnosis of the respiratory distress syndrome by amniocentesis. Am J Obstet Gynecol 109:440, 1971

22. Gluck L, Kulovich MV, Eidelman AI, Cordero L, Khazin AF: Biochemical development of surface activity in mammalian lung. IV. Pulmonary lecithin synthesis in the human fetus and newborn and etiology of the respiratory distress syndrome. Pediatr Res 6:81, 1972

23. Gluck L, Motoyama EK, Smits HL, Kulovich MV: The biochemical development of surface activity in mammalian lung. I. The surface-active phospholipids; the separation and distribution of surface-active lecithin in the lung of the developing rabbit fetus. Pediatr Res 1:237, 1967

24. Graven SM, Opitz JM, Harrison M: Respiratory distress syndrome–risk related to maternal factors. Am J Obstet Gynecol 96:969, 1966

25. Harrison VC, Heese H DeV, Klein M: The significance of grunting in hyaline membrane disease. Pediatrics 41:549, 1968

25a. Jones MD, Burd LI, Bowes WA, Battaglia FC, Lubchenco LO: Failure of association of premature rupture of membranes with respiratory distress syndrome. N Engl J Med 292:1253, 1975

26. Lieberman J: Clinical syndrome associated with deficient lung fibrinolytic activity. I. A new concept of hyaline-membrane disease. N Engl J Med 260:619, 1959

27. Liggins GC, Howie RN: A controlled trial of antepartum glucocorticoid treatment for prevention of the respiratory distress syndrome in premature infants. Pediatrics 50:515, 1972

28. Mathis RK, Freier EF, Hunt CE, Krivit W, Sharp HL: Alpha 1-antitrypsin in the respiratory-distress syndrome. N Engl J Med 288:59, 1973

29. Miller HC, Futrakul P: Birth weight, gestational age, and sex as determining factors in incidence of respiratory distress syndrome of prematurely born infants. J Pediatr 72:628, 1968

30. Moss AJ, Duffie ER, Fagan LM: Respiratory distress syndrome in the newborn: study on the association of cord clamping and the pathogenesis of distress. JAMA 184:48, 1963

31. Naeye R, Harcke H, Blanc W: Adrenal gland structure and the development of hyaline membrane disease. Pediatrics 47:650, 1971

32. Nelson NM: On the etiology of hyaline membrane disease. Pediatr Clin North Am 17:943, 1970

33. Stahlman M, Hedvall G, Dolandki E, Faxelius G, Burko H, Kirk V: A six-year follow-up of clinical hyaline membrane disease. Pediatr Clin North Am 20:433, 1973

34. Sundell H, Garrott J, Blankenship WJ, Shepard FM, Stahlman MT: Studies on infants with type II respiratory distress syndrome. J Pediatr 78:754, 1971

35. Usher R, McLean F, Maughan GB: Respiratory distress syndrome in infants delivered by cesarean section. Am J Obstet Gynecol 88:806, 1964

36. Wu PYK, Borer RC Jr, Modanlou H: Diagnosis of the respiratory distress syndrome (RDS) by the absence of phosphatidyl dimethylethanolamine (PDME)—tracheal effluents of low birth weight (LBW) infants. Pediatr Res 5:415, 1971

37. Yoon JJ, Harper RG: Observations on the relationship between duration of rupture of the membranes and the development of idiopathic respiratory distress syndrome. Pediatrics 52:161, 1973

PROLONGED RESPIRATORY DISTRESS

38. Anderson WR, Strickland M: Pulmonary complications of oxygen therapy in the neonate. Arch Pathol 91:506, 1971

39. Hodgman JE, Mikity VG, Tatter D, Cleland RS: Chronic respiratory distress in premature infants—Wilson-Mikity syndrome. Pediatrics 44:179, 1969

40. Krauss AN, Levin AR, Grossman H, Auld PAM: Physiologic studies on infants with Wilson-Mikity syndrome. J. Pediatr 77:27, 1970

41. Northway WH Jr, Rosan RC, Porter DY: Pulmonary disease following respirator therapy of hyaline membrane disease: bronchopulmonary dysplasia. N Engl J Med 276:357, 1967

42. Wilson MG, Mikity VG: A new form of respiratory disease in premature infants. Am J Dis Child 99:489, 1960

PRIMARY APNEA OF PREMATURITY

42a. Shannon DC, Gotay F, Stein IM, Rogers MC, Todres ID, Moylan FMB: Prevention of apnea and bradycardia in low birthweight infants. Pediatrics 55:589, 1975

42b. Uauy R, Shapiro D, Smith B, Warshaw J: Effect of theophylline on severe primary apnea of prematurity: A preliminary report. Pediatrics 55:595, 1975

PULMONARY HEMORRHAGE

43. Cole VA, Normand ICS, Reynolds EOR, Rivers RPA: Pathogenesis of hemorrhagic pulmonary edema and massive pulmonary hemorrhage in the newborn. Pediatrics 51:175, 1973

44. Fedrick J, Butler NR: Certain causes of neonatal death. IV. Massive pulmonary haemorrhage. Biol Neonate 18:243, 1971

45. McAdams AJ: Pulmonary haemorrhage in the newborn. Am J Dis Child 113:255, 1967

46. Parker JC, Brown AL, Harris LE: Pulmonary hemorrhages in the newborn. Mayo Clin Proc 43:465, 1968

MECONIUM ASPIRATION

47. Auld PAM, Rudolph AJ, Avery ME, Cherry RB, Drorbaugh JE, Kay JL, Smith CA: Responsiveness and resuscitation of the newborn: the use of the Apgar score. Am J Dis Child 101:713, 1961

48. Gooding CA, Gregory GA: Roentgenographic analysis of meconium aspiration of the newborn. Radiology 100:131, 1971

ASSISTED VENTILATION

49. Barrie H: Simple method of applying continuous positive airway pressure in respiratory distress syndrome. Lancet 1:776, 1972

50. Chernick V, Vidyasagar D: Continuous negative chest wall pressure in hyaline membrane disease: one year experience. Pediatrics 49:753, 1972

51. Coldiron J: Estimation of naso-tracheal tube length in neonates. Pediatrics 41:823, 1968

52. Daily WJ, Cave-Smith P: Mechanical ventilation of the newborn infant. Part I. Curr Probl Pediatr 1 (No. 8):3, 1971

53. Daily WJ, Cave-Smith P: Mechanical ventilation of the newborn infant. Part II. Curr Probl Pediatr 1 (No. 9):3, 1971

54. Fanaroff AA, Cha CC, Sosa R, Crumrine RS, Klaus MH: A controlled trial of continuous negative external pressure in the treatment of severe respiratory distress syndrome. J Pediatr 82:921, 1973

55. Gregory GA, Kitterman JA, Phibbs RH, Tooley WH, Hamilton WK: Treatment of the idiopathic respiratory distress syndrome with continuous positive airway pressure. N Engl J Med 284:1333, 1971

56. Harris TR: Continuous positive airway pressure applied by face mask (abst). Pediatr Res 6:410, 1972

57. Kattwinkel J, Fleming D, Cha CC, Fanaroff AA, Klaus MH: A device for administration of continuous positive airway pressure by the nasal route. Pediatrics 52:131 1973

58. Stahlman MT, Malan AF, Blankenship W, Young WC, Gray J: Negative pressure assisted ventilation in infants with hyaline membrane disease. J Pediatr 76:174, 1970

59. Woody NC, Person SM: An economical device for continuous positive airway pressure. Lancet 1:1301, 1973

7

Cardiovascular Disorders

CARL N. STEEG
WELTON M. GERSONY

INTRODUCTION

Approximately 20,000 infants (about 0.8% of live births) with congenital cardiac anomalies are born each year in the United States (11). It is estimated that 2:1000 neonates have heart disease significant enough to necessitate cardiac catheterization in the first year of life.

In a large series of patients with congenital heart defects reported by the Childrens Hospital Medical Center in Boston (12), ventricular septal defect was the most common lesion (20%), followed by patent ductus arteriosus (15%), coarctation of the aorta (8%), pulmonary stenosis (7.5%) and tetralogy of Fallot (6%). A review from The Hospital for Sick Children in Toronto reported similar incidence of these lesions, although atrial septal defect occurred somewhat more frequently (10).

In the neonatal period more complex lesions are more often encountered. The Childrens Medical Center study of patients in the first year of life who required cardiac catheterization indicates that ventricular septal defect (16.8%), transposition of the great arteries (11.8%) and the hypoplastic left heart syndrome (7.5%) are the most common defects studied.

CARDIOVASCULAR DEVELOPMENT AND FUNCTION

EMBRYOLOGY

The embryonic heart begins as a straight tube composed of four distinct chambers. Cephalad to caudad, these are: 1) the truncus arteriosus (forerunner of the aortic root and main pulmonary artery), 2) the bulbus cordis (forerunner of the right ventricle), 3) the primitive ventricle (forerunner of the left ventricle) and 4) the sinus venosus (forerunner of the atria). At about the third week of embryonic life, the primitive cardiac tube undergoes "looping" whereby it begins to bulge towards the right, bringing the bulbus cordis to the right of the ventricle and thereby establishing a normal relationship between what will become the two ventricles (2). This normal looping process has been called "D" looping (Fig. 7–1) to differentiate it from the abnormal "L" looping in which the ventricles become inverted. Should L looping take place, the bulbus cordis would orient itself to the left of the ventricle and thereby cause the anatomic and embryonic right ventricle to sit to the left of the anatomic and embryonic left ventricle (ventricular inversion).

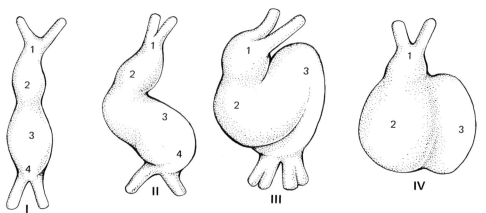

1—Truncus arteriosus
2—Bulbus cordis (embryologic right ventricle)
3—Ventricle (embryologic left ventricle)
4—Sinus venosus

FIG. 7–1. D looping of the ventricles. I, Primitive cardiac tube; II, D-looping begins with the primitive tube developing a convexity along its right border; III, With further looping, the bulbus cordis assumes the position of the right ventricle, to the right of the primitive ventricle; IV, The bulbus cordis and ventricle are now related to each other as right and left ventricle respectively. The sinus venosus has been eliminated in states III and IV to allow for clarity. (Modified from Langman J, Van Mierop LHS in Moss and Adams: Heart Disease in Infants, Children and Adolescents. Baltimore: Williams and Wilkins, 1968)

Atria and Pulmonary Veins

The sinus venosus becomes incorporated into what is to become the atria, primarily the right atrium. A good portion of the left atrium takes its origin from the incorporation of the primitive common pulmonary vein into which the four pulmonary veins drain during embryonic life. Failure to properly incorporate this structure results in a lesion known as cor triatriatum, or triatrial heart.

The primitive pulmonary veins are diffusely anastomotic with the cardinal system, as well as with the developing splanchnic venous system. Abnormalities in the development of the common pulmonary vein, such as hypoplasia or atresia, result in the further development of the cardinal or splanchnic connections and in abnormal pulmonary venous connections to the systemic venous circulation and right atrium.

The primitive atrium divides into left and right portions by the initial development of a septum primum. The septum primum grows towards the area of the atrioventricular groove and developing endocardial cushions. It fails to reach the groove and leaves a defect—the ostium primum. Simultaneously, multiple perforations that have developed in the upper portion of the septum primum coalesce to form a second interatrial communication, or ostium secundum.

The ostium primum is later closed by the development of the endocardial cushions, a portion of which grows to meet the lower end of the septum primum. If the cushion fails to close the ostium primum, a defect persists after birth. A septum secundum grows down from the medial portion of the right atrium and alongside the septum primum. This partially developed septum grows far enough to cover the ostium secundum, leaving a flaplike communication between the now-separated atria (foramen ovale). Maldevelopment of the second septum results in a secundum atrial septal defect.

Ventricles, Mitral and Tricuspid Valves

The ventricular canal forms its septum from a number of sources. The muscular portion of the septum originates from the expansion and growth of the medial walls of the two ventricles (bulbus cordis and ventricle). The upper portions of the septum develop from endocardial cushion tissue, from membranous structures and from the septal and parietal bands of the crista supraventricularis. In addition, the uppermost portion of the septum (just inferior to the semilunar valves) is composed of tissue derived from the lowermost portion of the primitive truncus arteriosus—the so-called conus portion of the septum. Failure of fusion or proper development of any of these structures results in a persistent communication between the two ventricles (ventricular septal defect).

The ventricular septal structure then shifts from right to left. Failure of this shift to occur results in atresia of the tricuspid valve, whereas too great a leftward shift may cause mitral valve atresia.

The mitral valve itself is derived from endocardial cushion tissue, as is the septal portion of the tricuspid valve. The remainder of the tricuspid valve develops from an invagination of the right ventricular endocardium. Improper or incomplete invagination of the endocardium causes the tricuspid valve to be abnormally formed and inferiorly malposed, lying within ventricular epicardium. This abnormality is referred to as Ebstein's malformation of the tricuspid valve.

Great Vessels

The truncus arteriosus also septates to form the ascending aorta and main pulmonary artery. Initially, the two vessels lie one behind the other in a parallel relationship, with the aorta being the anterior vessel and related to the bulbus cordis or right ventricle. The septated portions of the truncus arteriosus then spiral about one another and rotate 180° bringing the aorta over the posterior ventricle (left ventricle) and the pulmonary artery over the anterior ventricle (right ventricle, bulbus cordis). The inferiormost portion of the primitive truncus, the conus or conal ridges, is a muscular structure that will form the portion of the heart known as the infundibulum. The portion of the conus related to the left ventricle normally resorbs so that only the portion related to the right ventricle persists. The presence of the infundibulum in the right ventricle causes the pulmonary valve to be located superior to the aortic valve and creates muscular discontinuity between the pulmonary valve and the tricuspid valve.

The aortic valve and the mitral valve, on the other hand, are in fibrous continuity and have no interposing muscular infundibulum. The semilunar valves develop from the conal ridges (lower portion of the truncus arteriosus).

Improper spiraling and rotation of the septated primitive truncus results in a transposition of the great arteries and causes the aortic valve to be discontinuous with the mitral valve as well as the tricuspid valve (4). Different degrees of abnormalities in rotation of the aorta and pulmonary artery result in the many forms of aorta-pulmonary malrelationships that have been described. Should the truncus fail to septate at all, the condition known as truncus arteriosus or persistent truncus arteriosus will result. Should there be only partial septation of the truncus, a persistent communication between the aorta and the pulmonary artery will exist, referred to as an aortopulmonary window.

The arch of the aorta is the persistent left fourth aortic arch of the embryo's series of six bilateral arches. The two pulmonary arteries arise from the two sixth arches, and the ductus arteriosus is also derived from the sixth left aortic arch.

Full formation of the heart is completed by the eighth week of embryonic life, and no alteration of its architecture can be affected by intrauterine developments after that time.

PERINATAL CIRCULATION

The normal fetal circulation is characterized by a low-resistance systemic and placental circuit and a high resistance pulmonary arteriolar bed. This marked disparity results in the shunting of approximately 90% of venous return to the systemic arterial circulation via the patent foramen ovale and ductus arteriosus.

Flow patterns within the right atrium divert approximately 50% of the highly oxygenated umbilical venous return (Po_2 = 30 mm Hg) across the foramen ovale to the left atrium. This blood thus reaches the brachiocephalic vessels and perfuses the developing fetal brain. The less saturated superior vena caval blood (Po_2 = 15 mm Hg) eventually flows almost in its entirety across the ductus arteriosus to the lower trunk.

At birth the alveoli become distended with air, and pulmonary vascular resistance decreases dramatically. The low-resistance placental circulation is eliminated, resulting in a sudden marked increase in the systemic vascular resistance. As the ductus arteriosus constricts, the circulation rapidly assumes the normal postnatal course. The pulmonary and systemic circuits separate and their relative pressures become dependent on their respective resistances.

Closure of the ductus arteriosus is directly related to an increase in oxygen tension. Several agents (e.g., bradykinin, prostaglandins, cyclic AMP) have been considered as mediators in this interaction.

Although the foramen ovale remains anatomically patent for months or even years, right-to-left flow ceases immediately after birth as left atrial pressure exceeds right atrial pressure. Both fetal channels may assume important roles in the regulation of circulation in babies with various cyanotic heart defects.

INHERITANCE

In most instances, no distinct mendelian inheritance pattern can be implicated in the transmission of congenital heart defects. Rather, the pattern of inheritance follows a multifactorial trend, resulting from the apparent interaction of both genetic and environmental agents. According to Nora (13) this form of inheritance is confirmed when a disorder is: 1) common, 2) shows familial aggregates, 3) has a recurrence rate in siblings of from 1% to 5%, 4) is susceptible to

environmental influences and 5) is found much more commonly in both identical twins than in both nonidentical twins.

Edwards (7) has calculated that traits inherited in this multifactorial fashion appear in siblings and parents of affected individuals with a frequency approximating the square root of the population frequency. For example, if the frequency of an anomaly is 1:100 (1%) in the general population, it should be found in 1:10 (10%) of siblings. The expected incidence of similar defects in siblings has been shown to follow the multifactorial pattern for several of the more common acyanotic defects (e.g., atrial septal defect, patent ductus arteriosus, ventricular septal defect). A few studies carried out on the siblings of children with tetralogy of Fallot reveal a recurrence rate of congenital heart disease of 2% to 3%. This risk rate is suggestive of multifactorial inheritance. Of the affected siblings, 60 to 70% also had tetralogy of Fallot.

In rare instances, congenital cardiac defects follow a true mendelian pattern of inheritance. Cardiomyopathies, atrial septal defects, patent ductus arteriosus, hypoplastic left heart syndrome and others have been described in some families with more than two affected members.

NONGENETIC FACTORS

Chromosomal abnormalities

Many of the syndromes associated with chromosomal abnormalities include cardiac malformations. One-half of children with Down's syndrome (trisomy 21) have documented congenital heart disease. Endocardial cushion defects are the most common abnormalities seen in these children, although other lesions have also been reported. Congenital heart disease is even more common among infants with trisomy 18 and trisomy 13–15, occurring in 80% to 100% of cases. Ventricular septal defect is the lesion most frequently encountered in these infants. Among the sex chromosomal abnormalities, Klinefelter's syndrome and Turner's syndrome have been widely studied. The Klinefelter's (XXY) abnormality is not associated with congenital cardiac defects, whereas children with Turner's syndrome (XO) have an increased incidence of congenital heart disease (20% to 45%), predominantly coarctation of the aorta. Patients with Turner's phenotype, but normal sex chromosomes (Noonan's syndrome), have been found to have dysplasia of the pulmonary arteries or pulmonary valve, or both.

Maternal infection

The only congenital cardiovascular disorders known to be associated with specific maternal viral infection are those found with the congenital rubella syndrome (8). Patent ductus arteriosus and peripheral pulmonary artery stenosis are frequently occurring lesions associated with this syndrome, often appearing together. When maternal rubella occurs within the first six weeks of gestation, the incidence of fetal deformaties approaches 90%.

Some reports have implicated the mumps virus in the etiology of primary endocardial fibroelastosis (14). Others, however, have found no relationship between mumps virus and clinical fibroelastosis (7a).

THE NEONATAL ELECTROCARDIO-GRAM AND ARRHYTHMIAS

ELECTROCARDIOGRAM

The normal neonatal electrocardiogram (ECG) is distinctly different from that of an older child or adult, the differences being related to the relative dominance of the right ventricle in the neonatal period. Since the right ventricle has maintained systemic pressure during fetal life, the right ventricular myocardium is well developed as compared to the left. This is reflected in the ECG recorded during the first days of life by the normal findings of right axis deviation, large R waves and upright T waves in the right precordial leads (V_3R and V_1). When pulmonary resistance decreases and right ventricular pressure reaches its normal

level, the right precordial T waves become negative. In the great majority of instances, this occurs within the first 48 hours of life. Concomitantly, the QRS axis gradually shifts leftward and right ventricular forces slowly regress, as the left ventricle becomes dominant, and the ECG evolves to the adult pattern.

Two important principles must be emphasized: 1) the diagnosis of pathologic right ventricular hypertrophy (Fig. 7–2) is difficult in the first week of life, serial tracings often being necessary to determine if marked right axis deviation and abnormal right precordial forces or T waves, or both, will persist, and 2) a normal adult tracing is distinctly abnormal in the neonatal period. An adult ECG pattern seen in a neonate suggests left ventricular enlargement (Fig. 7–3). The premature baby, however, may display a more "mature" ECG than his full-term counterpart (Fig. 7–4) as a result of lower pulmonary resistance secondary to underdevelopment of the medial muscular layer of the pulmonary arterioles.

In the frontal plane leads of the standard ECG, the mean QRS axis normally lies in the range of $+110°$ to $+180°$. The right-sided chest leads reveal a larger positive (R) than negative (S) wave. This may persist for months or years since the positioning of the right precordial leads tend to be influenced to a greater extent by right ventricular depolarization. Left-sided leads (V_5 and V_6) also reflect right-sided dominance in the early neonatal period with RS ratio less than one. However, since left precordial leads are in direct proximity to the left ventricle, a dominant R wave reflecting left ventricular forces quickly becomes evident within the first few days of life. Criteria for the diagnosis of specific chamber enlargement are outlined in Table 7–1.

Aside from the diagnosis of hypertrophy and rhythm disorders, the neonatal ECG may be useful for the evaluation of electrolyte imbalance. Hyperkalemia results in tall, peaked T waves, especially in the left precordial leads. Increasing serum potassium levels result in QRS widening, PR prolongation and QT shortening. When hypokalemia

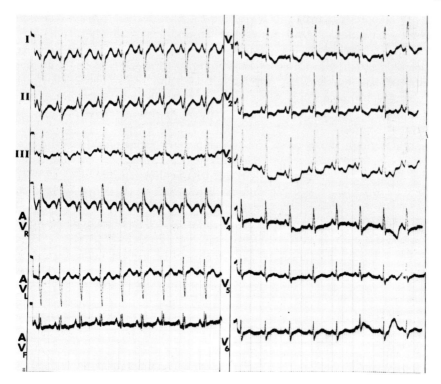

FIG. 7–2. Right ventricular hypertrophy in a newborn infant with severe valvular pulmonic stenosis. The precordial leads are recorded at one-half normal standardization. ST–T wave sagging and T wave inversion are seen in leads V_1–V_4, suggestive of right ventricular strain. Note also the peaked P waves in lead II, suggesting right atrial enlargement.

exists, T waves decrease markedly in amplitude, along with ST segment depression, and U waves may become prominent and merge with the T wave causing an apparent increase in the QT interval. Calcium is the other cation that directly affects cardiac depolarization. Under conditions of hypercalcemia, the QT interval shortens. When low calcium levels are present, a prolongation of the QT interval becomes evident.

ARRHYTHMIAS

The normal newborn infant has a sinus tachycardia with a range of 110 to 150 beats per minute. Variations with respiration (sinus arrhythmia) are frequent. The premature infant may exhibit intermittent sinus bradycardia and various forms of ectopic pacemaker activity, presumably secondary to an immature autonomic nervous system.

Specific rhythm disorders may be recognized in the neonate. On occasion, these may be life threatening and may require immediate treatment.

Supraventricular Tachycardia

Supraventricular tachycardia is generally manifested as an atrial tachycardia in excess of 200 beats per minute. In spontaneously occurring supraventricular tachycardia, e.g., not drug-induced, the arrhythmia is conducted to the ventricles in a 1:1 fashion and considered to be a "re-entrant" or "circus" tachycardia involving the atrioventricular node (15). Because sinus conduction is absent, normal P waves are not visible in the ECG. In the majority of instances, P waves cannot be discerned using standard ECG leads. Specialized techniques, e.g., using Lewis or Golub leads, may allow for P wave visualization. When P waves are visible, an

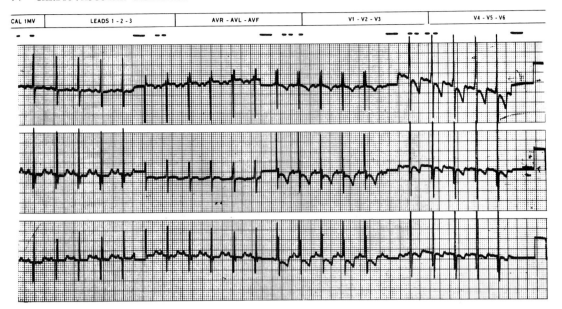

FIG. 7–3. Left ventricular hypertrophy in a newborn infant with endocardial fibroelastosis. The frontal plane axis of +60°, although normal for an adult, is leftward oriented for the neonate. Deep S waves in lead V_1 and tall R waves in lead V_6 are typical of left ventricular enlargement. T wave inversions are seen throughout the precordial leads and are secondary either to the abnormality or digitalis effect, or both.

FIG. 7–4. ECG of a normal premature infant. The tracing has a typically "mature" pattern seen in normal adults.

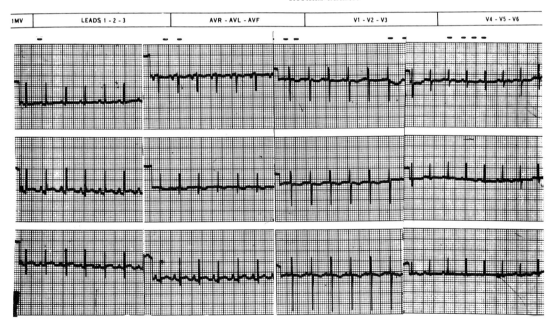

TABLE 7.1. Normal Precordial R and S Wave Amplitudes

Age	R Wave Mini-mum	5%	Mean	95%	Maxi-mum	S.D.	S Wave Mini-mum	5%	Mean	95%	Maxi-mum	S.D.
				Amplitudes in V_1								
0–24 hours	5.5	7.0	14.8	20.0	20.5	3.75	0	2.5	9.3	27.0	28.5	7.99
1– 7 days	5.5	9.0	18.2	27.4	29.5	5.44	1.5	4.6	10.4	18.8	25.5	4.70
8–30 days	2.5	4.2	11.4	19.8	26.5	4.97	0	2.5	5.0	12.8	18.5	3.73
				Amplitudes in V_2								
0–24 hours	11.5	13.0	20.1	28.1	29.5	3.81	5.0	9.0	20.3	33.8	37.0	6.73
1– 7 days	8.5	11.7	19.9	31.1	32.5	5.89	5.0	9.3	20.2	34.1	37.0	7.26
8–30 days	5.5	6.8	17.5	29.0	32.5	6.48	1.0	4.2	14.0	25.7	29.0	6.24
				Amplitudes in V_3								
0–24 hours	12.0	12.7	18.8	26.7	28.0	4.12	10.0	12.0	25.0	32.0	38.0	6.05
1– 7 days	4.0	8.8	18.1	30.0	40.0	6.55	0	2.6	17.1	33.0	38.0	8.37
8–30 days	0.0	8.3	18.8	33.8	36.0	7.50	2.0	4.2	12.4	20.0	26.0	5.47
				Amplitudes in V_4								
0–24 hours	8.0	9.0	17.4	26.0	32.0	5.97	2	4.0	21.8	36.0	42.0	9.08
1– 7 days	4.0	4.9	18.8	33.1	36.0	7.24	0	3.4	13.2	27.7	30.0	8.11
8–30 days	4.0	3.3	15.9	33.3	36.0	7.82	0	3.1	6.8	16.3	18.0	5.05
				Amplitudes in V_5								
0–24 hours	0.0	4.0	10.2	18.0	24.0	5.44	0	0.0	11.9	24.0	31.5	6.87
1– 7 days	0.0	3.4	10.7	19.3	28.0	5.54	0	3.6	6.8	16.2	19.5	4.73
8–30 days	0.0	3.5	11.9	27.0	36.0	7.28	0	2.7	4.8	12.3	13.5	3.50
				Amplitudes in V_6								
0–24 hours	0	2.3	3.3	7.0	7.5	2.10	0	1.6	4.5	10.3	14.0	2.78
1– 7 days	0	2.2	5.1	13.1	16.5	3.97	0	0.8	3.3	9.9	14.0	2.99
8–30 days	0	1.7	6,7	20.5	25.5	4.82	0	0.6	2.0	9.0	10.0	2.46
				Amplitudes in AVR								
0–24 hours	—	—	—	—	—	—	—	—	—	—	—	—
1– 7 days	0	0.5	2.8	6.4	7.5	1.80	3.0	3.7	7.9	13.9	15.0	3.11
8–30 days	0	1.0	2.0	4.0	6.5	1.39	5.0	5.6	10.1	14.6	15.0	2.81
				Amplitudes in AVL								
0–24 hours	—	—	—	—	—	—	—	—	—	—	—	—
1– 7 days	0	0.5	1.7	3.3	6.5	1.04	0	1.4	5.2	9.7	13.0	2.48
8–30 days	0	1.2	2.2	5.8	7.5	1.48	0	2.2	5.3	8.9	13.0	2.10
				Amplitudes in AVF								
0–24 hours	—	—	—	—	—	—	—	—	—	—	—	—
1— 7 days	1.0	1.9	5.4	10.5	13.0	2.43	0	0.6	0.7	3.1	3.5	1.10
8—30 days	1.0	1.4	6.1	12.4	15.0	3.39	0	0.6	0.6	3.8	5.5	1.20

(Hastreiter AR, Abella, JB: J Pediatr 78:346, 1971)

abnormality in the P wave vector or PR interval will differentiate this rhythm from a sinus tachycardia. This degree of tachycardia results in a rapid ventricular contraction and decreased ventricular filling time. If the arrhythmia is allowed to progress for 24 hours or more, congestive heart failure may ensue.

If the arrhythmia has been long standing and persistent at the time of initial examination, the infant may appear pale and irritable, with signs of cardiac decompensation. On auscultation a characteristic "tick-tock" rhythm is heard, and the rate will be difficult, if not impossible, to count. Rarely are murmurs audible.

The condition is only infrequently associated with structural cardiac anomalies (10% of cases). In some instances, with cessation of the arrhythmia and recurrence of sinus rhythm, a preexcitation pattern may become evident. This is most characteristically of the Wolf-Parkinson-White variety consisting of a short PR interval with a prolonged QRS complex (22, 24, 25). Patients with preexcitation syndromes may be prone to frequent recurrences of supraventricular tachycardias.

Digitalization by means of rapidly administered high doses of digoxin generally cause reversion to sinus rhythm (19, 23). Vagal maneuvers, e.g., eyeball pressure and carotid sinus massage, are rarely successful and may indeed be dangerous. Characteristically, in supraventricular tachycardia, conversion to a sinus rhythm is abrupt.

With acutely ill patients in whom time is of the essence, direct-current cardioversion at 10 Watt-seconds is indicated.

Atrial Flutter

This arrhythmia is less common than paroxysmal atrial tachycardia (21). The atrial rate is greater than 250 beats per minute and often as high as 300 to 400 beats per minute. The refractory period of the atrioventricular node will not permit such rapid conduction, and a 1:1 ventricular response in the higher flutter rates is rare. Flutter with variable degrees of atrioventricular block is the rule in such cases. The ECG is diagnostic and is characterized by the appearance of the "saw-toothed" flutter waves or F waves.

Clinical manifestations, when present, are similar to those observed in paroxysmal supraventricular tachycardia, and for the same reasons. Atrial tachycardias such as flutter or supraventricular tachycardia are one of the major causes of heart failure seen immediately at birth.

Digitalis may terminate the arrhythmia or increase the degree of atrioventricular block and thus retard the ventricular response. The addition of quinidine may occasionally be necessary for arrhythmia control. Cardioversion has been extremely effective and is the treatment of choice in markedly symptomatic patients.

CONGENITAL COMPLETE HEART BLOCK

Complete heart block occurs when all atrial impulses are blocked from entering the His-Purkinje system so that a slow ventricular pacemaker is substituted for the normally conducted ventricular responses. The condition may be diagnosed antenatally using a fetal ECG. The rhythm disturbance must be differentiated from fetal distress due to hypoxia.

The heart rates vary from 90 to as low as 30 per minute. At faster rates, the arrhythmia may go unrecognized since, even at very low rates, symptoms are usually absent. A loud left sternal border murmur may be audible, but this rarely indicates a structural cardiac anomaly and can be attributed to a flow phenomenon as a result of the high stroke volume associated with the bradycardia.

Associated congenital cardiac anomalies have been documented in about 30% of patients with complete heart block. Corrected transposition of the great vessels is the most common associated lesion. Familial incidence of heart block has been reported (29).

The ECG reveals a complete lack of association between atria and ventricles, with the atrial rates being greater than the ventricular (Fig. 7–5). In most patients with congenital heart block, the anatomic conduction defect is in the A-V node, and the site of impulse formation for the ventricles is usually in the bundle of His as evidenced by the relatively narrow normal appearance of the QRS complexes (31, 32). Since this pacemaker site is usually quite responsive to autonomic stimulation, it allows for relatively faster heart rates at rest and with exercise; hence, the general absence of signs in the congenital form of the disease, as opposed to acquired (postsurgical) heart block. However, signs may develop when there are significant associated cardiac defects. Only in extremely rare instances does congestive heart failure occur in the absence of anatomic deformities even with extremely low ventricular rates. However, the threat of Stokes-Adams attacks or ventricular arrhythmias, or both, is always present. Infants more prone to these complications often, but not invariably, have wide QRS complexes denoting the pacemaker site as being either in one of the bundle branches or in the ven-

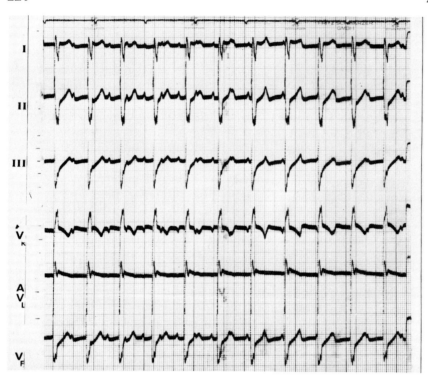

FIG. 7–5. Congenital complete heart block. A permanent ventricular pacemaker has been implanted, and each QRS complex is preceded by the pacemaker artefact. The P waves and the QRS waves are completely dissociated. Atrial rate: 166; ventricular (pacemaker) rate: 94.

tricular Purkinje system. Such pacemaker sites are relatively unstable and less responsive to autonomic stimulation. Heart block in these patients may be the result of abnormalities in all three major bundle branches (trifascicular block).

The vast majority of patients with congenital complete block are asymptomatic and require no therapy (28). Since clinical manifestations are rare and pacemaker implantation often involves significant morbidity and frequent reoperation, it is not recommended that this procedure be carried out on a prophylactic basis for infants with congenital heart block. However, if a Stokes-Adams episode is observed or a suggestive history of syncope is obtained, immediate pacemaker implantation is mandatory (33). In emergency situations insertion of a temporary IV pacing wire to the right ventricular outflow tract is required.

CONGESTIVE HEART FAILURE

Congestive heart failure results from the inability of the cardiac pump mechanism to supply the required cardiac output demanded by the body. Cardiac failure in the neonatal period occurs either on a direct cardiac basis or as a result of other disease processes that secondarily affect the circulatory system.

Congestive heart failure occurring immediately at birth is extremely rare and is most often not associated with structural cardiac malformations. Occasionally, a large cerebral arteriovenous fistula will cause profound high-output failure in the first day of life. Severe anemia, most often associated with erythroblastosis fetalis, fetal–placental bleeding or feto–fetal transfusions, may also result in early neonatal cardiac decompensation. Infants with the hypoplastic left heart syndrome or isolated tricuspid regurgitation are the only patients in whom primary heart disease causes congestive heart failure within the first 24 hours of life.

During the first week of life, cardiac defects are recognized with increasing frequency. Coarctation of the aorta, severe aortic stenosis, obstructed total anomalous pulmonary venous connection, severe pulmonary stenosis and transposition of the great arteries with a ventricular septal defect, along with the hypoplastic left heart syndrome, should be considered as diagnostic possibilities in this age group.

The large left-to-right shunts, such as ventricular septal defect and patent ductus arteriosus, generally do not cause decompensation until the patient has reached one to three months of life since this time is required for pulmonary vascular resistance to significantly decrease. Among premature babies, however, the cardiac failure secondary to left-to-right shunts, usually a patent ductus arteriosus, may occur much earlier. This is attributed to a lack of muscular development of the pulmonary arteriolar bed, which allows pulmonary vascular resistance to decrease almost immediately after birth.

A group of conditions classified as primary myocardial disease (congenital myocarditis, endocardial fibroelastosis a n d Pompe's cardiopathy) are also diagnostic considerations when congestive failure is encountered within the first two weeks of life. When failure occurs near the end of the first month of age, the diagnosis of the hypoplastic left heart syndrome becomes less likely, but the other diagnostic possibilities must still be considered.

Arrhythmias as a cause of cardiac decompensation can span the neonatal period, as well as older age groups. These are usually forms of tachyarrhythmias. Congenital heart block and other bradyarrhythmias are rarely associated with cardiac failure early in life. Congenital hyperthyroidism is another unusual cause of heart failure in the neonatal period.

PHYSIOLOGY

Left ventricular failure occurs when left ventricular volume or pressure work or primary myocardial dysfunction lead to a series of physiologic events resulting in pulmonary congestion. When the left ventricle can no longer eject the normal fraction of its end-diastolic volume, end-diastolic pressure rises; this is reflected in the left atrium, pulmonary venous and pulmonary capillary beds. When hydrostatic pressure exceeds colloid osmotic pressure, pulmonary congestion ensues. Accumulation of edema fluid in small bronchioles of newborn infants often leads to hypoventilation and poor gas exchange. In addition, alveolar collapse, possibly related to changes in surfactant activity, accounts for ventilation–perfusion imbalance and resultant arterial hypoxemia.

Right ventricular failure cannot be explained solely on the basis of elevated systemic venous pressures. Symptoms of right heart failure are seen with relatively low central venous pressures, and experimental evidence has shown that mechanical obstruction to systemic venous return does not result in the right ventricular failure syndrome. Increased blood volume always accompanies right heart failure and occurs on a renal basis. With significant right ventricular dysfunction, forward cardiac output to the lungs, left heart and arterial system is decreased. Although the exact mechanism is obscure, the kidney responds by decreasing renin production, which in turn leads to secondary hyperaldosteronism and salt retention. The release of antidiuretic hormone (ADH) by the pituitary gland is also increased, resulting in excess water reabsorption and further distention of the intravascular compartment.

CLINICAL AND LABORATORY MANIFESTATIONS

Left heart failure leads to signs of pulmonary congestion. Dyspnea with feeding is a cardinal feature, but with marked decompensation the infant is tachypneic and tachycardic, with a gallop rhythm even at rest. Respiratory distress interferes with feeding, and weight gain is inadequate. Cyanosis may be noted, even in the absence of a right-to-left intracardiac shunt since pulmonary congestion results in ventilation–perfusion inequality and decreased oxygenation of pulmonary venous blood. In

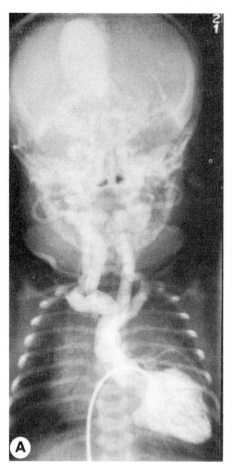

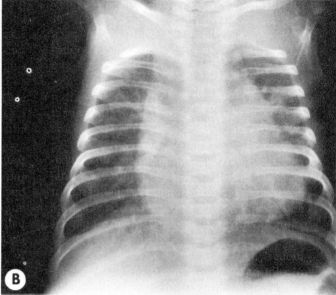

FIG. 7–6. A. Left ventricular angiocardiogram in a newborn with a large Vein of Galen malformation. Radio-opaque dye is injected into the left ventricle. There is marked dilatation of the carotid arteries. The large cerebral arteriovenous malformation is readily visualized. **B.** Frontal chest x ray of a newborn infant with congestive heart failure. There is significant cardiomegaly and a very prominent pulmonary circulatory pattern.

the most severe cases of left ventricular failure, pulmonary edema ensues, and cardiorespiratory collapse eventually results when the primary condition is unresponsive to treatment.

Left ventricular failure is almost never encountered as an isolated entity. Right ventricular decompensation will quickly occur, and hepatomegaly will be noted early in most cases. However, peripheral edema and neck vein distention, common in older patients with right ventricular failure, rarely occur in the neonate.

Pulses are normal in character unless cardiac output has markedly diminished. However, pulses may be bounding, even with signs of congestive heart failure, in patients with high-output decompensation (e.g., anemia, hyperthyroidism, arteriovenous fistulae) or in babies with an aortic diastolic "runoff" (e.g., patent ductus arteriosus, truncus arteriosus).

Congestive heart failure is frequently accompanied by mixed metabolic and respiratory acidosis. Arterial oxygen tensions are often decreased. Serum electrolytes are usually normal, but occasionally hyponatremia occurs. This represents the dilutional effect of excessive water retention, although total body sodium is increased.

Radiologic evidence of cardiomegaly is of importance in the diagnosis of congestive failure. In most cases, the heart is markedly enlarged, and the pulmonary vasculature appears engorged, secondary to either overcirculation or passive venous distention (Fig. 7–6B).

CONDITIONS ASSOCIATED WITH HIGH-OUTPUT FAILURE

Anemia

Anemia is a major cause of congestive heart failure observed within the first 24 hours of life (40). It most often occurs either as a result of severe erythroblastosis fetalis or because of fetal–maternal and feto–fetal transfusions. Profound anemia leads to increased demands on the heart for increased cardiac output to provide sufficient oxygen to the tissues. When the heart can no longer meet the needs of the body, high-output heart failure ensues. Clinical examination of infants with severe anemia reveals a high cardiac output state as evidenced by bounding peripheral pulses and distended neck veins. Murmurs are frequently audible, as the increase in cardiovascular dynamics causes excessive turbulence of blood flow through the heart. It may be difficult to differentiate murmurs that are secondary to anemia from those that are due to structural disorders. Management is directed towards eliminating the underlying cause of the anemia. Blood transfusions may be indicated. Partial exchange transfusion with high-hematocrit blood rapidly increases the hematocrit, but it protects the infant from pulmonary edema, which may result from the rapid overexpansion of the intravascular compartment that occurs in simple transfusion.

Peripheral Arteriovenous Fistulae

Arteriovenous fistulae may lead to massive, severe congestive failure in the early neonatal period. The most common sites of arteriovenous malformations are in the brain (Fig. 7–6A) and liver. These fistulae result in a massive diversion of the circulation from the arterial system during both systole and diastole, causing a significant drop in the diastolic pressure and a "steal" of oxygen from the peripheral tissues.

This causes a hyperkinetic, high cardiac output state and eventual congestive failure. In evaluating any infant who presents with congestive failure, especially within the first day or two of life, specific attention should be given to auscultation of areas other than the heart, such as the head and liver. A pronounced bruit over one of these areas in this context is virtually diagnostic of an arteriovenous malformation.

When a vein of Galen malformation is present, massive neck vein distention is observed—one of the few instances where this physical finding is commonly seen in the neonatal period. Cardiac murmurs are present, and it may be impossible to differentiate these flow murmurs from bruits that signify organic heart disease. The murmurs may be so pronounced that the rather unlikely possibility of an additional cardiac abnormality must be seriously considered. The chest x ray shows an enlarged heart with pulmonary plethora, and the ECG often indicates the presence of biventricular hypertrophy.

Once the diagnosis of an arteriovenous malformation is established, a trial of anticongestive measures should be initiated. Ligation of a large cerebral malformation is a hazardous and often unsuccessful procedure, but it may be attempted in desperate situations.

Diffuse hepatic arteriovenous malformations may respond to radiation therapy or administration of corticosteroids, or both. Once resolution begins, permanent cure may be expected.

Hyperthyroidism

Neonates with congenital hyperthyroidism (see section Hyperthyroidism, Ch. 11), may develop signs of high-output cardiac failure. Systolic murmurs are audible, and recurrent atrial tachycardias are not uncommon. Specific thyroid manifestations, such as a palpable neck mass or exophthalmos, may be observed.

Cardiac enlargement may be seen on chest x ray, and there is usually ECG evidence of right or biventricular enlargement.

Treatment of cardiac failure in congenital hyperthyroidism requires the use of cardiotonic agents together with specific antithyroid medications.

MANAGEMENT

The management of congestive heart failure consists primarily of administration of specific pharmacologic agents, maintenance of adequate Po_2 and modification of diet.

Rotating tourniquets, positive pressure oxygen and antibiotics may also be of value. However, elimination of the cause of congestive heart failure is the ultimate goal of treatment.

Pharmacologic Agents

Digitalis. Digitalis is the primary drug utilized in the management of congestive heart failure. Digitalis causes more vigorous myocardial contraction by increasing the amount of ionized calcium available to the contractile elements within the cardiac cells. This calcium release appears to be an indirect result of inhibition of the enzyme Na-K ATPase by cardiac glycosides.

Digitalis also exerts electrophysiologic effects on the heart. These are mediated predominantly by the vagus nerve as it influences the sinoatrial node and the atrioventricular junctional area. Although heart rate is decreased by the effect of digitalis on the sinoatrial node, this is not the primary explanation for the slowing of sinus tachycardia that occurs during the treatment of congestive heart failure. This slowing occurs as a result of the withdrawal of sympathetic stimulation of the heart which occurs during the decompensated state.

Digoxin is the most widely used glycoside preparation in pediatrics. The drug is absorbed quickly and has an intermediate duration of action. Digoxin can be utilized for rapid digitalization in an emergency situation as well as for maintenance therapy. Administration may be parenteral or by the oral route. On a practical basis, digoxin can serve as the single drug in a pediatric formulary, and allowing it to do so prevents the inadvertant substitution of another preparation with a different dosage scale.

This glycoside is excreted almost entirely by the kidneys without binding to other compounds. The rate of excretion depends on glomerular filtration, and there is no significant tubular reabsorption of the drug. Diuresis does not increase the rate of digoxin excretion. Approximately one-third of the total dose is excreted daily.

In most instances it is preferable to initiate digitalization of neonates by the parenteral route since regurgitation of the oral preparation is always possible. A lower dose is recommended for parenteral administration, since serum levels are higher than with the oral route (Table 7–2).

The recommended total digitalizing dose of digoxin is 40 to 60 μg/kg IM or IV given in three equally divided doses over a 16 to 24-hour period. One-quarter to one-third of the digitalizing dose serves as the daily maintenance dose. This regimen is modified according to individual circumstances. An infant with severe congestive heart failure may require more rapid digitalization. Premature babies are usually given smaller amounts of the drug (30 to 40 μg/kg). In patients with poor renal function, digitalization is initiated and maintained at a considerably lower dosage (approximately one-third to one-half of the usual dose). Serial serum digoxin levels are recommended in this situation. Digitalization is best carried out while the infant's rhythm is being continuously monitored.

It must be remembered that the recommended dosages serve only as a guideline. A decrease in heart rate, respiratory rate, liver size, as well as a general improvement in ability to feed and general disposition are indications of an adequate response to digitalis. The ECG offers no indication of the clinical effectiveness of the drug and is used only to evaluate toxicity.

Studies have been carried out among neonates concerning normal serum digoxin concentrations and serum levels in the presence of known or suspected digitalis toxicity (35). Knowledge of the serum digoxin level obtained after myocardial-serum equilibration (approximately six hours after a dose) is helpful in evaluating the state of digitalization.

Determination of the serum digoxin concentration may be helpful in a patient who is being given a rather large amount therapeutically without a reasonable clinical response. In this situation, if the serum digoxin level is found to be unusually low, dosage may be increased somewhat; whereas

TABLE 7–2. Serum Digoxin Levels in Nontoxic Infants:
Comparison by Mode of Administration

	Age	No. of Samples	Mean Dosage (mg/kg/day)	Mean Serum Level (ng/ml)
Intramuscular	1 wk–3 mo	11	0.023 ± 0.003	3.5 ± 1.3
Oral	1 wk–3 mo	20	0.023 ± 0.004	2.8 ± 1.4
	3 mo–11 mo	12	0.021 ± 0.004	2.2 ± 1.1

(Hayes CJ, Butler VP, Gersony WM: Pediatrics 52:561, 1973)

high serum concentrations probably indicate that the maximal effect of digitalization has already been attained.

Diuretics. Diuretics are also important in the management of congestive heart failure. The agents used most frequently for rapid diuresis are furosemide (Lasix) and ethacrynic acid (Edecrin). The former is preferred because of the absence of ototoxicity, which may occur when ethacrynic acid is used. These agents have largely replaced the once popular mercurial diuretics as they have been found to have a more potent effect and yet have no known nephrotoxic complications.

These agents work primarily by blocking the reabsorption of sodium in the loop of Henle. They are powerful drugs that are generally effective within minutes to a few hours. Care must be taken when they are administered, as marked fluid shifts may cause electrolyte imbalances. Potassium and chloride losses may become significant, causing a secondary contraction alkalosis with an increase in the serum-fixed base. Serum potassium levels should be carefully monitored when digitalis is being administered simultaneously. Insuring adequate potassium intake or promoting its renal reabsorption with aldosterone antagonists (spironolactone) is suggested. The salutory effects of the diuretics are best evaluated by the precise measurement of daily intake and output of fluids, as well as by daily weight determinations.

Furosemide and ethacrynic acid are administered intramuscularly or intravenously as a 1 mg/kg dose on a daily basis. Furosemide is also effective when given orally.

For long-term diuretic treatment, chloro-thiazide (Diuril) is recommended. This drug inhibits tubular reabsorption of sodium, chloride and potassium, resulting in the increased excretion of free water. Oral dosage is usually 20 to 35 mg/kg/day in two divided doses. Provisions for adequate potassium intake must be made.

The addition of the aldosterone antagonist spironolactone (Aldactone), 2 mg/kg/day, is often recommended when other diuretics are administered. This agent causes potassium retention and offsets the kaluresis resulting from the prolonged use of potent diuretics.

Oxygen

When arterial oxygen desaturation is on a pulmonary basis, oxygen therapy may result in some degree of symptomatic improvement. Oxygen is best administered in a head box and under humidification. The lowest concentration necessary to maintain an adequate Po_2 is indicated.

Diet

Low sodium formulas and fluid restrictions are indicated in severe cases. Some low sodium formulas are not palatable and may indeed be so deficient in sodium that they do not meet the requirements for normal growth and development. Total sodium intake should not be restricted to less than 1 to 2 mEq/kg/day.

Fluid intake may require restriction to a total of 80 ml/kg/day, depending on the degree of decompensation. The effectiveness of salt and water restriction is best evaluated on a day-to-day basis by the accurate measurement of daily weights, as well as by daily intake and output tallies. Proper caloric intake to insure adequate growth and development should be maintained.

Other Methods

Rotating Tourniquets. This technique is employed to retard venous return to the heart and thereby decrease the load on a decompensated myocardium. It is advocated in cases of severe pulmonary edema. Tourniquets are applied to three extremities and rotated every 15 minutes.

Positive Pressure. The use of positive pressure oxygen administration via nasotracheal intubation may be of great value in the acute treatment of pulmonary edema. Positive intrathoracic pressure overcomes secondary alveolar hypoventilation and fatigue. Its secondary effect of decreasing venous return to the heart is similar to that obtained by the application of rotating tourniquets. Under normal conditions, venous return increases with the negative intrathoracic pressure generated during inspiration. Positive pressure has the opposite effect.

Antibiotics. The inclusion of antibiotics in the therapeutic armamentarium for congestive heart failure is advocated when infection is documented or strongly suspected. The possibility of a superimposed pneumonic process cannot be positively eliminated when marked pulmonary overcirculation exists.

Specific Therapy

Elimination of the etiology of congestive heart failure is the goal of all treatment. Where congestive heart failure is secondary to noncardiac causes, e.g., anemia or thyrotoxicosis, specific therapy should obviously be carried out expeditiously. Cardiac lesions causing decompensation or severe hypoxia should undergo cardiac catheterization, and may require palliative or corrective surgery.

Neonates with potentially surgically correctable problems may require early operation if standard medical management to improve cardiac status fails to tide them over the early months. Specific surgical approaches will be discussed in the segments of this chapter dealing with specific lesions.

CONGENITAL ANOMALIES NOT ASSOCIATED WITH CYANOSIS

LEFT-TO-RIGHT SHUNTS

Intracardiac shunts may occur as a result of communications at the atrial, ventricular, great artery level or at multiple sites. When no obstruction to the right ventricular outflow tract is present, flow through the defect is always left-to-right. The degree of shunting depends on the size of the defect and, when a large defect is present, on the relationship betwen systemic and pulmonary vascular resistance. Rudolph (41) has divided left-to-right shunts into dependent and obligatory types.

Dependent Types

Dependent shunts are those in which flow is more directly dependent on pulmonary vascular resistance. Large defects that enter the right ventricle or pulmonary artery allow shunting of blood in direct proportion to the relationship of systemic to pulmonary vascular resistance; the greater the pulmonary vascular resistance, the smaller the left-to-right shunt. If pulmonary vascular resistance is greater than systemic, shunting is right-to-left.

Obligatory Types

Obligatory shunts occur in the presence of 1) abnormal venous connections or 2) a communication between an artery or ventricular chamber and a vein or atrium. Since blood is shunted directly into the low pressure venous system by virtue of the anatomic connection, this type of shunt is relatively independent of the pulmonary resistance, e.g., total anomalous pulmonary venous drainage, arteriovenous fistulae and left ventricle-to-right atrial shunts.

SPECIFIC DEFECTS

Ventricular Septal Defect

Ventricular septal defect, the most frequently occurring congenital heart lesion, accounts for 25% of all congenital cardiac defects. Ventricular septal defects can be classified anatomically with reference to the portion of septum involved. The septum, as visualized from the right ventricle, may be divided into: 1) subcristal, 2) subpulmonary, 3) membranous, 4) muscular and 5) endocardial cushion portions. Defects may occur at one or more levels. Muscular defects may be multiple.

Ventricular septal defects are best classified physiologically as simply being large or small. A large ventricular septal defect is defined as a defect of sufficient size to virtually eliminate a gradient of pressure between the left and right ventricles. All other defects may be regarded as small.

Pathophysiology. When a large ventricular septal defect is present, right ventricular and pulmonary artery pressures are at systemic levels. When pulmonary vascular resistance falls significantly, by four to six weeks of age, large left-to-right shunts are measured. Pulmonary to systemic flow ratios often reach 3:1. The increased pulmonary blood flow returns to the left ventricle, which, being thus "diastolically" loaded, must eject the excess blood back through the defect to the lungs. The right ventricle will require an elevated systolic pressure in order to eject its normal diastolic volume into the high pressure pulmonary artery.

When a small ventricular septal defect is present, a gradient of pressure exists across the defect, and the defect itself offers resistance to flow. In such lesions, flow is pressure dependent and is therefore always left to right. The shunts are small, and the pulmonary artery pressure is normal.

Clinical Features. Patients with small defects and small left-to-right shunts are generally asymptomatic, but when a large defect is present, congestive heart failure may develop at the time the shunt becomes maximal. These infants generally present with signs of fatigue with feeding and tachypnea. Failure to thrive becomes apparent with time. On physical examination, tachycardia and tachypnea (respiratory rate greater than 60 per minute), often associated with sternal retractions, are noted. The pulmonic component of the second heart sound is increased in intensity.

The hallmark of the infant with a ventricular septal defect is a systolic murmur at the mid and lower left sternal border. The intensity of the murmur is not directly related to the size of the left-to-right shunt. The murmur may be discovered on the first day of life, but more often it is initially heard later in the first month of life. With large shunts, a middiastolic mitral flow rumble is often audible at the apex, and signs of congestive heart failure may be present.

The ECG shows left ventricular or biventricular enlargement. The chest x ray reveals cardiomegaly with pulmonary vascular overcirculation. Arterial blood gases generally show a normal Po_2 but may show a decrease in the value if there is marked pulmonary congestion. Unless pulmonary edema is present, the Pco_2 is normal or slightly increased and the pH is normal.

Management. Patients with a ventricular septal defect who are symptomatic should be treated with a cardiotonic regimen consisting of digitalis, diuretics and a low salt diet. Cardiac catheterization is indicated to document the anatomic defect and to measure the size of the left-to-right shunt and the pulmonary artery pressure (44). The study should include a left ventricular angiocardiogram, and the additional presence of a patent ductus arteriosus should be ruled out by an aortic root angiocardiogram.

If medical management fails to control congestive heart failure and the infant fails to thrive, surgical management becomes necessary (47). Palliative pulmonary artery banding to restrict pulmonary blood flow and lower distal pulmonary artery pressure has been the surgical treatment of choice in the past. However, more recently, total anatomic correction employing cardiopulmonary bypass has been the preferred surgical procedure at many centers. If the infant does relatively well on medical management, recatheterization is advisable in the second year of life. If pulmonary artery hypertension remains, operative repair is carried out prior to two years of age in order to prevent late pulmonary vascular disease.

Small defects with small shunts often require no treatment. As many as 50% of these defects close spontaneously (43).

Patent Ductus Arteriosus

The ductus arteriosus is a muscular vessel that in fetal life directs blood flow from the pulmonary artery to the descending aorta. Prior to birth, patency is due to low arterial Po_2. Soon after delivery, the ductus arteriosus normally constricts. Functional flow via the ductus usually ceases during the first 24 hours of life. In some neonates, the ductus arteriosus remains patent. This occurs especially in premature infants who display significant hypoxemia. Patent ductus arteriosus represents 10% of congenital heart lesions. The incidence is known to be increased at higher altitudes where ambient Po_2 is lower than at sea level.

Pathophysiology. The hemodynamics of patent ductus arteriosus in a full-term infant without hypoxemia are similar to those of a ventricular septal defect; left-to-right shunting of blood occurs from the aorta through the ductus arteriosus into the pulmonary artery and lungs. Flow through a small defect is limited by the narrow ductal diameter. When a ductus arteriosus remains widely patent, shunting is of the dependent type and is regulated by the level of pulmonary vascular resistance. A large left-to-right shunt causes pulmonary overcirculation and left atrial and left ventricular diastolic overload similar to patients with ventricular septal defects. The left ventricle is more adversely affected by the volume load of a large patent ductus arteriosus than by an identical shunt through a ventricular septal defect since there is no intracardiac defect to provide a route of decompression during ventricular contraction.

When a patent ductus arteriosus exists in a premature infant with early RDS, shunting is right to left or bidirectional. Later in the clinical course, however, a large left-to-right shunt may become apparent.

Clinical Features. Congestive heart failure resulting from a large patent ductus arteriosus may occur earlier than it would when a large ventricular septal defect is present, especially in a premature infant. The classic murmur of the patent ductus arteriosus in the older patient is a continuous systolic and diastolic bruit beneath the left clavicle. In the neonatal period, however, the diastolic component of the murmur is likely to be absent. The systolic portion is described as having a "rolling dice" or "clicky" quality, which descriptive characteristic is rather specific for patent ductus arteriosus. If the shunt is large, the rumbling diastolic murmur of increased flow across the mitral valve may be audible at the apex.

Since in the presence of a large patent ductus arteriosus there is an aortic runoff of blood into the pulmonary artery during diastole, peripheral pulses are bounding, and the pulse pressure is widened. The ECG, chest x ray and arterial blood gases are similar to those seen in patients with ventricular septal defects.

Management. Patients with congestive heart failure should be managed medically (see section Congestive Heart Failure), but if failure is severe and intractable, surgical ligation is mandatory. Operative risk is low in the hands of experienced surgeons and expert pediatric anesthesiologists, even for a severely ill premature infant. Patients with classic findings on physical examination, ECG and chest x ray may not require diagnostic cardiac catheterization prior to surgical intervention. However, if any unusual or inconsistent findings are present, hemodynamic studies should be done.

The prognosis for full-term infants with patent ductus arteriosus is excellent. Surgery is feasible at any time and should be the eventual treatment of choice. Infants who can be managed medically or who are asymptomatic should have surgery deferred. However, the possibility of spontaneous closure is small among full-term infants. Premature infants with or without RDS are far more likely to close a patent ductus arteriosus spontaneously. Thus, among these patients, conservative management is indicated unless congestive heart failure cannot be controlled. Early closure of the patent ductus arteriosus in patients with severe RDS, when the pulmonary component is dominant, remains controversial.

Atrial Septal Defects and Atrioventricular Canal

Atrial septal defects consist of about 13% of all congenital heart disease and are more common in females. They are rarely recognized clinically during the neonatal period and generally remain undiagnosed until childhood or early adult life. There are two basic types of atrial septal defects: 1) secundum and 2) primum. The latter is an abnormality of the endocardial cushion and includes associated mitral and tricuspid valve clefts. If a ventricular septal defect is also present, the lesion is classified as a form of atrioventricular canal. Because of the additional hemodynamic abnormalities with this lesion, congestive heart failure may occur early in the first year of life. A strong association exists between atrioventricular canal and Down's syndrome (54). Atrial left-to-right shunts without other defects rarely cause problems in the neonate because significant pulmonary hypertension is not present and the right ventricle tolerates the extra volume load without difficulty.

Clinical Features. Most infants with atrial septal defects are asymptomatic and display normal growth and development. Physical examination reveals a right ventricular impulse over the precordium. The second heart sound is widely split and fixed because of constant right ventricular output during both inspiration and expiration. A systolic murmur caused by turbulence secondary to increased blood flow across the right ventricular outflow tract is best heard at the left base. An early diastolic tricuspid flow rumble may also be audible at the left middle and left lower sternal border.

The ECG shows a typical right ventricular conduction delay in leads V_3R and V_1. Right axis deviation and mild right ventricular enlargement are present with secundum atrial septal defects; primum lesions and atrioventricular canals are associated with a left superior axis. The chest x ray shows cardiomegaly and pulmonary overcirculation in the presence of a large shunt.

Management. If signs of congestive heart failure are present, a cardiotonic treatment with digitalis and diuretics is indicated. Cardiac catheterization should be carried out to define the presence and severity of the defect.

If congestive heart failure cannot be controlled medically, cardiac surgery may be necessary. In such a situation, complete correction using cardiopulmonary bypass is indicated, although with a large ventricular defect (atrioventricular canal), pulmonary artery banding may be an effective palliative procedure. If surgery is necessary during the neonatal period for defects, which include associated severe atrioventricular valve deformities, the risk is high. The prognosis for the vast majority of cases of primum and secundum atrial septal defects is excellent.

Coarctation of the Aorta

Coarctation of the aorta occurs as a localized constriction near the area of insertion of the ductus arteriosus (Fig. 7–7). In some instances a longer coarcted segment may be present, and in others, there is complete interruption of the aortic arch. It has been suggested that the angle of insertion of the ductus arteriosus may be related to the development of coarctation. The literature has tended to emphasize the site of the coarctation in relation to the ductus, i.e., preductal versus postductal. However, almost all coarctations are "juxtaductal" and therefore positional descriptions should be considered

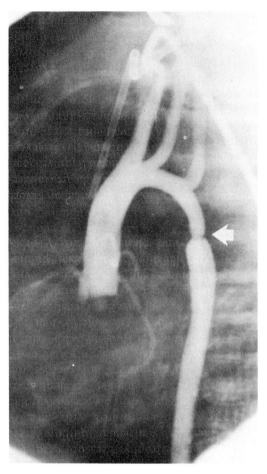

FIG. 7–7. Lateral projection of angiocardiogram in a newborn infant with coarctation of the aorta (arrow). The patient had an associated ventricular septal defect (not shown).

to be on a hemodynamic rather than strict anatomic basis.

Coarctation accounts for 6% of congenital cardiac lesions and is a frequent cause of congestive heart failure in the first month of life. However, the great majority of symptomatic cases have associated cardiac anomalies (50). The most frequent are patent ductus arteriosus, ventricular septal defect, anomalies of the aortic arch and ascending aorta and abnormalities of the aortic and mitral valves. Patients with isolated coarctation are more likely to remain asymptomatic during infancy and childhood.

Pathophysiology. Coarctation of the aorta is best classified hemodynamically depending on whether the right or left ventricle is responsible for providing the systemic output. When the patent ductus inserts relative to the coarctation in such a manner that blood flow to the lower trunk is provided by the right ventricle via the pulmonary artery, pulmonary artery hypertension is present at systemic level. An associated ventricular septal defect is extremely common. In order for significant blood to flow through the ductus, pulmonary vascular resistance must remain elevated. When pulmonary vascular resistance falls or the ductus narrows, hemodynamics significantly worsen, with increased pulmonary flow and decreased perfusion of the viscera, kidneys and lower body. The physiology is not dissimilar to the hypoplastic left heart syndrome and preductal coarctation is often classified within this group.

When left ventricular hypertension is observed, the ductus arteriosus inserts proximal to the coarctation. A patent ductus then results in aortic runoff of blood into the pulmonary artery (left-to-right shunt). The left ventricle must thus assume both an increased volume and pressure load, and early left ventricular failure is more likely. Bicuspid aortic valves may be recognized with coarctation, but associated severe aortic stenosis is uncommon.

Clinical Features. Early signs of congestive heart failure are universal when a preductal coarctation and associated lesions are present. Differential cyanosis is described, but in most instances, congestive heart failure and generalized cyanosis are present, and differential cyanosis is not clinically obvious. However, differential right brachial artery–femoral artery oxygen saturations may be documented. Femoral pulses are palpable and equal to the brachial pulse since the right ventricle supplies the lower extremities at systemic pressures via the ductus. When the left ventricle must pump blood through the coarctation, absent femoral pulses and differential blood pressures are observed.

An ejection systolic murmur is usually audible at the left base and back. Murmurs of associated defects are frequently heard. When severe coarctation with congestive failure is present, cardiomegaly with pulmonary overcirculation is present on the chest x ray. The ECG characteristically shows right ventricular enlargement or biventricular enlargement during infancy. With isolated coarctation and a high pressure left ventricle, the ECG evolves gradually to left ventricular enlargement.

Management. In symptomatic patients, cardiac catheterization is indicated to document associated defects and visualize the anatomic characteristics of the coarctation. Patients with congestive heart failure should be rapidly digitalized, and diuretic therapy and other cardiotonic agents should be administered as necessary. A fair number of patients with isolated postductal coarctation will improve, and surgical intervention may be deferred beyond the first year of life. In most instances of preductal coarctation, surgical resection of the lesion should be carried out following initial stabilization since prolonged improvement often does not occur when medical management alone is utilized (59).

When a patent ductus arteriosus is present, it is ligated at surgery. If an existent large ventricular septal defect with pulmonary hypertension is present, pulmonary artery banding is indicated at the time of coarctation resection.

Aortic Stenosis

Aortic stenosis, which occurs in approximately 4% of children with congenital heart disease, is most often valvular, but it may be subvalvular or supravalvular. When the aortic orifice is entirely absent (aortic valve atresia), the condition is classified under the hypoplastic left heart syndrome (discussed elsewhere in this chapter). Valvular aortic stenosis involves a commissural fusion of either a bicuspid or unicuspid valve. Subvalvular aortic stenosis occurs as a discrete obstruction, either membranous or muscular, or as a diffuse muscular process (idiopathic hypertrophic subaortic stenosis (62). Supravalvular aortic stenosis is most often associated with idiopathic hypercalcemia of infancy, and the syndrome also includes

peripheral pulmonic stenoses, elfin facies, mild to moderate mental retardation and dental anomalies (60).

Pathophysiology. The presence of significant aortic stenosis increases the pressure load on the left ventricle and results in left ventricular hypertrophy. Pressure gradients across the left ventricular outflow tract must always be interpreted with care. A severely ill infant with decreased cardiac output may have a smaller gradient than another patient in whom flow across the aortic valve is normal. Thus, only a 30 or 40 mm gradient may be present with critical aortic stenosis in the neonate. When left ventricular decompensation ensues, increased left ventricular end-diastolic pressure and volume will be measured, with concomitant elevation of left atrial, pulmonary venous and pulmonary artery pressures.

Clinical Features. In the absence of severe obstruction with congestive heart failure, the infant will display normal growth and development. When aortic stenosis is severe and left ventricular decompensation is present, signs of congestive heart failure will develop. Chest pain appears to occur in infants, but it may be interpreted as colic.

Physical examination of the heart reveals the second sound to be single or narrowly split. A systolic ejection murmur is audible at the right base and left midsternal border and transmits to the neck. A thrill at the right base, suprasternal notch or neck may be present, but this is rare in the neonate. The presence of a thrill generally denotes greater severity, but with critical stenosis the murmur may be less intense and thrills may be absent.

The ECG in aortic stenosis shows left ventricular enlargement. In severe cases, ST–T wave strain patterns are present over the left precordium (leads V_5 and V_6), and T waves may be inverted. However, it is not unusual for patients with severe obstruction to have normal ECGs.

The chest x ray may show a left ventricular configuration and a prominent aortic knob. Cardiomegaly and pulmonary venous distention are seen when left ventricular decompensation is present.

Management. If suspected left ventricular obstruction appears to be critical, urgent cardiac catheterization and surgical intervention are indicated. Digitalization should be carried out, but medical measures rarely control congestive heart failure secondary to severe aortic stenosis for prolonged periods of time. Although modern techniques have improved the chances for survival, operation for this lesion still carries considerable risk in a small infant. For operative survivors, significant residual stenosis or aortic insufficiency is common. In the infant age group, surgical repair should not be considered to be final and definitive. In cases of mild or moderate aortic stenosis, the prognosis during childhood is good.

Supravalvular or subvalvular stenoses rarely cause difficulties in infancy, and severe cases can be operated on with less risk later in childhood.

CONGENITAL DISORDERS ASSOCIATED WITH CYANOSIS

DISORDERS WITH INCREASED PULMONARY BLOOD FLOW

Transposition of the Great Arteries

Transposition of the great arteries is one of the most common cyanotic congenital cardiac disorders. It accounts for 9% of patients born with cyanotic congenital heart disease. Transposition of the great arteries may be defined as: 1) reversal of the anteroposterior relationship of the aorta and the pulmonary artery regardless of the proximal connection of these arteries and 2) origin of the aorta completely from the morphologic right ventricle with origin of the pulmonary artery completely from the morphologic left ventricle. Two parallel circulations exist (Fig. 7–8); one involves the aorta and the systemic circulation, and the other the pulmonary artery and the pulmonary circulation. This is opposed to normal hemodynamics in which the two circulations are

connected to one another in a series relationship.

The disorder occurs with intact ventricular septum, with a ventricular septal defect and with a ventricular septal defect and pulmonary stenosis. The viability of the patient who has two parallel circulations depends entirely on the number and size of communications between these two circulations. With an intact ventricular septum, mixing must occur at sites of fetal communication, namely the foramen ovale, and possibly at the ductus arteriosus. As these communications tend not to remain widely patent for long periods of time, such infants are in severe jeopardy soon after birth. Intense cyanosis associated with signs of hypoxia tend to occur within the first few days of life. Patients with a ventricular septal defect tend to display much better mixing of the pulmonary and systemic venous blood since a large mixing communication is present across the interventricular septum. Such patients, therefore, do not develop as severe cyanosis and may not be recognized until two to four weeks of age. They develop marked pulmonary overcirculation and hyperkinetic pulmonary hypertension with resultant congestive heart failure; dynamics are very similar to patients with large ventricular septal defects and normally positioned great arteries. Infants with a ventricular septal defect and pulmonary stenosis are fewer in number and display hemodynamics that are variable depending on the degree of pulmonary outflow tract obstruction. In most instances this obstruction is of a moderate degree. Heart failure is less evident since the presence of pulmonary outflow tract obstruction limits the amount of pulmonary blood flow and prevents significant pulmonary hypertension. In a minority of patients with transposition of the great arteries, ventricular septal defect and pulmonary stenosis, the pulmonary obstruction is so marked that the clinical presentation is similar to that of a patient with severe tetralogy of Fallot.

The patient with transposition of the great arteries may suffer from the lack of mixing of pulmonary and systemic venous blood, pulmonary overcirculation or de-

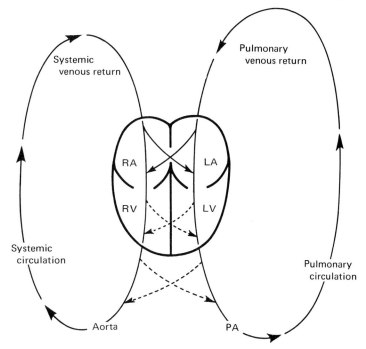

FIG. 7–8. Circulation in transposition of the great arteries. Two parallel circulations exist, and mixing must occur for survival. A mixing site is always present at the atrial level via a patent foramen ovale (solid arrows). Other potential sites of communication are via a 1) ventricular septal defect and 2) patent ductus arteriosus (dotted arrows). The two circulations differ in size, the pulmonary circulation almost always being greater than the systemic circulation. For circulation to be maintained, total left-to-right and right-to-left shunting must be identical, i.e., the net shunt must be zero.

creased pulmonary flow, either alone or in combination depending on the nature of the associated defects.

Clinical Features. The infant with an intact ventricular septum generally presents within the first few days of life with intense cyanosis and tachypnea and respiratory distress. Physical examination usually shows no evidence of congestive heart failure; pulses are of good quality, and there are no murmurs. The ECG reveals right ventricular hypertrophy that cannot be considered definitely abnormal for age. The chest x ray classically shows a normal-sized heart and relatively normal pulmonary vascular markings. Often, the cardiac silhouette is described as resembling an egg on side, and the superior mediastinal shadow is characteristically narrowed. This configuration is due to the abnormal parallel relationship of the great vessels as they emerge from the heart.

The infant who has an associated ventricular septal defect generally presents later, usually about the second week of life. The cardinal signs are cyanosis with congestive heart failure. The degree of cyanosis depends on how adequately the two circula-

tions mix. On physical examination the murmur of a ventricular septal defect is present. The chest x ray in these infants demonstrates significant cardiomegaly accompanied by marked pulmonary overcirculation. The ECG shows right axis deviation and right ventricular hypertrophy.

Acute Management. All neonates suspected of having transposition of the great arteries should undergo urgent catheterization. Once the diagnosis is confirmed, balloon atrial septostomy should be carried out in order to improve mixing of blood at the atrial level and, in patients with ventricular septal defects, to decrease left atrial hypertension by decompression of this chamber. Immediate improvement in arterial oxygenation should be noted in the infants with an intact ventricular septum if a successful septostomy has been achieved. Such procedures are best performed in centers accustomed to handling these patients on a 24-hour basis.

The neonate with an intact ventricular septum may continue to show arterial oxygen desaturation following the septostomy, but this will improve as compared to pre-septostomy levels. Most infants can be discharged from the nursery within seven to ten days. They will remain cyanotic but will be much less distressed and tachypneic; they should take feedings adequately at home. Caution must be taken to maintain adequate hemoglobin levels since relative anemia may lead to episodes of cerebral hypoxia.

In patients with ventricular septal defects, digitalis and diuretics are usually necessary, and their course in the initial stages is very similar to that of patients with isolated ventricular septal defects.

Long-Term Management. Patients with intact ventricular septums are candidates for complete correction. The Mustard procedure, which in effect reroutes atrial flow, directing systemic venous return into the left ventricle and pulmonary artery and directing pulmonary venous return into the right ventricle and aorta, may now be successfully carried out at one year of age, or even earlier if indicated by hypoxic manifestations.

Patients with ventricular septal defects must undergo banding of the pulmonary artery at three to six months of age as an elective procedure. Such patients are likely to develop pulmonary vascular obstructive disease early and banding is carried out to prevent this complication. Mustard procedures can then be electively performed along with ventricular septal defect closure and pulmonary artery debanding at approximately five years of age. Patients with ventricular septal defect associated with naturally occurring pulmonary stenosis are handled in the same way, although occa-

sionally a systemic-to-pulmonary artery shunt is necessary in infancy (65, 70).

Until the mid-1960s, the prognosis for patients born with transposition of the great arteries was universally poor; 90% of such patients did not survive the first year of life. The lesion is now considered correctable (66) and exemplifies the dramatic progress that has taken place in treating the infant born with a severe congenital cardiac defect.

Hypoplastic Left Heart Syndrome

Hypoplastic left heart syndrome encompasses a group of anomalies including mitral atresia, underdevelopment of the left ventricle and aortic valve, aortic atresia and hypoplastic ascending aorta. Preductal co-arctation of the aorta may be classified in this group. The syndrome accounts for approximately 1% of congenital defects and is one of the most common causes of severe congestive heart failure with cyanosis in the first weeks of life.

In the presence of hypoplastic left heart syndrome with little or no left ventricular output, pulmonary flow returning to the left atrium shunts via a dilated foramen ovale into the right atrium. Hence, virtually all of the systemic and pulmonary venous return leaves the heart via the pulmonary artery. If there is no flow across the aortic valve, blood flow is provided only through a patent ductus arteriosus. The coronary blood flow and brachiocephalic blood flow are maintained via retrograde filling of the aortic arch. Thus in this syndrome, patent fetal communications are necessary for survival. In addition, pulmonary vascular resistance must remain high in order to insure right-to-left ductal flow, i.e., flow from the pulmonary artery to aorta. High left atrial pressure as a result of limitation of the size of the foramen ovale causes pulmonary venous congestion and pulmonary edema.

Clinical Features. Most patients are critically ill with cyanosis and marked congestive heart failure within the first few days of life. Cyanosis may not be marked early in the course of the disease in some instances due to maintenance of high pulmonary blood flow. Usually, however, signs of congestive heart failure develop early. A hallmark is the absence of vigorous pulses in the extremities. Systolic murmurs are audible along the left sternal border, but these are nonspecific and not particularly helpful in diagnosis.

The chest x ray shows marked cardiomegaly and pulmonary vascular distention. The ECG shows marked right ventricular enlargement and decreased left ventricular forces over the precordial leads. An occasional patient will show equal RS patterns over the left precordium.

Catheterization should be carried out to exclude the diagnosis of coarctation of the aorta or aortic stenosis. However, echocardiography has been useful in diagnosing this disorder and may eliminate the need for invasive procedures.

Management. Medical management of congestive heart failure should be instituted but is rarely beneficial for a sustained period. These infants usually expire within a few days; rarely, a prolonged course will occur. Complex palliative operative procedures may lead to temporary improvement in some infants.

Single Ventricle

Single ventricle is a complex hemodynamic and embryologic abnormality that accounts for about 1% of congenital cardiac malformations. The abnormality is the result of the embryologic development of only one ventricle, either the left ventricle (type A) or the right ventricle (type B). The nondeveloped ventricle exists only as a rudimentary outflow tract. Rarely, the defect is the result of total absence of the ventricular septum, with adequate development of both ventricles (type C). The majority of cases of single ventricle (80%) are associated with transposition of the great vessels. Common atrioventricular valve, coarctation of the aorta, subaortic stenosis and pulmonary stenosis or atresia are other frequently associated defects.

Clinical Features. Infants with single ventricle who have no obstruction to pulmonary flow present with signs of congestive heart failure and mild cyanosis. In the presence of severe pulmonary stenosis or pulmonary atresia, cyanosis is more prominent and the presentation is similar to that seen in severe forms of tetralogy of Fallot. The chest x ray generally shows a large heart with variable pulmonary circulation, depending upon the presence of pulmonary outflow tract obstruction. The ECG may show either right ventricular enlargement or left ventricular enlargement (76). Q wave abnormalities across the right precordium are often observed.

Management. Treatment consists of digitalization and other measures to control congestive failure. In the presence of increased pulmonary blood flow with pulmonary artery hypertension, a pulmonary artery banding may be helpful. However, if there is a significant decrease in pulmonary blood flow, a surgical systemic to pulmonary arterial shunt may be required.

Truncus Arteriosus

Truncus arteriosus is defined as a single arterial vessel exiting from both ventricles with the pulmonary artery arising from the truncal vessel. The lesion is always associated with a ventricular septal defect. Various forms of the anomaly exist, based on the nature of origin of the pulmonary arteries from the truncus. However, the hemodynamics are basically the same.

Both ventricles eject into the common truncus, and consequently cyanosis must always be present. However, the degree of cyanosis depends entirely on the magnitude of pulmonary blood flow. During infancy pulmonary blood flow is almost always markedly increased, and cyanosis is rarely extreme. Since the pulmonary artery originates directly from the truncal vessel (or aorta), pulmonary hypertension at systemic levels occurs. In addition, the truncal valve may be deformed, resulting in truncal valve insufficiency (78). This increases the volume load of the left ventricle, and there is a greater possibility of congestive heart failure in early infancy.

Clinical Features. Signs of congestive heart failure may be manifest in the early neonatal period. Mild cyanosis is noted. Auscultatory findings include a harsh holosystolic murmur at the left sternal border and, occasionally, a decrescendo diastolic murmur caused by the truncal valve insufficiency. Continuous murmurs, similar to those heard with a patent ductus arteriosus, are occasionally described. The second heart sound is usually single, as would be anticipated, but "split" second sounds have been reported. The explanation for the presence of two components is not clear.

The chest x ray shows cardiomegaly and marked pulmonary overcirculation. The ECG most often reveals combined ventricular hypertrophy. Isolated right ventricular hypertrophy or even isolated left ventricular hypertrophy may also be seen.

Management. Following accurate diagnosis by cardiac catheterization, medical management with digitalis and diuretics is instituted for infants with congestive heart failure. Most patients respond to treatment, however, infants who have associated truncal valve insufficiency are more refractory to therapy and have a poorer prognosis. Pulmonary artery banding (79) may be attempted in order to control congestive heart failure if medical management fails. Should the infant survive, later total correction is feasible.

Total Anomalous Pulmonary Venous Connection

Total anomalous pulmonary venous connection is a malformation characterized by the absence of direct communication between the pulmonary venous return and the left atrium. It accounts for approximately 4% of congenital heart diseases. Drainage from the lung reaches the right atrium by various routes, depending on the type of anomalous connection. The only route by which oxygenated blood can reach the aorta is through a patent foramen ovale. The anomaly can be classified into three types: 1) supracardiac (approximately 50% of cases), in which the pulmonary veins drain into a left superior vena cava and flow into the right atrium via the innominate vein and superior vena cava; 2) intracardiac (25% of cases), in which the pulmonary veins drain either into the right atrium via the coronary sinus or, less frequently, directly into the right atrium; 3) infracardiac (25% of cases), in which the pulmonary veins connect into the inferior vena cava via the portal vein. Mixed forms of anomalous connection may also occur.

Pathophysiology. Pulmonary venous return enters the right atrium and mixes with the systemic venous return. The mixture enters the systemic circulation through a patent foramen ovale or atrial septal defect. If pulmonary blood flow is markedly increased, systemic arterial oxygen saturation may be relatively high, and cyanosis is only moderate. Patients with large pulmonary blood flow develop hyperkinetic pulmonary hypertension and behave similarly to patients with large left-to-right shunts.

Many infants, however, have significant pulmonary venous obstruction somewhere along the course of anomalous drainage, causing elevation of total pulmonary resistance and a resultant decrease in pulmonary blood flow. These children are more cyanotic and display greater elevation of pulmonary artery pressure. In some instances, obstruction to flow may occur at the level of the foramen ovale.

Clinical Features. In general, patients with marked pulmonary artery hypertension will present with congestive heart failure and respiratory distress in the neonatal period. Severe pulmonary venous obstruction is present in all cases of infradiaphragmatic drainage, and consequently, such infants will become severely ill within the first few days of life.

A hallmark of the infant with total

anomalous pulmonary venous connection and pulmonary artery hypertension is the marked degree of tachypnea. Respiratory rates not infrequently approach 90 to 100 per minute. Patients with elevated pulmonary blood flow may not become symptomatic for months or even years, surviving the immediate neonatal period without difficulty.

Auscultation of the chest reveals a short systolic ejection murmur at the left base. Not infrequently, an early diastolic murmur can be heard along the left sternal border. On occasion, continuous left upper sternal border murmurs are present. These represent venous flow through the anomalous connection. Left sternal border pansystolic murmurs that are secondary to tricuspid insufficiency may also be heard. This finding is related to the marked degree of pulmonary and right ventricular hypertension.

The chest x ray shows a large heart with significant pulmonary venous distension. The "snowman" or "figure eight" appearance of the cardiothymic image often described with supracardiac total anomalous pulmonary venous connection is rarely seen in the neonatal period. In patients with infradiaphragmatic drainage, the chest x ray typically shows a small heart with marked pulmonary venous distension and pulmonary edema. The film may be confused with that of RDS. The ECG in all types of total anomalous pulmonary venous connection demonstrates right axis deviation and marked right ventricular hypertrophy.

Management. Digitalization and other medical measures for infants with congestive heart failure secondary to total anomalous pulmonary venous connection are usually only temporizing measures and rarely obviate more-definitive therapy. The treatment of choice at several centers is primary surgical correction using cardiopulmonary bypass or inflow occlusion and hypothermia. Atrial balloon septostomy is used as an effective palliative measure at some institutions, and in a number of instances, surgical intervention can be delayed for several months.

DISORDERS WITH DECREASED PULMONARY BLOOD FLOW

Tetralogy of Fallot

This combination of defects consists of: 1) a large ventricular septal defect, 2) infundibular or valvular pulmonary stenosis, or both, 3) an over-riding aorta and 4) right ventricular hypertrophy. In the extreme form of this lesion the pulmonary outflow tract is completely atretic. Tetralogy of Fallot accounts for approximately 10% of all congenital cardiac anomalies and is the most common cyanotic lesion. In most cases, however, severe cyanosis is not present until after the neonatal period (85).

A marked degree of right ventricular outflow tract obstruction must be present to cause clinical signs in the neonate. Most of the blood entering the right ventricle is shunted from the right ventricle to the aorta through the ventricular septal defect, bypassing the lungs. In the extreme form, all right ventricular inflow exits via the aorta, pulmonary blood flow being supplied by a patent ductus arteriosus or bronchial collaterals, or both.

Clinical Features. Patients with severe tetralogy of Fallot present with cyanosis within the first month of life. The earlier the presentation, the greater the right ventricular outflow tract obstruction and, generally, the more likely the need for surgical intervention. Otherwise, the clinical course may be characterized by hypoxemia and syncopal spells.

On auscultation, a short systolic ejection murmur is evident at the left upper sternal border. The less impressive the murmur, the worse the right ventricular outflow tract obstruction. In cases with pulmonary atresia there may be absence of a murmur. When a patent ductus arteriosus or significant bronchial collateral flow is present, a continuous murmur may be audible. The second sound is generally single and loud and represents aortic closure.

The ECG shows marked right ventricular hypertrophy and right axis deviation. The chest x ray (Fig. 7-9) shows a heart that is normal-to-decreased in overall size. The pulmonary vasculature is markedly diminished, as is the main pulmonary artery segment, giving the overall "dutch shoe" configuration.

Treatment. The symptomatic infant with tetralogy of Fallot is an urgent candidate for surgery. A Waterston shunt should be carried out as soon as the diagnosis is confirmed. Long-term management with propranolol is not recommended. With advanced surgical techniques, the eventual outcome for these patients is good. Should they survive the neonatal period, complete surgical correction is carried out in early childhood (86). Early open-heart correction is gradually replacing the palliative procedures after the first few months of life for patients who are not severely hypoxic as neonates.

Pulmonary Stenosis

In valvular pulmonary stenosis, the pulmonary valve leaflets are partially fused, causing obstruction to right ventricular emptying. In severe cases, right-to-left shunting occurs across the patent foramen ovale, and for this reason, severe valvular pulmonary stenosis is often classified with the cyanotic disorders in the neonate. The lesion accounts for approximately 7% of patients with congenital heart disease.

With more severe degrees of right ventricular outflow obstruction, the right ventricle must produce greater systolic pressures in order to eject an adequate blood volume. Thus, a pressure gradient exists between the right ventricle and the pulmonary artery. Among older patients, severity is classified by the degree of the right ventricle–pulmonary artery peak systolic gradient. However, in the neonate, this value must always be interpreted along with the clinical course (87, 88). If obstruction is severe enough to cause congestive heart failure and cyanosis, flow across the pulmonary valve may be decreased, and the gradient will be misleadingly small. Blood flow is directed away from the right ventricle and the lungs, and severe cyanosis ensues.

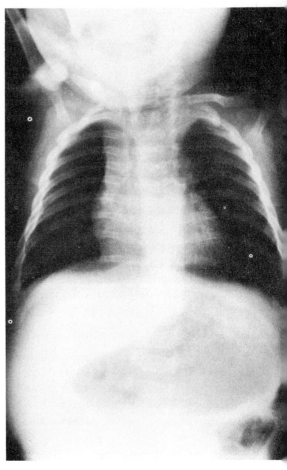

FIG. 7–9. Frontal chest x ray of infant with tetralogy of Fallot. The heart appears small. There is marked pulmonary undercirculation. The mild concavity along the upper portion of the left heart border is secondary to relative hypoplasia of the pulmonary artery segment.

Clinical Features. Pulmonary stenosis is only rarely severe enough to cause significant difficulties in the neonatal period. The infants are generally asymptomatic and have a systolic ejection murmur audible at the left base. A variable systolic click may also be heard at the mid-left sternal border.

In critical pulmonary stenosis, congestive heart failure and cyanosis may be present, but severe obstruction may also be present in the totally asymptomatic baby. In this situation, cardiac findings of a loud, late-peaking murmur and an ECG allow the degree of severity to be assessed.

The ECG shows right axis deviation and

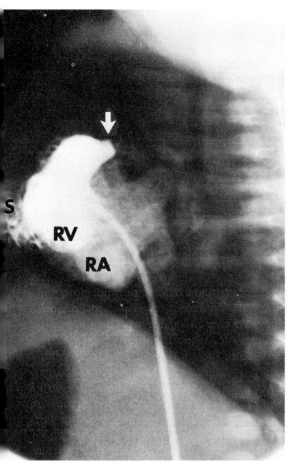

FIG. 7–10. Lateral projection of right ventricular angiocardiogram in a patient with pulmonary atresia and intact ventricular septum. The pulmonary outflow tract ends blindly (arrow). Insufficiency of the tricuspid valve has caused filling of the right atrium (RA). Coronary sinusoids (S) opacify secondary to marked hypertension in right ventricle (RV).

right ventricular hypertrophy. In severe cases, right ventricular strain and right atrial enlargement will be present. The x ray in mild or moderate pulmonary stenosis is usually normal. In cases of severe obstruction, accompanied by congestive heart failure, the heart will be increased in size. With the additional presence of an atrial right-to-left shunt, the pulmonary vascular markings will be decreased.

Management. When mild or moderate pulmonary stenosis is present, no special diag-

nostic tests or specific treatment need be undertaken. Cardiac catheterization may be deferred. If severe stenosis is suspected, cardiac catheterization should be carried out on an emergency basis (89). A Brock valvotomy is the treatment of choice for the very young infant. Infants over two to three months of age are candidates for correction using cardiopulmonary bypass. Results are generally excellent, although occasionally reoperation may be required later.

Pulmonary Atresia with Intact Ventricular Septum

In pulmonary atresia with intact ventricular septum there is no outflow from the right ventricle, which often is a diminutive, functionless blind pouch, hence the alternate designation of hypoplastic right ventricle syndrome. Occasionally, however, a normal-sized right ventricle is encountered. Pulmonary atresia with intact ventricular septum accounts for 1% of congenital heart defects.

Blood flow to the lung is limited (Fig. 7–10) and occurs via a patent ductus arteriosus or bronchial collateral circulation, or both. In the presence of pulmonary atresia, blood entering the right ventricle may regurgitate to the right atrium or be diffused directly into the coronary sinusoids and thence retrograde into the coronary arteries and aorta. The latter occurs when the obstructed right ventricle develops suprasystemic pressure and the tricuspid valve maintains a reasonable degree of competence. In addition, there is a tendency for the thick, overburdened right ventricle to infarct.

Clinical Features. Infants with pulmonary atresia and intact ventricular septum become markedly cyanotic as the patent ductus arteriosus narrows or closes soon after birth. Marked dyspnea is present, and marked acidemia may rapidly develop. A systolic murmur is usually audible at the left sternal border and may be continuous at the left base. The murmurs are usually attributed to the patent ductus or to tricuspid insufficiency. The second heart sound is single. Hepatomegaly may be present. The arterial pulses are good as long as cardiovascular collapse has not developed.

The ECG shows a frontal plane axis that can range from superior to right inferior. The majority fall in the range of $+30°$ to $+120°$. Left ventricular preponderance is usually present, but in cases with large right ventricular chambers, right ventricular enlargement may be seen. The x ray shows moderate to marked cardiomegaly and a marked decrease in pulmonary vasculature.

Management. Following initial stabilization of the acidemia, urgent cardiac catheterization and angiocardiography are mandatory to document the size of the right ventricle and the avenue of pulmonary blood flow. Following catheterization the infant should undergo a combined surgical procedure including a Waterston shunt (between the right pulmonary artery and ascending aorta) and a Brock transventricular pulmonary valvotomy. The shunt allows an immediate increase in pulmonary blood flow, and the valvotomy may allow enough forward flow to cause the right ventricle to decompress and develop in size with time (92, 93). However, in some instances a valvotomy alone is sufficient.

Congestive heart failure may occur following surgery as a result of marked increase in the pulmonary blood flow from the Waterston procedure. Digitalization is then necessary, and even shunt revision has been required at times.

The prognosis for infants with pulmonary atresia with intact ventricular septum is guarded, but palliation has been increasingly successful in some centers, and in recent years, later total correction has been carried out in a few patients using valve homografts or artificial prostheses.

Tricuspid Atresia

Tricuspid atresia accounts for 3% of patients with congenital heart disease. In this disorder there is total absence of the tricuspid orifice with consequent hypoplasia of the right ventricle. The right ventricular cavity is rarely more than a small remnant of an outflow tract. Several variations exist, but in all cases a patent foramen ovale or an atrial septal defect is present; 85% also have a ventricular septal defect. In the remaining 15%, pulmonary blood flow is supplied solely by a patent ductus arteriosus. Of patients with tricuspid atresia, 30% have associated transposition of the great vessels, and these are invariably associated with large ventricular septal defects.

Venous blood returning to the right atrium from the superior vena cava and inferior vena cava passes into the left atrium via the interatrial communication and subsequently mixes with pulmonary venous return as it flows into the left ventricle. However, blood flow enters the pulmonary artery by way of the ventricular septal defect, so that pulmonary blood flow is most often limited by the size of the ventricular septal defect or the degree of right ventricular outflow tract obstruction, or both. When no ventricular septal defect is present, blood reaches the pulmonary artery via a patent ductus arteriosus.

In approximately 25% of cases, pulmonary blood flow is increased in early infancy, but in most instances pulmonary obstruction increases with time. Among patients with tricuspid atresia, transpostion of the great vessels and a large ventricular septal defect, pulmonary blood flow is increased.

Clinical Features

Cyanosis is usually recognized within the first few weeks of life; the more severe the cyanosis, the greater is the degree of obstruction to pulmonary blood flow. Patients with large pulmonary blood flow may rarely present with findings of congestive heart failure at one to three weeks of age.

A systolic murmur is generally present along the left sternal border and left base and may be secondary to either the ventricular septal defect or a patent ductus arteriosus. The second heart sound is most often single. Hepatomegaly is inconstant; a pulsating liver or prominent neck veins occur rarely, and if present, are accounted for by inadequate interatrial communication.

The ECG (Fig. 7–11) is of great diagnos-

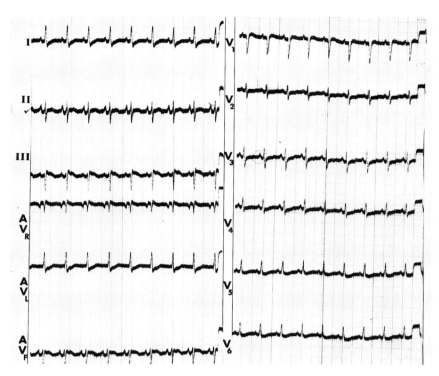

FIG. 7–11. ECG of an infant with tricuspid atresia. The frontal plane QRS axis is −30°. The precordial leads are compatible with relative right ventricular hypoplasia and left ventricular hypertrophy. Peaked P waves in lead II suggest right atrial enlargement.

tic importance in this lesion (96). In 80% of cases there is a superior axis with a counter-clockwise rotation of the frontal plane QRS vector loop. This is accompanied in most instances by left ventricular hypertrophy. Tall and notched P waves may be evident. Radiologic features generally include a heart that is normal to slightly enlarged and decreased pulmonary vascular markings. However, the x-ray findings vary depending on pulmonary blood flow.

Management. Management of tricuspid atresia during the neonatal period depends on the pulmonary blood flow. When flow is inadequate and either severe cyanosis with hypoxic episodes or growth failure occur, the creation of a surgical pulmonary-to-systemic shunt is mandatory. During the first six months of life, a Waterston (right pulmonary artery-to-ascending aorta) anastomosis is utilized. Eventual management is simplified if the infant can reach the age where this approach can be avoided. Later, a Glenn (superior vena cava-to-right pulmonary artery) procedure is the operation of choice. Recently an operation has been devised that allows right atrial blood to flow directly into the pulmonary artery by means

of a conduit (Fontan procedure). This can only be attempted in older patients.

Ebstein's Anomaly of the Tricuspid Valve

This anomaly consists of a downward displacement of a portion of the tricuspid valve into the right ventricle. The tricuspid valve itself is markedly deformed and insufficient, and there is, secondarily, marked hypertrophy of the right atrium with dilatation of the foramen ovale. The lesion is quite rare, accounting for 0.6% of congenital cardiac abnormalities.

The major hemodynamic feature is tricuspid regurgitation with subsequent right atrial enlargement. The right atrium often contracts poorly, consequently causing poor right ventricular filling and atrial right-to-left shunting with decreased pulmonary blood flow.

Clinical Features. Not all patients with Ebstein's anomaly are recognized during the neonatal period. Symptomatic cases generally present with cyanosis only and occasionally with tachypnea. A loud systolic murmur of tricuspid insufficiency is audible along the left sternal border. The second heart sound is normal. Characteristically, third and fourth heart sounds are audible, resulting in a triple or quadruple rhythm. A diastolic murmur of relative tricuspid stenosis may also be audible.

Of clinical interest is the apparent decreasing cyanosis in surviving infants. This feature has been attributed to the increasing pulmonary blood flow that occurs with the fall in pulmonary vascular resistance.

Atrial arrhythmias are a major clinical problem. Atrial flutter, supraventricular tachycardias and the Wolff-Parkinson-White syndrome are not infrequent.

The ECG classically demonstrates large P waves and a right ventricular conduction delay. The PR interval is often prolonged. The chest x ray characteristically shows severe cardiomegaly, often of such magnitude as to totally obscure the lung fields. The pulmonary vascular markings are usually decreased.

Management. Treatment is often directed towards control of the arrhythmias. When congestive heart failure occurs secondary to the tricuspid insufficiency, anticongestive measures are employed. Surgical palliation of the cyanosis has not met with much success in the neonatal period. In older infants a Glenn shunt may be successful. Replacement of the tricuspid valve has been employed in older infants and children (97) but has not been successfully carried out in the neonatal period.

CARDIOMYOPATHIES

GLYCOGEN STORAGE DISEASE OF THE HEART

Glycogen storage disease of the heart is an inborn error of metabolism that results in the abnormal deposition of glycogen in the heart as well as in other bodily tissues

(101). The disorder is familial, transmitted by a single autosomal recessive gene. The type II form (Pompe's disease), which is related to a biochemical aberration of the enzyme acid maltase (α-1,4-glucosidase), primarily affects the heart. The myocardium becomes laden with glycogen deposits that interfere with proper function. Congestive heart failure resulting from myocardial pump failure presents within the neonatal period and is associated with clinical signs indistinguishable from other forms of cardiac failure.

Clinical examination reveals a large heart, weak pulses and absence of murmurs. Generalized hypotonia and lethargy often accompany the syndrome. The x ray shows an enlarged heart with evidence of pulmonary congestion. The ECG may be of considerable help, as one often sees significantly increased voltage over the left precordium associated with ST–T wave alterations. Abbreviated PR intervals are commonly present and are an excellent diagnostic sign. The diagnosis is confirmed definitively by means of muscle biopsy.

The condition is not amenable to therapy, and most infants are dead prior to the end of the first year of life, most often as a result of sudden arrhythmias. Antiarrhythmic drugs may be useful in the management of some infants.

ANOMALOUS LEFT CORONARY ARTERY

Anomalous origin of the left coronary artery from the pulmonary artery is a rare congenital cardiac defect. In most cases, blood flows from the aorta and the normally originating right coronary artery into the left coronary artery and pulmonary artery via myocardial intercoronary anastomoses. Hence, improper perfusion of a major portion of the left ventricular myocardium and myocardial infarction may occur (infantile type). In some instances, extensive collaterals from the right coronary artery supply the left ventricular myocardium, thus averting decreased myocardial perfusion, and no signs are observed. However, the majority of patients have some, but not total, decrease in myocardial oxygenation. If the myocardium is spared, the patient may present later with signs of a coronary artery–pulmonary artery fistula and no myocardial damage. This is often referred to as the "adult type" (103).

The neonate may have anginal pain manifested by crying during feedings, but this history is difficult to interpret. Most often, the infants become diaphoretic and markedly tachypneic, and physical examination discloses signs of congestive heart failure. Pansystolic apical murmurs are not infrequent and are secondary to mitral regurgitation induced by papillary muscle infarction. Later, short systolic or even continuous murmurs may be heard due to the coronary artery–pulmonary artery shunt.

The ECG is of considerable help in the diagnosis of this abnormality in symptomatic infants. Marked T wave inversions and deep Q waves in standard leads I and AV_L and the left precordial leads (V_5 to V_6) are seen as well, suggesting an anterolateral myocardial infarction. The chest x ray shows significant cardiomegaly and pulmonary venous congestion.

Following demonstration of left coronary to pulmonary artery flow by cardiac catheterization, surgical treatment of the anomaly must be undertaken (102). In most centers this is accomplished by ligation of the anomalous vessel, allowing collateral blood flow from the right coronary to reach the lateral left ventricular myocardium. However, if severe damage has occurred, the prognosis remains guarded. Detaching the aberrant vessel from the pulmonary artery and anastomosing it to the aorta provides a more physiologic approach. However, for technical reasons, this techique has been generally limited to the older child with an adult type fistula.

ENDOCARDIAL FIBROELASTOSIS

Endocardial fibroelastosis is a defect in which there is marked endocardial thickening due to proliferation of subendocardial fibroelastic tissue. A rather typical shiny grayish white appearance of the endocardial surface is noted pathologically. This disorder primarily involves the left ventricular myocardium, but on occasion, atrial and right ventricular involvement are noted. A primary and secondary type have been identified, the latter being associated with severe left ventricular deformity or hypertension (hypoplastic left heart syndrome, aortic stenosis, coarctation of the aorta). The etiology of the disorder is unclear, but several viruses have been implicated (100). Primary endocardial fibroelastosis in the neonatal period may be a residual of fetal myocarditis. However, a definitive cause and effect relationship has never been clearly documented.

The hemodynamic consequences that lead to symptomatology with this lesion are entirely secondary to left ventricular muscle failure and resultant left atrial and pulmonary venous hypertension. The condition may simulate severe mitral stenosis if either the mitral valve or its apparatus is significantly involved.

The disease should be considered as a diagnostic possibility in a neonate presenting with marked congestive failure in the absence of significant murmurs.

The ECG reveals significantly increased left ventricular forces with T wave abnormalities in V_5 and V_6. The chest x ray shows a dilated, enlarged heart and pulmonary venous distension.

The classic findings at cardiac catheterization include significantly elevated left ventricular end-diastolic, left atrial and pulmonary venous pressures. Left ventricular ejection fractions are significantly decreased, and angiography shows a poorly contracting left ventricular myocardial wall.

The differentiation of primary endocardial fibroelastosis from other cardiomyopathies is histologic, and therefore, definitive diagnosis can be made only on a pathologic basis. If the infant recovers with apparently complete resolution of disease, the original diagnosis of endocardial fibroelastosis must remain in doubt. The infants are managed medically with the standard cardiotonic regimen, including digitalis preparations and diuretics. A number of these patients initially respond to therapy only to exacerbate and succumb at a later time.

INFECTIOUS MYOCARDITIS

A number of infectious agents have been implicated in the etiology of neonatal myocarditis (100). These have been primarily viral and include group B coxsackie viruses, mumps, influenza, cytomegalovirus, h. simplex and rubella. Epidemics have been described. Sporadic cases have been attributed to psittacosis, infectious mononucleosis, toxoplasmosis and others.

The infection is generally transmitted in utero, and the neonate usually develops signs within the first week of life. Murmurs are rarely present, but congestive failure and gallop rhythms are common.

The chest x ray shows evidence of significant cardiomegaly and pulmonary vascular congestion. The ECG typically shows low QRS voltage and flat T waves over the left precordial leads. Arrhythmias are commonly noted and may occur as a terminal event.

Attempts should be made to recover the etiologic agent by culturing of stool, urine, throat and blood. Blood samples for antibody titers should be collected during an acute illness and six weeks later. Treatment should be instituted with digitalis and other agents. Care must be taken in administering digitalis preparations since infants with myocarditis may be especially sensitive to the drug. Antibiotics should be reserved for those instances when the possibility of bacterial sepsis is high or when specific etiologic agents have been recovered. In unresponsive cases, corticosteroids have been employed with questionable success. Neonatal myocarditis carries a guarded prognosis.

ASPLENIA AND POLYSPLENIA SYNDROMES

Asplenia, congenital absence of the spleen, and polysplenia, the presence of multiple small spleens, are usually associated with complex cardiac defects, most often involving abnormalities of the cardiac situs, e.g., dextrocardia and atrial situs inversus. Common atrium or single ventricle, or both, occur often and are found in combination with other defects, including total anomalous pulmonary venous drainage, left superior vena cava and common atrioventricular valve. Pulmonary valve stenosis or atresia, and transposition of the great arteries are more likely with asplenia. Absence of the inferior vena cava is to be expected in cases of the polysplenia syndrome. The multiplicity of the cardiac abnormalities signifies what appears to be a form of arrest of normal cardiovascular development in all aspects.

The hemodynamics and consequent clinical features of congestive heart failure or hypoxia, are dependent on the defects involved. In most instances signs appear early in infancy and are severe. The liver, both clinically and radiologically, is frequently noted to be transverse in the midline. When asplenia is present, the peripheral blood smear contains Howell-Jolly bodies. The chest x ray often shows abnormalities of abdominal and cardiac situs and cardiac enlargement. The EKG is quite variable. Abnormalities in Q wave progression may be seen, as may right ventricular enlargement. A left superior frontal plane QRS axis is common.

Surgical treatment, when possible, is palliative and is directed at control of pulmonary blood flow via either a surgical systemic-pulmonary artery shunt or pulmonary artery banding, depending on the anatomy. The overall outlook for these infants has been poor, but some patients may be amenable to correction with the advent of more sophisticated surgical techniques.

CARDIAC CATHETERIZATION

INDICATIONS

Cardiac catheterization is indicated in the infant who demonstrates either congestive heart failure or marked cyanosis considered secondary to a cardiac malformation. However, clinical diagnostic possibilities must be carefully considered prior to the study in order to avoid the possibility that a sick infant with pulmonary or CNS disease will undergo the additional risk of unnecessary hemodynamic study.

If cardiac catheterization is to be done in a critically ill infant with congenital heart disease, a surgical team should be alerted in the event that an operation must follow immediately. In general, catheterization studies on neonates should be done at a medical center with the capabilities for providing total pediatric and surgical care. The surgical group should be experienced with the specific palliative and definitive cardiac surgical procedures that may be required.

In most situations, catheterization should be done when an infant is in the most optimal condition possible, after a clinical diagnosis of heart disease has been made, and hypothermia, hypoxia, acidosis and congestive heart failure have been evaluated and treated. The procedure should be done before the physiologic sequelae of the cardiac defect leads to irreversible deterioration despite medical therapy.

A key factor in the initial differential diagnosis of congenital heart disease and, hence, in the timing of cardiac catheterization is the magnitude of pulmonary blood flow as determined by x ray. Medical treatment offers little or nothing in the management of marked hypoxia secondary to decreased effective pulmonary blood flow. Although initial improvement may occur after treatment of hypothermia and acidosis, the situation only worsens with time. In some instances, a patent ductus arteriosus (which may be the only significant source of pulmonary blood flow) suddenly narrows or closes, rapidly causing terminal hypoxemia and acidosis. Since balloon septostomy or emergency surgical intervention for a palliative shunt or valvotomy may be lifesaving, infants with decreased or normal pulmonary vascularity are likely to require immediate cardiac catheterization. Similarly, there are times when left ventricular obstructive disease with pulmonary congestion (e.g., aortic stenosis, coarctation of the aorta) is present to such a severe degree that catheterization and operation may not be safely postponed

for even a few hours. On the other hand, when pulmonary vascularity is increased because of ventricular volume overload, digitalization and other anticongestive measures for 24 to 72 hours may improve the patient's condition considerably and reduce the risk of cardiac catheterization and subsequent surgery. On occasion, among older infants with large left-to-right shunts, the improvement may be so striking that surgical intervention may not be necessary during early infancy.

RISKS

The risk of cardiac catheterization is higher among seriously ill infants than among older patients. One cooperative study on cardiac catheterization (105) collected data from 16 institutions and found a death rate of 6% among small infants as compared to a 0.44% overall mortality. Ho et al (106) reported a mortality rate of 3% for each of the first two months of life during cardiac catheterization. Of 27 deaths, 13 occurred within the first 48 hours of life. Some degree of increased mortality may be expected for infants, but these statistics also reflect the fact that infants are often studied when in extremely poor condition, even in extremis, and that some will have cardiac lesions that are incompatible with viability. Cardiac catheterization mortality figures thus include many patients for whom death reflects the natural history of the disorder, rather than a procedural complication.

The risk of hemodynamic study depends to a great degree on the experience and technical skill of the physician carrying out the procedure, but factors related to environmental conditions and the cardiac catheterization team's readiness to deal with complications are also of major importance in lowering morbidity and mortality.

ASSOCIATED PROCEDURES

Balloon Septostomy

In 1966 Rashkind and Miller (107) reported a method for increasing the mixing of blood at the atrial level in patients with transposition of the great vessels. A balloon-tipped catheter is inserted into the femoral vein

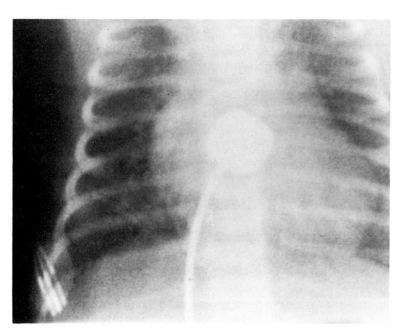

FIG. 7–12. Frontal frame of cineangiocardiogram during a balloon atrial septostomy. The balloon was inflated with contrast material following placement of the catheter into the left atrium via the patent foramen ovale. The catheter is then vigorously withdrawn into the right atrium, fracturing the interatrial septum in the process.

and advanced to the right atrium and across the foramen ovale into the left atrium. The balloon is then inflated and the catheter vigorously withdrawn to the right atrium. The balloon fractures the atrial septum, thereby enlarging the interatrial communication (Fig. 7–12). This procedure has now found use in other lesions in which obstruction to free flow across the atrial septum is detrimental, e.g., pulmonary atresia, tricuspid atresia, total anomalous pulmonary venous connection and hypoplastic left heart syndrome.

Angiocardiography

Angiocardiograms should be performed with the greatest of care and should be limited only to those that are essential for accurate diagnosis and management. Since the number of angiocardiograms which may be safely carried out is limited, the sites of injection must be carefully selected.

COMPLICATIONS

Major complications associated with cardiac catheterization include: 1) development of arrhythmias, 2) hypothermia and acidosis, 3) myocardial perforation and 4) venous or arterial hemorrhage, or both (108).

Particular care must be taken in observing sick infants after cardiac catheterization, and it is suggested that they be carefully observed and monitored in intensive care facilities for 12 to 24 hours following study.

ECHOCARDIOGRAPHY

Echocardiography is a useful noninvasive method of evaluating structural cardiac abnormalities in the neonate (Fig. 7–13). A beam of high-frequency sound waves (ultrasound) is directed at intracardiac structures in a standardized fashion. The reflected waves, or echoes, are then displayed on an oscilloscope to be utilized in the evaluation of cardiac anatomy and physiology. The most common form of echocardiographic display is the single plane M scan. More recently, two dimensional displays (B scan) have also been devised. Methods using multiple beams of sound (multiscan) are also presently being evaluated.

Echocardiography has been useful principally in the evaluation of left atrial size, mitral valve motion and size of the ventricular septum. In the neonate, a principal application has been in the diagnosis of the hypoplastic left heart syndrome. The inability to record a mitral valve echo in a newborn infant is highly suggestive, if not diagnostic, of mitral valve atresia. When this is associated with the additional findings of left ventricular and left atrial hypoplasia, the diagnosis of hypoplastic left heart syndrome is virtually assured. In some

centers, the echocardiographic diagnosis of this syndrome may be considered sufficiently firm so as to preclude the necessity of cardiac catheterization since most of these patients are not operable. Echocardiography has also been useful in the assessment of various other forms of severe congenital heart disease in infants.

CARDIAC SURGERY IN THE NEONATE

The great strides in pediatric cardiology and particularly in neonatal cardiology are in large part due to the surgical procedures devised to either totally correct or palliate otherwise fatal lesions. Total correction of all lesions carried out at whatever age necessary is the goal, but although much progress has been made towards this ideal, palliative

FIG. 7–13. Echocardiogram of: **A.** Normal infant. **B.** Infant with hypoplastic left heart syndrome. In B, only a large right ventricular cavity is well visualized; the tricuspid valve can be seen; the left ventricular cavity is significantly diminished; and mitral valve motion is markedly attenuated. CW = Chest wall; RV = Right ventricular cavity; VS = Ventricular septum; Arrows (in A) = Anterior leaflet of mitral valve; Closed arrows (in B) = Tricuspid valve; and Open arrows (in B) = Mitral valve.

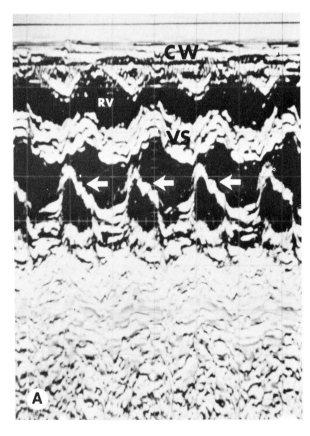

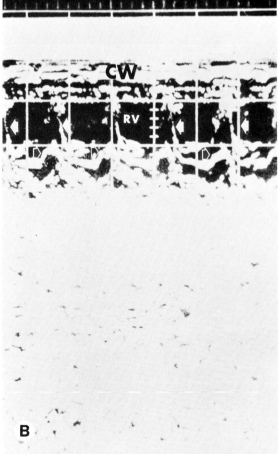

procedures are still necessary for many lesions (123).

PALLIATIVE PROCEDURES

Lesions with Decreased Pulmonary Blood Flow

In 1945 Dr. Alfred Blalock (114) performed the first "blue-baby" operation. Pulmonary blood flow was augmented in patients with tetralogy of Fallot and other defects in which there is decreased pulmonary blood flow by anastomosing the subclavian artery to the pulmonary artery. The advantage of the Blalock-Taussig procedure over other types of systemic to pulmonary artery anastomoses is that systemic pressure is not transmitted to the lungs and excess pulmonary blood flow rarely leads to congestive heart failure. However, this operation has not been feasible in the neonate because of the small caliber of the subclavian artery.

The Potts' anastomosis (122) joins the descending aorta to the left pulmonary artery, and the Waterston procedure (124) joins the ascending aorta to the right pulmonary artery. Both serve the same purpose as the Blalock-Taussig shunt and are utilized primarily for small infants. The latter shunt is the procedure of choice because of its easy accessibility during later repairative surgery. The size of the aortopulmonary communication in these side-to-side anastomoses is totally dependent on surgical judgment. Great care must be taken so as not to create a shunt which is too large, with subsequent congestive heart failure, or too small, resulting in inadequate palliation. Large shunts are not uncommon, and congestive heart failure occurred in approximately one-third of patients in a large series of Waterston and Potts' shunts.

The Glenn (117) procedure is a shunt operation that diverts flow from the right side of the heart by anastomosing the superior vena cava directly to the right pulmonary artery. It is also reserved for older infants and children for technical reasons. Since the Glenn shunt is at present considered a permanent operation, it is gen-erally performed only in those patients in whom eventual total correction is not considered to be feasible.

Lesions with Increased Pulmonary Blood Flow

The pulmonary artery banding procedure was devised for those infants with pulmonary hypertension secondary to increased pulmonary blood flow associated with congestive heart failure who could not be successfully managed medically through infancy. A ligature, or "band," is placed about the pulmonary artery just distal to the pulmonary valve (118, 121). The ligature is tightened so that the pulmonary artery systolic pressure, measured directly at surgery, falls to approximately one-third to one-half of the systemic systolic pressure. This limits the size of the left-to-right shunt and protects the pulmonary arteriolar bed from damage due to overcirculation at high pressure. The placement of an acute obstruction to right ventricular outflow may cause the ventricle to fail suddenly in the absence of an interventricular communication. Thus, the procedure is recommended only for patients in whom a large ventricular septal defect is present, either as an isolated defect or as part of a more complex malformation. The banding may be carried out later as part of a corrective open heart operation.

Procedures to Increase Mixing

The Blalock-Hanlon (113) procedure is a partial atrial septectomy carried out under inflow occlusion. It allows for increased mixing of the pulmonary and systemic venous circulations in transposition of the great vessels. The procedure has been largely replaced by the balloon atrial septostomy, which is performed at the time of cardiac catheterization.

The Edwards (116) procedure is a modification of the Blalock-Hanlon whereby a portion of the pulmonary venous return is directed into the right atrium by repositioning of the atrial septum.

TOTAL CORRECTION

Certain corrective procedures do not require open-heart techniques. Coarctation of the aorta, patent ductus arteriosus and severe pulmonic stenosis can be corrected by a closed-heart procedure. The latter is accomplished by a transventricular pulmonary valvotomy (Brock procedure) (115). In critical situations this operation is lifesaving, although reoperation using open-heart techniques may be required at a later date.

Total correction is now performed in a number of major centers on infants less than six months of age with various congenital heart defects including ventricular septal defect, aortic stenosis, pulmonary stenosis, transposition of the great vessels, atrial septal defect and total anomalous pulmonary venous connection. The youngest patient to receive a successful open-heart

procedure (at the Columbia-Presbyterian Medical Center) was a child two weeks of age with total anomalous pulmonary venous connection (119). These procedures should be attempted only after definitive catheterizations have been obtained and at centers specializing in this type of surgical care.

Total cardiopulmonary bypass using normothermia or deep hypothermia has been successfully utilized in the neonatal age group (112, 120). Postsurgical management of these infants is of extreme importance. Airway problems, acid-base disturbances and arrhythmias can cause rapid demise if optimal intensive care management is not maintained in the critical immediate postoperative period. Mechanical positive pressure endotracheal ventilation is utilized in

FIG. 7–14. Recovery area adapted for the infant who has undergone operative repair of an intracardiac lesion using cardiopulmonary bypass.

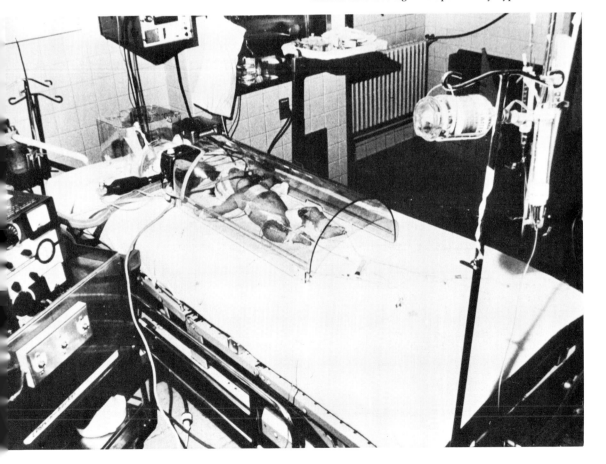

virtually all infants after open-heart surgery for 24 to 72 hours in order to avoid the early complication of fatigue, hypoventilation, acidosis and subsequent respiratory arrest.

In general, if surgical intervention has successfully corrected or palliated the hemodynamic abnormality, the later postoperative period is one of rapid improvement of cardiac function to well beyond the preoperative status, without undue difficulties in management.

The essential prerequisite for a successful outcome following surgery for infants with congenital heart disease is an operation that achieves anatomic correction or palliation of the basic hemodynamic abnormality. In addition, however, careful perioperative medical management is required to prepare the critically ill infant for surgery and to allow him to benefit from its technical accomplishment (Fig. 7–14).

The goals during the preoperative period are twofold: to attain optimal cardiorespiratory status and to obtain an accurate diagnosis. Following surgery, physiologic data is meticulously monitored, and intensive supportive care is instituted.

REFERENCES

EMBRYOLOGY

1. Duckworth JWA: Embryology of congenital heart disease. In Heart Disease in Infancy and Childhood. Edited by JD Keith, RD Rowe, P Vlad. New York, Macmillan, 1967
2. Goor DA, Dische R, Lillehei CW: The conotruncus. I. Its normal inversion and conus absorption. Circulation 46:375, 1972
3. Langman J, Van Mierop LHS: Development of the cardiovascular system. In: Heart Disease in Infants, Children, and Adolescents. Edited by AJ Moss, FH Adams. Baltimore, Williams & Wilkins, 1968, p 3
4. Van Mierop LHS, Alley RD, Kausel HW, Stranahan A: Pathogenesis of transposition complexes. I. Embryology of the ventricles and great arteries. Am J Cardiol 12:216, 1963

PERINATAL CIRCULATION

5. Gessner I, Krovetz LJ, Benson RW, Prystowsky H, Stenger V, Eitzman DV: Hemodynamic adaptations in the newborn infant. Pediatrics 36:752, 1965
6. Rudolph AM: The effects of postnatal circulatory adjustments in congenital heart disease. Pediatrics 36:763, 1965

INTRODUCTION AND INHERITANCE PATTERNS

7. Edwards JH: Simulation of Mendelism. Acta Genet (Basel) 10:63, 1960
7a. Gersony WM, Katz SL, Nadas AS: Endocardial fibroelastosis and the mumps virus. Pediatrics 37:430, 1966
8. Gibson S, Lewis KC: Congenital heart disease following maternal rubella during pregnancy. Am J Dis Child 83:317, 1952
9. Jackson BT: The pathogenesis of congenital cardiovascular anomalies. N Engl J Med 279:25, 1968
10. Keith JD, Rowe RD, Vlad P: Heart Disease in Infancy and Childhood, 2nd ed. New York, Macmillan, 1967
11. Mitchell SC, Korones SB, Berendes HW: Congenital heart disease in 56,109 births. Incidence and natural history. Circulation 43:323, 1971
12. Nadas AS, Fyler DC: Pediatric Cardiology, 3rd ed. Philadelphia, Saunders, 1972
13. Nora JJ: Multifactorial inheritance hypothesis for the etiology of congenital heart diseases. The genetic-environmental interaction. Circulation 38:604, 1968
14. Noren GR, Adams P, Anderson RC: Positive skin reactivity to mumps virus antigen in endocardial fibroelastosis. J Pediatr 62:604, 1963

THE NEONATAL ELECTROCARDIOGRAM AND ARRHYTHMIAS

15. Bigger JT, Goldreyer BN: The mechanism of supraventricular tachycardia. Circulation 42:673, 1970
16. Emmanouilides GC, Moss AJ, Adams FH: The electrocardiogram in normal newborn infants: correlation with hemodynamic observations. J Pediatr 67:578, 1965
17. Hastreiter AR, Abella JB: The electrocardiogram in the newborn period. I. The normal infant. J Pediatr 78:146, 1971
18. Hastreiter AR, Abella JB: The electrocardiogram in the newborn period. II. The infant with disease. J Pediatr 78:346, 1971
19. Linde LM, Turner SW, Awa S: Present status and treatment of paroxysmal supraventricular tachycardia. Pediatrics 50:127, 1972
20. Lundberg A: Paroxysmal tachycardia in infancy: follow-up study of 47 subjects ranging in age from 10 to 26 years. Pediatrics 51:26, 1973
21. Moller JH, Davachi F, Anderson RC: Atrial flutter in infancy. J Pediatr 75:643, 1969
22. Narula OS: Wolff-Parkinson-White syndrome. A review. Circulation 47:872, 1973

23. Rutkowski MM, Doyle EF, Cohen SN: Drug therapy of heart disease in pediatric patients. III. The therapeutic challenge of supraventricular tachyarrhythmias in infants and children. Am Heart J 86:562, 1973

24. Schiebler GL, Adams P, Anderson RD: The Wolff-Parkinson-White syndrome in infants and children. Pediatrics 24:585, 1959

25. Swiderski J, Lees MH, Nadas AS: The Wolff-Parkinson-White syndrome in infancy and childhood. Br Heart J 24:561, 1972

CONGENITAL COMPLETE HEART BLOCK

26. Ayers CR, Boineau JP, Spach MS: Congenital complete heart block in children. Am Heart J 72:381, 1966

27. Campbell M, Thorne MG: Congenital heart block. Br Heart J 18:90, 1956

28. Corne RA, Mathewson FAL: Congenital complete atrioventricular block. A 25-year follow-up study. Am J Cardiol 29:412, 1972

29. Griffith GC, Zinn WJ, Vural IL: Familial cardiomyopathy. Heart block and Stokes-Adams attacks treated by pacemaker implantation. Am J Cardiol 16:267, 1965

30. Griffiths SP: Congenital complete heart block. (editorial) Circulation 43:615, 1971

31. Kelly DT, Brodsky SJ, Mirowski MD, Krovetz LJ, Rowe RD: Bundle of His recordings in congenital complete heart block. Circulation 45:277, 1972

32. Lev M, Silverman J, Fitzmaurice FM, Paul MH, Cassels DC, Miller RA: Lack of connection between the atria and the more peripheral conduction system in congenital atrioventricular block. Am J Cardiol 27:481, 1971

33. Liu L, Griffiths SP, Gerst PH: Implanted cardiac pacemakers in children. A report of their application in five patients. Am J Cardiol 20:639, 1967

CONGESTIVE HEART FAILURE

34. Goldring D, Hernandez A, Hartmann AF Jr: The critically ill child: care of the infant in cardiac failure. Pediatrics 47:1056, 1971

35. Hayes CJ, Butler VP, Gersony WM: Serum digoxin studies in infants and children. Pediatrics 52:561, 1973

36. Lees MH: Heart failure in the newborn infant. Recognition and management. J Pediatr 75:139, 1969

37. Rudolph AM: Cardiac failure in children: a hemodynamic overview. Hosp Prac 5:44, 1970

38. Shaffer AB, Katz LN: Hemodynamic alterations in congestive heart failure. N Engl J Med 276:853, 1967

39. Tikoff, G, Kuida H: Pathophysiology of heart failure in congenital heart disease. Mod Concepts Cardiovasc Dis 41:1, 1972

40. Varat MA, Adolph RJ, Fowler NO: Cardio-vascular effects of anemia. Am Heart J 83:415, 1972

LEFT-TO-RIGHT SHUNTS

41. Rudolph AM: The changes in the circulation after birth. Their importance in congenital heart disease. Circulation 41:343, 1970

VENTRICULAR SEPTAL DEFECT

42. Edwards JE: The pathology of ventricular septal defect. Semin Roentgenol 1:2, 1966

43. Hoffman JIE, Rudolph AM: The natural history of ventricular septal defects in infancy. Am J Cardiol 16:634, 1965

44. Hoffman JIE, Rudolph AM: Increasing pulmonary vascular resistance during infancy in association with ventricular septal defect. Pediatrics 38:220, 1966

45. Rose V, Collins G, Kidd L, Keith J: Clinico-hemodynamic correlations in ventricular septal defect in childhood. J Pediatr 69:359, 1966

46. Spach MS, Boineau JP, Canent RV Jr: Defects of the ventricular septum. In: Heart Disease in Infants, Children, and Adolescents. Edited by AJ Moss, FH Adams. Baltimore, Williams & Wilkins, 1968

47. Sigmann JM, Stern AM, Sloan HE: Early surgical correction of large ventricular septal defects. Pediatrics 39:4, 1967

PATENT DUCTUS ARTERIOSUS

48. Kitterman JA, Edmunds LH Jr, Gregory GA, Heymann MA, Tooley WH, Rudolph AM: Patent ductus arteriosus in premature infants. Incidence, relation to pulmonary disease and management. N Engl J Med 287:473, 1972

49. Ziegler RF: Patent ductus arteriosus. In: Heart Disease in Infants, Children, and Adolescents. Edited by AJ Moss, FH Adams. Baltimore, Williams & Wilkins, 1968

ATRIAL SEPTAL DEFECT AND ATRIOVENTRICULAR CANAL

50. Dimich I, Steinfeld L, Park SC: Symptomatic atrial septal defect in infants. Am Heart J 85:601, 1973

51. Hunt CE, Lucas RV Jr: Symptomatic atrial septal defect in infancy. Circulation 47:1042, 1973

52. Nakamura FF, Hauck AJ, Nadas AS: Atrial septal defect in infants. Pediatrics 34:101, 1964

53. Shah CV, Patel MK, Hastreiter AR: Hemodynamics of complete atrioventricular canal and its evolution with age. Am J Cardiol 24:326, 1969

54. Tandon R, Edwards JE: Atrial septal defect in infancy. Common association with other anomalies. Circulation 49:1005, 1974

COARCTATION OF THE AORTA

55. Becker AE, Becker MJ, Edwards JE: Anomalies associated with coarctation of aorta. Particular reference to infancy. Circulation 41:1067, 1970

56. Hartmann AF Jr, Goldring D, Staple TW: Coarctation of the aorta in infancy. Hemodynamic studies. J Pediatr 70:95, 1967

57. Malm JR, Blumenthal S, Jameson AG, Humphreys GH II: Observations on coarctation of the aorta in infants. Arch Surg 86:110, 1963

58. Rudolph AM, Heymann MA, Spitznas U: Hemodynamic considerations in the development of narrowing of the aorta. Am J Cardiol 30:514, 1972

59. Tawes RL Jr, Aberdeen E, Waterston DJ, Bonham-Carter RE: Coarctation of the aorta in infants and children. A review of 333 operative cases, including 179 infants. Circulation 39–40 (Suppl I):173, 1969

AORTIC STENOSIS

60. Antia AU, Wiltse HE, Rowe RD, Pitt EL, Levin S, Ottesen OE, Cooke RE: Pathogenesis of the supravalvular aortic stenosis syndrome. J Pediatr 71:431, 1967

61. Hastreiter AR, Oshima M, Miller RA, Lev M, Paul MH: Congenital aortic stenosis syndrome in infancy. Circulation 28:1084, 1963

62. Lakier JB, Lewis AB, Heymann MA, Stanger P, Hoffman JIE, Rudolph AM: Isolated aortic stenosis in the neonate. Natural history and hemodynamic considerations. Circulation 50:801, 1974

63. Mody MR, Nadas AS, Bernhard WF: Aortic stenosis in infants. N Engl J Med 276:832, 1967

64. Ongley PA, Nadas AS, Paul MH, Rudolph AM, Starkey GWB: Aortic stenosis in infants and children. Pediatrics 21:207, 1958

TRANSPOSITION OF THE GREAT ARTERIES

65. Baker F, Baker L, Zoltun R, Zuberbuhler JR: Effectiveness of the Rashkind procedure in transposition of the great arteries in infants. Circulation 43–44 (Suppl I):1, 1971

66. Clarkson PM, Barratt-Boyes BG, Neutze JM, Lowe JB: Results over a ten year period of palliation followed by corrective surgery for complete transposition of the great arteries. Circulation 45:1251, 1972

67. Goor DA, Edwards JE: The spectrum of transposition of the great arteries. With specific reference to developmental anatomy of the conus. Circulation 48:406, 1973

68. Mair DD, Ritter DG: Factors influencing systemic arterial oxygen saturation in complete transposition of the great arteries. Am J Cardiol 31:742, 1973

69. Noonan JA, Nadas AS, Rudolph AM, Harris GBC: Transposition of the great arteries. A correlation of clinical, physiologic and autopsy data. N Engl J Med 263:592, 1960

70. Plauth WH Jr, Nadas AS, Bernhard WF, Gross, RE: Transposition of the great arteries. Clinical and physiological observations on 74 patients treated by palliative surgery. Circulation 37:316, 1968

71. Shaher RM: What is transposition of the great arteries? (editorial) Am Heart J 87:541, 1974

HYPOPLASTIC LEFT HEART SYNDROME

72. Krovetz LJ, Rowe RD, Schiebler GL: Hemodynamics of aortic valve atresia. Circulation 42:953, 1970

73. Noonan JA, Nadas AS: The hypoplastic left heart syndrome: an analysis of 101 cases. Pediatr Clin North Am 5:1029, 1958

74. Saied A, Folger GM Jr: Hypoplastic left heart syndrome. Clinico-pathologic and hemodynamic correlation. Am J Cardiol 29:190, 1972

SINGLE VENTRICLE

75. Lev M, Liberthson RR, Kirkpatrick JR, Eckner FAO, Arcilla RA: Single (primitive) ventricle. Circulation 39:577, 1969

76. Quero-Jiminez M, Casanova-Gomez M, Castro-Gussoni C, Moreno-Granado F, Perez-Martinez V, Merino-Batres G: Electrocardiographic findings in single ventricle and related conditions. Am Heart J 86:449, 1973

77. Van Praagh R: Single (common) ventricle. In: Heart Disease in Infancy and Childhood, 2nd ed. Edited by JD Keith, RD Rowe, P Vlad. New York, Macmillan, 1967

TRUNCUS ARTERIOSUS

78. Gelband H, Van Meter S, Gersony WM: Truncal valve abnormalities in infants with persistant truncus arteriosus: a clinico-pathologic study. Circulation 45:397, 1972

79. Kreidberg MB, Fisher JH, DeLuca FG, Chernoff HL: Pulmonary artery banding for persistent truncus arteriosus. J Pediatr 64:557, 1964

80. McNamara DG, Sommerville RJ: Truncus arteriosus. In: Heart Disease in Infants, Children, and Adolescents. Edited by AJ Moss, FH Adams. Baltimore, Williams & Wilkins, 1968

TOTAL ANOMALOUS PULMONARY VENOUS CONNECTION

81. El-Said G, Mullins CE, McNamara DG: Management of total anomalous pulmonary venous return. Circulation 45:1240, 1972

82. Gathman GE, Nadas AS: Total anomalous pulmonary venous connection. Clinical and physiologic observations of 75 pediatric patients. Circulation 42:143, 1970

83. Gersony WM, Bowman FO Jr, Steeg CN, Hayes CJ, Jesse MJ, Malm JR: Management of total anomalous pulmonary venous drainage in early infancy. Circulation 43 (Suppl I). 19, 1971

84. Snellen HA, Van Ingen HC, Hoefsmit ECM: Patterns of anomalous pulmonary venous drainage. Circulation 37:45, 1968

TETRALOGY OF FALLOT

85. Bonchek LI, Starr A, Sunderland CO, Menashe VD: Natural history of tetalogy of Fallot in infancy. Clinical classification and therapeutic implications. Circulation 48:392, 1973

86. Sunderland CO, Matarazzo RG, Lees MH, Menashe VD, Bonchek LI, Rosenberg JA, Starr A: Total correction of tetralogy of Fallot in infancy. Postoperative hemodynamic evaluation. Circulation 48:398, 1973

PULMONARY STENOSIS

87. Anderson IM, Nouri-Moghaddam S: Severe pulmonary stenosis in infancy and early childhood. Thorax 24:312, 1969

88. Freed MD, Rosenthal A, Bernhard WF, Litwin SB, Nadas AS: Critical pulmonary stenosis with a diminutive right ventricle in neonates. Circulation 48:875, 1973

89. Gersony WM, Bernhard WF, Nadas AS, Gross RE: Diagnosis and surgical treatment of infants with critical pulmonary outflow obstruction. Circulation 35:765, 1967

90. Luke MJ: Valvular pulmonic stenosis in infancy. J Pediatr 68:90, 1966

PULMONARY ATRESIA

91. Bowman FO Jr, Malm JR, Hayes CJ, Gersony WM, Ellis K: Pulmonary atresia with intact ventricular septum. J Thorac Cardiovasc Surg 61:85, 1971

92. Dhanavaravibul S, Nora JJ, McNamara DG: Pulmonary valvular atresia with intact ventricular septum: problems in diagnosis and results of treatment. J Pediatr 77:1010, 1970

93. Khoury GH, Gilbert EF, Chang CH, Schmidt R: The hypoplastic right heart complex. Clinical, hemodynamic, pathologic and surgical considerations. Am J Cardiol 23:792, 1969

94. Shams A, Fowler RS, Trusler GA, Keith JD, Mustard WT: Pulmonary atresia with intact ventricular septum: report of 50 cases. Pediatrics 47:370, 1971

TRICUSPID ATRESIA

95. Diehl AM, Lauer RM, Shankar KR: Tricuspid atresia. In: Heart Disease in Infants, Children, and Adolescents. Edited by AJ Moss, FH Adams. Baltimore, Williams & Wilkins, 1968

96. Gamboa R, Gersony WM, Nadas AS: The electrocardiogram in tricuspid atresia and pulmonary atresia with intact ventricular septum. Circulation 34:24, 1966

EBSTEIN'S ANOMALY OF THE TRICUSPID VALVE

97. Barnard C, Schrire V: Surgical correction of Ebstein's malformation with a prosthetic tricuspid valve. Surgery 54:302, 1963

98. Bialostozky D, Horwitz S, Espino-Vela J: Ebstein's malformation of the tricuspid valve. A review of 65 cases. Am J Cardiol 29:826, 1972

99. Kumar AE, Fyler DC, Miettinen OS, Nadas AS: Ebstein's anomaly. Clinical profile and natural history. Am J Cardiol 28:84, 1971

CARDIOMYOPATHIES

100. Abelmann WH: Virus and the heart. Circulation 44:950, 1971

101. Hohn AR, Lowe CU, Sokal JE, Lambert EC: Cardiac problems in the glycogenoses with specific reference to Pompe's disease. Pediatrics 35:313, 1965

102. Nora JJ, McNamara DG, Hallman GL, Sommerville RJ, Cooley DA: Medical and surgical management of anomalous origin of the left coronary artery from the pulmonary artery. Pediatrics 42:405, 1968

103. Wesselhoeft H, Fawcett JS, Johnson AL: Anomalous origin of the left coronary artery from the pulmonary trunk. Its clinical spectrum, pathology, and pathophysiology based on a review of 140 cases with seven further cases. Circulation 38:403, 1968

ASPLENIA AND POLYSPLENIA SYNDROMES

104. Van Mierop LHS, Gessner IH, Schiebler GL: Asplenia and polysplenia syndrome. Congenital Cardiac Defects—Recent Advances. National Foundation: March of Dimes 8:74, 1972

CARDIAC CATHETERIZATION

105. Braunwald E, Swan HJC: Cooperative study on cardiac catheterization. American Heart Association Monograph No. 20. Circulation 37 (Suppl III):1, 1968

106. Ho CS, Krovetz LJ, Rowe RD: Major complications of cardiac catheterization and angiography in infants and children. Johns Hopkins Med J 131:247, 1972

107. Rashkind WJ, Miller WW: Creation of an atrial septal defect without thoracotomy. A palliative approach to complete transposition of the great arteries. JAMA 196:991, 1966

108. Stanger P, Heymann MA, Tarnoff H, Hoffman JIE, Rudolph AM: Complications of cardiac

catheterization of neonates, infants, and children. A three-year study. Circulation 50:595, 1974

109. Varghese PJ, Celermajer J, Izukawa T, Haller JA, Rowe RD: Cardiac catheterization in the newborn: experience with 100 cases. Pediatrics 44:24, 1969

ECHOCARDIOGRAPHY

110. Feigenbaum H: Echocardiagraphy. Philadelphia, Lea & Febiger, 1972

111. Meyer RA, Kaplan S: Non-invasive techniques in pediatric cardiovascular disease. Prog. Cardiovasc Dis 15:341, 1973

SURGERY

112. Barratt-Boyes BG, Simpson M, Neutze JM. Intracardiac surgery in neonates and infants using deep hypothermia with surface cooling and limited cardiopulmonary bypass. Circulation 43,44 (Suppl I):25, 1971

113. Blalock A, Hanlon CR: Surgical treatment of complete transposition of the aorta and pulmonary artery. Surg Gynecol Obstet 90:1, 1950

114. Blalock A, Taussig HB: Surgical treatment of malformations of the heart in which there is pulmonary stenosis or pulmonary atresia. JAMA 128:189, 1945

115. Brock RC: Pulmonary valvulotomy for the relief of congenital stenosis: report of three cases. Br Med J 1:1121, 1948

116. Edwards WS, Bargeron LM Jr: More effective palliation of transposition of the great vessels. J Thorac Cardiovasc Surg 49:790, 1965

117. Glenn WWL, Ordway NK, Talner NS, Call EP: Circulatory bypass of the right side of the heart. VI. Shunt between superior vena cava and distal right pulmonary artery: report of clinical application in thirty-eight cases. Circulation 31:172, 1965

118. Hunt CE, Formanek G, Levine MA, Castaneda A, Moller JH: Banding of the pulmonary artery. Results in 111 children. Circulation 43:395, 1971

119. Malm JR, Bowman FO Jr, Jesse MJ, Hayes CJ, Steeg CN, Gersony WM: Technics in management of infants requiring cardiopulmonary bypass. Birth Defects 8:51, 1972

120. Mohri H, Dillard DH, Crawford EW, Martin WE, Merendino KA: Method of surface-induced deep hypothermia for open heart surgery in infants. J Thorac Cardiovasc Surg 58:262, 1969

121. Muller WH Jr, Dammann JF Jr: Treatment of certain congenital malformations of the heart by the creation of pulmonic stenosis to reduce pulmonary hypertension and excessive pulmonary blood flow. Surg Gynecol Obstet 95:213, 1952

122. Potts WJ, Smith S, Gibson SJ: Anastomosis of aorta to pulmonary artery: certain types in congenital heart disease. JAMA 132:627, 1946

123. Truccone NJ, Bowman FO Jr, Malm JR, Gersony WM: Systemic-pulmonary arterial shunts in the first year of life. Circulation 49:508, 1974

124. Waterston DJ: Treatment of Fallot's tetralogy in children under one year of age. Rozhl Chir 41:181, 1962

8

Hematologic Patterns and Bilirubin Metabolism

PERINATAL HEMATOLOGY

Normal hematologic function is vital for the survival of both fetus and newborn infant. In the transition from fetal to extrauterine life, numerous hematologic disorders, many potentially treatable, occur. The clinician must be able to recognize the various signs of hematologic disease, make a prompt and accurate diagnosis based on both clinical judgment and laboratory results and institute specific therapy before an irreversible process ensues. He must also be conversant with the normal hematologic values uniquely observed during the first days of life so as to avoid misinterpretation of laboratory data.

FETAL HEMATOLOGY

PHYSIOLOGY

Red Blood Cell Formation and Hemoglobin Synthesis

Synthesis of red blood cells (RBCs) begins in the yolk sac during the first month of gestation; by the sixth week the liver begins to assume this function. Medullary hematopoiesis, which does not begin until the fifth month of gestation, progressively assumes a

dominant role during the third trimester. The spleen, lymph nodes and thymus are also blood-forming organs during gestation.

In the first trimester the volume of RBCs is almost twice that at term, and the cells are predominantly nucleated. The hemoglobin concentration, which may be as low as 6 g/100 ml at 10 weeks, rises to about 14 g/100 by 24 weeks. The rate of increase in hemoglobin concentration during the third trimester is relatively slow, although the largest proportion of iron is transmitted from the mother to fetus during this period.

During gestation, three types of hemoglobin are synthesized by the fetus. Gower hemoglobins 1 and 2 predominate during the first six weeks (2). The former is composed of four ε polypeptide chains and the latter of two ε and two α chains. Fetal hemoglobin, which replaces them, contains two α and two γ chains, and has a stronger affinity for oxygen than does adult hemoglobin (hemoglobin A) (see section Oxygenation of the Fetus and Newborn Infant, Ch. 3). Fetal hemoglobin predominates throughout the remainder of pregnancy. Hemoglobin A, which contains two α and two β chains, begins to appear early in the second trimester (although β-chain synthesis has been detected as early as the 55th day of gestation) (5). By the 34th to 36th week of gestation, 5% to 10% of hemoglobin is the adult type, and this proportion increases to as much as 30% at term.

White Blood Cell Formation

Extramedullary production of leukocytes begins at about the seventh week of gestation, and it is not until about the fifth month that the marrow takes over this function. A marked rise in the number of circulating leukocytes occurs during the third trimester.

Lymphocyte production begins by the end of the second month of gestation, with the number of circulating lymphocytes reaching a maximum during the middle of pregnancy and slowly declining thereafter.

Platelet Formation

Megakaryocytes are first observed in the yolk sac by the sixth week of gestation, and by the third month they are consistently present in the bone marrow.

DISORDERS

Hemolytic Disease

Of the hematologic disorders affecting the fetus, the most important clinically is severe hemolytic anemia secondary to Rh incompatibility. This is discussed in the section Hemolytic Disease of the Newborn.

Intertwin Transfusions

The intertwin transfusion syndrome (see section Multiple Pregnancy, Ch. 2), which may result in either fetal anemia or polycythemia, cannot be diagnosed antenatally.

Disorders of Hemoglobin Synthesis

Sickle cell anemia and hemoglobin C disease, in which abnormal β chains are produced, and thalassemia major, in which there is decreased β-chain production, do not cause clinical illness in the fetus or newborn infant because of the low concentration of adult hemoglobin normally present

at this time. However, methods that enable the sampling of small quantities of fetal blood have made it possible to diagnose these disorders during the second trimester (4).

The presence of Barts hemoglobin (in which α chains have been replaced by γ chains in the hemoglobin molecule) affects the fetus only when the condition is present as a homozygous trait, e.g., α thalassemia, (6). Fetal death, secondary to erythroblastosis and hydrops fetalis usually occurs early in the third trimester. Most reported cases have occurred among infants of oriental extraction.

Maternal Factors

A number of maternal diseases and exposure of the mother to certain drugs may affect the hematologic status of the fetus.

Hemolytic anemia and thrombocytopenia may be present in such fetomaternal infections as syphilis, toxoplasmosis, rubella, h. simplex and cytomegalovirus. Maternal idiopathic thrombocytopenic purpura and systemic lupus erythematosus may be responsible for fetal thrombocytopenia.

Maternal ingestion of barbiturates and salicylates may prolong the prothrombin time of the fetus. Thiazides and quinine may lead to thrombocytopenic purpura, while ingestion of a variety of drugs may lead to hemolytic anemia in G-6-PD deficient fetuses (see Ch. 21, Pharmacology).

NEONATAL PERIOD

Hematologic adaptation from fetal to neonatal life involves a decline in the hemoglobin concentration, adjustment of blood volume, physiologic and morphologic changes in the cellular elements of the blood and maturation of coagulation factors.

NORMAL VALUES

Hemoglobin Concentration

At birth, the normal mean cord blood hemoglobin concentration is about 17 g/100 ml, and the hematocrit 50% to 55%, with a wide

TABLE 8-1. Hemoglobin and Hematocrit Values and Reticulocyte Counts (Venous Blood)

		Cord Blood	First 24 Hrs	24–72 Hrs	1 Week
Hb*	(g/100 ml)	17–18	18–19	17–18	17
Hematocrit*	(%)	50–55	55–60	50–55	50
Reticulocytes	(%)	3–5	3–5	1–3	0–1

* These values are increased by 5% to 10% if peripheral blood is used. In premature infants, the cord blood hemoglobin concentration may be as low as 15 g/100 ml and hematocrit 45%.

range of normal values (Table 8–1). Both hemoglobin and hematocrit determinations obtained from heel-prick samples are usually 5% to 10% higher than those of venous blood because of peripheral vasoconstriction.

The volume of placental transfusion influences these values, and infants whose umbilical cords have been clamped "late" have higher hemoglobin concentrations and hematocrit levels than those infants whose cords have been clamped "early" (7, 13). There is normally an increase in these values during the first day of life, followed by a steady decline over the first months of life.

Blood Volume

Blood volumes shortly after birth vary from 50 to 100 ml/kg of body weight in the full-term infant, with a mean of about 85 ml/kg of body weight. Like hemoglobin concentrations, these are higher in those infants whose cords have been clamped late. Premature infants tend to have slightly higher values due to increased plasma volume. A decrease in blood volume to normal adult levels of 75 to 80 ml/kg occurs by the second month of life.

Erythrocytes

The erythrocyte of the fetus and newborn infant is larger than that of the older infant, child, or adult. The average diameter at birth is between 8.0 and 8.5 μ, which declines to 7.5 μ by age six months and remains so for the rest of life. A variation in the size of neonatal erythrocytes (anisocytosis) is commonly observed, however.

The reticulocyte count, is usually about 3% to 5% during the early days of life, de-

clines to 1% or less by the end of the first week. Elevation of the reticulocyte count during the early neonatal period is usually a reflection of either blood loss or a hemolytic process. The relative paucity of reticulocytes usually seen in the late neonatal period reflects decreased erythropoiesis accompanying the poor erythropoietin production at this time of life (8).

Premature infants and those with hemolytic disease have more nucleated RBCs than normal full-term infants. In prematures, the range is usually between 1000 and 1500/mm^3, while in normal full-term infants the count is usually about 500/mm^3. A dramatic decline occurs by age 48 hours, with an increased number indicating a hemolytic process.

Aside from qualitative differences in the biochemical structure of the hemoglobin molecule, several differences exist between fetal and neonatal RBCs and those of the older child and adult.

The mechanical fragility of fetal and neonatal erythrocytes is usually increased. These cells have a shorter life span and a higher degree of metabolic activity (with higher glucose consumption) than adult cells. Concentrations of ADP and ATP are increased, as is the activity of a variety of intracellular enzymes (10). The cell membrane differs from that of the adult erythrocyte, which contains less sphingomyelin, but more lecithin and linoleic acid. Potassium influx is greater in the fetal and neonatal erythrocyte than in its adult counterpart. On phase microscopy, about one-half of the erythrocytes of premature infants are noted to have crater-like indentations (or pock marks) of the cell membrane. This is present in about one-fourth of the erythrocytes of normal full-term infants, compared to an in-

TABLE 8–2. Total White Blood Count and Differential in Neonates

		First Day	One Week
WBCs	(mm³)	18,000–20,000	12,000
PMNs	(%)	55–60	45–50
Lymphocytes	(%)	30	40
Monocytes	(%)	10	5–10
Eosinophils	(%)	2	2

cidence of 2.6% in adult erythrocytes. The reason for this finding is unknown, but a tentative explanation is that these pock marks may be related to splenic hypofunction (3).

White Blood Cells

The total white blood cell (WBC) count of the newborn infant is usually higher than that of the older child and adult, with an average value of about 18,000 to 20,000 cells/mm³ in cord blood (Table 8–2). This declines to about 12,000/mm³ after the second or third day of life and remains at this level throughout early infancy. The differential count is marked by an initial preponderance of polymorphonuclear leukocytes (PMNs), about 60% of the total count. By the end of the first week of life, PMNs declines to about 45%, while the lymphocyte count increases from 30% to 40%. About 10% of the WBCs in cord blood are monocytes. This ratio falls to about 6% by the second or third day. The normal full-term infant has about 2% eosinophils, but lower levels are found among premature infants, and these cells do not appear until about the second day of life.

It is difficult to interpret the total WBC and differential counts in newborn infants because of the extremely wide range of normal values and the considerable unexplained variations that occur spontaneously. Very low total counts (below 5000/mm³ during the first week of life) may be of greater diagnostic significance than those that appear to be elevated, especially in the presence of an overwhelming gram-negative bacterial infection associated with endotoxin release. Leukopenia may also be associated with maternal drug ingestion or the pres-

ence of maternal antibodies formed against fetal leukocytes. Disappearance of eosinophils from the peripheral blood is usually associated with terminal illness in premature infants.

Leukocytes of newborn infants have a higher degree of metabolic activity than those of older children or adults. They have twice the oxygen consumption of maternal leukocytes and an enhanced ability to phagocytize foreign matter (as demonstrated by the large proportion of nitroblue tetrazolium positive leukocytes present in the newborn infant) (11).

Platelets

The platelet count following delivery varies from 150,000 to 350,000; lower levels may normally be seen among premature infants. Normal values vary to some extent with the laboratory method utilized.

Bone Marrow

The bone marrow of newborn infants is initially hypercellular, with a myeloid to erythroid ratio of about 1.5:1. This hypercellularity decreases during the first week of life, and by the age of eight days, the myeloid to erythroid ratio is about 6:1.

TABLE 8–3
Normal percentile values for micro–ESR in 100 low-birth-weight infants 3 days of age or less

Percentile	ESR (mm/hr)	
	Male*	Female†
10	1.0	1.0
25	1.8	1.8
50	2.5	3.0
75	3.3	4.0
90	4.0	6.0
95	6.0	6.0
99	8.8	8.3

* Hematocrit: median 57%, range 43% to 78%
† Hematocrit: median 54%, range 41% to 77%
(Evans et al: J Pediatr 76:448, 1970)

TABLE 8-4
Normal percentile values for micro-ESR in 30 low-birth-weight infants, median age 28 days, range 9-56 days

Percentile	ESR (mm/hr)
10	3.0
25	3.8
50	5.5
90	9.5
95	11.0

Hematocrit: median 35%, range 25% to 58%
(Evans et al: J Pediatr 76:448, 1970)

Erythrocyte Sedimentation Rate

The erythrocyte sedimentation rate (ESR) is usually less than 6 mm/hour during the first three days of life (Table 8-3) and less than 11 mm/hour (Table 8-4) after the first week of life. Elevations, using a micromethod, have been shown to be associated with systemic bacterial infections (1).

Coagulation Factors

Under normal circumstances, transient deficiencies of certain coagulation factors occur during the neonatal period. Those factors whose synthesis depends on the presence of vitamin K, prothrombin, factor VII (proconvertin), factor IX (PTC) and factor X (Stuart-Prower) usually reach their lowest concentrations by the third or fourth day of life and attain normal adult levels after several weeks of life. Factors V (labile factor) and VIII (AHF), which are not vitamin K dependent, are also present in lower-than-adult concentrations (Table 8-5).

DIAGNOSIS OF HEMATOLOGIC DISORDERS

Many signs observed in the neonatal period, occurring either alone or in conjunction with disorders of other systems, may suggest a hematologic problem. Pallor, jaundice, petechiae, bleeding from the umbilicus or from circumcision or needle puncture site, GI bleeding, hepatosplenomegaly, tachycardia, tachypnea, apathy and anorexia should lead the clinician to suspect hematologic disease.

These may range from early and minimal to severe and grave findings. There are few illnesses of the neonatal period in which hematologic involvement does not occur. Signs of one disease entity may overlap with those of others, hence detailed laboratory studies are often required to provide a clear-cut diagnosis. However, in the face of life-threatening illness, diagnostic studies may necessarily have to be abbreviated, with treatment being directed to save the patient's life.

History Taking

Maternal and Obstetric History. Maternal and obstetric history may provide important clues in establishing a hematologic diagnosis. Certain malignancies, collagen diseases, maternal infectious disease (e.g., rubella and cytomegalovirus) and ingestion of drugs such as thiazides, salicylates and sulfonamides, may all lead to hematologic disorders in the neonate.

Family History. A positive family history, in which siblings have had either hemolytic disease, a coagulation disorder or an inborn error of erythrocyte metabolism, such as G-6-PD deficiency, may narrow the diagnostic possibilities.

Intrapartum History. The intrapartum history may also contribute significantly to the diagnosis of neonatal hematologic disorders. Placenta previa, for example, may be associated with fetal blood loss. Obstetric trauma may lead to subdural hematoma, adrenal hemorrhage (especially with a breech presentation) and rupture of the liver with intraabdominal bleeding. The use of a vacuum extractor may be associated with subaponeurotic bleeding, which can lead to severe anemia. Severe perinatal asphyxia or amnionitis may lead to disseminated intravascular coagulation.

Postnatal History. Postnatally, the time of onset, nature and severity of signs are all vital in correctly diagnosing an hematologic disorder. A very early onset (within the first 48 hours of life) may suggest that maternal

TABLE 8–5. Coagulation factor in normal pregnant women and newborn infants

| Category | Fibrinogen (mg/100 ml) | Factors | | | | | | | | | Euglobulin lysis time (min) | Partial thrombo-plastin time* (sec) | Prothrombin time (sec) | Thrombin time (sec) |
		II (%)	V (%)	VII (%)	VIII (%)	IX (%)	X (%)	XI (%)	XII (%)	XIII (titer)				
Normal adult or child	190–420	100	100	100	100	100	100	100	100	1/16	90–300	37–50	12–14	8–10
Term pregnancy	483	92	108	170	196	130	130	69	—	1/16	278	44	13	8.0
Premature (1500–2500 g) cord blood	233	25	67	37	80	Dec†	29	—	—	1/8	214	90	17(12–21)	14(11–17)
Term infant cord blood	216	41	92	56	100	27	55	36	—	1/8	84	71	16(13–20)	12(10–16)
Term infant, 48 hours	210	46	105	20	100	Dec	45	39	25	—	105	65	17.5(12–21)	13(10–16)

Note: All levels expressed as means or ranges
* Kaolin PTT
† Dec = decreased
(Hathaway: Pediatr Clin North Am 17:929, 1970)

and intrapartum factors are involved. Bleeding observed in premature infants during the first days (usually associated with RDS or infection) raises the possibility of disseminated intravascular coagulation (DIC). A significant fall in the hemoglobin concentration after several days or weeks of repeated blood sampling suggests an iatrogenic origin of the anemia.

Physical Examination

Physical examination includes both the infant's general appearance and specific signs. Severe pallor, rapid respirations and a rapid, thready pulse are suggestive of an acute blood loss. A few petechiae limited to the conjunctivae and face in vertex presentations and over the thigh and buttocks in breech deliveries are usually normal findings; if petechiae are present over the entire body, thrombocytopenia may be suspected. Hepatosplenomegaly and jaundice may be suggestive of either hematologic disease, infection or both. The presence of a laceration may suggest blood loss secondary to the trauma of either amniocentesis or cesarean section, if these procedures have been performed.

Laboratory Diagnosis

The extent of laboratory examination required will vary with each case. The minimum number of diagnostic tests include a hematocrit or hemoglobin concentration, total WBC and differential count. These determinations can be performed on a peripheral blood sample. More sophisticated laboratory procedures are discussed in individual sections on specific hematologic disease.

HEMATOLOGIC DISORDERS

ANEMIA

An abnormally low number of circulating RBCs (anemia) is a relatively common finding among newborn infants. Causes of anemia in the neonatal period include blood group incompatibility, intertwin transfusion, fetomaternal bleeding, acute hemorrhage, infection, removal of blood for diagnostic purpose, metabolic defects of the RBC, anemia of prematurity, folic acid deficiency and vitamin E deficiency. Prompt recognition and treatment are imperative since untreated anemia may lead to unnecessary morbidity or even mortality.

Blood Group Incompatability

Hemolytic disease, secondary to a blood group incompatibility, may cause severe and even life-threatening anemia in the fetus and newborn infant. Diagnosis and treatment are discussed in the section Neonatal Jaundice and Hemolytic Disease.

Intertwin Transfusions and Fetomaternal Bleeding

The intertwin transfusion syndrome (see section Multiple Pregnancy, Ch. 2) occurs in monochorionic twins. The donor twin appears pale and often undergrown, while the recipient twin is quite ruddy. In order to make this diagnosis, there must be a hemoglobin concentration difference of at least 5 mg/100 ml of blood between the twins. Since a velamentous insertion of the cord may occur more frequently in monochorionic twins than in singleton deliveries, an acute blood loss secondary to a torn blood vessel must be excluded in these cases. A similar type of chronic blood loss occurs in the presence of a fetomaternal transfusion (14). In both of these types of chronic blood loss the infant generally appears quite pallid, but distress is mild, if present at all. Occasionally, the blood loss may be so great that the infant is severely anemic and has generalized edema. The diagnosis of chronic blood loss, into either the circulation of the mother or twin, is made by the presence of an anemia that is usually hypochromic and microcytic. Hepatosplenomegaly is absent; the Coombs' test is negative. In fetomaternal bleeding, fetal RBCs can be detected in the maternal circulation by the acid elution technique of Kleihauer et al (15). The clinical course of these infants is usually uneventful. A small, carefully administered transfusion of packed RBCs will usually raise the infant's hemoglobin concentration to satisfactory levels. Because of the anemia, venous pressure may be high, and there is always some danger of producing congestive heart failure when administering even small quantities of packed RBCs. A partial exchange transfusion may sometimes be necessary in the presence of an increased venous pressure. If the chronic anemia is mild, iron therapy alone will often be satisfactory.

Hemorrhage

Acute blood loss during the intrapartum period requires prompt recognition and treatment. At worst, severe hemorrhage may lead to fetal death. If the fetus survives, he will appear pale with irregular gasping, often rapid respirations. Retractions of the chest wall are usually absent unless there is concurrent lung disease. The cardiac rate is usually rapid, and both arterial and venous blood pressures are low. The hemoglobin concentration, while often quite low (in the range of 5 to 10 g/100 ml), may be in the normal range because of one of two reasons. The infant may be in shock with peripheral vasoconstriction resulting in peripheral pooling of RBCs. In this case, a hemoglobin or hematocrit determination on venous blood gives a truer picture of hemoglobin concentration than if the test had been performed on capillary blood. If the bleeding has been of very recent onset, equilibration of hemoglobin concentration to a lower level may not yet have occurred.

Treatment of acute blood loss in the neonatal period is the same as at any other time of life: administration of whole blood. If this is not immediately available, either plasma, dextran or saline may be used as a temporary measure to combat signs of shock. If the infant appears pale at birth, is in no distress and has a normal hemoglobin or hematocrit level, determinations of hemoglobin or hematocrit must be performed at four to eight-hour intervals. If there is evi-

dence of a falling hematocrit (below 45%) or hemoglobin (below 15 g/100 ml), transfusion is usually indicated.

Pallor secondary to blood loss may occur at any time following delivery. Bleeding into the liver, adrenal gland or subdural space (which may be secondary to obstetric trauma) may not become apparent until sometime after delivery. Usually, the severity of the infant's illness outweighs the degree of the anemia in these cases.

Infection

Hemolytic anemia may accompany both bacterial and nonbacterial infections. If the etiology of an anemia is not apparent, an evaluation for the presence of infection should be undertaken.

Coagulation Disorders

A fall in hematocrit or hemoglobin concentration in sick newborn infants may be the first sign of DIC. This is most likely to occur in the first 24 to 48 hours of life.

Thrombocytopenia, which may be secondary to isoimmunization, infection, maternal drug administration or maternally produced antiplatelet antibodies, may cause bleeding and anemia. The site of bleeding is usually superficial and the degree of anemia mild. The association of petechiae and pallor warrants a diagnostic evaluation for thrombocytopenia.

The routine administration of vitamin K has made blood loss secondary to hemorrhagic disease of the newborn a rarity. This occurs typically on the third or fourth day of life in infants who are otherwise well. These entities are discussed in the section Coagulation Disorders.

Removal of Blood for Diagnostic Purposes

A common cause of anemia and pallor in the sick low-birth-weight infant is the removal of blood for diagnostic purposes. While microtechniques have greatly reduced the quantities of blood necessary for most diagnostic procedures, repeated blood sampling significantly lowers the number of circulating RBCs. Frequent determinations of hemoglobin or hematocrit are necessary in these infants.

Hemolytic Anemia

Postnatal hemolysis, secondary to metabolic defects of the RBC (most often G-6 PD deficiency), may result in anemia. This may or may not be accompanied by hyperbilirubinemia.

Anemia of Prematurity

The normocytic, normochromic anemia of prematurity is often encountered in infants of very low birth weight prior to their discharge from the nursery. Folic acid deficiency may also be rarely responsible for anemia in this group of infants (18). Iron deficiency anemia is almost never a consideration during the neonatal period.

Vitamin E Deficiency and Hemolytic Anemia

Low serum concentrations of tocopherol (vitamin E) have been associated with hemolytic anemia and edema in six to ten-week-old infants who had been born prematurely. This substance, which is an antioxidant, protects the RBC against hemolysis by a variety of oxidizing agents. Formulas rich in linoleic acid and fortified with supplementary iron appear to potentiate this hemolytic process (18a).

Ritchie et al (17) have been able to correct this anemia by oral administration of 75 to 100 IU alpha tocopherol acetate per day to affected infants. Oski and Barness (16) have observed higher hemoglobin concentrations and lower reticulocyte counts in premature infants treated prophylactically with 15 IU vitamin E orally per day than in untreated controls.

Late Anemia Following Isoimmunization

An anemia occurring either during the late neonatal period or after the first month of life may be seen in infants with hemolytic disease. This is due to persistent slow hemolysis of sensitized RBCs. In infants who have been treated with exchange transfusion, it is due also in part to the relatively low hematocrit of donor blood.

Routine determinations of hemoglobin and hematocrit concentrations must be performed at regular intervals on low-birth-weight infants and on those infants who have had hemolytic disease.

POLYCYTHEMIA

The newborn infant normally has a hematocrit and hemoglobin concentration higher than that of older children and adults. However, when the venous hematocrit rises above 60% to 65%, or the hemoglobin above 20 to 22 g/100 ml (capillary blood generally gives higher values), blood viscosity begins to increase sharply. This may lead to a variety of abnormal clinical signs that, left untreated, may lead to permanent neurologic damage (19).

Etiology

Often the cause of polycythemia can be easily explained. The intertwin transfusion syndrome (see section Multiple Pregnancy, Ch. 2), which can occur in monochorionic twins, may result in one anemic and one polycythemic infant. Maternofetal transfusion and a delay in clamping the umbilical cord may also lead to polycythemia.

Intrauterine oxygenating disorders may lead to an increased RBC mass to compensate for the decreased arterial oxygen tension (Pao_2). Polycythemia has been reported in Down's syndrome (mongolism), Beckwith's syndrome, infants of diabetic mothers, neonatal thyrotoxicosis and adrenogenital syndrome (20). It may also occur in the absence of a known underlying cause.

Clinical Manifestations

The polycythemic infant may appear extremely ruddy yet have no abnormal signs. On the other hand, the decreased flow of blood to vital organs due to increased viscosity may cause respiratory distress, cardiomegaly with congestive heart failure (sometimes leading to a mistaken diagnosis of congenital heart disease), cyanosis (usually peripheral), tremors, irritability and even seizures. Hyperbilirubinemia, which is caused by a breakdown of an increased number of RBCs, is a frequent finding, as is a decreased platelet count. An increased incidence of hypoglycemia has been reported.

Infants with venous hematocrits below 60% may also have increased viscosity of their blood and develop similar clinical manifestations. This is thought to be due to decreased deformability of RBCs.

Diagnosis and Treatment

The definitive diagnosis depends not only on finding an increased hemoglobin or hematocrit concentration, but also on actually measuring an increase in viscosity of the blood (19–21).

The treatment of symptomatic polycythemia consists of partial exchange transfusion with fresh frozen plasma in an attempt to lower the venous hematocrit to about 60%. (The risk of neurologic sequelae in infants with asymptomatic polycythemia is not known and therefore the need for treatment is not certain.)

Simple phlebotomy reduces blood volume without reducing either the hematocrit or viscosity and should therefore not be employed as a therapeutic measure.

Oski and Naiman (9) propose the following formula for calculating the volume of the exchange transfusion:

Volume of exchange (ml) = Blood volume × of infant

$$\frac{\text{(observed hematocrit} - \text{desired hematocrit)}}{\text{observed hematocrit}}$$

Abnormal signs should disappear when the hematocrit is lowered to a normal level.

COAGULATION DISORDERS

HEMORRHAGIC DISEASE OF THE NEWBORN

Hemorrhagic disease of the newborn is a disorder of the second phase of coagulation (the conversion of prothrombin to thrombin) due to a deficiency of vitamin K. Its incidence in infants not receiving vitamin K supplementation is probably between 1:200 and 1:400. Although it was apparently recognized by the ancient Hebrews (who delayed circumcision until the eighth day of life, when the risk of this disorder is rare), it was not until 1894 that Townsend (28) coined the name by which this entity is still known today.

The mechanism of hemorrhagic disease of the newborn was discovered in the late 1930s (26). Since that time, the routine administration of vitamin K to all newborn infants has led to the virtual disappearance of this disorder in the United States.

Etiology

Vitamin K, which is synthesized by bacteria in the small intestine, is necessary for the synthesis of prothrombin and of factors VII, IX and X by the liver. Since the fetal intestine is sterile, vitamin K is derived from the maternal circulation. Thus, the vitamin K dependent factors are essentially normal at the time of birth but tend to become depleted by the second or third day of life. This depletion is accompanied by a prolongation of the prothrombin time, and during this period hemorrhagic disease of the newborn can occur. With bacterial colonization of the GI tract, which begins after oral feedings have been started, vitamin K can be synthesized by the infant. By the end of the first week of life, the prothrombin time returns to normal.

During the critical period when vitamin K is not being synthesized in the gut, the infant's only source (if he is not given a supplement at birth) is dietary. Human breast milk contains only about 1.5 μg/100 ml; therefore breast-fed infants who do not receive a vitamin K supplement are at highest risk for developing hemorrhagic disease (27).

Reduced levels of the vitamin K dependent clotting factors have been reported in infants of mothers receiving diphenylhydantoin therapy for convulsive disorders

(25). These infants are especially prone to hemorrhagic disease.

Clinical Manifestations

The initial presenting signs are either localized or generalized bleeding, usually on the second or third day of life. Continued oozing of blood may be noted following an IM injection or heel prick. An enlarging cephalhematoma may be an early manifestation. Bleeding into the skin or from an umbilical stump or circumcision site may be noted. Gastrointestinal bleeding or hemorrhage into either the brain or another internal organ may be associated with significant anemia.

Diagnosis and Treatment

It is vital that hemorrhagic disease of the newborn be differentiated from DIC since both the treatment and prognosis are completely different (23).

Some of the features differentiating the two disorders are listed in Table 8–6. The most constant abnormality of coagulation seen in hemorrhagic disease is a markedly prolonged prothrombin time, which may be as high as 60 seconds.

The best treatment of hemorrhagic disease of the newborn is its prevention by administration of vitamin K following delivery, as suggested by the Committee on Nutrition of the American Academy of Pediatrics (24). Although Aballi (22) has found that 25 μg vitamin K is sufficient to prevent hemorrhagic disease, the average dosage is 1.0 mg IM. This is administered as vitamin K_1. The use of water-soluble analogues of vitamin K, e.g., menadione, in moderate or large doses may lead to a hemolytic anemia and hyperbilirubinemia. However, when given in a proper dosage, they are safe and effective.

Active treatment of the disease consists of the IV injection of 1 to 2 mg vitamin K. In the absence of moderate or severe anemia, this therapy brings about a decrease in prothrombin time within two to four hours. If bleeding is severe and significant anemia is present, administration of fresh whole blood is desirable. This will not only replace the lost blood but will immediately provide some of the missing clotting factors.

DISSEMINATED INTRAVASCULAR COAGULATION (DIC)

With the virtual elimination of hemorrhagic disease in the United States, most of the perinatal hemorrhage now observed is due to DIC. This disorder was termed "secondary hemorrhagic disease of the newborn" by Aballi and de Lamerens (23) in 1962 since it was not amenable to treatment with vitamin K.

TABLE 8–6. Differential Diagnosis of the Bleeding Infant

Condition	Platelets	Partial thrombo-plastin time	Pro-thrombin time	Thrombin time	Fibrin split products
Hemorrhagic disease of new-born (vit. K deficiency)	N	Inc	Inc	N	N
Hemophilia A or B	N	Inc	N	N	N
Congenital factor VII deficiency	N	N	Inc	N	N
Isolated thrombocytopenia	Dec	N	N	N	N
Disseminated intravascular coagulation* (DIC)	Dec	Inc	Inc	Inc	N or Inc
Prolonged hypoxia or liver disease	N or Dec	Inc	Inc	Inc	N or Inc

Dec = decreased; Inc = increased; N = normal for newborn infant
* Factor VIII level is Dec in DIC and N in liver disease
(Hathaway: Pediatr Clin North Am 17:929, 1970)

While hemorrhagic disease of the new-born is usually first observed on the second or third day of life and is associated with no underlying disorder except for a vitamin K deficiency, DIC may occur at any time from intrauterine life to the late neonatal period and is always secondary to a severe predisposing illness. It is most frequently seen during the first two days after birth.

Etiology

Several conditions, such as hypoxia, acidosis and bacterial and nonbacterial infections, may lead to intravascular clotting, with the consumption (and subsequent decreased blood concentrations) of such factors as platelets, fibrinogen and factors II (pro-thrombin), V (proaccelerin) and VIII (anti-hemophiliac globulin). In cases of pre-eclampsia, eclampsia, abruptio placentae and death of a twin, thromboplastic material may cross the placenta into the fetal circulation and initiate the intravascular clotting process. Liver damage or necrosis, secondary to infection or hypoxia causing a release of thromboplastic factors into the circulation, may also precipitate DIC (30). The formation of fibrin microthrombi in the blood vessels tends to activate fibrinolysins, often causing the presence of split products of fibrin in the blood (31).

The consumption of clotting factors by intravascular coagulation predisposes the infant to severe bleeding and hemorrhage into the brain and other vital organs.

This disorder is most common among premature infants, especially those with RDS, hypoxia or systemic infection.

Clinical Manifestations

The hemorrhagic phenomenon accompanying DIC is superimposed on a predisposing illness and is usually quite severe. However, there is a wide spectrum of disease, and DIC may infrequently occur in the absence of overt bleeding.

The most common clinical findings are oozing from venipuncture or heel-prick sites, petechiae, purpura, bleeding from the umbilical cord stump and hemorrhage into the brain, lung, adrenal glands and other organs. A decline in the hemoglobin concentration and hematocrit level accompanies this bleeding.

Diagnosis

Besides the clinical manifestations of hemorrhage in an already compromised newborn infant, there are several laboratory tests that will facilitate the diagnosis.

Hemolytic anemia with fragmentation of RBCs is frequently encountered. Thrombocytopenia (a platelet count of less than $100,000/mm^3$) along with decreased levels of factors II, V, VIII and fibrinogen are seen. The thrombin, prothrombin and partial thromboplastin times are abnormally prolonged. Split products of fibrin may be present in low concentrations in newborn infants with DIC; however, not too much reliance can be placed on the measurement of this factor. Because of the low levels of fibrinogen, the ESR is extremely low.

Treatment

Treatment begins with an attempt to control the underlying disease. This includes the administration of antimicrobial therapy for sepsis, correction of hypoxia and acidosis, maintenance of fluid and electrolyte balance and establishment of a thermoneutral environment. Since the actual mechanisms for the initiation of hypercoagulability are unknown, specific therapy is not available.

The most successful therapeutic agent in this disorder is heparin, an anticoagulant that is operative at several points in the coagulation process. Heparin is an antithrombin substance that inhibits the activation of factor IX by factor XI and the activation of factor VIII by factor IX.

Heparin may be administered in one of two ways: 1) rapid IV injection in doses of 50 to 100 U/kg every four to six hours for an average of two to three days or 2) exchange transfusion using freshly collected heparinized blood. Using the former technique, Whaun et al (32) were able to improve the survival rate in DIC from 50% to 69%; Gross and Melhorn (29) successfully used the exchange transfusion technique in four full-term infants with DIC. This therapeutic modality has the advantage not only of introducing heparin into the infant's circulation, but of supplying depleted factors as well. It may also serve to remove factors that have initiated or are perpetuating intravascular clotting.

Heparin therapy should be instituted only if there is definite generalized bleeding or evidence of thrombosis with a laboratory diagnosis of DIC.

Fresh frozen plasma or platelets should not be administered until the infant is adequately heparinized since further consumption of clotting factors will ensue. When platelets are administered, the dosage is 1 U/5 kg of body weight.

Two laboratory tests may be used as guidelines to determine the adequacy of therapy. The whole blood clotting time should be maintained in the range of 20 to 30 minutes, and the activated partial thromboplastin time maintained at 60 to 70 seconds. The efficacy of therapy is most effectively monitored by daily platelet counts. Since treatment is directed towards both the underlying disease and DIC, evaluation of the efficacy of therapy is often difficult.

In very immature, severely hypoxic infants the presence of widespread hemorrhage is associated with a grave prognosis even with intensive therapy. On the other hand, in more mature infants with a potentially manageable problem, such as bacterial sepsis, both heparin and other forms of therapy may well effect a reversal of the process and lead to gradual improvement and recovery.

THROMBOCYTOPENIA

Thrombocytopenia is an important cause of bleeding in newborn infants. A decreased number of platelets, due either to decreased production, increased destruction, or both, may be secondary causes. Qualitative deficiencies of platelet function have also been described in newborn infants (35).

Infection

Infection is a major cause of neonatal thrombocytopenia. Decreased platelet counts ranging from 10,000 to 50,000 may be seen in congenital rubella, accompanied by purpura and petechiae. There is a decreased number of megakaryocytes in the bone marrow, and hepatosplenomegaly is usually an accompanying sign. Although this usually resolves spontaneously, an exchange transfusion or platelet transfusion may occasionally be required. In cytomegalovirus infection, the thrombocytopenia is associated with an absence of megakaryocytes. In congenital syphilis, megakaryocytes are usually normal, and the thrombocytopenia that is sometimes encountered is probably due to increased platelet destruction.

A markedly decreased platelet count with clinical manifestations of petechiae and purpura may also be seen in congenital toxoplasmosis, h. simplex and rubella.

Immune Thrombocytopenia

Immune thrombocytopenia may either be due to passively acquired antibodies or involve an active, or isoimmune process. In the former category, maternal antiplatelet antibodies may be transmitted to the fetus across the placenta in the presence of maternal systemic lupus erythematosus, idiopathic thrombocytopenia or following the ingestion of such drugs as thiazides by the mother (36). In the latter situation fetal platelets are antigenically different from maternal platelets. (There are four different types of platelet antigens: Pl^{A_1}, Pl^{A_2}, Pl^{B_1} and Pl^{B_2}. Of these, Pl^{A_1} is by far the most common, occurring in about 97% of the population). If fetal platelets different from these of the mother cross the placenta into the maternal circulation, they stimulate antibody formation against themselves. When these antibodies enter the fetal circulation, they lead to platelet destruction and thrombocytopenia. This condition may occur in conjunction with hemolytic disease of the newborn or may be an isolated entity.

With hemolytic disease of the newborn, treatment with exchange transfusion is usually adequate. In isolated neonatal immune purpura, the mortality rate is 10% to 15%, usually secondary to intracranial hemorrhage. Treatment consists of infusing compatible platelets (33, 34). Corticosteroids, which improve capillary integrity, may be of value. Exchange transfusion can be employed if platelets are unavailable.

Other Conditions

Congenital thrombocytopenia, with megakaryocytic hypoplasia, may occur either as an isolated entity or together with other congenital anomalies, such as absence of the radii or Fanconi's syndrome (multiple congenital anomalies and pancytopenia).

In the inherited forms of thrombocytopenia, such as Aldrich's syndrome, the presence of signs in the neonatal period is rare.

In the Kasabach-Merritt syndrome, sequestration of platelets by giant hemangiomas may lead to thrombocytopenia and bleeding during the first month of life. The severity of the disease is usually reflected by the size of the tumor.

Thrombocytopenia is also an accompanying finding in congenital leukemia.

OTHER DEFECTS OF COAGULATION

Several congenital defects of the coagulation mechanism may lead to bleeding in the newborn infant. These include absence of factors VII, VIII (AHG) and IX (PTC). Neonatal hemorrhage may also occur secondary to severe liver disease.

LEUKEMIA

Although leukemia is rare in the neonatal period, it is nonetheless a leading cause of deaths due to neoplasia at this time of life. A distinction must be made between congenital leukemia, noted on the first day of life, and neonatal leukemia, which is initially observed after the first day.

While most acute leukemias of childhood are either of the lymphoblastic or stem-cell type, leukemia seen in the neonatal period is usually myelogenous. As is true in later life, there is an unusually high association with mongolism (36b). None of the mothers of leukemic infants have had leukemia themselves.

The presenting findings are pallor, thrombocytopenic purpura, hemorrhagic diathesis, subcutaneous nodules, and hepatosplenomegaly. The white blood count is usually extremely high, and neutropenia is extremely rare.

Caution must be exercised in making the diagnosis of congenital or early neonatal leukemia. A marked elevation of the white blood count, along with hepatosplenomegaly, may occur in the presence of erythroblastosis or certain infections, such as syphilis. Leukemia may be diagnosed only if there is an infiltration of nonhematopoietic tissues by immature white blood cells. The prognosis is very poor, for both forms of the disorder and most affected infants die several months after the diagnosis is made. However, spontaneous remissions are occasionally observed in mongoloid infants with congenital leukemia (36a).

NEONATAL JAUNDICE AND HEMOLYTIC DISEASE

Unconjugated bilirubin, the major substance responsible for neonatal jaundice, is a potent CNS toxin capable of producing death or severe neurologic disability. Measuring its concentration in serum, correlating its clinical and biochemical effects and determining therapy to prevent encephalopathy, or kernicterus, are major activities in the newborn nursery.

Numerous advances have been made in

prevention, diagnosis and treatment during the 1960s and early 1970s. However, important problems remain, among which is our inability to evaluate the precise risk of bilirubin encephalopathy at a given age and serum bilirubin concentration in a particular infant. The value and long-term effects of certain types of treatment, such as phototherapy, must also be more closely evaluated. This additional knowledge will enable the clinician to treat neonatal jaundice in a more rational manner.

BILIRUBIN METABOLISM

Approximately 75% of the bilirubin present in the fetus and newborn infant is derived from the breakdown of RBCs. Hemoglobin, the parent compound of bilirubin, is comprised of a protein, globin, that is combined with heme, an iron-porphyrin complex. After RBCs are lysed within cells of the reticuloendothelial system, the heme ring opens, and carbon monoxide is released. This reaction depends on the presence of the enzyme heme oxygenase. Iron is broken off and stored as ferriten, while the globin portion is broken down into amino acids. The porphyrin moiety is degraded to biliverdin, which is then rapidly reduced to bilirubin. Regardless of the chemical structure of the globin molecule (which changes both during gestation and after birth), 1 g hemoglobin yields 34 mg bilirubin, since the heme portion, which is the forerunner of bilirubin, remains chemically the same throughout gestation.

The remaining 25% of bilirubin is derived from non-erythrocyte-containing heme proteins, such as myoglobin, peroxidase, catalase and cytochromes. There is also some direct synthesis of bilirubin from porphyrins.

The bilirubin thus formed is of the unconjugated type, which is nonpolar and insoluble in water, but soluble in lipids and chloroform. This is the same as indirect-reacting bilirubin described by van den Bergh (94) on the basis of its reaction with diazotized sulfanilic acid. This form of bilirubin is soluble in the cell membrane and responsible for damage to brain cells. To be transported in plasma prior to its excretion from the body, it must be bound to albumin. One mole of albumin is theoretically capable of binding two moles of unconjugated bilirubin. The first binding site is a strong one; the second is considerably weaker. In a one to one molar ratio (each molecule of albumin binding one molecule of bilirubin), 1 g albumin is capable of binding 16 mg unconjugated bilirubin, at a pH of 7.40.

FETAL ASPECTS

While the newborn infant excretes bilirubin via the GI tract, the fetus, who produces approximately 1000 mg of unconjugated bilirubin during a 40-week gestation, must have an alternate mechanism for excretion. This is accomplished by the transfer of unconjugated bilirubin across the placenta from fetal to maternal circulation. The maternal liver then clears and excretes this bilirubin. A small proportion of the bilirubin produced by the fetus is conjugated by the fetal liver and excreted into the GI tract. Because of the high concentration of the enzyme β-glucuronidase in the mucosal cells of the fetal small intestine, a considerable portion of this conjugated bilirubin is decomposed into unconjugated bilirubin and reabsorbed into the circulation. Bilirubin appears in the amniotic fluid by the 12th week of gestation, peaks during the second trimester and disappears by the 36th week of gestation. The mechanisms involved are not known.

In order for transplacental passage of bilirubin to occur in the fetus, it must remain in its lipid-soluble (or unconjugated) form. For postnatal excretion to occur, it must be converted to its water-soluble (or conjugated) form. To efficiently excrete the bilirubin it produces, the fetus must therefore be deficient in the mechanism for conjugation. To prepare for extrauterine life, there must be a rapid maturation during the perinatal period of the processes that allow the liver of the newborn infant to take up, conjugate and excrete bilirubin.

NEONATAL ASPECTS

Hepatic Uptake

The unconjugated bilirubin that circulates in the plasma bound to albumin is selectively removed from the blood by liver cells (Fig. 8–1). This process appears to be mediated by two cytoplasmic organic anion-binding proteins present in the hepatocyte (Y and Z

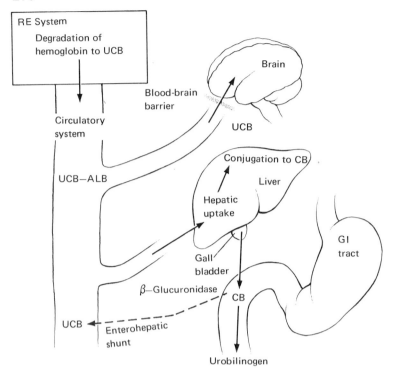

FIG. 8–1. Normal bilirubin metabolism. In the reticuloendothelial (RE) system, hemoglobin and other heme-containing pigments are broken down into unconjugated bilirubin (UCB), which is transported in the blood bound to albumin molecules (UCB-AlB); when albumin-binding sites are saturated, UCB may enter the brain and cause bilirubin encephalopathy. UCB is converted to conjugated bilirubin (CB) in the liver and excreted via bile into the GI tract. Bacteria then convert it into urobilinogen, which is excreted in the urine and stool. The enzyme β-glucuronidase, present in cells lining the wall of the small intestine, may convert CB into UCB that is ultimately reabsorbed into the systemic circulation (enterohepatic shunt).

proteins). Levi et al (68) have demonstrated that the Y protein, which is the major acceptor of indirect bilirubin, is deficient in rhesus monkeys during the perinatal period and reaches adult levels by the age of ten days. Z protein, the less important of the hepatocyte protein receptors, is present in adult levels in late fetal life. Gartner and Lane (55) have demonstrated that the cumulative hepatic uptake of bilirubin in the newborn rhesus monkey (during the first 36 hours of life) is 35% of the adult capacity. In monkeys who are born two weeks postterm, this mechanism is fully mature by age four hours.

Glucuronidation

Once the unconjugated bilirubin is incorporated into the hepatocyte, it must be converted into a more polar water-soluble form capable of being excreted into the GI tract via the bile.

The mechanism by which unconjugated bilirubin is converted to conjugated bilirubin was discovered simultaneously by Billings and Lathe (41), Schmid et al (85) and Talefant in 1956 (92). In this reaction, two moles of glucuronic acid, derived from uridine diphosphate glucuronic acid (UDPGA), become attached to the carboxyl groups of the side chains of unconjugated bilirubin. Since UDPGA is formed from glucose, this reaction may be impaired by the presence of hypoglycemia. Glucuronidation occurs in the presence of glucuronyl transferase, an enzyme associated with the endoplasmic reticulum of the hepatocyte. There is experimental evidence that this reaction is depressed during the early neonatal period (55).

The conjugation of bilirubin can be depicted by the following set of equations:

1. Glucose = 1 = PO_4 + Uridine = 1 = $(PO_4)_3$ $\xrightarrow{\text{Uridyl transferase}}$ Uridine diphosphoglucose (UDPG) + Pyrophosphate

2. UDPG + DPN+ $\xrightarrow{\text{UDPG dehydrogenase}}$ Uridinediphosphoglucuronic acid (UDPGA) + DPNH

3. Unconjugated bilirubin + UDPGA $\xrightarrow{\text{Glucuronyl transferase}}$ Bilirubin diglucuronide

Excretion

The water-soluble bilirubin diglucuronide thus formed is excreted into the bile canaliculus via an energy-dependent process and then through the bile ducts and gall bladder into the intestine. There is evidence that in newborn animals the ability of the hepatocyte to excrete conjugated bilirubin is decreased during the first days of life.

In the older child and adult, most of the conjugated bilirubin is then reduced by bacterial flora of the GI tract to urobilinogens. About 75% of the urobilinogen is reabsorbed in the ileum and subsequently excreted by the kidney and liver. The urobilinogen may be oxidized by bacteria in the GI tract and excreted in the stool.

During the first days of life, when bacterial colonization of the GI tract is being established, the conversion of conjugated bilirubin to urobilinogen may be markedly decreased. Relatively large amounts of bilirubin may therefore remain within the GI tract. Since β-glucuronidase activity is still present in intestinal mucosal cells during the neonatal period, conjugated bilirubin may be reconverted to unconjugated bilirubin by the uncoupling of two moles of glucuronide from the former compound. The unconjugated bilirubin can then be reabsorbed across the intestinal mucosa into the infant's circulation (enterohepatic shunt) or excreted in the stool.

CAUSES OF NEONATAL HYPERBILIRUBINEMIA

Causes of early onset of hyperbilirubinemia in the neonate include: isoimmunization (Rh or ABO incompatibility); physiologic jaundice; G-6-PD deficiency; unusual RBC abnormalities (e.g., hereditary spherocytosis, pyruvate kinase deficiency, hereditary elliptocytosis); reabsorption of blood; infection; and inadequate circulatory adjustment (e.g., patent ductus venosus). Late onset neonatal hyperbilirubinemia may be caused by galactosemia; alpha 1-antitrypsin deficiency; breast milk jaundice; hypothyroidism; surgical disorders (e.g., biliary atresia, choledochol cysts, annular pancreas, intestinal obstruction); and Crigler-Najjar syndrome (may appear early).

PHYSIOLOGIC JAUNDICE

Since the ability of all newborn infants to conjugate and excrete bilirubin is at least somewhat limited, serum concentrations of unconjugated bilirubin are universally elevated during the first days of life when compared to adult levels. Clinical jaundice becomes evident when serum bilirubin levels exceed 4 mg/100 ml. There is evidence that RBC breakdown is slightly accelerated in the neonatal period (fetal RBCs have a relatively short half-life, and hemoglobin concentrations decrease considerably from their high intrauterine levels during the first weeks of life). However, it is unlikely that this is a major factor in the production of jaundice.

In the gestationally mature (or postmature) infant, in whom there is no active hemolytic process nor any other reason for a major destruction of RBCs, the functional ability of systems involved in hepatic uptake, conjugation and excretion of bilirubin increases during the first few days of life, and the problem is rapidly overcome. In the infant who is gestationally immature, even without increased RBC destruction, a prolongation of the inability to remove bilirubin may be seen. With this, there may be a moderate or marked accumulation of bilirubin in the infant. This "physiologic" jaundice of prematurity is apparently due to the functional immaturity of one or more of the steps in the metabolic pathway of bilirubin from incorporation into the hepatocyte to excretion via the GI tract.

The peak elevation of serum bilirubin occurs earlier (about the third day) and is usually lower in full-term than in premature infants (about the fifth day). Although elevated levels usually fall rapidly in healthy full-term infants, they may persist into the second week of life in premature babies. For jaundice to be physiologic, the maximum daily increase in the concentration of unconjugated bilirubin must not exceed 5 mg/100 ml per day and the peak bilirubin level should not exceed 12 mg/100 ml in a full-term or 15 mg/100 ml in a premature infant.

HEMOLYTIC DISEASE OF THE NEWBORN

Increased hemolysis of RBCs (hemolytic disease of the newborn) is the most important underlying cause for significant neonatal jaundice and its neurologic sequelae. In the case of a maternofetal blood group incompatibility, fetal and neonatal RBCs are destroyed by an antibody of maternal origin. The antibody formed in the mother against an antigen that is present in the fetal RBCs (but absent in the mother's) crosses the placenta into the fetal circulation, with a resultant increased hemolysis of fetal and neonatal RBCs. The two major groups of antigens responsible for hemolytic disease of the newborn are the Rh and ABO groups. Since Rh antigens are found only in RBCs, prior sensitization in a pregnant Rh negative woman (due either to a previous completed pregnancy, abortion or transfusion with Rh positive blood) is usually necessary before a fetus can become sensitized in utero. On the other hand, A and B antigens are universal, and antibodies are usually found in women who do not have these antigens in their red cells.

Therefore, it is highly unlikely for the first Rh positive fetus of an Rh negative woman to be affected by Rh hemolytic disease unless the mother has been previously sensitized by Rh positive blood. On the other hand, the first fetus of a type O mother may develop hemolytic disease.

Of the two, Rh incompatibility is by far the more severe. It has been responsible for significant fetal morbidity and mortality and severe neurologic damage secondary to bilirubin encephalopathy. Hemolytic disease secondary to AO or BO incompatibility is generally more benign, with little fetal morbidity and no fetal mortality.

Rh Incompatability

The past quarter century has witnessed one of the significant series of advances in perinatal medicine: first, treatment of the infant affected by Rh hemolytic disease, then the treatment of the affected fetus and finally the ability to almost completely eradicate this disease by preventative means.

The discovery of the Rh factor by Landsteiner and Wiener (67) and Levine et al (69) paved the way to understanding erythroblastosis fetalis and rationally approaching its management. Several Rh antigenic substances on the red blood cell have a mendelian dominant mode of inheritance. The most important of these, accounting for about 93% of cases of Rh incompatibility, is the Rh_o (or D) antigen.

The pathogenesis of erythroblastosis is straightforward. Rh negative mothers are capable of producing Rh positive fetuses if the father is heterozygous or homozygous Rh positive. Fetal RBCs will therefore contain an antigenic substance not present in maternal cells. Since the human placenta contains a single syncitial layer separating the villi containing fetal blood vessels and maternal sinuses, the thinning out of the expanding placental surfaces and the presence of small leaks in the placental barrier facilitate passage of RBCs from fetal to maternal circulation. At the time of delivery or abortion, larger volumes of blood enter the maternal circulation, with about 0.03 to 0.07 ml necessary to initiate a maternal antibody response. The antibody produced by the mother is usually of the IgG class and is able to cross the placenta back into the fetal circulation. These antibodies attach to fetal RBCs and cause hemolysis. During the first pregnancy of an Rh negative mother, the fetus is usually unaffected (unless the mother has had a previous transfusion with Rh positive blood) because the quantity of fetal blood entering the maternal circulation during pregnancy is insufficient to stimulate an initial antibody response. However, the larger volume of blood that enters the maternal blood at parturition or abortion can initiate this response.

If an Rh negative woman has been previously sensitized and is pregnant with an Rh positive fetus, an anamnestic response will occur when very small amounts of fetal blood enter the maternal circulation during the course of pregnancy. The anti-Rh antibody thus produced will then enter the fetal circulation with subsequent hemolysis of fetal RBCs.

Several factors may influence the presence or severity of the hemolytic disease caused by Rh incompatibility. The father may be either Rh negative or heterozygous Rh positive. In all of the former and about one-half of the latter cases, fetal red cells are antigenically similar to the mother's. In many cases, where the fetus has Rh positive cells, the mother may not be stimulated to produce antibody in spite of exposure to the fetal antigen.

There are two types of Rh antibodies. The "complete," or saline-active type, do not cross the placenta and are therefore not involved in the etiology of erythroblastosis. The second type, which crosses the placenta, is active in plasma, serum or albumin and is "incomplete." "Blocking" antibodies are a variety of the incomplete type. The incomplete antibodies are determined by either a direct or indirect test. Both employ Coombs' serum (rabbit anti-human gamma globulin) and the test is conducted either on the infant's red cells (direct test) or on the serum (indirect test). The extent of positivity of the test usually correlates with the severity of the disease.

In Caucasian populations the prevalence of Rh negativity is about 15%; Rh incompatible marriages occur in about 13% of the population, and erythroblastosis occurs in 1:150 to 1:200 full-term pregnancies (prior to the institution of immunoprophylaxis). This low prevalence reflects the inability of most Rh negative mothers to produce Rh antibodies; even among those who are Rh negative and have been previously sensitized, about 10% fail to respond to further stimulation. Among the black population, the prevalence of Rh negativity is about 5%; when disease occurs, it is usually milder than among Caucasians. Rh negativity is almost nonexistent among people of Oriental background.

ABO Incompatability

About 20% to 25% of infants born to mothers with type O blood have either type A or B red cells. Hemolytic disease secondary to this type of incompatibility occurs in about 10% of these cases. While the clinical picture may resemble that seen with Rh hemolytic disease, hyperbilirubinemia is usually the major problem; anemia, if present, is rarely life threatening.

The presence of anti A and B antibodies in the serum of group O mothers is almost universal and therefore of limited diagnostic or prognostic value. Unlike Rh disease, in which the severity increases with succeeding pregnancies, no such trend is consistently observed in ABO incompatibility. About 50% of all cases occur among first-born infants, in contrast to almost none with Rh incompatibility.

An infant may be icteric for reasons other than ABO isoimmunization even when this incompatibility is present. The presence of a positive direct Coombs' test and microspherocytes on peripheral blood smear help establish a presumptive diagnosis.

This disorder is managed in essentially the same way as Rh isoimmunization, except that it is usually milder and rarely associated with severe cardiovascular problems.

Occasionally Rh and ABO incompatibility occur simultaneously. Because of the greater antigenicity of A and B antigens, Rh isoimmunization may be suppressed. Since type A or B red cells entering the maternal circulation are hemolyzed by maternal antibodies already present, fewer cells may be available for Rh isoimmunization. Mild hemolytic disease therefore often ensues if there is a double incompatibility.

GLUCOSE-6-PHOSPHATE DEHYDROGENASE DEFICIENCY

The reduction or absence of RBC glucose-6-phosphate dehydrogenase (G-6-PD) activity occurs in a group of sex-linked recessive traits found among black, Mediterranean and certain Asiatic populations. The defect is usually most severe in the Mediterranean group.

Newborn male infants with this disorder have red blood cells that are especially prone to hemolysis by a variety of chemical agents and by such perinatal factors as hypoxia and acidosis (75). The hyperbilirubinemia resulting from the hemolysis may lead to bilirubin encephalopathy.

The exact mechanism causing hemolysis in G-6-PD deficient individuals is not completely understood. This enzyme is necessary for the regeneration of reduced nicotinamide adenine dinucleotide (NADH), which in turn is required as the source of hydrogen ions for the production of reduced glutathione (GSH). This latter compound protects the RBC from oxidation and subsequent hemolysis.

In populations with a high incidence of G-6-PD deficiency, agents capable of inducing hemolysis, e.g., sulfonamides, water-soluble analogues of vitamin K, certain antimalarials, nitrofurans, salicylates, fava beans and mothballs, must be scrupulously avoided during both pregnancy and the neonatal period.

When hyperbilirubinemia secondary to this disorder occurs, it should be approached in the same manner as other varieties of hemolytic disease.

OTHER CAUSES OF NEONATAL JAUNDICE

RBC Abnormalities

A variety of intrinsic abnormalities of the RBC may be responsible for increased hemolysis during the neonatal period. Hereditary spherocytosis, pyruvate kinase deficiency and hereditary elliptocytosis have been implicated as unusual etiologic factors.

Reabsorption of Blood

Mobilization of blood that has accumulated in a closed space of the body, e.g., skin, adrenal glands, cephalhematoma and liver, may be responsible for an unusually large load of unconjugated bilirubin that the liver is not able to completely clear from the blood, conjugate and excrete into the bile. This is a fairly frequent cause of neonatal jaundice. Ingestion of large quantities of maternal blood during the intrapartum period with GI absorption has also been implicated as a cause of neonatal jaundice (57).

Infection

Infection may also be associated with neonatal jaundice. Hyperbilirubinemia is often a presenting sign in rubella, toxoplasmosis, h. simplex, cytomegalovirus and infectious hepatitis. In bacterial sepsis, increased hemolysis may play a role in the pathogenesis of the jaundice.

Inadequate Circulatory Adjustment

Inadequate circulatory adjustment in the premature infant may lead to an increase in the concentration of unconjugated bilirubin. If the ductus venosus remains patent for a prolonged period after birth, portal vein blood may largely bypass the liver, thus preventing clearance of unconjugated bilirubin.

Metabolic Disorders

Certain metabolic disorders, such as galactosemia and α_1-antitrypsin deficiency, may have jaundice as a presenting sign.

Breast Milk Jaundice

The observation of prolonged jaundice in some breast-fed infants has led to the isolation of an icterogenic factor, pregnane-3α, 20β-diol, from their mothers' milk (38, 39). Discontinuation of breast feeding leads to an amelioration of the jaundice. Whether this is the only substance in "icterogenic milk" causing hyperbilirubinemia has been seriously questioned. It has been suggested that there may be more than one inhibitory substance leading to this condition (61).

Mongolism and Hypothyroidism

Hyperbilirubinemia may be associated with mongolism and congenital hypothyroidism. The reason for this is not completely understood.

Surgical Disorders

Certain surgical conditions of the neonate are also associated with an increased incidence of jaundice. With intestinal obstruction, the hyperbilirubinemia may be secondary to increased enterohepatic shunting of bilirubin. Choledochal cysts (a cystic dilatation of the common bile duct) and annular pancreas are associated with in increase in the concentration of conjugated bilirubin. Biliary atresia is usually not evident in the early neonatal period. Increased accumulations of both conjugated and unconjugated bilirubin may be encountered in this disorder. Hyperbilirubinemia may also accompany pyloric stenosis. This may be due, at least in part, to the compression of the ampulla of Vater by the pyloric tumor.

Crigler-Najjar Syndrome

The Crigler-Najjar syndrome (congenital absence of the enzyme glucuronyl transferase) may be mistaken for physiologic jaundice, at least in the early neonatal period (47). However, prolonged and unremitting jaundice, often causing bilirubin encephalopathy, may lead to the suspicion of this diagnosis.

BILIRUBIN ENCEPHALOPATHY (KERNICTERUS)

Kernicterus (literally "nuclear staining") is the deposition of unconjugated bilirubin in cells of the CNS. Bilirubin is a toxin that interferes with vital cellular functions; the exact mechanism of action within the cell is not known. In the test tube it uncouples mitochondrial oxidative phosphorylation. However, Diamond and Schmid (49) were unable to demonstrate deranged oxidative phosphorylation in parts of the most highly stained brains of guinea pigs with bilirubin encephalopathy.

The areas of the brain most affected by bilirubin are the globus pallidus, lenticular nucleus of the corpus striatum, the subthalamic nucleus of the hippocampus, mamillary bodies on the flood of the fourth ventricle and the cerebellar nuclei. The thalamus and putamen are less often involved, as is the gray matter of the cerebral cortex. After the acute episode of entry of bilirubin into brain cells, the pigment gradually disappears (in surviving infants), and neuronal atrophy and gliosis may be seen. Microscopic changes (pyknotic and degenerated nuclei) may be seen as early as 24 hours after the acute insult.

Since unconjugated bilirubin is cleared by the placenta, kernicterus does not occur in utero in the human fetus. Hirata et al (62) were able to induce kernicterus in fetal rats by intraperitoneal injection of unconjugated bilirubin. They were able to worsen the kernicterus risk with concurrent injection of hyaluronidase and to decrease the risk with epinephrine, suggesting that vascular permeability of the blood-brain barrier is involved in the pathogenesis of kernicterus.

CLINICAL MANIFESTATIONS

The classic manifestations of kernicterus usually occur between the second and fourth days of life, but they may develop at any time until the beginning of the second week. In children with persistent unconjugated hyperbilirubinemia (Crigler-Najjar syndrome), however, bilirubin encephalopathy is not limited to the neonatal period and may occur during infancy or childhood.

Kernicterus usually occurs in neonates with hemolytic disease, most often due to a blood group incompatibility in which serum unconjugated bilirubin levels have risen above 20 mg/100 ml. It may occur at much lower levels in small premature infants, especially those who have been asphyxiated (37, 56) or acidotic and those who have RDS. In these infants, the classic signs of kernicterus may not be seen, and the diagnosis is not made until either postmortem examination or manifestation of neurologic signs in survivors.

The initial signs are lethargy, poor suck and a sluggish Moro reflex with incomplete flexion. The infant may assume an opisthotonic position, especially when startled. At first the infant is hypotonic, but this is soon replaced by generalized rigidity. Paresis of the extraocular muscles may occur, and a "setting sun" sign may appear. Twitching, oculogyric crises and frank convulsions may be seen. Some infants become hyperpyrexic. Gastric, CNS and pulmonary hemorrhages may occur terminally. Occasionally, the signs in full-term infants may be quite subtle, and only lethargy is seen. Here, the diagnosis of kernicterus is made retrospectively when the classic sequelae subsequently appear. About one-half of full-term and at least 75% of premature infants who shows signs of kernicterus do not survive the neonatal period.

LONG-TERM EFFECTS

Among survivors, there may be a latent period of up to three months when neurologic signs disappear. In later infancy and childhood, choreoathetosis and rigidity are frequently seen, and in less severely affected infants there may be hypotonia. High-frequency deafness is common, along with faulty tooth enamel formation. Mental retardation is seen frequently and is often severe.

There is growing evidence that unconjugated hyperbilirubinemia may adversely affect psychomotor development without frank kernicterus and at levels that had not been previously considered toxic. In a collaborative study of 23,000 infants, Boggs et al (42) found evidence of psychomotor retardation (using the Bayley Infant Developmental Scale) at age eight months in infants whose peak serum bilirubin levels in the neonatal period (16 to 19 mg/100 ml) are not ordinarily associated with kernicterus. Hardy and Peeples (60) found that as unconjugated bilirubin levels in the neonatal period rose over 10 mg/100 ml, the association with psychomotor retardation became progressively stronger, especially with regard to the Bayley Scale. Hymen et al (63) showed that serum concentrations as low as 15 mg/100 ml had an adverse effect on the functional development of the CNS. However, other studies have suggested that the availability of albumin binding sites rather than peak serum bilirubin concentrations are correlated with the development of encephalopathy (see section Diagnosis and Treatment of Hemolytic Disease and Neonatal Jaundice).

PATHOGENESIS

There is evidence demonstrating that unconjugated bilirubin bound to albumin is nontoxic and does not enter nerve cells. Diamond and Schmid (49) have demonstrated that when C^{14} bilirubin bound to human albumin is infused into newborn guinea pigs or adult Gunn rats, bilirubin does not accumulate in the brain, and neurotoxicity is absent. When bilirubin is infused unbound to albumin, clinical manifestations similar to human kernicterus occur. When this latter group of animals is subsequently infused with human albumin, almost all of the bilirubin dissolved in the brain is removed, with a marked decrease in morbidity and mortality. Silberberg et al (86) demonstrated that albumin binding of unconjugated bilirubin prevents damage to cerebellar cells in vitro. Odell et al (79) have indirectly demonstrated that decreased binding of bilirubin by plasma albumin in human infants is significantly related to the development of brain damage.

Other factors besides the total concentration of albumin affect the binding of bilirubin. Odell (77) has demonstrated that with decreasing blood pH, unconjugated bilirubin becomes less tightly bound to albumin and that conversely with rising pH, the bond is strengthened.

Silberberg et al (86) demonstrated in rat cerebellar tissue cultures that at a constant bilirubin to albumin molar ratio, a decrease in the pH of the medium resulted in proportionately greater cytotoxicity. At pH 7.6, cytotoxicity did not occur, even in the presence of a relatively high bilirubin to albumin ratio.

Organic anions in the blood can decrease albumin binding of bilirubin. Such drugs as salicylates and sulfisoxazole compete with bilirubin for albumin-binding sites (see Ch. 21, Pharmacology). Free fatty acids, which may be elevated in the presence of cold stress, hypoglycemia or starvation, also tend to compete for these sites. Increased concentrations of heme, secondary to hemolysis of RBC may also do this. Whether photodegradation products of bilirubin are bound to protein remains to be determined.

It is therefore apparent that measurement of the bilirubin concentration in a given jaundiced infant is inadequate in predicting the danger of encephalopathy. Acid-base balance, albumin concentration, the infant's maturity and drugs that have been administered must all be taken into consideration.

DIAGNOSIS AND TREATMENT OF HEMOLYTIC DISEASE AND NEONATAL JAUNDICE

During the 1960s two major advances in fetal medicine occurred in the areas of prevention and treatment of hydrops fetalis. Intrauterine diagnosis of fetal hemolytic disease by examination of amniotic fluid and development of techniques to perform intrauterine blood transfusions led to increased perinatal survival of affected fetuses (51, 53, 72). Passive immunization against the Rh antigen, which became widely available in the late 1960s, led to a marked reduction in the incidence of isoimmunization (54).

MANAGEMENT OF THE RH$_0$ NEGATIVE GRAVIDA

Maternal blood type must be determined at the first prenatal visit. If it is Rh$_0$ negative and there has been either a previous pregnancy or transfusion with Rh$_0$ positive blood, the possibility of fetal isoimmunization must be borne in mind, and the father's blood type must be determined. If it is Rh$_0$ negative, the fetus is in no danger. More likely, the father will be Rh$_0$ positive. In this case, maternal blood specimens should be obtained to determine antibody titers during the first trimester. These should be repeated monthly during the second trimester and every two weeks during the third trimester. If antibody is detected, closer surveillance is necessary, and measurements should be made at one to two-week intervals.

There is only an approximate correlation between the level of anti-Rh$_0$ antibodies in maternal serum and the severity of the hemolytic process in the fetus. If the antibodies are primarily of the complete or saline-agglutinating type, the disorder may be less severe than if the antibodies are predominantly of the incomplete (albumin-agglutinating) type.

If the titer of anti-Rh$_0$ antibody is 1:32 or greater, amniocentesis is indicated (fetal death secondary to hydrops fetalis is rarely if ever seen if the antibody titer is 1:16 or less).

If a gravida has been sensitized during a previous pregnancy, a high antibody titer may be observed even if the present fetus is not sensitized. Fixed high titers may be present and may rise even when the fetus is Rh$_0$ negative. Amniocentesis should be performed in the presence of a fixed titer of 1:32 or greater, even though it may actually represent sensitization that has occurred in a previous pregnancy.

The initial amniocentesis may be performed as early as the 24th week of preg-

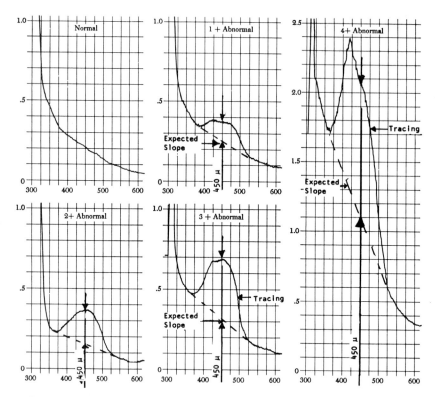

FIG. 8–2. Serial tracings on amniotic fluid specimens demonstrating the progressive development of the abnormal curve. (Freda VJ, Am J Obstet Gynecol 92:341, 1965)

nancy and is repeated as indicated at one to two-week intervals.

Interpretation of Amniocentesis

Amniotic fluid is examined by a spectrophotometric method that detects the presence of bile pigments (primarily bilirubin) that have accumulated because of increased hemolysis of fetal RBCs.

The normal smooth spectrophotometric curve of amniotic fluid at the wave lengths of visible light and departures from normal, in the region of 450 nm are due to bile pigments (Fig. 8–2).

Interpretation of results is based both on the difference in optical density (Δ OD) between expected and observed reading at a wave length of 450 nm and on the total bilirubin concentration of amniotic fluid.

With a normal reading, the fetus is judged to be safe for the next two weeks and may even be Rh₀ negative. In this case, amniocentesis should be repeated in two weeks.

With a 1+ curve, the fetus is in no immediate danger, and amniocentesis should be repeated in ten days.

If the curve is 2+, abnormal hemolytic disease is known to exist, but the fetus is safe for at least one more week at which time amniocentesis is repeated.

A 3+ curve indicates that immediate treatment must be undertaken to save the life of the fetus. Treatment may consist of intrauterine transfusion or immediate delivery and is dependent on the degree of fetal pulmonary maturity, i.e., on the ability of the fetus to survive in an air-breathing environment. Fetal maturity is assessed by determining the quantity of surface active phospholipids in amniotic fluid (see section Respiratory Distress Syndrome, Ch. 6). If there is a minimal or moderate risk of RDS (usually in fetuses of 32 or more weeks' gestation), immediate delivery is indicated.

If the risk of severe RDS is high, intrauterine transfusion is the treatment of choice. Caution is advised, however, in the interpretation of these tests of fetal maturity, since both false positive and false negative results may be encountered.

If there is a 4+ curve, the fetus is either moribund or already dead, and immediate delivery is indicated.

Since such contaminants of amniotic fluid as blood and meconium may lead to inaccurate results, the curves must be interpreted with caution.

Intrauterine Transfusion

The basic principle of intrauterine transfusion is the treatment of the profound anemia with packed RBCs to prevent fetal death. Liley (71) found that packed RBCs injected into the fetal peritoneal cavity could be absorbed into the circulation, thus increasing the hemoglobin concentration.

Prior to transfusion, a radiopaque dye is injected into the amniotic cavity, where it mixes with amniotic fluid. The fetus swallows the amniotic fluid, outlining the GI tract. In order to inject RBCs, a 17-gauge needle is inserted into the fetal peritoneal cavity. A polyethylene catheter is threaded through the needle, and the needle then removed. Packed, fresh type O, Rh$_0$ negative RBCs are then injected through the catheter. Freda (52) suggests an RBC volume of 50 ml at 23 weeks' gestation, with increments of 20 ml for each additional 2 weeks of gestation. Transfusion should be repeated at two-week intervals until there is biochemical evidence of fetal pulmonary maturity, at which time the fetus should be delivered. If the fetus is born alive, one or more exchange transfusions may be anticipated.

Complications of this procedure are premature induction of labor, bleeding and fetomaternal infection. Trauma to such fetal organs as the kidney and liver may occur if they have been inadvertently pierced by the needle. In fetuses of up to 25 weeks' gestation, the mortality rate associated with this procedure is 90% to 100%. This decreases from 50% to 80% between 25 and 30 weeks'

gestation and is below 50% after the 30th week.

Prevention of Isoimmunization

It has been well recognized for many years that active immunization is suppressed in the presence of passive immunization. Since active immunization occurs in the Rh$_0$ negative mother when fetal Rh$_0$ positive RBCs enter her circulation either at parturition or following abortion, it follows that administration of Rh$_0$ immunoglobulin at this time suppresses the synthesis of Rh$_0$ antibody. Gorman et al (59) tested this hypothesis in adult male Rh$_0$ negative subjects who received Rh$_0$ positive erythrocytes intravenously. When Rh$_0$ immunoglubulin was administered within three days to these subjects, 100% protection against the formation of Rh$_0$ antibodies was afforded with no harmful side-effects noted.

Clinical trials in pregnant women demonstrated the efficacy and safety of this mode of therapy (54, 96) and showed conclusively that Rh$_0$ positive erythrocytes were destroyed by Rh$_0$ immunoglobulin administered to the mother.

NEONATAL PERIOD

Hydrops Fetalis

The incidence of hydrops fetalis has been markedly reduced. However, it is occasionally encountered in clinical practice.

The major immediate threat to the newborn infant who has been hemolyzing red blood cells in utero (almost always secondary to Rh incompatibility) is severe anemia. The most severely affected infants are hydropic. If born alive they are usually premature, often less than 34 weeks' gestational age, with severe pallor, subcutaneous edema, hepatosplenomegaly, congestive heart failure and ascites. Survival is uncommon in this group, and most die shortly after birth without much spontaneous respiratory activity. Emergency treatment in the delivery room with a partial exchange transfusion with blood of high hematocrit may increase survival. In spite of the very high venous pressure, the blood volume may not be elevated, and phlebotomy without replacement may present certain dangers. Nathan (76) has found the use of peritoneal dialysis and positive pressure ventilation, along with exchange transfusion, to be of some value in increasing survival rates. Usually, these infants have severe anemia with cord blood hemoglobin levels of less than 6 to 7 g/100 ml. They represent cases that should have been followed carefully by amniocentesis and treated with either early delivery or intrauterine transfusion.

Severe Anemia Without Hydrops

Another group requiring prompt therapy consists of infants with severe anemia (cord blood hemoglobin less than 12 g/100 ml, but greater than 6 to 7 g/100 ml). While Rh isoimmunization accounts for most of these infants, severe ABO incompatibility may also occasionally produce this picture. These infants, who generally have cord blood unconjugated bilirubin levels of 3 to 5 mg/100 ml are usually vigorous, with mild edema, pallor and hepatosplenomegaly. Hypoglycemia, secondary to pancreatic beta-cell hypertrophy may occur. The reason for this phenomenon has not been fully explained. In the first few hours of life exchange transfusion is necessary to remove sensitized RBCs (which are likely to hemolyze and serve as a source of unconjugated bilirubin) and to increase the hemoglobin concentration, thereby ameliorating or preventing congestive heart failure. This group usually consists of infants identified as being moderately affected by amniocentesis and delivered after 37 weeks' gestation.

Jaundice With Mild or No Anemia

A third group consists of less severely affected infants whose cord blood hemoglobin concentrations are above 12 g/100 ml and whose unconjugated bilirubin is below 3 mg/100. Immediate therapy is not required in this group. Amniocenteses are usually normal or show only mild peaks; hence, there would have been no interruption of pregnancy. In some, levels of hemoglobin may be almost normal, and bilirubin levels may be at 2 mg/100 ml or less in the cord blood. Among this latter group are those in whom the risk of hemolytic disease is high (mother Rh negative and infant Rh positive, or mother O and infant A or B), and a direct Coombs' test on the infant's red cells should be performed. A positive result confirms the presence of Rh sensitization. If the hemolytic process is secondary to AO or BO incompatibility, the Coombs' test is usually, but not necessarily, positive.

In the presence of hyperbilirubinemia secondary to hemolytic disease, serum bilirubin determinations should be performed once every four to eight hours; a very rapid rise in the level of serum bilirubin during the first day of life is a clear-cut indication for performing an exchange transfusion. An unconjugated bilirubin level, whether secondary to Rh or ABO incompatibility of over 6 mg/100 ml in the first 6 hours, or 10 mg/100 ml in the first 12 hours, or a rate of increase of serum indirect bilirubin concentration of 0.75 to 1.0 mg/hr, are indications for immediate exchange transfusion.

While the clinical course of the infant is being closely followed, preparations for a possible exchange transfusion should be made.

It is in the group of infants whose increment in serum bilirubin is not extremely rapid that the dilemma concerning management arises. If there were a definitive method of determining which infants were at risk of developing bilirubin encephalopathy, then only those infants would have to undergo exchange transfusion. There would, therefore, be a minimal number of unnecessary exchange transfusions (the mortality rate is almost 1%) (95), and no infant would escape exchange transfusion if any real danger of bilirubin encephalopathy existed.

As a general rule, unconjugated serum bilirubin concentrations of over 20 mg/100 ml are associated with a risk of bilirubin encephalopathy. At this level a 1:1 molar ratio of unconjugated bilirubin to albumin is approached in normal infants with serum albumin concentrations of 3.0 to 3.5 g/100 ml. There are so many exceptions to this that the level of 20 mg/100 ml can only be used as an approximation. In full-term infants, lower levels may be associated with psychomotor retardation or minimal cerebral dysfunction (42, 60, 65); and in very small and gestationally immature infants, especially those who have been asphyxiated, acidotic or have a low serum albumin level, kernicterus may occur at levels below 10 mg/100 ml (37, 56). On the other hand, infants with serum bilirubin levels of 25 to 30 mg/100 ml have been known to escape neurologic sequelae.

DIAGNOSIS

Management begins with careful and close observation of all newborn infants during the first 48 hours of life and identification of those who appear jaundiced. If a sensitized fetus is identified during pregnancy, the pediatrician should be notified prior to delivery and preparations made for emergency treatment after the infant is born. Fresh Rh negative blood should be available in the delivery room since immediate exchange transfusion may be necessary. Testing of the infant's blood type, serum bilirubin level, direct Coombs' test, hemoglobin (or hematocrit) and peripheral blood smear should be performed even if the jaundice is not yet visible. The cord blood specimen should be used for initial testing. We have made it a practice to save the cord blood of every neonate for four to five days since jaundice secondary to ABO incompatibility may not become evident until after the first day of life.

When jaundice first becomes apparent, the serum bilirubin concentration must be determined. A micromethod using just a few drops of serum (70) should be available so that frequent determinations can be made without lowering the blood volume or subjecting the infant to the trauma of repeated venipunctures. We have found this to be an excellent screening device for monitoring total bilirubin concentrations. When a level of total bilirubin is reached at which it is felt

there may be an impending risk of neurologic damage, unconjugated bilirubin concentrations are also measured. In addition, hemoglobin (or hematocrit) concentrations are routinely followed. It should be noted that hemoglobin concentrations often increase under ordinary circumstances during the first day or two after birth. Reticulocyte counts and inspection of the peripheral blood smear for nucleated RBCs are also of value in determining if a hemolytic process is occurring.

An attempt must be made to determine the etiology of the jaundice. In many cases, especially in the presence of a positive Coombs' test, the specific diagnosis of a blood group incompatibility can be made. The presence of microspherocytes on a peripheral smear is usually indicative of an ABO group incompatibility. However, this finding may also occur in congenital spherocytosis, an infrequent cause of neonatal jaundice that should nonetheless be considered. In many instances, the diagnosis may be more obscure. If there is a positive Coombs' test and no evidence of a major blood group incompatibility, then a less commonly encountered cause of isoimmunization must be sought. Unexplained jaundice in the face of a falling hemoglobin may be due to systemic infection or bleeding into an internal organ, and these possible causes should be investigated. Jaundice not infrequently accompanies pyelonephritis; therefore, a urinalysis should be a routine part of the investigation. The hepatitis associated with congenital syphilis, rubella, toxoplasmosis, cytomegalovirus and h. simplex may be a cause of jaundice. The hepatosplenomegaly usually present in hemolytic disease may also suggest sepsis. If the infant is of black, Mediterranean or Chinese ancestry, G-6-PD deficiency may be seriously considered. A screening test for G-6-PD should be performed when deficiency is suspected. Jaundice secondary to ingestion of breast milk, hypothyroidism, neonatal hepatitis or biliary atresia are rare in the early neonatal period.

In the premature infant, especially one who is sick, a specific cause for the jaundice may not be ascertained. Many small and relatively immature infants have bruising with leakage of blood into subcutaneous tissues. The inability of the liver to conjugate and excrete the bilirubin formed from this blood often contributes to the jaundice seen in these infants.

Since both blood pH and albumin concentration are important in the binding of unconjugated bilirubin, it is particularly necessary to make these measurements in compromised or premature infants with jaundice. Determinations can be performed on very small quantities of blood, the former by the Astrup technique and the latter by use of a total solute refractometer.

Tests of Albumin Binding

Porter and Waters (83) described a test that measures the reserve bilirubin-binding sites of albumin utilizing an organic dye, 2(4'-hydroxybenzeneazo) benzoic acid. Using this technique, Johnson and Boggs (65) have shown that jaundiced infants with relatively few available binding sites (binding capacity less than 50%) have a significantly higher incidence of psychomotor retardation at age four years than those jaundiced infants with a greater availability of binding sites (capacity greater than 50%). The availability of binding sites was not necessarily related to the peak bilirubin level.

Odell et al (79) have devised a technique utilizing salicylate binding of albumin to determine the availability of binding sites. They, too, were able to correlate deficiency of binding sites with neurologic damage, irrespective of peak bilirubin concentrations. The in vitro test is carried out at a pH of 7.40, whereas the infant's actual blood pH may be considerably lower. Therefore, interpretation of the test may pose difficulties.

The use of Sephadex columns to determine the presence in the serum of unconjugated bilirubin not bound to albumin has been suggested (64). A possible disadvantage to this method is that when unbound bilirubin is detected in the serum, some of it may have already entered brain cells.

These measurements hold promise as additional laboratory tools in evaluating the potential risk of bilirubin toxicity. However, further trials are required before the efficacy of these techniques in clinical practice can be determined.

Treatment

Three general methods can be employed to decrease serum bilirubin levels. The first is removal of both sensitized red cells and bilirubin by exchange transfusion. This is the only method that has been conclusively shown to be of value in the prevention of bilirubin encephalopathy. The second, rarely used in clinical practice, is acceleration of normal physiologic processes (such as with phenobarbital) that may either enhance hepatic uptake of bilirubin or increase glucuronyl transferase activity. The experimental use of agar, which stabilizes conjugated bilirubin in the intestine and prevents its hydrolysis and reabsorption into the circulation, may fall into this category. The third method consists of providing alternate pathways for the degradation of bilirubin, such as with phototherapy.

In addition there are many nonspecific measures that may decrease the risk of bilirubin encephalopathy (such as maintenance of a thermoneutral environment, adequate oxygenation, treatment of acidosis and early administration of IV fluids or oral feedings).

Suggested therapeutic guidelines are shown in Table 8–7.

Exchange Transfusion

The purposes of exchange transfusion are the removal of sensitized RBC and unconjugated bilirubin, the correction of anemia and the provision of albumin in the plasma of donor blood that is capable of binding the bilirubin already diffused into body tissues.

While this procedure is usually safe in the hands of experienced operators, it is not without hazards; mortality rates of up to 1% may occur as a direct result of exchange transfusion (95). With the number of exchange transfusions being performed declining (because of prophylaxis against isoim-

TABLE 8–7. Suggested Treatment of Neonatal Jaundice

Unconjugated Bilirubin (mg/100 ml)	Day 1	Day 2	>Day 2	Comments
5–10	Phototherapy			In infants with birth weights <1500 g (especially in the presence of RDS, asphyxia, hypothermia, hypoproteinemia or acidosis) exchange should be performed in 10–15 mg/100 ml range.
10.1–15	Phototherapy (exchange in presence of hemolysis)	Phototherapy	Phototherapy	
15.1–20	Exchange	Exchange (occasionally phototherapy may be effective)	Phototherapy	With larger premature infants, exchange is usually necessary at levels >15 mg/100 ml regardless of circumstances.
>20	Exchange	Exchange	Exchange	Infants may be treated with phototherapy in 20–22 mg/100 ml range following an exchange transfusion or if albumin-binding sites are adequate.

munization, a declining birth rate and phototherapy), some expertise in performing the procedure may be lost through lack of experience. This could increase the risk associated with exchange transfusion.

Once the decision to perform an exchange transfusion has been made, the sequence of events must proceed smoothly and efficiently. The situation must be carefully explained to the parents, and operative consent obtained. A sample of maternal blood is required for cross matching since the blood used during the procedure must be compatible with the mother's blood. (If the blood used were the same type as the infant's, antibodies already present in the infant's circulation would cause rapid hemolysis of the infused blood.) If the mother is known to be sensitized, the blood bank should be alerted prior to delivery so that blood is immediately available.

Acid Citrate Dextrose. The ideal anticoagulant is still controversial. Acid citrate dextrose (ACD), which has been commonly used as an anticoagulant, has the advantage of allowing the blood to be stored for many days. The principal disadvantages of ACD blood are its very low pH (6.8 or less) and its markedly decreased concentrations of ionized calcium and magnesium (secondary to binding of these ions by citrate). Vigorous full-term infants can tolerate the low pH and, in fact, metabolize the citrate to bicarbonate, so that immediately after ex-

change transfusion there is a significant elevation of blood pH. Many small and sick infants, who are already acidotic, may not be able to tolerate the increased acid load of ACD blood (40, 44). In these infants, adding sodium bicarbonate or THAM [Tris (hydroxymethyl) aminomethane] buffer to the blood (to raise the pH to 7.40) may be necessary (81).

During exchange transfusion with ACD blood, the infant's ionized calcium concentration is extremely low, despite the routine administration of 10% calcium gluconate at intervals during the procedure.

Since the blood pH and 2,3-diphosphoglycerate (2,3-DPG) content of RBCs (see Ch. 3, Oxygenation) falls and potassium concentration rises with age following collection of the blood, it is usually inadvisable to use ACD blood that is more than two or three days old.

Heparin. Heparin has several major advantages as an anticoagulant. Among these are a normal pH, normal concentrations of ionized calcium and magnesium and normal red blood cell 2,3-DPG content. Possible disadvantages are that heparinized blood must be freshly collected and that heparin may elicit an increase in blood concentrations of nonesterified fatty acid in the infant (84). Since nonesterified fatty acid competes with unconjugated bilirubin for albumin-binding sites, the ability of albumin to bind bilirubin may be impaired. Heparin interferes with coagu-

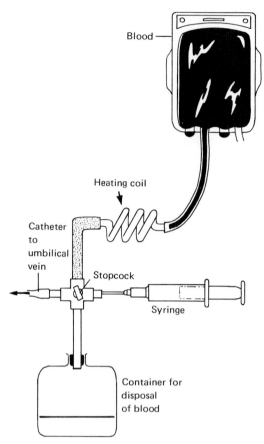

Blood

Heating coil

Catheter
to
umbilical
vein

Stopcock

Syringe

Container for
disposal
of blood

FIG. 8–3. Exchange transfusion via umbilical venous catheter. Blood is withdrawn from the infant into syringe and injected into the disposal container. Warmed, fresh blood is then drawn into the syringe and injected into the infant. Process is repeated until the desired amount of blood has been exchanged.

lation of the infant's blood, and when heparinized blood is used, 5 mg protamine should be administered intravenously (in a 3 kg full-term infant) following the transfusion.

Procedure. The infant should not be fed for at least four hours prior to an exchange transfusion since vomiting and aspiration may occur. A nasogastric tube should be inserted into the infant's stomach, and gastric contents removed.

If the infant is not anemic and has a normal venous pressure, salt-poor albumin (1 g/kg of body weight) may be administered intravenously approximately two

hours prior to exchange transfusion. This maneuver significantly increases the quantity of bilirubin removed from the infant during the transfusion (45).

An exchange transfusion must be carried out with precautions comparable to those of a surgical procedure. A portion of the nursery should be set aside as a treatment room for this purpose. Prior to the transfusion the operators must see to it that resuscitative equipment is in working order and that oxygen and suction are available. Heart rate should be monitored carefully, preferably with an electronic cardiac monitor. A thermoneutral environment should be maintained with a radiant heater.

Classically, exchange transfusions have been performed through an umbilical venous catheter, with blood being withdrawn and injected through this one route (Fig. 8–3). Concurrent use of both the umbilical vein (for withdrawal of blood) and artery (for its injection) has been advocated. Cropp (48) has successfully used a continuous isovolumetric exchange technique using a roller infusion pump to both remove blood from the umbilical vein and inject it into the umbilical artery.

The quantity of blood used in an exchange transfusion is usually twice the infant's blood volume (about 180 ml/kg). In this way, approximately 87% of the infant's original blood volume is removed. The transfusion should not be performed too rapidly. At least one hour should be allowed so that unconjugated bilirubin can diffuse out of the tissues into the vascular space. To avoid cold stress the blood should be warmed to body temperature, preferably by a heating coil, prior to its injection into the infant.

Blood should be removed for bilirubin determinations both before and after the transfusion. The postexchange unconjugated bilirubin concentration is usually about one-third that of the pre-exchange level, but the concentration rises rapidly when bilirubin reenters the circulation from peripheral tissues and becomes bound to the albumin of donor blood. Within an hour after completion of the transfusion, the bilirubin level is usually about two-thirds of that of the pre-exchange value.

Criteria for performing a second exchange transfusion vary with the infant's age, weight, clinical condition and serum bilirubin concentration. In a full-term infant an unconjugated bilirubin of 20 mg/100 ml is not as dangerous as a similar level prior to the transfusion, since much bilirubin has been removed from the tissues. If the unconjugated bilirubin level stabilizes at about 20 mg/100 ml or less following the procedure, repeat exchange transfusion is unnecessary. If it continues to rise above the 20 mg/100 ml level, the procedure should be repeated.

Continuous careful monitoring of the infant is required until the infant's clinical condition has stabilized and the serum bilirubin concentration is declining.

Chemotherapy

Certain drugs, when administered either to the mother or neonate or both, are associated with decreased levels of unconjugated bilirubin in the infant (91, 93). The most important is phenobarbital. This type of therapy has never been shown to have any effect in preventing neurologic damage, and its clinical use for prevention of hyperbilirubinemia or lowering of serum bilirubin levels is not advocated.

Another interesting, but still experimental, method of dealing with the bilirubin problem has been described by Poland et al (82). Administration of agar to neonates appears to stabilize conjugated bilirubin in solution in the lumen of the small intestine, preventing its breakdown by β-glucuronidase to unconjugated bilirubin, and therefore preventing the enterohepatic shunting of bilirubin. This phenomenon has never been confirmed, however.

Phototherapy

Cremer's (46) observation in 1958 that exposure to sunlight ameliorates neonatal jaundice led to the introduction of phototherapy as a means of lowering serum bilirubin concentrations in newborn infants. Exposure of jaundiced infants to fluorescent light was first used clinically on a large scale in Europe and South America during the early 1960s and proved successful in decreasing the number of exchange transfusions required. No apparent deleterious side-effects were immediately evident. However, there were no systematic long-term follow-up studies to evaluate the efficacy or hazards of therapy.

Phototherapy was introduced into the United States in the late 1960s. In 1968 Lucey et al (74) published the first controlled study demonstrating that phototherapy significantly decreases serum bilirubin concentrations in premature infants with physiologic jaundice. Subsequently, phototherapy was shown to be of value in decreasing serum bilirubin concentrations in mild to moderate hemolytic disease secondary to ABO incompatibility (89).

Although follow-up studies evaluating the long-term effects of phototherapy were underway in the early 1970s, there is no available evidence that phototherapy modifies neurologic development (either beneficially or adversely) in infants treated with this therapeutic regimen. In spite of this, phototherapy is undoubtedly the most popular means of treating neonatal jaundice in the United States.

Physiologic Basis of Phototherapy. Unconjugated bilirubin is photolabile at certain wave lengths (420 to 470 nm, but maximally in the blue range of 450 to 460 nm) in the presence of singlet oxygen (molecular oxygen in its first excited state). Unconjugated bilirubin is slowly degraded to more polar, more water-soluble compounds. Although the exact nature of the breakdown products is not known, there is evidence that the four pyrrole rings that make up the bilirubin molecule are broken down, first into biliverdin and then into fragments containing two pyrrole rings linked by a methane bridge.

Diamond and Schmidt (50) have demonstrated that injection of these breakdown products into experimental animals is not associated with bilirubin encephalopathy and that these substances were harmlessly excreted into the bile and urine. Silberberg et al (87) showed that photodegradation products of unconjugated bilirubin are non-toxic to newborn rat cerebellum tissue cultures. In an in vivo study involving infants with Crigler-Najjar syndrome, Callahan et al (43) demonstrated that the breakdown products are excreted primarily in bile and to a lesser extent in urine.

There is also experimental evidence that phototherapy may somehow alter the hepatic excretory pathways for bilirubin. Ostrow (80) noted that in Gunn rats exposed to phototherapy there is a markedly increased excretion of unconjugated bilirubin in the bile. This mechanism has also been demonstrated in newborn infants treated with phototherapy.

Odell et al (78) have found that the bilirubin-binding capacity of albumin is decreased when serum is exposed in vitro to 2000 footcandles of light. However, this finding has never been substantiated in living subjects.

There is some evidence that erythrocytes become photosensitized in the presence of unconjugated bilirubin, with a loss of cations, especially potassium, occurring across the altered cell membranes.

Other biologic effects of phototherapy in the human neonate are poorly understood. There is evidence, for example, that newborn piglets whose eyes remain unshielded while exposed to fluorescent lighting incur pathologic retinal changes including hemorrhage (88). No known visual changes have been described, however, in newborn infants being treated with phototherapy. However, in clinical practice the eyes always are shielded.

Animal studies have also shown that exposure to light affects circardian rhythms, weight of gonads, time of onset of puberty and ovulation.

Clinical Considerations. Although countless thousands of newborn infants have been treated with phototherapy, there are still no absolute guidelines for the institution of therapy, duration of treatment and types of light that should be used. The potential risks of bilirubin encephalopathy must clearly outweigh any potential side-effects of this method of treatment. As a rule, phototherapy should not be used prophylactically in the nonjaundiced infant.

Phototherapy should be instituted in physiologic jaundice or mild to moderate hemolytic disease only when the serum concentration of unconjugated bilirubin exceeds 10 mg/100 ml. In the presence of mild to moderate hemolytic disease, phototherapy may be used during the first 24 hours of life if the bilirubin concentration is in the range of 5 to 10 mg/100 ml. In the presence of moderately severe or severe hemolytic disease, when unconjugated bilirubin concentrations are rising rapidly and significant anemia is present, phototherapy should not be used in place of a necessary exchange transfusion.

A variety of phototherapy units are commercially available for use in the nursery. White, daylight, blue and narrow spectrum blue fluorescent bulbs have all been used in these units. The effectiveness of the bulb in lowering the serum bilirubin concentration depends on the amount of energy it emits in the blue spectrum (Fig. 8–4). While daylight bulbs have been used with a considerable degree of success, Sisson et al (90) found a narrow spectrum (420 to 470 nm) blue bulb to be more effective than either standard blue or daylight bulbs in lowering serum bilirubin concentrations. It should be noted that the effectiveness of the bulb (as measured by microwatts) is not related to the intensity of the light it emits (as measured by footcandles). While four to six days of continuous therapy is usually necessary when daylight bulbs are used, Sisson et al have been able to significantly decrease the treatment time by using the special blue bulbs. However, because of the rapid decay of the effective energy output in commercially available blue bulbs, daylight bulbs are still being used (as of 1975), on a clinical basis.

An alternate approach to phototherapy has been suggested by Giunta et al (58). Exposure of premature infants to relatively high-intensity overhead daylight fluorescent

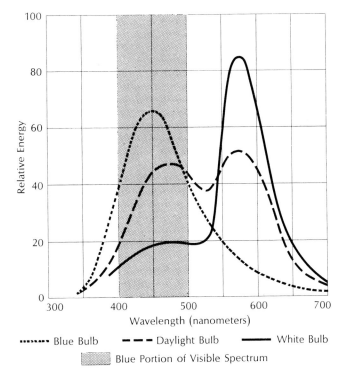

FIG. 8-4. Light emissions in the blue part of the visible spectrum decompose serum bilirubin most effectively. Although the blue fluorescent generates more radiant energy in the blue band than other types, the daylight bulb with its mixed wavelengths also contains a substantial amount. (Giunta F: Hosp Pract 6:87, 1972)

lighting beginning on the first day of life was associated with significantly decreased peak serum bilirubin levels when compared to a control group. Skin pigmentation does not appear to modify the response to phototherapy, which is equally effective in black and white children.

Before phototherapy is begun, a thorough medical evaluation of the infant must be carried out, and an etiology of the jaundice established. A pattern of rising serum bilirubin concentrations should be established. In those infants in whom an exchange transfusion is clearly indicated, a trial of phototherapy should not be attempted; however, the use of phototherapy following an exchange transfusion may prevent the necessity of subsequent transfusions. Serum bilirubin concentrations must be determined at regular intervals during the course of therapy since the disappearance of unconjugated bilirubin from cutaneous tissue usually does not reflect the serum bilirubin concentration. A plateauing or slight decrease in the bilirubin concentration is usually noted within the first 12 to 24 hours of

therapy. If there is a brisk hemolytic process occurring, mild to moderate increments in the bilirubin concentration may be noted in spite of phototherapy.

The eyes of the infant should be carefully shielded from the bright light with eye patches. These should be changed daily, so that a developing conjunctivitis is not overlooked.

Since the lights exert a distinct thermal effect, care must be taken to avoid hyperthermia. Vasodilatation with increased insensible water loss may occur in some infants, and adequate fluids should be provided.

Because the photodecomposition of bilirubin takes place in cutaneous capillaries, a maximum amount of exposed surface area is necessary for optimal results. Clothing, therefore, should be restricted to a diaper, and the infant should be nursed in an incubator to maintain thermal balance.

Loose stools are frequently noted in infants receiving phototherapy. This may be due to the laxative effect of the breakdown products of bilirubin that are excreted in the bile. Darkened urine may be due to the presence of some breakdown products that are excreted through the kidney.

Phototherapy increases the rate of platelet production and shortens platelet life span. Monitoring platelet counts during a course of phototherapy is therefore advisable (75a).

A darkening of the skin ("bronze baby syndrome") has been reported following phototherapy in an infant with obstructive jaundice (66). The mechanism involved here is not known.

Following completion of phototherapy, continued hematologic evaluation of the infant is mandatory. Some infants with mild to moderate hemolytic disease who have been treated with phototherapy continue to hemolyze their RBCs following discharge from the nursery and occasionally require transfusions of packed RBCs.

Although phototherapy has markedly reduced the number of exchange transfusions in jaundiced infants, its long-term effects can only be determined by prospectively planned and carefully performed clinical trials (50a).

SUPPORTIVE TREATMENT OF THE JAUNDICED INFANT

All jaundiced infants should be raised under conditions of thermoneutrality since sub-thermoneutral environmental conditions are associated with increased blood levels of free fatty acids (which displace bilirubin from albumin-binding sites). Early feedings appear to help prevent excessively high peak serum bilirubin levels (probably due to lessening of the enterohepatic shunting of bilirubin). If the infant is unable to tolerate oral feedings, an IV infusion of 10% dextrose and water should be started since both starvation and hypoglycemia increase levels of nonesterified fatty acids in the blood, which compete with unconjugated bilirubin

for albumin-binding sites. Glucose is also necessary as a precursor of UDPGA, which is required for the glucuronidation of unconjugated bilirubin.

Specific measures, such as antimicrobial therapy for the treatment of infection should be utilized. In rare instances, hemolytic disease of the newborn may be manifested only by anemia and splenomegaly, with minimal elevations of serum unconjugated bilirubin. In these instances, a simple transfusion of packed RBCs may be necessary.

The question of administering albumin without subsequent exchange transfusion has been raised. While the use of this procedure would theoretically increase the binding capacity of the blood for unconjugated bilirubin, it has never been shown in a clinical trial to decrease the incidence of neurologic sequelae of jaundice. One possible deleterious side-effect, in the presence of an already elevated venous pressure, would be the onset of congestive heart failure.

REFERENCES

HEMATOLOGIC DISORDERS

1. Evans HE, Glass L, Mercado C: Erythrocyte sedimentation rate in the newborn. J Pediatr 76:448, 1970
2. Hecht F, Motulsky AG, Lemire RJ, Shepard TE: Predominance of hemoglobin Gower 1 in early human embryonic development. Science 152:91, 1966
3. Holroyde CP, Oski FA, Gardner FH: The pocked erythrocyte: red-cell surface alterations in reticuloendothelial immaturity of the neonate. N Engl J Med 281:516, 1969
4. Kan WY, Valenti C, Carnazza, V: Fetal blood sampling in utero. Lancet 1:79, 1974
5. Kazazian HH, Woodhead AP: Hemoglobin synthesis in the developing fetus. N Engl J Med 289:58, 1973
6. Lehmann H: Different types of alpha-thalassemia and significance of hemoglobin Bart's in neonate. Lancet 2:78, 1970
7. Moss AJ, Monset-Couchard M: Placental transfusion: Early vs late clamping of the umbilical cord. Pediatrics 40:109, 1967
8. O'Brien RT, Pearson HA: Physiologic anemia of the newborn infant. J Pediatr 79:132, 1971
9. Oski FA, Naiman JL: Hematologic Problems in the Newborn, 2nd ed. Philadelphia, Saunders, 1972

10. Oski FA, Smith C, Brigandi E: Red cell metabolism in the premature infant. III. Apparent inappropriate glucose consumption for cell age. Pediatrics 41:473, 1968
11. Park BH, Holmes BH, Good RA: Metabolic activities in leukocytes of newborn infants. J Pediatr 76:237, 1970
12. Smith CH: Blood Diseases of Infancy and Childhood, 3rd ed. St. Louis, Mosby, 1972
13. Usher R, Shephard M, Lind J: The blood volume of the newborn infant and placental transfusion. Acta Paediatr Scand 52:497, 1963

Anemia

14. Durkin CM, Finn R: Foetal haemorrhage into the maternal circulation. Lancet 2:100, 1961
15. Kleihauer E, Braun H, Betke K: Demonstration von fetalem Hamoglobin in den Erythrocyten eines Blutausstrichs. Klin Wschr 35:637, 1957
16. Oski FA, Barness LA: Vitamin E deficiency: previously unrecognized cause of hemolytic anemia in premature infant. J Pediatr 70:211, 1967
17. Ritchie JH, Fish MB, McMasters V, Grossman M: Edema and hemolytic anemia in premature infants. A vitamin E deficiency syndrome. N Engl J Med 279:1185, 1968
18. Roberts PM, Arrowsmith DE, Rau SM, Monk-Jones ME: Folate status of premature infants. Arch Dis Child 44:637, 1969
18a. Williams ML, Shott RJ, O'Neal PL, Oski, FA: Role of dietary iron and fat on vitamin E deficiency anemia of infancy. N Engl J Med 292:887, 1975

Polycythemia

19. Gross GP, Hathaway WE, McGaughey HR: Hyperviscosity in the neonate. J Pediatr 82:1004, 1973
20. Kontras SB: Polycythemia and hyperviscosity syndromes in infants and children. Pediatr Clin North Am 19:919, 1972
21. Wells RE, Denton R, Merrill EW: Measurement of viscosity of biologic fluids by cone-plate viscometer. J Lab Clin Med 57:646, 1961

COAGULATION DISORDERS

Hemorrhagic Disease of the Newborn

22. Aballi AJ, DeLamerens S: Coagulation changes in neonatal period and early infancy. Pediatr Clin North Am 9:785, 1962
23. Aballi AJ: The action of vitamin K in the neonatal period. South Med J 55:48, 1965
24. Committee on Nutrition, American Academy of Pediatrics: Vitamin K compounds and the water-soluble analogues: use in therapy and prophylaxis in pediatrics. Pediatrics 28:501, 1961
25. Mountain CR, Hirsch J, Gallus AS: Neonatal coagulation defect due to anticonvulsant drug treatment in pregnancy. Lancet 1:265, 1970
26. Nygaard KK: Prophylactic and curative effect of vitamin K in hemorrhagic disease of the newborn. Acta Obstet Gynecol Scand 19:361, 1939
27. Sutherland JM, Glueck HZ, Gleser G: Pathogenesis of hemorrhagic disease of the newborn. Am J Dis Child 119:524, 1967
28. Townsend CW: The hemorrhagic disease of the newborn. Arch Pediatr 11:559, 1894

Disseminated Intravascular Coagulation

29. Gross S, Melhorn DK: Exchange transfusion with citrated whole blood for DIC. J Pediatr 78:415, 1971
30. Hathaway WE, Mull MM, Pechet GS: Disseminated intravascular coagulation in the newborn. Pediatrics 43:233, 1969
31. Stiehm ER, Clatanoff DV: Split products of fibrin in the serum of newborns. Pediatrics 43:770, 1969
32. Whaun JM, Urmson J, Oski FA: One year's experience with disseminated intravascular coagulation in a children's hospital (abstr). Pediatr Res 5:647, 1971

Thrombocytopenia

33. Adner MM, Fisch GR, Starobin SG, Aster RH: Use of "compatible" platelet transfusions in treatment of congenital isoimmune purpura. N Engl J Med 280:244, 1969
34. McIntosh S, O'Brien RT, Schwartz AD, Pearson HA: Neonatal isoimmune purpura: response to platelet infusions. J Pediatr 82:1020, 1973
35. Mull MM, Hathaway WE: Altered platelet function in newborns. Pediatr Res 4:229, 1970
36. Rodriguez SU, Leikin SL, Hiller MC: Neonatal thrombocytopenia associated with ante-partum administration of thiazide drugs. N Engl J Med 270:881, 1964

LEUKEMIA

36a. Behrman RE, Sigler AT, Patchefsky AS: Abnormal hematopoiesis in 2 of 3 siblings with mongolism. J Pediatr 68:569, 1966
36b. Krivit W, Good RA: Simultaneous occurrence of mongolism and leukemia. Am J Dis Child 94:289, 1957

NEONATAL JAUNDICE AND HEMOLYTIC DISEASE

37. Ackerman BC, Dyer GY, Leydorf MM: Hyperbilirubinemia in small premature infants. Pediatrics 45:918, 1970
38. Arias IM, Gartner LM: Production of unconjugated hyperbilirubinemia in full-term new-

born infants following administration of pregnane-3 (alpha) 20 (beta)-diol. Nature 203:1292, 1964

39. Arias IM, Gartner LM, Seifter S, Furman M: Prolonged neonatal unconjugated hyperbilirubinemia associated with breast feeding and a steroid, pregnane-3 (alpha), 20 (beta)-diol, in maternal milk that inhibits glucuronide formation in vitro. J Clin Invest 43:2037, 1964

40. Barrie H: Acid-base control during exchange transfusion. Lancet 2:712, 1965

41. Billing BH, Cole PG, Lathe GH: The excretion of bilirubin as a diglucuronide giving the direct Van den Bergh reaction. Biochem J 65:774, 1957

42. Boggs TR Jr, Hardy JB, Frazier TM: Correlation of neonatal serum total bilirubin concentrations and developmental status at age eight months. J Pediatr 71:553, 1967

43. Callahan EW Jr, Thaler MM, Karon M, Bauer K, Schmid R: Phototherapy of severe unconjugated hyperbilirubinemia: formation and removal of labelled bilirubin derivatives. Pediatrics 46:841, 1970

44. Calladine M, Gairdner D, Naidoo BI, Orrell DH: Acid-base changes following exchange transfusion with citrated blood. Arch Dis Child 40:626, 1965

45. Comley A, Wood B: Albumin administration in exchange transfusion for hyperbilirubinemia. Arch Dis Child 43:151, 1968

46. Cremer RJ, Perryman PW, Richards DH: Influence of light on the hyperbilirubinemia of infants. Lancet 1:1094, 1958

47. Crigler JF Jr, Najjar VA: Congenital familial nonhemolytic jaundice with kernicterus. Pediatrics 10:169, 1952

48. Cropp GJA: A continuous isovolumetric exchange transfusion technique. J Pediatr 77:881, 1970

49. Diamond I, Schmid R: Experimental bilirubin encephalopathy. The mode of entry of bilirubin-^{44}C into the central nervous system. J Clin Invest 45:678, 1966

50. Diamond I, Schmid R: Neonatal hyperbilirubinemia and kernicterus. Experimental support for treatment by exposure to visible light. Arch Neurol 18:699, 1968

50a. Final Report of the Commiteee on Phototherapy in the Newborn. National Academy of Science, Washington, DC, 1974

51. Freda VJ: The Rh problem in obstetrics and a new concept of its management using amniocentesis and spectrophotometric scanning of amniotic fluid. Am J Obstet Gynecol 92:341, 1965

52. Freda V: Hemolytic disease. Clin Obstet Gynecol 16:72, 1973

53. Freda VJ, Adamsons K: Exchange transfusion in utero. Am J Obstet Gynecol 89:817, 1964

54. Freda VJ, Gorman JG, Pollack W: Suppression of the primary Rh immune response with passive Rh IgG immunoglubulin. N Engl J Med 277:1022, 1967

55. Gartner LM, Lane D: Hepatic metabolism and transport of bilirubin during physiologic jaundice in the newborn Rhesus monkey (abstr). Pediatr Res 5:413, 1971

56. Gartner LM, Snyder RN, Chabon RS, Bernstein J: Kernicterus: high incidence in premature infants with low serum bilirubin concentrations. Pediatrics 45:906, 1970

57. Gessner IH: Neonatal hyperbilirubinemia associated with ingestion of maternal blood. Pediatrics 43:896, 1969

58. Giunta F, Rath J: Effect of environmental illumination in prevention of hyperbilirubinemia of prematurity. Pediatrics 44:162, 1969

59. Gorman JG, Freda VJ, Pollack W: Prevention of Rhesus haemolytic disease. Lancet 2:181, 1965

60. Hardy JB, Peeples MO: Serum bilirubin levels in newborn infants. Distribution and association with neurological abnormalities during the first year of life. Johns Hopkins Med J 128:265, 1971

61. Hargreaves T, Piper RF: Breast milk jaundice. Effect of inhibitory breast milk and 3αC, 20β-pregnanediol on glucuronyl transferase. Arch Dis Child 46:195, 1971

62. Hirata Y, Matsuo T, Shibata M, Takatera Y, Nakamura K: Experimental studies in kernicterus. Biol Neonate 12:371, 1968

63. Hymen CB, Keaster J, Hanson V, Harris I, Sedgwick R, Wursten H, Wright HR: CNS abnormalities after neonatal hemolytic disease or hyperbilirubinemia. Am J Dis Child 117:395, 1969

64. Jirsova V, Jirsa M, Heringova A, Koldovsky O, Weirichova J: The use and possible diagnostic significanuce of sephadex gel filtration of serum from icteric newborn. Biol Neonate 11:204, 1967

65. Johnson LH, Boggs TR: Failure of exchange transfusion to prevent minimal cerebral damage when employed so as to maintain serum bilirubin concentrations below 18 and 20 mg/100 ml. Soc Ped Res Program and Abstracts, Atlantic City, 1970, p 107

66. Kopelman AE, Brown RS, Odell GB: The "bronze baby," a complication of phototherapy. J Pediatr 81:466, 1972

67. Landsteiner K, Wiener AS: An agglutinable factor in human blood recognized by immune sera for Rhesus blood. Proc Soc Exp Biol Med 43:223, 1940

68. Levi AJ, Gatmaitan Z, Arias IM: Deficiency of hepatic organic anion-binding protein, impaired organic anion uptake by liver and "physiologic" jaundice in newborn monkeys. N Engl J Med 283:1136, 1970

69. Levine P, Katzin E, Burnham L: Isoimmunization in pregnancy. JAMA 116:825, 1941

70. Levkoff AH, Westphal MC, Finklea JF: Evaluation of direct reading spectrophotometer for neonatal bilirubinometry. Am J Clin Pathol 54:562, 1970

71. Liley AW: Intrauterine transfusion of foetus in haemolytic disease. Br Med J 2:1107, 1963

72. Liley AW: Amniocentesis and fetal transfusion in erythroblastosis. Pediatrics 35:836, 1965

73. Lopez R, Cooperman JM: Glucose 6 phosphate dehydrogenase deficiency and hyperbilirubinemia in the newborn. Am J Dis Child 122:66, 1971

74. Lucey J, Ferreiro M, Hewitt J: Prevention of hyperbilirubinemia of prematurity by phototherapy. Pediatrics 41:1047, 1968

74a. Lund HT, Jacobsen J: Influence of phototherapy on the biliary bilirubin excretion pattern in newborn infants with hyperbilirubinemia. J Pediatr 8:262, 1974

75. Maisels MJ: Bilirubin—on understanding and influencing its metabolism in the newborn infant. Pediatr Clin North Am 19:447, 1972

75a. Maurer HM, Fratkin MJ, Haggins JC, McWilliams NB: Effect of phototherapy on thrombopoiesis (abst). Pediatr Res 9:368, 1975

76. Nathan E: Severe hydrops fetalis treated with peritoneal dialysis and positive pressure ventilation. Lancet 1:1393, 1968

77. Odell GB: Studies in kernicterus. I. The protein binding of bilirubin. J Clin Invest 38:823, 1959

78. Odell GB, Brown RS, Holtzman NA: Dye-sensitized photo-oxidation of albumin associated with a decreased capacity for protein-binding of bilirubin. In: Bilirubin Metabolism in the Newborn. Birth Defects. Edited by D Bergsma. Original Article Series 6:31, 1970

79. Odell SB, Cohen SN, Kelly PC: Studies in kernicterus. II. The determination of the saturation of serum albumin with bilirubin. J Pediatr 74:214, 1969

80. Ostrow JD, Branham RV: Photodecay of bilirubin in vitro and in the jaundiced (Gunn) rat. In: Bilirubin Metabolism in the Newborn. Birth Defects. Edited by D Bergsma. Original Article Series 6:93, 1970

81. Pierson WE, Barrett CT, Oliver TK: The effect of buffered and non-buffered ACD blood on electrolyte and acid-base homeostasis during exchange transfusion. Pediatrics 41:802, 1968

82. Poland RD, Odell GB: Physiologic jaundice: the enterohepatic circulation of bilirubin. N Engl J Med 284:1, 1971

83. Porter EG, Waters WJ: A rapid micromethod for measuring the reserve albumin binding capacity in serum from newborn infants with hyperbilirubinemia. J Lab Clin Med 67:660, 1966

84. Schiff D, Aranda JV, Chan G, Colle E, Stern L: Metabolic effects of exchange transfusion. I. Effect of citrated and of heparinized blood on glucose, nonesterified fatty acids, 2-(4 hydroxybenzeneazo) benzoic acid binding, and insulin. J Pediatr 78:603, 1971

85. Schmid R, Hammaker L, Axelrod J: The enzymic formation of bilyirubin glucuronide. Arch Biochem Biophys 70:285, 1957

86. Silberberg DH, Johnson L, Ritter R: Factors influencing toxicity of bilirubin in cerebellum tissue culture. J Pediatr 77:386, 1970

87. Silberberg DH, Johnson L, Schutta H, Ritter L: Effects of photo-degradation products of bilirubin on myelinating cerebellum cultures. J Pediatr 77:613, 1970

88. Sisson TRC, Glauser SC, Glauser EM, Tasman W, Kuwabara T: Retinal changes produced by phototherapy. J Pediatr 77:221, 1970

89. Sisson TRC, Kendall N, Glauser SC, Knutson S, Bunyaviroch E: Phototherapy of jaundice in newborn infants. I. ABO blood group incompatibility. J Pediatr 79:904, 1971

90. Sisson TRC, Kendall N, Shaw E, Kechavarz-Olai L: Phototherapy of jaundice in the newborn. II. Effect of various light intensities. J Pediatr 81:35, 1972

91. Stern L, Khanna NN, Levy G, Yaffe SJ: Effect of phenobarbital on hyperbilirubinemia and glucuronide formation in newborns. Am J Dis Child 120:26, 1970

92. Talafant E: Properties and composition of the bile pigment giving a direct diazo reaction. Nature 178:312, 1956

93. Trolle D: A possible drop in first-week mortality rate for low-birthweight infants after phenobarbitone treatment. Lancet 2:1123, 1968

94. Van den Bergh AAH, Muller P: Uber eine direkte und eine indirekte Diazoreaktion auf Bilirubin. Biochem Z 77:90, 1916

95. Weldon VV, Odell GB: Mortality risk of exchange transfusion. Pediatrics 41:797, 1968

96. Woodrow JC, Clarke CA, McConnell RR, Towers SH, Donohoe WTA: Prevention of Rh hemolytic disease: Results of the Liverpool "low risk" clinical trial. Br Med J 2:610, 1971

9

Neuroskeletal and Neuromuscular Diseases

DEVELOPMENT OF THE CENTRAL NERVOUS SYSTEM

Normal postnatal life depends primarily on an intact central nervous system (CNS). Since most brain growth occurs during fetal life and early infancy, any insult during this time may lead to permanent impairment.

FETAL DEVELOPMENT

The CNS is derived from a primitive neural plate that is transformed into a neural tube prior to the fourth week of gestation. The rostral half enlarges to form the primitive forebrain, midbrain and hindbrain; the distal portion retains its tubelike appearance and forms the spinal cord.

Forebrain

During the fourth week of gestation, the forebrain subdivides into the telencephalon (which will differentiate into the cerebral hemispheres and lateral ventricle) and the diencephalon (which forms the choroid plexus of the third ventricle, pineal body, posterior commisure, pituitary gland, thalamus and hypothalamus). By the sixth week, the cerebral hemispheres begin to attain the prominence that they will have for the remainder of fetal and postnatal life.

Midbrain

The midbrain becomes the mesencephalon, which gives rise to the nuclei of the tro-

chlear and oculomotor nerves, the nucleus of Edinger-Westphal, several long tracts (such as the corticospinal, corticobulbar and corticopontine tracts), the anterior and posterior colliculi, the substantia niger and nucleus ruber.

Hindbrain

By the fifth week, the hindbrain differentiates into the metencephalon and myelencephalon. The metencephalon has a dorsal portion, which becomes the cerebellum, and a ventral portion, which becomes the pons. The most distal portion of the brain, the myelencephalon, becomes the medulla oblongata. Various motor nuclei, such as those of the glossopharyngeal, vagus and accessory nerves, arise from the medulla, as do several sensory relay nuclei and nuclei of various somatic afferent nerves, such as the bulbospinal portion of the trigeminal nerve. The medulla also gives rise to the pia mater, covering of the brain and spinal cord; the choroid plexus; and the two lateral foramina of Luschka and the medial foramen of Magendie.

Neuronal Development

The formation of new nerve cells occurs primarily between the 10th and 18th week of gestation. Interference with brain growth during this period, which can occur in the presence of such intrauterine infections as rubella, cytomegalovirus, h. simplex and toxoplasmosis, may lead to a permanent reduction in the number of brain cells and microcephaly. Exposure to intensive radiation during the first half of pregnancy (such as in the atomic bomb explosions at Hiroshima and Nagasaki) can also lead to a reduced nerve cell number and microcephaly. Chromosomal abnormalities are another cause of a defective brain growth during the first half of gestation.

Congenital Anomalies

Major congenital anomalies of the CNS (meningoceles, myelomeningoceles and encephaloceles) are due to osseous and neurogenic maldevelopment early in the first trimester. These are discussed in the section Neurosurgery, Chapter 23.

Anencephaly represents failure of closure of the cephalic portion of the neural tube. The cranial vault is absent, and only rudimentary brain tissue is present. There is a deficiency of pituitary tissue, and along with this there is marked hypoplasia of the adrenal cortex. There are several antenatal diagnostic signs of this condition. Hydramnios develops because of the inability of the fetus to swallow amniotic fluid; fetal x ray shows absence of the skull, and concentrations of α-fetoprotein are elevated in the amniotic fluid and maternal plasma (2). In addition, maternal serum and urinary concentrations of estriol are markedly decreased because of adrenocortical hypoplasia. The diagnosis may be made antenatally by ultrasonic examination (2a).

Anencephaly invariably leads either to fetal death or demise within several hours after birth.

Late Fetal Brain Growth

Brain growth begins to rapidly accelerate during the second half of pregnancy. While active division of neuronal elements is decelerating, glial cells are appearing, myelinization is beginning and synapses are rapidly forming between nerve cells. It is during this critical period that fetal malnutrition most severely affects brain development (see section Intrauterine Growth Retardation, Ch. 4).

PERINATAL TRAUMA

During the perinatal period, hypoxia may lead to permanent CNS damage (see section Perinatal Asphyxia and Resuscitation, Ch. 3). Other insults to the CNS during this period, such as hypoglycemia, hypocalcemia, infection, intracranial bleeding and hyperbilirubinemia may all lead to impaired psychomotor development. The neurologic examination of the newborn infant is discussed in Chapter 17, History, Physical, and Neurologic Examination.

NEONATAL SEIZURES

Seizures observed during the neonatal period may be due to a variety of causes; in clinical appearance they are usually unlike the typical grand mal convulsions seen in older infants and children and are therefore often difficult to identify. Elements of the history that are helpful in identifying neonatal seizures are

- I. Obstetric Aspects
    - A. Preeclampsia
    - B. Diabetes mellitus
    - C. Use of addictive drugs (narcotics, barbiturates)
    - D. Hyperparathyroidism
    - E. Previous infant with neonatal convulsion (e.g., pyridoxine dependency, maple syrup urine disease, kernicterus)
    - F. Infection (e.g., rubella, toxoplasmosis, CMV)
- II. Intrapartum
    - A. Antenatal signs of fetal distress (fetal bradycardia, passage of meconium, decreasing urinary estriol levels)
    - B. Prolonged rupture of membranes with amnionitis
    - C. Anesthetics and other medications administered during labor
    - D. Birth trauma
- III. Neonatal
    - A Apgar score
    - B. Birth weight and gestational age
    - C. Nature, time of onset and duration of CNS signs

D. Abnormal physical findings (e.g., pallor, jaundice, cyanosis, petechiae, microcephaly)

E. Abnormal biochemical findings (e.g., hypoglycemia, hypocalcemia, abnormally low Pa_{O_2})

The etiology of neonatal seizures is as follows:

I. Biochemical
 A. Hypocalcemia
 B. Hypoglycemia
 C. Hypomagnesemia
 D. Hyponatremia and hypernatremia
 E. Pyridoxine dependency
 F. Abnormalities of amino acid metabolism (e.g., maple syrup urine disease)
II. Infection
 A. Bacterial
  1. Sepsis
  2. Meningitis
  3. Gastroenteritis
 B. Viral meningoencephalitis
 C. Other (toxoplasmosis)
III. Perinatal asphyxia
IV. Traumatic (e.g., subdural hematoma)
V. Hematologic
 A. Intracranial bleeding (secondary to to asphyxia, DIC, or hemorrhagic disease)
 B. Kernicterus (usually secondary to blood group incompatibility)
VI. Congenital CNS malformations
 A. Microcephaly
 B. Porencephaly
 C. Hydrocephaly
 D. Hydrancephaly
 E. Arteriovenous fistulas
VII. Withdrawal from addictive drugs (narcotics, barbiturates)

The underlying disease process that led to the seizure activity may have previously caused some brain damage (often irreversible) by the time the seizure is recognized. In other cases, the seizure may be caused by a process potentially capable of producing permanent brain damage, but in which prompt recognition and treatment of the underlying illness may be associated with

intact survival of the infant. It is therefore important to be able to recognize all manifestations of seizure activity in newborn infants and to perform an orderly and rapid evaluation to identify and treat potentially curable illness.

Typical grand mal convulsions are not often encountered in newborn infants, probably because cerebral cortical function is poorly organized. The neonate functions essentially on a subcortical level, and the type of noxious stimulus that would spread through the cortex and result in a grand mal seizure in an older child does not do so in the newborn infant. Most evident seizure activity in neonates appears to result from noxious stimuli affecting subcortical structures and causing abnormal discharges from these areas. A wide variety of signs appear as clinical manifestations of neonatal seizures. Among these are tremors, sudden changes in muscle tone, apneic episodes, cyanosis, eye blinking, nystagmus, opisthotonos, chewing movements of the jaw, twitching of facial muscles, changes in vasomotor activity, an abnormal or high-pitched cry and clonic movement of one or more extremity. Any one or more of these, occurring either alone or together with rarely encountered grand mal activity may be the manifestation of any of the pathologic conditions causing neonatal seizures.

HYPOCALCEMIA (see Section Calcium and Phosphorus Metabolism, Ch. 10)

Decreased serum calcium concentrations may lead to seizure activity in the newborn infant. Since recognition and treatment usually result in a good prognosis, measurements of both serum calcium and phosphorus concentrations must be made in any infant who appears to be having seizures. At the same time, blood pH and total protein concentration should be measured in order to evaluate the level of ionized calcium. Even if another diagnosis appears obvious, it is still advisable to make these determinations since hypocalcemia may occur concurrently with another seizure-provoking condition, such as hypoglycemia or perinatal asphyxia. Serum calcium levels below 8.0 mg/100 ml in the presence of clinical signs can usually be accepted as the underlying cause of the seizures. However, many infants may have these low levels without clinical manifestations. If the hypocalcemia is caused by phosphate overload secondary to cow's milk feeding (seventh day hypocalcemia) or maternal hyperparathyroidism, serum phosphate concentrations may be elevated (above 8 mm/100 ml in a nonhemolyzed specimen). The prolongation of the $Q_{-o}T_c$ (5) interval (measured from origin of the Q wave to origin of the T wave) on an electrocardiogram (ECG) in the presence of both clinical signs and a decreased serum calcium level confirms the diagnosis.

Intravenous injection of 10% calcium gluconate solution (5 to 10 ml given over a 10-minute period) will halt seizure activity due to hypocalcemia. The $Q_{-o}T_c$ interval, if prolonged, returns to normal with correction of the hypocalcemia, and any abnormalities seen on the ECG should disappear. Following initial therapy, the infant should receive 1 to 2 ml of 10% calcium gluconate/kg body weight per day by IV drip for several days, until asymptomatic. For the next four weeks, supplementary calcium gluconate (3 to 4 g/day in three divided doses), should be administered along with the formula. In addition, oral feedings of a formula with a low phosphate content and a favorable calcium to phosphate ratio (e.g., Similac PM 60/40) should be started and continued until normal calcium levels have been stabilized. If the signs are equivocal and the serum calcium levels are borderline, treatment for hypocalcemia is justified.

If marked hypocalcemia accompanied by convulsions persists in spite of seemingly adequate therapy, congenital absence of the parathyroid glands and thymus (DiGeorge's syndrome) may be suspected (11). In this condition, which has a poor prognosis, the thymic shadow is not seen on the chest x ray and lymphocyte function is found to be decreased by in vitro testing. Subse-

quently, the infant will show a wide range of clinical and laboratory signs of immunologic deficiency.

HYPOGLYCEMIA

Central nervous signs caused by decreased concentrations of blood glucose are often difficult to identify since lethargy, poor suck, cyanosis and apneic spells appear to be more common in this condition than tremulousness or frank convulsions. Maternal diabetes mellitus, intrauterine growth retardation and perinatal asphyxia are conditions commonly associated with neonatal hypoglycemia. However, any infant showing abnormal neurologic signs should have a blood glucose determination so that treatment may be started before clinical manifestations become apparent. The treatment for hypoglycemia (see section Carbohydrate Metabolism, Ch. 12) should be instituted promptly in any symptomatic infant with low blood glucose concentrations (regardless of whether the hypoglycemia is actually the underlying cause for the abnormal signs). As is the case with hypocalcemia, it is often difficult to correlate the degree of biochemical abnormality with the clinical picture.

INFECTION

Although lethargy and apnea are common presenting signs of neonatal sepsis and meningitis, demonstrable seizure activity may not appear in either bacterial meningitis or sepsis until the disease process is fairly well advanced. Gastroenteritis, in the absence of systemic infection, may also be accompanied by seizures. The onset of lethargy, apneic spells or any other sudden change in neurologic behavior warrants a lumbar puncture and blood culture; by the time frank convulsions appear, the prognosis worsens considerably. Disseminated intravascular coagulation (DIC), which often accompanies sepsis, may lead to the intracranial bleeding that is itself one cause of seizure activity.

Encephalitis secondary to nonbacterial infections may also cause seizures. These include maternofetal infections (e.g., rubella, toxoplasmosis, cytomegalovirus and h. simplex) and postnatally acquired infections (e.g., group B coxsackie viruses). Although there is no available treatment for rubella, cytomegalovirus or group B coxsackie viruses, certain semiexperimental therapeutic agents are of some value in the treatment of h. simplex and toxoplasmosis. Therefore, a definitive diagnosis should be made at the earliest possible time.

HYPOMAGNESEMIA

Hypomagnesemia, which is relatively uncommon, presents with the same clinical signs as hypocalcemia and is usually accompanied by decreased levels of serum calcium (8). If an infant treated for symptomatic hypocalcemia shows little or no response to apparently adequate treatment, determination of the serum magnesium level is indicated. If serum magnesium concentrations can be measured easily on small quantities of serum, this determination should be performed whenever the serum calcium level is measured. Serum magnesium levels below 1.5 mEq/l associated with seizure activity strongly suggest hypomagnesemia as the etiology. The two most common causes of this disorder are probably an inborn error of metabolism and exchange transfusion with citrated blood. Treatment of hypomagnesemic seizures consists of an IV infusion of 2 to 6 ml of 2% or 3% magnesium sulfate solution, followed by a daily maintenance dose of 1 ml of 50% magesium sulfate given IM.

HYPONATREMIA AND HYPERNATREMIA
(see Ch. 10, Renal Function and Fluid and Electrolyte Balance)

Abnormally low or high concentrations of serum sodium may cause neonatal seizures. Hyponatremia may occur secondary to excessive administration of hypotonic IV fluids or inappropriate antidiuretic hormone (ADH) secretion (dilutional hyponatremia).

This latter circumstance may be a consequence of either perinatal asphyxia or neonatal meningitis. In these instances, the hyponatremia should be treated with restriction of water. If in the presence of diarrhea there is excessive sodium loss in the stool, hyponatremia may occur. In this case, the lost sodium should be replaced.

Elevated serum sodium levels in the neonate (above 150 mEq/l) may occur either following diarrhea in which proportionately more water than sodium is lost in the stool or following administration of an excessive amount of sodium. In the past this has occurred when salt instead of sugar was inadvertently added to the formula; at present, it is more likely to be due to the infusion of a hypertonic sodium bicarbonate solution.

PYRIDOXINE DEPENDENCY

Pyridoxine-dependent seizures are extremely rare in the neonate but nonetheless treatable (5). This familial inborn error of metabolism may occur in utero or may be manifested first during the nearly neonatal period. This syndrome, which seems to be due to a defect in the binding of the coenzyme pyridoxal phosphate to glutamic transcarboxylase, may be treated by administration of large doses of pyridoxine to the mother of the convulsing fetus or to the infant who is convulsing. The history of a previous sibling with this disorder strongly suggests the diagnosis. The amount of pyridoxine required to treat the convulsion varies from case to case. If the fetus is convulsing, the mother usually requires about 100 mg of pyridoxine orally daily; in a convulsing neonate with pyridoxine dependency, 25 to 50 mg IV usually stops the convulsion. A large but variable daily dose of pyridoxine is required to maintain a convulsion-free state thereafter.

In the presence of convulsions of undetermined etiology, 25 to 50 mg of pyridoxine may be given as a therapeutic trial if all other modes of therapy have been ineffective.

PERINATAL ASPHYXIA (see Section Perinatal Asphyxia and Resuscitation, Ch. 3)

Seizures are often sequelae of severe perinatal asphyxia. Hypoxemia adversely affects all areas of the brain: cortex, cerebellum, basal ganglia and brain stem, both gray and white matter. Petechial hemorrhages, intracellular and extracellular edema and infarction may occur. The insult may be so severe as to cause fetal death. When the infant is born alive following severe intrauterine asphyxia, he is usually extremely depressed, often with absent respiratory effort and bradycardia. Following resuscitation, seizures may occur because of the anoxic insult to the brain. These are usually of the tonoclonic variety often accompanied by eye rolling.

Apneic spells are sometimes noted as a manifestation of seizure activity. The treatment of these infants consists of routine supportive measures (e.g., adequate oxygenation, temperature control, IV glucose and correction of acid-base aberrations) and the judicious use of phenobarbital to control the seizures. Diazepam (Valium) is effective in controlling seizures resistant to phenobarbital; however, its duration of action is relatively short, and it cannot be used for maintenance therapy. Corticosteroids have been administered in an attempt to reduce the cerebral edema that accompanies perinatal asphyxia, but there have been no controlled studies that support the efficacy of this mode of treatment.

Surviving infants in this group have an extremely high incidence of severe neurologic sequelae, including convulsive disorders. They must be followed carefully after discharge from the nursery and should be maintained on anticonvulsant therapy through infancy and childhood.

INTRACRANIAL BLEEDING

Subdural hematomas are a potentially treatable cause of neonatal seizures. This condition must be suspected in any infant (usually full term) whose delivery was traumatic and in whom seizure activity appears. A bulging anterior fontanelle and separation of sutures alert the clinician to the presence of subdural bleeding. When suspected, bilateral subdural taps should be performed, and if the diagnosis is confirmed, the procedure may be repeated at intervals.

Intraventricular and subarachnoid bleeding, seen primarily in premature infants, can precipitate seizures. Since there is no specific therapy available, medical care must be supportive. Phenobarbital may be used for control of seizures.

MISCELLANEOUS CAUSES

Withdrawal from Drugs of Abuse

Convulsions and other abnormal neurologic manifestations are frequently observed in neonates whose mothers are addicted to opiates, barbiturates and tranquilizers. Diagnosis and treatment is fully discussed in Chapter 15, Drug Abuse.

CNS Anomalies

In certain developmental anomalies of the CNS (e.g., cerebral dysgenesis with microcephaly, porencephaly, hydrocephalus, hydranencephaly and arteriovenous fistulas), the primary pathology may at least be partially correctable. The remainder can only be treated symptomatically with anticonvulsant therapy.

Others

There are numerous other causes of neonatal seizures. Abnormalities of amino acid metabolism exert a toxic effect on the CNS. Although phenylketonuric seizures appear well after the neonatal period, those of other disorders such as maple syrup urine disease appear shortly after birth.

Diagnostic and therapeutic measures for the prevention and treatment of neonatal jaundice have made kernicterus a relatively uncommon cause of neonatal seizures. Unfortunately, once the signs of bilirubin encephalopathy appear, there is nothing to offer in the way of therapy, except for supportive care.

PROGNOSIS

The long-term outlook for infants who have had neonatal seizures is guarded. Figures vary from one series to another (7, 9, 10); this may be due at least in part to varying proportions of underlying causes for the convulsions. About one-half to two-thirds of these infants die in early infancy or have long-term neurologic sequelae. The best overall prognosis is among those infants whose seizures have been secondary to hypocalcemia or hypoglycemia. Seizures due to other causes, such as perinatal asphyxia or meningitis, tend to have a much poorer prognosis.

In a prospective follow-up study of 144 infants who had neonatal seizures, Rose and Lombroso (9) found about 50% of their patients normal and 30% with neurologic sequelae; about 20% had died. They were able to correlate, with a fair degree of accuracy, the neonatal EEG with ultimate prognosis. With a normal EEG, there was an 86% chance of normal neurologic development at age four years. This did not appear to be related to the severity of clinical signs during the neonatal period. Those with grossly abnormal EEGs had only a 7% chance of normal neurologic development. With unifocal abnormalities (primarily due to hypocalcemia) the long-term prognosis was variable.

It cannot be overemphasized that in the treatment of neonatal seizures, a specific etiologic diagnosis must be sought as rapidly as possible in order to institute specific therapy. Delays in beginning specific therapy may lead to a worsening long-term prognosis. Nonspecific anticonvulsant therapy (phenobarbital or diazepam) should be limited to those infants in whom no specific treatable etiology (such as perinatal asphyxia) can be found.

INTRACRANIAL BLEEDING

Significant bleeding into the subdural or subarachnoid spaces, the ventricular system or, less commonly, into the substance of the brain may occur during the perinatal period (Table 9–1). A high mortality rate accompanies intracranial bleeding, and neurologic sequelae are common among survivors. Premature delivery is the most common antecedent; obstetric trauma, which in an earlier era accounted for a good deal of intracranial bleeding, is rarely implicated today. In the presence of hypoxia (often encountered in premature infants), DIC may play a role in the pathogenesis of the bleeding. Cerebral venous congestion, which is associated with hypoxemia and hypercapnea in poorly ventilated infants with RDS, may predispose to bleeding. Less commonly observed hemorrhagic disorders, such as thrombocytopenia or hemorrhagic disease of the newborn, may also lead to CNS bleeding.

Since medical and surgical therapy are of limited value, prevention of conditions capable of causing CNS bleeding must be a goal of physicians caring for both mother and newborn infant.

SUBDURAL HEMATOMA

Etiology

In the full-term infant, subdural bleeding is more common than hemorrhage in the other three areas. Obstetric trauma and molding of the head that may cause tears of the falx cerebri or tentorium cerebelli are most likely to occur in difficult deliveries and with large infants (such as infants of diabetic mothers). If blood vessels are involved in these tears, bleeding into the subdural space will occur. Tears of blood vessels bridging the surface of the brain with the dura or dural sinuses also lead to subdural bleeding. Most subdural bleeding involves the supratentorial areas; however, tentorial tears may occasionally lead to subtentorial (retrocerebellar) subdural bleeding.

Although improved obstetric technique, and specifically a reduction in the use of midforceps, has led to a marked reduction in the incidence of subdural bleeding, early recognition of this condition is of utmost importance since proper therapy usually leads to a total cure.

TABLE 9–1. Intracranial Bleeding

Site of Bleeding	Blood Vessels Involved	Etiology	Clinical Manifestations	Infants at Risk	Diagnostic Work-up	Treatment
Subdural space	Falx cerebri and tentorium cerebelli	Obstetric Trauma	Lethargy, irritability, hypotonia, poor suck, bulging anterior fontanelle separation of sutures, convulsions	Full-term	Subdural tap, lumbar puncture, echoencephalogram, transillumination	Repeated subdural taps
Intraventricular, subarachnoid, intracerebral	Subependymal	Hypoxia, hypercapnea, DIC	Apnea, hypotonia, convulsions	Preterm, often together with RDS	Lumbar puncture blood sugar and calcium coagulation studies	Symptomatic heparin or exchange transfusion with heparinized blood if DIC is present

Clinical Manifestations

Symptoms of subdural bleeding may become apparent from any time immediately after birth to several days after delivery. Abnormal neurologic signs, such as lethargy, hypotonia, poor suck and irritability, may be accompanied by labored or decreased respirations, cyanosis and—occasionally—apneic episodes. A shrill high-pitched cry may be present. Tremors and generalized convulsions may also occur. The most important diagnostic sign accompanying supratentorial subdural bleeding is a bulging anterior fontanelle, often with a separation of sutures. A rapid increase in head circumference may occur if the condition remains untreated. Pallor and a decrease in the hemoglobin concentration may accompany the bleeding. Retinal hemorrhages may also be present, but these can be seen frequently among normal neonates even in the absence of intracranial pathology.

Diagnosis and Treatment

Transillumination of the infant's head and echoencephalography may be of value in confirming the diagnosis. However, diagnostic subdural taps must be performed whenever there is the slightest suspicion of subdural bleeding (Fig. 9–1). After the head is shaved and surgically cleansed, a blunt spinal needle is introduced into each coronal suture at the most lateral aspect of the anterior fontanelle and advanced 2 to 3 mm. Under normal conditions a very small quantity of clear fluid (less than 0.5 ml) may be found in the subdural space. If there is fresh subdural bleeding, gross blood will flow out of the needle once the subdural space is entered. If the bleeding has occurred several days before the subdural tap, the blood is partially decomposed and has a dark color, with a xanthochromic supernatant fluid. If subdural hematomas are found, bilateral subdural taps should be performed every other day until the bleeding has stopped completely. With early and adequate treat-

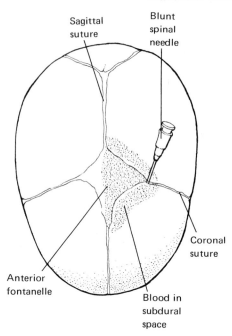

FIG. 9–1. Technique of subdural tap. After the head is shaved and cleansed, a blunt spinal needle is introduced into each coronal suture at the most lateral aspect of the anterior fontanelle and advanced 2 to 3 mm. In the presence of subdural bleeding, blood flows out of the needle once the subdural space is entered.

ment, formation of a membrane (and the need to excise it surgically) is extremely rare.

HEMATOMAS OF THE POSTERIOR FOSSA

Subdural hematomas of the posterior fossa are much more difficult to diagnose in the neonatal period than supratentorial hematomas. Although clinical manifestations of both conditions are similar (lethargy, vomiting, gasping respirations, loss of Moro and sucking reflexes), bulging of the anterior fontanelle and separation of sutures are absent. Both Pitlyk et al (16) and Gilles and Shillito (14) have demonstrated that an internal hydrocephalus, secondary to compression of the fourth ventricle by the hematoma, exists in this condition. Hydrocephalus, with dilatation of the third ventricle, aqueduct of Sylvius and upper portion of the fourth ventricle, is demonstrable with ventriculography. Early recognition and diagnosis of this condition, together with craniotomy and evacuation of the hematoma, may be curative and may preclude the need for a future shunting procedure.

CNS BLEEDING IN PREMATURE INFANTS

Etiology and Pathogenesis

Although subdural bleeding is most commonly seen in full-term infants, premature infants are more prone to intraventricular and subarachnoid hemorrhage. Isolated subarachnoid bleeding may be occasionally noted, but it usually occurs secondary to intraventricular bleeding. The etiology of intracranial bleeding in premature infants has been a subject of debate for many years. However, it now appears that hypoxia is a predisposing event. Disseminated intravascular coagulation, present in many of these infants, is probably related to the hypoxia.

Intracranial bleeding is an extremely common cause of death in premature infants. Harcke et al (15) found that in premature infants with gestational ages of less than 29 weeks who died on the first day of life, the incidence of intraventricular hemorrhage was 23%; among those infants in this group who died on the second and third day of life, the incidence of intraventricular hemorrhage was 73%. In infants over 29 weeks' gestation, 12% who died during the first day of life had intraventricular hemorrhage, whereas 17% of those dying on days 2 and 3 had this type of bleeding. These authors found that RDS, intrauterine growth retardation and intrauterine infection predisposed to intraventricular bleeding.

Fedrick and Butler (13) found that the most important factors predisposing to intraventricular bleeding were immaturity and intrauterine growth retardation. Illegitimacy, severe maternal preeclampsia and maternal infection also predisposed to this lesion. Males outnumbered females by 2:1. Unlike the findings of Harcke et al (15) no relationship was found to RDS.

It is now generally recognized that blood vessels lying in subependymal tissue in the lateral wall of the lateral ventricles are the source of bleeding in intraventricular hemorrhage. Towbin (17) has studied the pathogenesis of this disorder in premature infants. Severe hypoxia in the fetus or neonate predisposes to circulatory failure with venous stasis. This is followed by stasis thrombosis of deep cerebral veins, leading to infarction of germinal matrix tissue in the subependymal zones of the cerebral hemispheres. When these lesions become hemorrhagic, intraventricular hemorrhage ensues. Towbin also postulates that infarctional damage to the germinal matrix without the advent of hemorrhage is probably a major cause of the subsequent psychomotor retardation seen in expremature infants subjected to hypoxia during the perinatal period.

Clinical Manifestations

The clinical signs of intraventricular bleeding (labored respirations, hypoventilation, cyanosis, apnea, high-pitched cry and convulsions) overlap those of such treatable CNS disorders as meningitis, hypocalcemia and hypoglycemia. A full diagnostic workup, including lumbar puncture, is indicated in the presence of these findings. If a lumbar puncture indicates the presence of fresh blood in the cerebrospinal fluid (CSF), a tentative diagnosis of intraventricular bleeding that has extended into the subarachnoid space can be made. This is often accompanied by a falling hematocrit.

Treatment

Once intraventricular bleeding begins, it is virtually impossible to control, and hence the mortality rate is extremely high. Among the few who survive, long-term morbidity is nearly universal. Therefore, prevention is much more important than treatment. From the obstetric point of view, delivery of a nonasphyxiated fetus is vital. Once delivered, every effort must be made to keep the infant adequately oxygenated, especially in the presence of respiratory distress. Maintenance of a thermoneutral environment, administration of IV fluids and maintenance of a normal acid-base balance are essential. Of special importance in this area is prevention of carbon dioxide retention, which may in itself predispose to intracranial bleeding. Coagulation studies in infants with RDS may detect the earliest clotting defects associated with DIC, and treatment with heparin or exchange transfusion with heparinized blood may play some role in preventing intraventricular hemorrhage. With very extensive intraventricular bleeding, a ventricular tap may be attempted to decrease the elevated pressure that is secondary to the bleeding. This, however, is rarely of much avail. Infants who survive require comprehensive follow-up care because of the high incidence of neurologic sequelae.

OTHER TYPES OF INTRACRANIAL BLEEDING

Bleeding of any consequence into the substance of the brain is relatively uncommon. Petechial hemorrhages often accompany the congestion and edema seen in the brains of newborn infants, usually full-term, who succumb to severe perinatal cerebral hypoxia; more severe bleeding is unusual. Since this diagnosis is not made antemortem, the treatment is the same as that given to the severely asphyxiated newborn infant.

Epidural hemorrhage is extremely rare in the neonatal period. This type of bleeding may accompany a skull fracture.

NEUROMUSCULAR DISORDERS

HYPOTONIA

The most usual clinical manifestation of disturbed neuromuscular function in the neonate is hypotonia, which is commonly secondary to perinatal asphyxia, maternal analgesia and systemic infection. Hypotonia is also a typical finding in Down's syn-

drome. Certain metabolic disorders, such as glycogen storage disease and disturbances of amino acid metabolism, may also lead to hypotonia.

In addition to the above disorders, several unusual congenital neuromuscular disorders may be apparent in the newborn infant.

Myasthenia Gravis

Myasthenia gravis, a disorder of the neuromyal junction, may occur in one of two forms in the neonate (19). It is encountered most often in infants of myasthenic mothers and is apparently due to transplacental transmission of some unknown substance. In this type, clinical manifestations usually disappear by one month of age. A congenital form, in which the infant is affected for life, is rarely encountered.

Clinical manifestations vary in severity and are similar to those found in neonates whose hypotonia is due to other causes. The diagnosis is not difficult to make in the presence of maternal myasthenia, but it may be easily overlooked if there is a negative maternal history. Confirmation of the diagnosis is made by improvement of muscular activity within ten minutes following an IM injection of 0.1 to 0.2 mg of neostigmine.

Werdnig-Hoffmann Disease

Werdnig-Hoffmann disease is a degenerative disorder of the anterior horn cells having an autosomal recessive mode of transmission. The progressive hypotonia, which usually leads to death of the infant, may be initially observed during the neonatal period. There is no specific therapy, and treatment is supportive.

Arthrogryposis Multiplex Congenita

Arthrogryposis multiplex congenita is a rare congenital disorder in which one or more joints is frozen in a position of either flexion or extension (18). The limbs may appear shortened, with the joints thickened and knobby. Hypotonia is usually present. The etiology of this disorder is uncertain, but it may be due to a primary anterior horn cell or muscle defect. There is no treatment except for physical therapy (which is of little value), and the prognosis is extremely poor.

SKELETAL SYSTEM

Skeletal abnormalities of the fetus and newborn infant may be due to several causes, including genetic and metabolic defects, infection and trauma.

FETAL DEVELOPMENT

The bony skeleton is formed in two ways. Long bones are derived from a cartilagenous framework that begins to calcify at about the eighth week of gestation, whereas the skull develops by membranous bone formation. With advancing gestational age, the mineral and collagen content of the bone increases, and the water content decreases. In long bones, calcium and phosphorus deposition increases progressively with advancing gestational age; in the skull, however, mineral deposition is essentially complete by the beginning of the third trimester. The increasing hardness of the skull noted during the third trimester may be due to deposition of carbonate ions during this period.

Intrauterine abnormalities of bone development, especially those occurring early in gestation, may have profound effects on long-term growth and development.

CONGENITAL BONE DISORDERS

Several congenital disorders of bone formation may be apparent at birth.

Osteogenesis Imperfecta

In the congenital form of osteogenesis imperfecta (26), which has an autosomal recessive mode of inheritance, the incidence of fetal wastage is relatively high. The very fragile long bones with poorly developed cortices appear ribbon-like on x ray. They fracture easily, following a minimum amount of trauma, and healing is usually prompt, but the bone replacing the callus is defective, and new fractures may occur. Varying degrees of deformity are relatively common. Serum calcium, phosphorus and alkaline phosphatase levels are normal.

The bone fragility observed in this disorder is apparently secondary to an imbalance between the laying down and resorption of bone. Calcification is poor, and immature tissue lacking architectural strength is present.

Besides bone, other connective tissue is involved. The sclerae are thin and may have a bluish cast; dental deficiencies and otosclerosis are also common.

Except for the avoidance of trauma as much as possible and orthopedic management whenever fractures occur, there is no specific treatment for this disorder.

Achondroplasia

Achondroplasia is the most widely recognized bone disorder observed in the neonatal period. It has an autosomal dominant mode of inheritance and is observed in about 1:10,000 deliveries. The long bones, especially the femurs and humeri, are the most severely shortened, whereas the trunk and skull are of relatively normal size (Fig. 9–2).

The basic defect is the inability of the epiphyseal plates to produce enough cartilage for adequate ossification. However, subperiosteal bone formation is normal, giving the long bones a short, thick appearance.

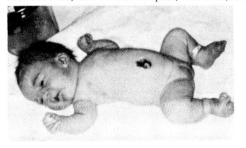

FIG. 9–2. Newborn infant with classic achondroplasia, showing relatively long trunk and short extremities. (Schaffer AJ, Avery ME: Diseases of the Newborn, 3rd ed. Philadelphia, Saunders, 1971)

The diagnosis in the neonatal period is based on parental history of the disorder, shortened extremities and a fairly typical x-ray picture of short, broadened, long bones with irregular epiphyses and "mushrooming" of the ends of the shafts.

If the mother is the achondroplastic parent, her abnormally shaped pelvis may necessitate delivery by cesarean section.

Chondroectodermal Dysplasia

Chondroectodermal dysplasia (Ellis–van Creveld syndrome) is an autosomal recessive disorder that resembles achondroplasia in its bony manifestations. In addition, polydactyly, dystrophic nails and—often—congenital heart disease are associated findings.

Thanatophoric Dwarfism

Thanatophoric dwarfism is a condition that resembles achondroplasia and is uniformly fatal in the first days of life (23). The limbs and fingers are extremely short, the thorax narrow, with marked hypotonia present. The cause of the early death is respiratory failure. The mode of inheritance of this disorder is not known.

Asphyxiating Thoracic Dystrophy

Asphyxiating thoracic dystrophy is a rare familial condition that radiologically and clinically bears a resemblance to chondroectodermal dysplasia (21). Severe constriction of the thorax (associated with short horizontal ribs) and poor chest expansion lead to an early onset of respiratory distress. This disorder is fatal in its more severe form. Survival beyond the neonatal period is possible with death delayed until the second or third year of life.

Diastrophic Dwarfism

Diastrophic dwarfism is another form of chondrodystrophy that has an autosomal recessive mode of inheritance. The short extremities are similar to those seen in achondroplasia. In addition, ear deformities and club feet point to this diagnosis in the neonatal period.

Hypophosphatasia

Hypophosphatasia is a rare inborn error of metabolism characterized by the inability of osteoblasts to secrete alkaline phosphatase (22). Calcification of bone is poor, and skeletal deformities may be present in utero in severe cases. Almost complete lack of mineralization of bone in the fetus has been reported in this condition. This is associated with either fetal or early neonatal death.

Clinical manifestations are failure to thrive, vomiting, hypotonia, drowsiness, the appearance of a "rachitic rosary" and an enlargement of wrists and ankles similar to that seen in rickets.

Characteristic laboratory findings are decreased serum alkaline phosphatase, increased serum calcium concentrations and the presence in the urine of an abnormal metabolite, ethanolamine phosphate.

There is no specific therapy available for this disorder.

Bony Defects of the Head

A number of bony defects of the head are seen in the newborn infants. Among the most important of these are encephalocele, choanal atresia, cleft palate and craniosynostosis, which are discussed in Chapter 23, Surgical Problems.

Micrognathia

Micrognathia, or congenital mandibular hypoplasia, may occur either as an isolated finding or together with a variety of other congenital defects. It is often associated with cleft palate and glossoptosis (Pierre Robin syndrome). In micrognathia, the tongue, which is too large for the small oral cavity, tends to fall backwards, causing respiratory obstruction. Often a suture must be placed through the tip of the tongue to hold it in a forward position.

Mandibulofacial Dysostosis

In mandibulofacial dysostosis (Treacher-Collins' syndrome), mandibular hypoplasia is associated with external ear deformities, antimongoloid slanting of the eyes and coloboma of the lower eyelids.

Wormian Bones

Wormian bones, which can only be detected radiologically, are small accessory bones found along sutural lines of the skull or within the fontanelles. Their presence may be associated with osteogenesis imperfecta, cleidocranial dysostosis, cretinism and hydrocephalus.

Pryles and Khan (25) have observed a 96% correlation between the presence of Wormian bones and serious neurologic disorders in pediatric patients. They have also noted a 71% incidence of Wormian bones in mongoloid children.

Since this finding can usually be detected in the neonatal period, it may prove to be an early prognosticator of CNS abnormalities.

Rickets

Nutritional rickets is rarely seen today in the developed countries because of addition of vitamin D to milk and the widespread use of vitamin supplements.

Rickets has been reported among premature infants whose vitamin D intake averaged about 50 IU/day. Lewin et al (24) suggest that all low-birth-weight infants receive 400 IU of vitamin D daily in addition to a vitamin D–enriched formula. Congenital rickets secondary to severe maternal malabsorption has been reported by Begum et al (20).

Osteomyelitis

Infections of bone may occur either antenatally or postnatally. Rubella and congenital syphilis are typical examples of infections that can involve bones during intrauterine life, and a wide variety of bacteria may be responsible for postnatally acquired osteomyelitis (see Ch. 19, Bacterial Infections).

Other Skeletal Deformities

Orthopedic deformities, such as fractures, congenital dislocation of the hip and club foot are discussed in Chapter 23, Surgical Problems.

AMNIOTIC CONSTRICTION RINGS

Amniotic constriction rings, which occur in about 1:10,000 deliveries, are circular soft tissue depressions of any portion of the body (but most often digits and extremities) frequently associated with congenital amputations, lymphedema distal to the constriction, syndactyly, club foot and areas of denudation and abrasions over the body. The deformities are asymmetric, often unilateral, and unassociated with internal malformations. Fibrous strings of tissue, or amniotic bands, may be attached to the infant or may float freely in the amniotic fluid. Fetal swallowing of one of these bands may be associated with cleft lip or palate. The sex distribution is approximately equal, and familial predilection has not been reported.

The pathogenesis of this syndrome remained unclear until Torpin (28) demonstrated that rupture of the amnion early in gestation was a prerequisite for its occurrence. Following a tear in the amniotic membrane, fibrous bands tend to form from both the outer surface of the amniotic membrane and the denuded area of the chorion. Entanglement of fetal parts in these bands leads to the formation of constriction rings, which may cause a compromise in the arterial circulation leading to autoamputation of the encircled part. The free edges of the amnion may also encircle and form a constriction ring around a fetal part. In addition, a portion of the fetus may rub against the exposed area of the chorion, with resultant adhesions or abrasions.

The maternal factors leading to this condition remain vague. Baker and Rudolph (27) have observed maternal urinary tract infection and second trimester bleeding in several cases. The role of trauma, including diagnostic amniocentesis, has not been fully evaluated.

This syndrome can be easily distinguished from one caused by either a genetic disorder or the teratogenic effect of a maternal drug by the asymmetry of the observed deformities.

REFERENCES

DEVELOPMENT OF THE CNS

1. Brock DJH, Bolton AE, Scrimgeour JB: Prenatal diagnosis of spina bifida and anencephaly through maternal plasma-alpha-fetoprotein measurement. Lancet 1:767, 1974
2. Brock DJH, Sutcliffe RG: Alpha-fetoprotein in the antenatal diagnosis of anencephaly and spina bifida. Lancet 2:197, 1973
2a. Campbell S, Pryse-Davies J, Coltart TM, Seller MI, Singer JD: Ultrasound in the diagnosis of spina bifida. Lancet 1:1065, 1975
3. Timiras PS, Vernadakis AV, Sherwood NM: Development and plasticity of the nervous system. In: Biology of Gestation vol II. Edited by MS Assali. New York, Academic Press, 1968, p 261

NEONATAL SEIZURES

4. Bejsovec M, Kulenoa Z, Ponca E: Familial intrauterine convulsions in pyridoxine dependency. Arch Dis Child 42:201, 1967
5. Colletti RB, Pan MW, Smith EWP, Genel M: Detection of hypocalcemia in susceptible neonates: the Q-$_o$T$_c$ interval. N Engl J Med 290:931, 1974
6. Freeman JM: Neonatal seizures—diagnosis and management. J Pediatr 77:701, 1970
7. McInerny TK, Schubert WK: Prognosis of neonatal seizures. Am J Dis Child 117:261, 1969
8. Paunier L, Radde IC, Kooh SW, Conen PE, Fraser D: Primary hypomagnesemia with secondary hypocalcemia in an infant. Pediatrics 41:385, 1968
9. Rose AL, Lombroso CT: Neonatal seizure states: a study of clinical, pathological and electroencephalographic features in 137 fullterm babies with long-term follow-up. Pediatrics 45:404, 1970
10. Schulte FJ: Neonatal convulsions and their relation to epilepsy in early childhood. Dev Med Child Neurol 8:381, 1966
11. Taitz LS, Zarate-Salvador C, Schwartz E: Congenital absence of the parathyroid and thymus glands in an infant (III and IV pharyngeal pouch syndrome). Pediatrics 38:412, 1966

12. Volpe J: Neonatal seizures. N Engl J Med 289:413, 1973

INTRACRANIAL BLEEDING

13. Fedrick J, Butler NR: Certain causes of neonatal death. II. Intraventricular hemorrhage. Biol Neonate 15:257, 1970
14. Gilles FH, Shillito J: Infantile hydrocephalus: retrocerebellar subdural hematoma. J Pediatr 76:529, 1970
15. Harcke HT, Naeye RL, Storch A, Blanc WA: Perinatal cerebral intraventricular hemorrhage. J Pediatr 80:37, 1972
16. Pitlyk PJ, Miller RH, Stagura LA: Subdural hematoma of the posterior fossa: report of a case. Pediatrics 40: 436, 1967
17. Towbin A: Cerebral intraventricular hemorrhage and subependymal matrix infarction in the fetus and premature newborn. Am J Pathol 52:121, 1968

NEUROMUSCULAR DISORDERS

18. Blattner RJ: Arthrogryposis multiplex congenita. J Pediatr 71:367, 1967
19. Namba T, Brown SB, Grob D: Neonatal myasthenia gravis: report of two cases and review of the literature. Pediatrics 45:488, 1970

SKELETAL SYSTEM

20. Begum R, de L Coutinho M, Dormandy TL, Yudkin S: Maternal malabsorption presenting as congenital rickets. Lancet 1:1048, 1968
21. Hanissian AS, Riggs WW, Thomas DA: Infantile thoracic dystrophy—a variant of Ellis–Van Creveld syndrome. J Pediatr 71: 855, 1967
22. James W. Moule B: Hypophosphatasia. Clin Radiol 17: 368, 1966
23. Langer LO, Spranger JW, Greenacher I, Herdman RC: Thanatophoric dwarfism: condition confused with achondroplasia in the neonate, with brief comments on achondrogenesis and homozygous anchondroplasia. Radiology 92: 285, 1969
24. Lewin PK, Reid M, Reilly BJ, Surjer PR, Fraser D: Iatrogenic rickets in low-birth-weight infants. J Pediatr 78:207, 1971
25. Pryles CV, Khan AJ: Wormian bones: radiologic warning of abnormal nervous system (abst). Pediatr Res 8:189, 1974
26. Remigio PA, Grinvolsky HT: Osteogenesis imperfecta congenita. Am J Dis Child 119:524, 1970

AMNIOTIC CONSTRICTION RINGS

27. Baker CJ, Rudolph AJ: Congenital ring constrictions and intrauterine amputations. Am J Dis Child 121:393, 1971
28. Torpin R: Fetal Malformations Caused by Amnion Rupture During Pregnancy. Springfield, Charles C Thomas, 1968

10

Renal Function and Fluid and Electrolyte Balance

RENAL DEVELOPMENT

EMBRYOLOGY

The kidneys begin to differentiate during the fifth week of fetal life, deriving from several sources (Fig. 10–1). The ureteric bud, a diverticulum of the wolffian (mesonephric) duct, gives rise to the collecting system (ureter, renal pelvis, calyces and collecting ducts). Initial branching of this bud leads to the development of the primary cranial and caudal bud tubules, which give rise to the major and minor calyces and the collecting ducts of renal pyramids. As this branching occurs, there is simultaneous proliferation and differentiation of glomeruli and tubules, which derive from mesenchyme, or metanephric blastema, and develop in close apposition to the collecting system.

A nephric vesicle is formed when a lumen develops within the condensed mesenchyme. The blind or free end forms the glomerulus; the other end establishes continuity with the collecting system. Capillaries enter the free end, forming glomerular vessels. A basement membrane becomes interposed between endothelial and epithelial layers and gradually thickens with age. The elongation and coiling of the vesicle forms the proximal and distal convoluted tubules and loops of Henle.

The most recently formed glomeruli are located peripherally in the cortex. The loops of Henle associated with these cortical nephrons do not reach the medulla. Older glomeruli are located nearer the corticomedullary junction, and their loops of Henle dip into the medulla. The latter glomeruli are larger than those found peripherally and undergo sclerosis, involution and reabsorbtion shortly after birth. Nephrogenesis therefore follows a centrifugal pattern of development, with medullary and juxtamedullary nephrons being more mature than peripheral ones. Hence, at birth medullary height is five times that of the cortex. In adults, the ratio is 2.4:1.

About 20% of the nephrons are formed at 3 months' gestation and 30% at 5 months; all are present by 32 weeks. About 1,000,000 nephrons are present in each kidney at birth, but the glomeruli are only about one-half their ultimate size. While the neonatal basement membrane is only one-half the thickness of the adult membrane, its filtering capacity is as well developed as the latter's.

Factors influencing postnatal renal growth are not well understood. Among premature infants further growth occurs following delivery, but to a lesser degree than would have occurred in utero. Generally, kidney growth is directly proportional to both age and body surface area,

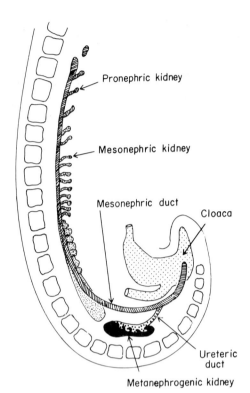

Pronephric kidney

Mesonephric kidney

Mesonephric duct

Cloaca

Ureteric duct

Metanephrogenic kidney

FIG. 10–1. Relationships of the three embryonic kidneys in the human fetus. (Crocker JFC, Brown DM, Vernier RL: Pediatr Clin North Am 18:355, 1971)

with most of this growth representing proximal renal tubular development.

Fetal development may progress normally in the absence of the kidneys, since the placenta serves as the fetus' excretory organ. While renal function is present during intrauterine life, low renal-plasma flow and high resistance limit urinary output. By the end of the first trimester, urine production begins. The fluid is hypotonic to plasma, reflecting a decreased concentration of urea and electrolytes. Animal studies indicate that glomerular filtration rates (GFRs) gradually increase, but that urinary output decreases as gestation advances. This latter phenomenon is due to maturation of the loop of Henle, where salt and water is reabsorbed.

Following delivery, renal blood flow increases, reflecting decreased renal arteriolar resistance, with subsequent improvement in renal function. Postnatal maturation of

renal function is discussed in the section Fluids and Electrolytes.

RENAL DYSPLASIA

Renal dysplasia is a general term for any congenital malformation of either the nephrons or collecting system. Involved kidneys (Fig. 10–2) have a primitive or fetal appearance. This abnormal embryonic organization results in: disorganization of epithelial structures; abnormal presence of cartilage, fibrous tissue and cysts (hence the name multicystic kidneys); and primitive ducts with tall columnar epithelium, which is sometimes ciliated. In the great majority of cases these findings are associated with urinary tract anomalies. The more generalized the dysplasia, the more severe the anomalies.

Along with aplastic kidneys (total absence of renal tissue), multicystic kidneys are most often unilateral and may appear in all age groups. When present bilaterally, manifestations of renal disease become apparent during the neonatal period, and the process is often lethal.

In unilateral multicystic disease, males are more frequently affected than females, and the involved kidney is usually on the left. Hypertension is absent, and the mass that is palpated may sometimes be confused with a Wilms' tumor. The deformed kidney may become insufficient, with infection supervening in about two-thirds of the cases.

POLYCYSTIC DISEASE

Polycystic disease of the kidneys is a group of disorders, usually familial, which may first appear clinically either during infancy or adult life.

Two types are seen in infancy. In Potter type I, which has an autosomal recessive mode of inheritance, the kidneys are spongy, secondary to dilatation of the collecting tubules. Gross landmarks of the kidney are preserved. Cystic changes are also noted in the liver and pancreas. This condition is so severe that it frequently results in either fetal or neonatal death. Marked en-

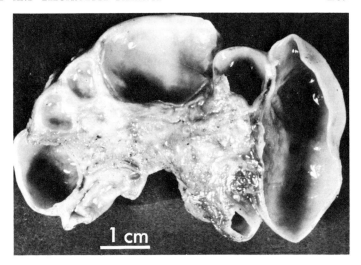

FIG. 10–2. Multicystic dysplasia. The kidney has been hemisected to show the peripheral arrangement of cysts and the central solid area above the hilus. The pelvis is occluded, and calyces cannot be identified. The solid core is relatively fibrous, and renal parenchyma is not grossly recognizable. (Bernstein J: Pediatr Clin North Am 18:395, 1971)

largement of the kidneys during fetal life may lead to dystocia.

In a second variety of polycystic kidney, which is usually discovered after the neonatal period, there is no familial pattern. Histologically, there is a marked increase in connective tissue, in contrast to the first type where this finding is not evident. Along with renal tubular medullary dilatation hepatic fibrosis and portal hypertension are present.

FLUIDS AND ELECTROLYTES

The development of safe and easy techniques of administering fluids intravenously has allowed major advances in the medical management of low-birth-weight and other compromised infants. Use of the disposable scalp vein needle, for example, has made cannulation of both scalp and peripheral veins an easily learned, routine nursery procedure. Increasing skill in catheterization of the umbilical vessels (especially the umbilical artery) has made this a popular route for IV administration of fluids, and methods by which protein hydrolysate or amino acid solutions could be administered either through a deep or peripheral vein have opened up new therapeutic possibilities. It is now possible not only to administer IV fluids on a short-term basis, but also to provide complete or nearly complete protein

and caloric requirements by this route for weeks or even months with an apparently normal growth in height, weight and head circumference.

Postpartum IV administration of fluids is mandatory for infants in whom immaturity or illness, or both, make it impossible to meet fluid, caloric and electrolyte requirements through the oral route and for those in whom abnormalities of acid-base balance require correction by IV infusions of alkali. The goals of parenteral therapy in the neonate are:

Maintenance of fluid and electrolyte requirements

Replacement of body fluids and electrolytes in the presence of vomiting, diarrhea or drainage from GI tract

Correction of metabolic acidosis

Correction of hypocalcemia

Correction of hypoglycemia

Provision of calories (as glucose and protein hydrolysate or amino acid solution)

Administration of antibiotics and other therapeutic medications

In most infants of very low gestational age who can tolerate some oral feedings, a supplementary IV infusion must be used to meet minimum caloric and fluid requirements until the infant is able to tolerate approximately 100 ml of fluid/kg/day by the oral route.

Special problems of fluid and electroyte balance and caloric intake occur in neonates requiring major GI surgery or in whom the alimentary tract may be nonfunctional for a prolonged period of time. Since IV solutions containing a 5% or 10% concentration of glucose provide only marginally for ongoing energy requirements and not at all for growth, the prolonged deprivation of an adequate protein and caloric intake may have permanently deleterious effects. Total parenteral alimentation has had its greatest clinical success among these infants.

Another group requiring IV therapy consists of those who are well in the days immediately after birth, but in whom subsequent illness, e.g., vomiting or diarrhea, necessitates IV therapy.

CLINICAL CONSIDERATIONS

In all infants treated with IV fluids, evaluation of the clinical condition is vital (Table 10–1) and should be performed several times daily. Special attention must be paid to any evidence of either dehydration or edema. Measurements of urine volume and GI drainage, when present, are also important. Infants should be weighed at least once a day to complement the clinical impression of the state of hydration. When an arm or leg board is used, the infant should be weighed before and after starting the infusion so that changes in weight can be assessed at regular intervals.

Laboratory examinations are essential in managing fluid therapy. Determinations of hemoglobin concentration and plasma osmolarity are guides to the state of hydration, as are the specific gravity and osmolarity of the urine. Measurements of blood constituents, e.g., sodium, potassium, urea nitrogen, chloride, calcium, phosphate and glucose, are vital, and the acid-base status must be frequently evaluated, especially in infants with poor pulmonary and renal function.

TABLE 10–1. Evaluation of Neonates Receiving Parenteral Therapy

Clinical
  Daily weight
  Evidence of overhydration (edema) or under-
    hydration (poor skin turgor, dry mucous mem-
    branes or depressed anterior fontanelle)
  Measurement of urinary output and GI drainage
Laboratory
  Hemoglobin concentration or hematocrit
  Plasma osmolarity
  Biochemical measurements of blood constituents
    (sodium, potassium, urea nitrogen, chloride,
    calcium, phosphate, glucose)
  Blood acid-base studies
  Urinary osmolarity or specific gravity
  Urinary glucose

Perhaps the most important consideration in calculating parenteral fluid requirements for the neonate is the fact that there is very little room for error. Because of the small size of the neonate (especially the low-birth-weight infant) and his limited renal capacity to excrete excessive water and solute loads, what would be small excesses of fluid in the older child or adult may be sufficient to cause overhydration in the infant. Likewise, osmotic diuresis may be induced by the administration of concentrated glucose solutions, and this can lead to blood glucose levels exceeding the renal tubular threshold, with a resultant glycosuria.

It is important not only to order the proper quantity of parenteral fluids, but also to ascertain that the infant actually receives the fluids ordered.

PHYSIOLOGIC BASIS FOR INTRAVENOUS FLUID THERAPY

The rational use of IV fluids in the neonate is based on several factors:

1. Appreciation of the infant's body composition (both actual tissue and water distribution)
2. Estimated daily energy expenditures and growth requirements
3. Renal, pulmonary, adrenal, parathyroid and pituitary function
4. Anticipated loss of fluid, electrolyte and base in certain disease conditions

BODY COMPOSITION

The body composition of the newborn infant differs significantly from that of both the older child and adult (Fig. 10–3). Among neonates there are also marked differences dependent on gestational and postnatal age, intrauterine growth rate and route of delivery. Differences exist both in the total amount and the distribution of body water.

As gestation progresses, there is a steady decline in the water content of the fetus, due largely to the normal decrease in the amount of extracellular water. Cassady (7) noted that extracellular fluid comprised about 37.5% of the weight of normally grown full-term infants immediately after delivery. Normally grown premature infants (33 to 36 weeks' gestation) had extracellular fluid compartments averaging about 42% of body weight, while the extracellular volumes in infants with intrauterine growth retardation were comparable to those in premature infants having similar birth weights, rather than similar gestational ages. Those infants with the most severe growth failure had the greatest expansion of their extracellular volumes. The expanded extracellular volume associated with intrauterine malnutrition might thus be analogous to the expansion of this compartment observed in postnatal malnutrition.

Much of the excessive extracellular fluid seen in the true premature infant at birth as edema fluid is lost after the first week of life. Contrary to opinions popular several decades ago, this water is minimally utilized in meeting the fluid requirements of these infants.

Glycogen stores comprise about 0.5% of body weight in premature infants. They are quickly exhausted during the intrapartum and early neonatal periods, especially during hypoxia and cold stress. In undergrown infants with intrauterine malnutrition, glycogen stores may also be negligible or nonexistent. Both groups of infants are deficient in body fat and have little reserve to meet energy requirements in the face of either partial or total starvation. Therefore, providing adequate calories in parenteral fluids is vital.

CALORIC EXPENDITURES AND GROWTH REQUIREMENTS

In calculating parenteral caloric requirements, it is necessary to know the anticipated caloric expenditure of the infant. The basal caloric expenditure depends on the infant's gestational and postnatal age, but it is higher in infants who have experienced chronic intrauterine malnutrition (see Ch. 13, Thermoregulation). It is usually between 35 and 50 calories/kg/day, with the lower figure applying to premature infants on the first day of life. Up to 15 additional calories/kg/day should be allowed for intermittent activity. In the low-birth-weight infant

FIG. 10–3. Body composition of premature and full-term infants, children and adults. (Heird WC et al: J Pediatr 80:351, 1972)

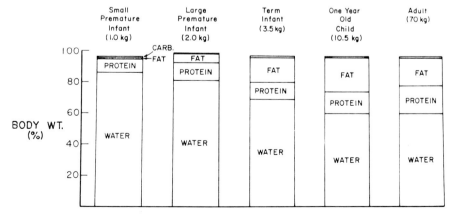

raised under thermoneutral conditions, the caloric expenditure secondary to occasional cold stress is negligible; otherwise, up to 10 calories/kg/day can be assumed to be required to offset the cold-induced increment in metabolic rate.

It is therefore obvious that the calories provided in a standard IV infusion containing 10% glucose are inadequate to meet the daily metabolic requirements of the infant.

ROLE OF ORGAN SYSTEMS IN FLUID AND ELECTROLYTE BALANCE

Water, electrolyte and acid-base homeostasis are regulated primarily by the lung and the kidney, with some evaporative water loss occurring via the skin. The adrenal cortex plays a major role in electrolyte metabolism, while the parathyroids regulate calcium and phosphate homeostasis (see section Calcium and Phosphorus Metabolism; also Adrenal Cortex, Ch. 11).

Lungs

About one-third of the evaporative water loss in newborn infants occurs via the lungs; with an increase in the relative humidity of the incubator, this loss decreases. The lungs also play a very important role in acid-base homeostasis. Hypoxia (whether secondary to pulmonary or CNS disease) often precedes a metabolic acidosis. Carbon dioxide retention, which may be secondary to hypoventilation or primary pulmonary disease, is associated with respiratory acidosis.

Kidney

The kidney plays the major role in maintaining water, electrolyte and acid-base homeostasis in the newborn infant. This capability is limited, however, during the early neonatal period because of immature glomerular and tubular function (11). These limitations of renal function require that care be taken in the preparation and administration of IV fluids.

Anatomic development of the renal cortex is incomplete at birth, with juxtamedullary nephrons being more completely developed than cortical ones. This immaturity is most marked in infants of low gestational age.

The decreased neonatal GFR appears to be due both to an increased intrarenal vascular resistance and to the pore size of the glomerular membrane being significantly smaller in the neonate than in the older child. The more developed juxtamedullary glomeruli appear to be more permeable than the cortical glomeruli during this period.

In the neonatal period the functioning of the renal tubules is even more limited than that of the glomeruli. With this glomerulotubular inbalance, there is a decreased ability of the tubules to reabsorb sodium, bicarbonate, glucose, amino acids and phosphate. The infant's difficulty in excreting an acid urine is at least partially due to the low renal tubular threshold for bicarbonate. Although in older children and adults bicarbonate concentration of the blood ranges from about 26 to 28 mEq/l, the low tubular threshold for reabsorption of bicarbonate in the neonate will usually permit blood levels of about 22.5 mEq/l. In addition, the ability to excrete titratable acid and ammonia is limited.

Perhaps the most important reason for care in the administration of IV fluids to newborn infants is the limitation of their kidneys in excreting either a concentrated or dilute urine. The maximum concentrating ability of the newborn kidney is about 700 mOsm/l, as compared to about 1200 mOsm/l for the normal older child or adult. This is probably due more to the low rate of urea excretion than to any other factor, since newborn infants fed high-protein formulas soon become capable of excreting a concentrated urine. Secretion of antidiuretic hormone (ADH) appears to be limited in neonates, but this is probably unimportant as regards the ability to excrete a concentrated urine.

During the first days of life the ability to excrete a dilute urine during overhydration is limited. With maturation of juxtamedullary nephrons (in whose long loops of Henle sodium reabsorption is most marked), this ability to excrete a water load usually improves by the end of the first week of life.

The ability of the renal tubules to excrete a phosphate load determines to a large degree the serum calcium and phosphate concentrations, but these also depend on parathyroid function (see section Calcium and Phosphorus Metabolism).

Adrenal Cortex

Maintaining a normal serum sodium concentration depends largely on normal aldosterone secretion. Deficiency of the enzyme 21-hydroxylase, which occurs in the adrenogenital syndrome, may be associated with hyponatremia and hyperkalemia ("salt-losing" syndrome). Adrenal hemorrhage may also affect sodium and potassium concentrations.

Parathyroids

The action of parathyroid hormone on the renal tubules and bone regulates serum concentrations of calcium and phosphate. The role of calcitonin in the neonatal period remains unclear.

Pituitary

An intact anterior pituitary gland is necessary to maintain normal adrenocortical function. The secretion of ADH by the posterior pituitary plays some role in water balance in the newborn infant; inappropriate ADH secretion, secondary to severe asphyxia or meningitis, may be associated with water retention and dilutional hyponatremia.

LOSS OF WATER, ELECTROLYTE AND BASE

In certain conditions an excessive loss of water, electrolyte and bicarbonate requires their replacement at regular intervals. Among these conditions are infectious and surgical diseases of the GI tract in which vomiting, diarrhea and postoperative GI drainage are present. Pyloric stenosis, a special situation with predominant loss of hydrogen, chloride and potassium ions, is rare in the early neonatal period.

INTRAVENOUS FLUID THERAPY IN LOW-BIRTH-WEIGHT INFANTS

The presence of the respiratory distress syndrome (RDS) is the most common cause among premature infants of inability to tolerate oral feedings during the first few days of life. These infants usually receive their entire fluid requirements by the IV route until their primary illness subsides to the extent that some oral feedings can be tolerated. While the number of calories received in the infusion may not be enough to meet all of their energy requirements, it may be adequate to tide them over the first critical days of life. The infusion also administers alkali to correct the metabolic acidosis accompanying RDS.

For the infant whose only source of fluid is through the parenteral route, the average amount necessary on the first day of life is approximately 75 ml/kg of body weight (Table 10–2). There are, of course, individual variations; adjustments must be made on the basis of changes in daily weight, osmolarity of the serum and urine, body temperature and clinical evidence of either dehydration or overhydration. Increased insensible water loss through thin and permeable skin in some infants of low gestational age may increase their daily water requirement. Advancing postnatal age also increases daily fluid requirements, and

TABLE 10–2. Early Neonatal Water and Electrolyte Maintenance

Supplement	Amount Usually Administered
Water	75 ml (range 40–100 ml) /kg/day, based on daily weights
Sodium	2 mEq/kg/day (given as sodium bicarbonate if infant is acidotic)
Potassium	2 mEq/kg/day (withheld on first day of life in presence of acidosis or hyperkalemia)
Chloride	2 to 4 mEq/kg/day

by the end of the first week the infant should be receiving approximately 120 ml/kg/day. Once oral feedings have started, the total amount of IV fluid is reduced proportionately. This is discussed in the section Feeding the Low-Birth-Weight Infant, Ch. 12.

CALORIC CONTENT OF THE INFUSION

Infusion of 5% glucose solution provides 20 calories/100 ml of solution; a 10% solution provides 40 calories/100 ml. A 15% glucose solution, often used to provide added calories for energy metabolism and to correct hypoglycemia, is associated with high osmolarity, making it difficult to maintain such an infusion in a peripheral vein for prolonged periods. In infants of very low gestational age (with poor insulin production), this concentration of glucose in the IV fluids may lead to glycosuria. Therefore, the urine of these infants must be carefully examined for the presence of glucose.

ELECTROLYTE REQUIREMENTS

The usual maintenance requirement for sodium, potassium and chloride in the neonate is 0.5 to 2.0 mEq/kg/day. If the infant is not acidotic, 2 mEq/kg of sodium and potassium and 2 to 4 mEq/kg of chloride may be infused daily. Infusion of potassium should be withheld on the first day of life (when urinary flow is ordinarily diminished) and in the presence of acidosis (when the concentration of intracellular potassium may be elevated). In the latter condition, the entire sodium requirement may be given as sodium bicarbonate.

The need for calcium during the first days of life in infants who are being fed intravenously and in whom normal serum calcium concentrations are present (above 8 mg/100 ml) has not been established. Calcium supplements should be given with long-term parenteral alimentation. Calcium that is administered to correct hypocalcemia should not be mixed with a bicarbonate-containing solution (a calcium carbonate precipitate will form).

CORRECTION OF ACIDOSIS

There is evidence that the correction of blood pH in acidotic low birth weight infants, especially those with RDS, is associated with decreased morbidity and possibly decreased mortality. However, treatment of the acidosis must be approached with caution. If the acidosis is primarily respiratory (carbon dioxide retention), administration of bicarbonate will lead to further accumulation of carbon dioxide. Hypercapnea should be treated with assisted ventilation (either bag and mask or respirator). An acidosis that is primarily metabolic probably represents a redistribution of bicarbonate ion in the body rather than an absolute loss, as seen in diarrhea. An overly vigorous correction may lead to the development of a metabolic alkalosis. Rapid correction is needed only in the presence of a severe acidosis. Otherwise, a cautious slow correction over a 24-hour period is justified.

The following is an easily used formula for administering alkali to the acidotic low-birth-weight infant during the early neonatal period:

$$\text{mEq of } HCO_3^- \text{ required} = \text{Wt in kg} \times (-\text{ base excess}) \times 0.4$$

The factor 0.4 represents the proportion of the body of a low-birth-weight infant that is extracellular water. A lower value (0.35) can be used for full-term infants. Although there is some intracellular distribution of bicarbonate ion, this formula is useful for practical purposes. When calculating for a period of 24 hours, about one-half of the sodium bicarbonate may be given over the first 8 hours and the other half over the next 16 hours. This may be modified depending on repeated pH and P_{CO_2} determinations.

The rapid infusion of fluid having a very high osmolarity should be approached with caution, but this type of therapy may be necessary to maintain homeostasis, e.g., the infusion of a 25% or 50% glucose solution for the correction of hypoglycemia or a 7.5% or 8.4% sodium bicarbonate solution for the correction of a severe metabolic acidosis. Finberg (12) has pointed out that a rapid increase in the osmolarity of the blood may expand the extracellular compartment by "pulling" water out of the cells and result in intracellular dehydration, particularly in the CNS. If this increase exceeds 40 mOsm/kg of water over a period of a few hours, renal, CNS and metabolic damage may ensue. The maximum safe tolerance for a normally hydrated newborn infant is about 25 mOsm/kg of water over a four-hour period.

An infusion of 3 mEq of sodium bicarbonate/kg of body weight causes an increase of 7.5 mOsm/kg of body water, and 1 ml of 50% glucose solution contains 2.75 mOsm of solute.

SPECIAL CLINICAL SITUATIONS

DIARRHEA

Diarrhea is usually associated with an acute infectious process and often requires discontinuation of oral feedings and total reliance on IV alimentation. Every attempt must be made to isolate the etiologic agent and treat the primary illness. However, the correction of dehydration, electrolyte and acid-base disturbances is of primary importance since passage of only a few diarrheal stools in the newborn infant may cause moderate or severe dehydration and a metabolic acidosis (secondary to loss of bicarbonate in the stool).

Intravenous therapy must satisfy maintenance water requirements and replace diarrheal water losses. The degree of dehydration is assessed by changes in the infant's weight, loss of skin turgor, dryness of mucous membranes and depression of the anterior fontanelle. The success of the rehydration process may be assessed by changes in the infant's clinical condition and change in weight. Measurement of the osmolarity of blood and urine is also useful.

Fever, occasionally occurring in infected full-term infants, requires additional fluids to compensate for the associated increased metabolism. Newborn infants with diarrhea who have developed a metabolic acidosis often hyperventilate to lower their arterial P_{CO_2} and thus raise their blood pH. This pulmonary water loss may also require additional fluid replacement.

Blood concentrations of sodium, potassium and chloride should be carefully followed. Excessively low concentrations of sodium in an infant who had been previously well raises the suspicion of congenital adrenal hyperplasia (salt-losing type; 21-hydroxylase deficiency). Hyperkalemia is usually associated with the hyponatremia, and must be corrected rapidly to avoid a potential fatality.

Elevated serum sodium concentrations (above 150 mEq/l) may be encountered if proportionately more water than sodium is lost in the diarrheal fluid. In correcting this type of dehydration, the concentration of sodium in the IV fluid should not exceed 30 mEq/l. Since there has been a loss of sodium in the stool, sodium-free solutions are contraindicated in the treatment of this condition. In addition, correction of hypernatremia should proceed slowly to avoid cerebral hemorrhage due to sudden osmotic shifts.

Because of the metabolic acidosis that is almost universally present in neonatal diarrhea, most or all of the sodium that is administered initially can be given as bicarbonate. Potassium should be withheld until there has been a good urinary flow and the acidosis has at least been partially corrected.

SURGERY

The neonate with a surgical problem requires parenteral fluid therapy prior to surgery to correct fluid, electrolyte and acid-base imbalance.

The catabolic response observed postoperatively in older children and adults appears to be attenuated following surgery in the neonate. Similarly, postoperative sodium and water retention may be a milder problem than in older age groups. Therefore, postoperative fluid and electrolyte therapy in the neonate must be based on individual clinical and laboratory observations (see Ch. 23, Surgical Problems).

In the infant who has undergone major GI surgery, prolonged parenteral therapy may be required. Since standard IV therapy provides suboptimal calories and no protein, its protracted use may seriously impair the infant's growth potential. Over the past several years total parenteral alimentation has been used successfully to promote growth in infants who cannot be adequately fed. This is especially useful after major GI surgery (see section Long-term Parenteral Therapy). Where surgery does not involve the GI tract, oral feedings can usually be resumed early in the postoperative period, and standard IV therapy may be successfully used on a short-term basis.

TECHNIQUES OF ADMINISTERING IV FLUIDS

The peripheral veins of the neonate can be easily cannulated with a No. 23 or 25 scalp vein needle. An ample number of scalp veins, as well as veins of the antecubital fossa and dorsa of the foot and hand are accessible. When cannulating a scalp vein, caution must be taken to avoid inadvertantly placing the needle in an artery. With proper care, a peripheral vein may be usable for several days, but the sclerosing effect of a relatively hypertonic solution may shorten this time.

It should be realized that the pH of a glucose-containing solution ranges from 4.0 to 4.5, acidification being necessary to prevent carmelization of the glucose during the sterilization process. This low pH may also be responsible for shortening the time a vein may be used for IV infusion, but raising the pH to about 8.5 by adding a small amount of sodium bicarbonate may lengthen the vein's usability.

The umbilical vein should be used for the infusion of fluids only in a life-threatening situation (e.g., the severely asphyxiated infant in the delivery room). The umbilical artery should only be used when an umbilical arterial catheter is being used to obtain blood samples or for blood pressure measurements.

Peripheral venous cutdowns may be necessary under certain circumstances, such as during an operative procedure, when the patency of a vein must be assured.

Cannulation of a central vein becomes necessary when long-term total parenteral venous alimentation is used.

The rate of infusion, which may be exceedingly slow, can usually be controlled by a microdrop infusion mechanism. Careful nursing observation, however, is important. Infusion pumps can usually maintain a slow, steady rate of flow, but even if the infusion infiltrates, the pump will continue to drive fluids into the subcutaneous tissue unless the site of the infusion is carefully watched. In delivering fluids into an arterial channel (e.g., the abdominal aorta) where there is a high head of pressure, use of the infusion pump is mandatory.

The infusion of very caustic solutions, such as undiluted sodium bicarbonate, into a peripheral vein may result in severe tissue necrosis if the fluids infiltrate into the local tissues. Such injections must be made with utmost caution.

Subcutaneous injection of fluid containing saline and glucose (hypodermoclysis) is never indicated. This fluid distributes itself poorly in the extracellular space, where it is needed. Even worse, it may act as a third fluid compartment and draw off water from the extracellular space.

LONG-TERM PARENTERAL THERAPY

The IV administration of a 5% or 10% glucose solution to a newborn infant receiving no other source of nutrition provides too few calories for basal metabolic requirements plus energy expenditure and insufficient nutrient for growth requirements. Therefore, when a glucose infusion is the sole source of calories, catabolism of body tissues is usually necessary to help meet energy requirements, and the smaller the infant, the smaller the total amount of fat, protein and glycogen available for catabolism during a period of total or semistarvation (Fig. 10–4). Heird et al (14) estimate

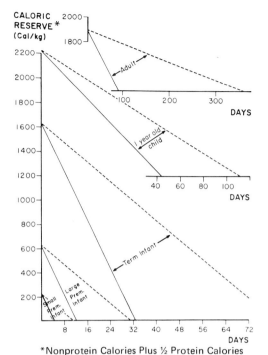

CALORIC RESERVE* (Cal/kg)

DAYS

*Nonprotein Calories Plus ½ Protein Calories

FIG. 10–4. Duration of survival expected in starvation (solid line) and semistarvation (broken line). (Heird et al: J Pediatr 80:351, 1972)

that the 1-kg premature infant, whose body contains approximately 1% fat and 8.5% protein, has a total caloric reserve (including liver glycogen) of about 450 calories. With increasing size, the proportion of metabolically active tissue (fat and protein) in the infant's body rises, so that the full-term infant with a 16% fat and 11% protein body content has a caloric reserve of about 2000 calories/kg. Therefore, the smaller the infant, the shorter the period during which he can be kept alive solely with an IV infusion of glucose and water. Because of this, a caloric intake in excess of that provided by a 5% or 10% IV glucose solution must be provided for low-birth-weight infants within a very short time after birth. Usually, this supplementation consists of increasing the amount of formula (see section Feeding the Low-Birth-Weight Infant, Ch. 12). When the infant is unable to tolerate feedings via the GI tract, alternate routes must be found.

Oral feedings may be contraindicated for a prolonged period of time in cases of GI surgery and severe medical illness (such as uncontrollable diarrhea). With prolonged infusion of a glucose solution as the sole source of calories, these infants will eventually succumb, their length of survival depending on their energy stores.

Dudrick et al (10) approached the problem of delivering enough calories and protein to newborn infants whose GI tracts were unavailable for alimentation over a prolonged period by infusing a protein hydrolysate and hypertonic glucose solution through a central venous catheter; they were able to establish normal growth in beagle puppies from whom oral feedings were withheld. This technique was soon successfully used in newborn infants with severe surgical problems of the GI tract, in whom oral feedings had to be withheld for periods up to 400 days (20). This approach has been widely accepted in centers performing neonatal GI surgery. Since many hazards and side effects complicate this therapy, it must be approached with caution, attention being paid to the most minute details.

CLINICAL APPROACH

For an infant to receive his full daily caloric and protein intake by the IV route in a quantity of water not exceeding his daily requirement, an extremely hypertonic solution (up to 1500 mOsm/l) must be used. This solution must be diluted rapidly once it enters the body; therefore infusion must be into a major blood vessel of relatively large caliber. In the newborn infant, a silastic catheter is usually inserted into the superior vena cava through the internal or external jugular vein under strict aseptic conditions (Fig. 10–5). The other end of the catheter is tunneled through the skin of the neck and scalp, so that it exits from the skin posterior and superior to the ear. The area around the entrance of the catheter must be kept sterile; an antibiotic or iodine-containing ointment should be applied whenever the dressing is changed (about three times weekly). If sterile conditions are maintained and if the catheter is not used for delivery of medication or for blood sampling, it can re-

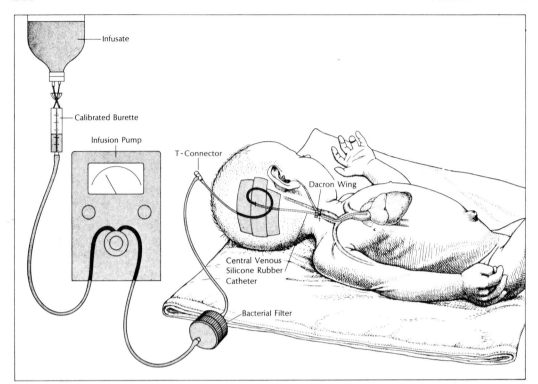

FIG. 10–5. The "lifeline system" provides complete IV nutrition for infants unable to take food orally or by gastric tube. The amino acid–glucose formula is administered at a uniform, slow rate by means of a constant infusion pump. The system includes a bacterial filter to eliminate any contaminants in the infusate and a T-connector to administer IV drugs. The central venous catheter is coiled once after exiting from the scalp and is held in place by a sterile dressing (Filler RM: Hosp Pract 7:79, 1972)

main in place for several weeks without infection or thrombosis. At the first signs of infection, the catheter should be removed, the tip cultured and a blood culture taken. To insure equal flow, a constant infusion pump should be used to deliver the fluid. The use of a 0.22-μm Millipore filter in the infusion line is generally recommended to decrease the possibility of infection.

The solutions used for total parenteral alimentation contain hypertonic glucose (usually about 20%) and either a protein hydrolysate or a mixture of L-amino acids. The commonly used protein hydrolysate solutions are Aminosol (derived from fibrin) and Amigen or Hyprotigen (derived from casein). Mixtures of synthetic L-amino acids (FreAmine and Neoaminosol) have a more reproducible amino acid composition than the protein hydrolysates.

The usual daily dosage of protein in the hydrolysate is about 4 g/kg/day; when using the L-amino acid solutions, Heird et al (14) have administered 2.5 g/kg/day of amino acids as FreAmine and 3.25 g/kg/day as Neoaminosol. The very hypertonic solution (about 1500 mOsm/1) contains about 90 to 100 calories/100 ml and is administered at the rate of 120 to 130 ml/kg/day. Sodium, potassium, calcium, magnesium and phosphate should be added to the nutrients, along with an IV multivitamin preparation (Table 10–3). Although IV lipid preparation is being used outside of the United States, its clinical use has not yet (1975) been approved in this country; therefore essential fatty acids cannot be given parenterally to the infant, except as very small quantities present in whole blood or plasma. Vitamins K and B_{12} and folic acid may also be given as a regular supplement.

TABLE 10-3. Electrolyte and Vitamin Supplements in Total Parenteral Alimentation

Electrolytes	Daily intake/kg/day (mEq)
Sodium	4.0
Potassium	2.6
Calcium	2.25
Phosphate	1.5
Magnesium	0.6
Chloride	4.5

Vitamins	Requirements/24 hours
Vitamin A	70–200 IU
Thiamine	0.2 mg/1000 calories
Riboflavin	0.3 mg/1000 calories
Pyridoxine	9 μg/g protein
Ascorbic acid	10 mg
Vitamin D	100–200 IU
Vitamin E	0.34–0.45 IU
Niacin	4.4 mg/1000 calories
Folic acid	5–50 μg
Vitamin K	5 μg
Vitamin B_{12}	<1 μg

(Modified from Shaw JCL: Pediatr Clin North Am 20:333, 1973, and Heird WC, et al: J Pediatr 80:351 1972)

COMPLICATIONS AND DANGERS

This method appears ideal for alimenting all newborn infants incapable of receiving nutrition through the GI tract. However, there are many associated complications and dangers: systemic infection, venous thrombosis, extravasation of fluid into tissues, plugging of catheter, hyperglycemia and glycosuria, unphysiologic serum levels of certain amino acids, hyperammonemia, hypophosphatemia and metabolic acidosis. Some of these are secondary to the placement of indwelling catheters in deep venous sites over a prolonged period of time, while others are related to the composition of the solution infused.

The presence of a deep venous catheter over a long period of time may predispose a debilitated newborn infant to systemic bacterial or fungal infection (5). Other problems are thrombosis, plugging of the catheter and extravasation of fluid out of the vein.

The high concentration of glucose may not be fully metabolized, especially by those infants of low gestational age whose pancreatic islet cell function is not fully devel-

oped. An osmotic diuresis, with glycosuria and dehydration may ensue. Often, these infants must be started on solutions with glucose concentrations of less than 20%; after several days, they may be able to tolerate the more highly concentrated solution. Protein hydrolysates contain concentrations of certain amino acids that may cause unphysiologically high blood levels (13). Since elevated levels of various amino acids, e.g., phenylalanine, leucine and isoleucine, may damage the neonatal brain (15), the question has been raised about potentially deleterious effects of hydrolysate solutions on the CNS (see section Feeding the Low-Birth-Weight Infant, Ch. 12). The use of synthetic amino acid solutions may circumvent this problem. Hyperammonemia may also be observed in infants receiving protein hydrolysates or synthetic amino acid mixtures.

Another undesirable side effect noted with the use of FreAmine and Neoaminosol has been a hyperchloremic metabolic acidosis (8). This has been attributed to a "cation gap," an excess of positively charged metabolizable amino acids that are a source of hydrogen ion. Use of solutions with an "anion gap" eliminates this problem, since hydrogen ions are not liberated when amino acids are converted to protein.

Depletion of adenosine triphosphate (ATP), possibly due to a relative deficiency of phosphate ions, may lead to erythrocyte damage, with impairment of sodium and potassium pump mechanisms (19).

INDICATIONS FOR USE

The clinical, physiologic and biochemical status of infants receiving total parenteral nutrition must be carefully evaluated since severe metabolic derangements, ultimately leading to death of the patient, may ensue if abnormalities are left uncorrected.

Because of side effects, total parenteral alimentation should be used only under circumstances in which death is likely without its use (e.g., GI malformations that preclude oral feedings and some cases of severe, unremitting diarrhea). Its use in very low-birth-weight infants with intact GI tracts in whom oral feedings are possible (but limited) is under investigation. Preliminary data show that these infants are capable of achieving normal growth with this regimen (9).

PERIPHERAL INTRAVENOUS ALIMENTATION

Because of problems associated with the use of deep venous sites, peripheral veins have been used for the infusion of hypertonic glucose and amino acid solutions. Extremely hypertonic solutions cannot, however, be infused through peripheral veins, and the caloric content of these solutions being thus limited, they cannot be used as a complete source of calories. Several groups of investigators (4, 6, 16) have found that oral feedings (with the attendant risk of aspiration) can be delayed in low-birth-weight infants receiving this regimen. Weight gain in these infants was satisfactory, and the infusion could be maintained in a peripheral vein for approximately two days.

At our institution we use a solution containing 1.7% FreAmine and 12% glucose for peripheral IV alimentation; the caloric value is 55 calories/100 ml.

ACID-BASE METABOLISM

Normal fetal and neonatal homeostasis depend on blood and tissue pH values being maintained within fairly narrow limits, and to a large extent, these in turn depend on adequate oxygenation. Fetal acid-base balance is maintained by a properly functioning placenta and the buffering capacity of the blood. In extrauterine life, the lungs and kidneys assume the functions of the placenta.

To maintain a normal blood pH, a balance must be maintained between the respiratory component (CO_2) and "metabolic" components. The latter, whose purpose it is to buffer excess hydrogen ions (H^+), is comprised of extracellular bicarbonate ions

(HCO_3) and intracellular proteins (primarily hemoglobin). The following relationship (Henderson-Hasselbach equation) expresses this buffering action.

$$\text{Blood pH} = 6.1 + \log\frac{[HCO_3^-]}{[CO_2]}$$

Under normal circumstances, the ratio of bicarbonate to carbon dioxide is approximately 20:1. Any alteration of this ratio is met by an attempt to rebalance it (Table 10–4). If, for example, there is a decrease in bicarbonate concentration secondary to accumulation of hydrogen ions (metabolic acidosis), the lungs, if functioning normally, will attempt to compensate by increasing carbon dioxide excretion. If, on the other hand, there is carbon dioxide retention secondary to hypoventilation or primary lung disease, there is a tendency for the kidney to conserve bicarbonate (which may be limited in the neonatal period).

In the presence of hyperventilation and respiratory alkalosis, compensatory renal bicarbonate loss occurs to maintain the normal ratio. With an excess of bicarbonate (metabolic alkalosis), the lungs will conserve carbon dioxide. With severe neonatal pulmonary insufficiency, there may be a combined metabolic and respiratory acidosis, and compensation may be impossible.

Technologic advancements during the 1960s and 1970s have greatly simplified the measurement of pH, carbon dioxide tension (Pco_2) and oxygen tension (Po_2) in very small quantities of blood (0.2 ml or less). Hence, serial determinations can be made at regular intervals to guide parenteral therapy and ventilatory assistance.

The popularly used Astrup method (21,

TABLE 10–4. Normal Values of Arterial pH and Pco_2 in the Neonate

Age	pH	Pco_2(mm Hg)
Umbilical artery (at birth)	7.25	50–55
1 hour	7.30	40
4 hours	7.33	38
24 hours	7.38	33–35
4 days	7.39	36

23, 30) for measuring blood pH and Pco_2 is based on the observation that the carbon dioxide titration curve of whole blood in vitro plotted logarithmically against the pH is a straight line. The pH of two samples of blood is measured after they have been equilibrated in vitro with two known carbon dioxide tensions. A straight line is drawn through these points. The pH of a third nonequilibrated sample of blood is determined and plotted on the straight line that has been drawn. In this way the actual Pco_2 of the infant's blood is derived from the graph. Once the pH and Pco_2 are known, values for the base excess, bicarbonate ions and carbon dioxide can be derived from the Siggaard-Anderson Alignment Nomogram (Fig. 10–6). Fully automated analyzers (such as the Radiometer ABLI Acid-Base Laboratory*) are also available for clinical use, and provide a direct printout of all acid-base and blood gas data.

FETAL PHYSIOLOGY

Normal acid-base balance in the fetus depends on adequate uptake of oxygen and release of carbon dioxide across a functioning placenta. Little is known about the transfer of hydrogen (H^+) and bicarbonate (HCO_3^-) ions. There is some evidence that slow diffusion of these ions does occur and that a maternal acidosis, e.g., diabetic acidosis, may be reflected in the fetus. In the normal state, carbon dioxide diffuses across the placenta very readily, and there is a very small differential in Pco_2 between maternal and fetal blood. Other factors besides easy diffusibility enhance transfer of carbon dioxide from fetus to mother. Fetal blood has a lesser affinity than maternal blood for carbon dioxide. An increase in oxygenation of the fetus (as oxygen is transferred across the placenta) decreases the affinity of hemoglobin for carbon dioxide (Haldane effect). In the same manner, as maternal blood loses oxygen, it takes up carbon dioxide more readily.

The Pco_2 of a pregnant woman nearing the end of gestation is somewhat lower than that of the nonpregnant adult (about 33 mm Hg). The fetal Pco_2 is slightly higher, and the pH slightly lower. The negatively charged bicarbonate ion, which appears to be relatively nonpermeable across the placenta, has the same concentration in both mother and fetus. The hydrogen ion also has an electrical charge and is relatively impermeable across the placenta.

Pathologic States

Aberrations in fetal acid-base balance are usually caused by an interference with the normal diffusion of oxygen and carbon dioxide across the placenta. With a decrease in fetal oxygenation, both a metabolic (lactic acid) and respiratory acidosis occur. Lactic acid accumulates as a by-product of anaerobic glycolysis, and carbon dioxide accumulates because of poor placental diffusion of this gas. With acidosis, the fetal oxyhemoglobin dissociation curve shifts to the right to provide fetal tissues with more oxygen (see section Fetal Oxygenation, Ch. 3). However, with poor placental transfer of oxygen, this mechanism is unable to compensate completely, and the infant becomes progressively more hypoxic and acidotic. Lactate is ordinarily capable of crossing the placenta into the maternal circulation when high levels accumulate in fetal serum. However, poor placental function often precludes this.

Knowing fetal acid-base values and being able to perform reliable measurements on fetal scalp blood during the intrapartum period (24) are of great value in the clinical evaluation of a fetus compromised prior to delivery (see section Fetal Oxygenation, Ch. 3).

NEONATAL PERIOD

Following delivery the kidneys and lungs regulate acid-base homeostasis. During delivery, and prior to the onset of spontaneous respirations, placental separation results in a temporary disruption of normal gaseous exchange. The supine position of the

* Radiometer A/S, 72 Emdrupvej, DK 2400 Copenhagen NV, Denmark.

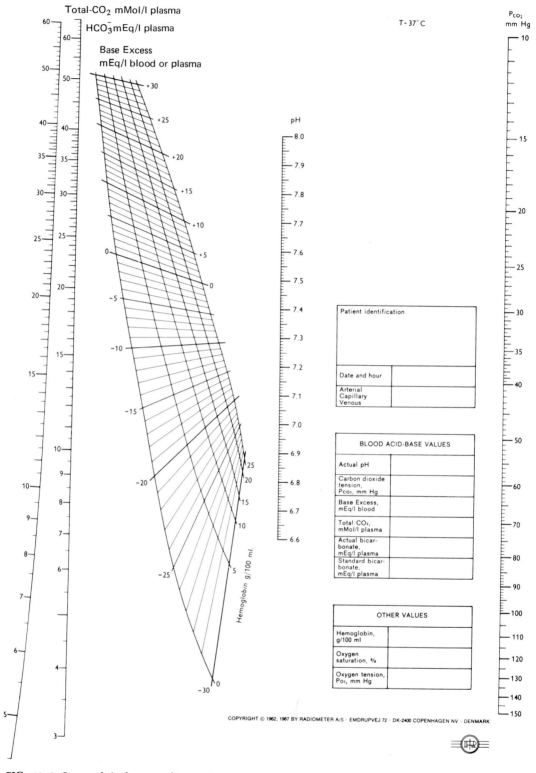

FIG. 10–6. Siggaard-Andersen alignment nomogram. (Radiometer A/S, Copenhagen, Denmark)

mother (which may lead to hypotension and umbilical cord compression), decreased uterine blood flow, uterine contractions, maternal hypoventilation and blood loss all tend to compound this disruption of gas exchange, which invariably results in a combined respiratory and metabolic acidosis.

If placental function has been normal throughout labor, and pulmonary function is normal or near normal following delivery, the acid-base status invariably returns to normal within one to three hours after birth.

If fetal asphyxia has been present, abnormalities of acid-base metabolism persist for a longer period of time following delivery (29). Fetal asphyxia compounded by postnatal respiratory failure may result in profound respiratory and metabolic acidosis.

Acid-base values during the immediate postnatal period have been extensively studied in normal infants. James et al (23) have observed a mean pH of 7.26 and a mean Pco_2 of 55 mm Hg in umbilical arterial blood of normal full-term infants at the moment of birth. Koch and Wendel (28) found the mean umbilical artery pH to be 7.24 and the Pco_2 50 mm Hg, while concurrent umbilical venous values at birth were pH 7.32 and Pco_2 38 mm Hg.

During the first five to ten postpartum minutes, there is a progression of the respiratory and metabolic acidosis that may be due to continued tissue hypoxia and carbon dioxide retention during a period of hypoventilation; this may also be partially due to the deposition by tissues of the breakdown products of anaerobic metabolism into the systemic circulation.

By one hour of age, the arterial pH has usually risen to a level slightly above 7.30, and the Pco_2 is about 40 mm Hg. The base excess at this time usually ranges from -6 to -2 mEq/l. Over the first 24 hours of life, further changes in the infant's acid-base status are noted, so that by the end of the first day, the pH is usually about 7.38, and the Pco_2 has dropped to between 33 and 35 mm Hg (31). This mild metabolic acidosis and respiratory alkalosis persists for the first three or four days postpartum. While the reason for low Pco_2 values during this

period has not been explained, these values may reflect the levels of pH and Pco_2 to which the fetus was exposed in utero. It is also possible that the metabolic acidosis is secondary to a low renal threshold of bicarbonate ion and that the infant compensates by hyperventilating and blowing off carbon dioxide.

After the first few days of life, acid-base values tend to stabilize at a level near that of the normal adult's. Koch and Wendel (28), who studied umbilical arterial blood samples in healthy full-term infants, found that by the end of the first week of postnatal life, the lower limit of normal adult Pco_2 and bicarbonate values had been attained.

Acid-Base Disturbances (Table 10–5)

Combined Acidosis. Acid-base disturbances during the early neonatal period have several etiologies. Intrauterine asphyxia is responsible for a combined metabolic and respiratory acidosis. This phenomenon was described in full-term infants by James et al (23) in 1958 and in premature infants by Kildeberg (25) in 1964. In adults the metabolic response to severe and protracted hypoxia is an accumulation of nonvolatile acids, e.g., lactic acid, in the blood. However, the levels of excess organic acids in acidotic neonates do not completely account for the degree of acidosis observed. The most likely explanation for this phenomenon is that an internal redistribution of bicarbonate ions occurs when excessive carbon dioxide (accumulated in the fetus because of placental failure) combines with water and buffer (predominantly hemoglobin) to form bicarbonate ions and H^+ ions and a hydrogen ion buffer–complex. The newly formed bicarbonate is probably redistributed from the vascular compartment to the extracellular fluid. There is subsequently a decreased buffering capacity of the blood (or increased negative base excess). If the lung functions normally after birth and the infant is well oxygenated, a correction towards normality is made, primarily by elimination of carbon dioxide from the lungs and also by the

TABLE 10–5. Acid-Base Diagnostic Terms

ACIDOSIS: A pathochemical condition resulting from *primary* accumulation of acid in (or primary loss of base from) the body or some specified fluid compartment

ALKALOSIS: A pathochemical condition resulting from *primary* accumulation of base in (or primary loss of acid from) the body or some specified body fluid compartment

NONRESPIRATORY ACIDOSIS (metabolic acidosis: Acidosis resulting from primary accumulation of nonvolatile acid (or primary loss of base)

NONRESPIRATORY ALKALOSIS (metabolic alkalosis): Alkalosis resulting from primary accumulation of basic (or primary loss of nonvolatile acid)

COMPENSATED NONRESPIRATORY ACIDOSIS: Nonrespiratory acidosis with *secondary* alveolar hyperventilation bringing about a reduction below normal, of plasma Pco$_2$

COMPENSATED NONRESPIRATORY ALKALOSIS: Nonrespiratory alkalosis with *secondary* alveolar hypoventilation bringing about a rise, above normal, of plasma Pco$_2$

RESPIRATORY ACIDOSIS: Acidosis resulting from primary alveolar hypoventilation bringing about a rise in Pco$_2$

RESPIRATORY ALKALOSIS: Alkalosis resulting from primary alveolar hyperventilation bringing about a fall in Pco$_2$

COMPENSATED RESPIRATORY ACIDOSIS: Respiratory acidosis with secondary renal adjustments in base retention (leading to an elevated base excess)

COMPENSATED RESPIRATORY ALKALOSIS: Respiratory alkalosis with secondary renal adjustments resulting in H$^+$ retention (leading to a low base excess)

COMBINED or MIXED ACIDOSIS: A pathochemical condition characterized by the simultaneous presence of respiratory and nonrespiratory acidosis

COMBINED or MIXED ALKALOSIS: A pathochemical condition characterized by the simultaneous presence of respiratory and nonrespiratory alkalosis

(Kildeberg P: Clinical Acid-Base Physiology. Baltimore, Williams & Wilkins, 1968)

metabolism of retained organic acids. Renal excretion of hydrogen ion does not play a major role at this age. In the presence of hypoventilation and continued tissue anoxia, this combined acidosis may persist. This type of picture is most commonly associated with RDS.

Respiratory Acidosis. An isolated respiratory acidosis that persists past the first few days of life is usually self-limiting and secondary to hypoventilation. However, the persistent hypercapnea sometimes noted in infants of very low birth weight may be due to a ventilation-perfusion imbalance, a condition in which atelectatic alveoli are perfused or well-aerated alveoli are not perfused.

Metabolic Acidosis. A predominantly metabolic acidosis may be observed in RDS over the first few days of life. In these cases, pulmonary ventilation is adequate to maintain carbon dioxide levels at or near normal, and the acidosis is secondary to tissue hypoxia accompanying inadequate oxygenation.

The treatment of these types of acid-base disturbances is discussed in the section Fluids and Electrolytes; also Respiratory Distress Syndrome, Ch. 6.

Diarrhea. Another major cause of primary metabolic acidosis in the newborn infant is diarrhea. Here, the acidosis is due to loss of bicarbonate ion in the stool (see section Fluids and Electrolytes).

Vomiting. An intestinal obstruction below the ampulla of Vater, vomiting is accompanied by loss of bicarbonate ion with a consequent metabolic acidosis. If obstruction is proximal to the ampulla of Vater (hypertrophic pyloric stenosis), hydrogen and potassium ions are lost in the acidic vomitus, and a primary hypokalemic metabolic alkalosis occurs. This condition is sometimes clinically confused with the salt-losing type of adrenal hyperplasia. In the latter condition, there is hyperkalemia along with a metabolic acidosis.

Respiratory Alkalosis. A primary respiratory alkalosis is observed in infants of heroin-addicted mothers who show signs of acute withdrawal. This alkalosis is secondary to the hyperventilation seen in these infants.

Late Metabolic Acidosis. Otherwise healthy one to three-week-old premature infants may develop a metabolic acidosis that is associated with poor weight gain (26). The cause of this appears to be at least partially a high-protein catabolism with retention of nonvolatile acids (secondary to a decreased renal capacity for hydrogen ion excretion). This may be accompanied by an increased serum chloride concentration, and mild respiratory compensation may occur. A spontaneous remission usually occurs within several weeks if the condition remains untreated. If several milk feedings are withheld and the infant is fed an oral solution containing glucose and sodium bicarbonate as a substitute, the blood pH usually returns to normal within a relatively short time.

CALCIUM AND PHOSPHORUS METABOLISM

FETAL PHYSIOLOGY

During intrauterine life, the growing fetus requires increasing amounts of calcium and phosphorus for normal skeletal development. The phosphorus content of the fetus is greater than its calcium content during the earliest weeks of pregnancy; however, by the end of the first trimester, the quantity of calcium in the fetal circulation begins to exceed that of phosphorus, and by term the ratio of calcium to phosphorus in the fetus is about 1.75:1.

Both calcium and phosphorus concentrations, until the time of delivery, are higher in the fetal than in the maternal circulation. It is therefore assumed that both enter the fetal circulation via an active placental transport mechanism.

In utero disturbances of calcium and phosphorus metabolism have not been described. However, certain antenatal conditions predispose the infant to neonatal hypocalcemia, usually within the first 48 hours of life. The most common of these are abruptio placentae, placenta previa, maternal diabetes mellitus and perinatal asphyxia (35, 41, 42, 44). True prematurity is related to the postnatal development of hypocalcemia, while intrauterine growth failure is not (40). When hypocalcemia is observed in infants with intrauterine growth retardation, it is usually secondary to either perinatal asphyxia or IV bicarbonate therapy (44a).

Such rare maternal disorders as osteomalacia and hyperparathyroidism also predispose to neonatal hypocalcemia (36). Congenital absence of the thymus and parathyroid glands leads to a severe, unremitting and sometimes fatal neonatal hypocalcemia (39).

NEONATAL HYPOCALCEMIA (Table 10–6)

Neonatal hypocalcemia may be defined as a total serum calcium concentration below 8 mg/100 ml. Decreased serum calcium concentrations may lead to a variety of clinical signs associated with increased neuromuscular irritability and may culminate in generalized convulsions.

While umbilical venous concentrations of calcium are usually higher than maternal concentrations, they tend to decline following delivery. In normal full-term infants, the serum calcium concentration invariably stabilizes at normal levels in the days following delivery; however, in premature and other compromised infants, hypocalcemia during the first two days of life is not unusual.

Another type of hypocalcemia, usually seen at one week to ten days of age, occurs in otherwise normal infants fed cow's milk formulas (32). An iatrogenic form of hypocalcemia, in which total calcium concentrations are normal but ionized calcium levels are extremely low, may occur in infants undergoing exchange transfusion with citrated blood (34).

Etiology and Pathogenesis

The underlying mechanisms that predispose the infant to hypocalcemia during the early neonatal period are poorly understood. Parathyroid gland hypofunction, especially in the presence of prematurity or perinatal asphyxia (in which tissue breakdown has added an additional phosphate load to the circulation), may lead to a decreased ability to excrete phosphate in the urine, with subsequent hypocalcemia. Another factor that may temporarily suppress neonatal parathyroid function is the normally increased fetal serum concentration of ionized calcium (43). Stress during the neonatal period may

TABLE 10–6. Neonatal Hypocalcemia

Etiologic Factors

Abruptio placentae
Placenta previa
Maternal diabetes mellitus
Prematurity
Maternal hyperparathyroidism
Congenital absence of parathyroid glands
Perinatal asphyxia
Stress
Dietary intake of phosphate
Exchange transfusion with citrated blood
Rapid correction of acidosis

Clinical Manifestations

Tremulousness
Apnea
Cyanosis
Vomiting
Abdominal distension
Convulsions
Carpodeal spasm
Laryngospasm

Diagnostic evaluation

Serum calcium (ionized calcium, if available)
Serum magnesium
Serum phosphorus (nonhemolyzed specimen)
Serum total protein
Blood pH
ECG for $Q-_0T_c$ interval

Treatment

Symptomatic
  5–10 ml of 10% calcium gluconate given IV
    over a 10-minute interval
Asymptomatic (and after initial manifestations
    have been treated)
  1–2 ml of 10% calcium gluconate/kg/day given
    IV until serum calcium concentration has
    stabilized
  Formula with low-phosphate content and high
    Ca :P ratio
  Following IV therapy, 3–4 g of calcium
    gluconate/day (orally) for four weeks

also be associated with decreased serum calcium levels.

In maternal diabetes mellitus, there is ordinarily an increased maternal serum calcium concentration. Tsang et al (41) suggest that this may suppress the fetal parathyroid gland in much the same way as maternal hyperparathyroidism. In this latter condition, unexplained neonatal hypocalcemia may, on rare occasion, lead to the diagnosis of an unsuspected parathyroid adenoma in the mother.

Hypocalcemia secondary to the excessive phosphorus load present in cow's milk formulas ("seventh-day hypocalcemia") was for many years a major cause of neonatal tetany in formula-fed infants. Cow's milk contains 1220 mg calcium and 900 mg phosphorus/l (Ca to P ratio of 1.35:1), while breast milk contains 340 mg calcium/l and 150 mg phosphorus/l (Ca to P ratio of 2.25:1). The very high phosphate load of cow's milk may overwhelm the immature neonatal parathyroid gland and lead to hypocalcemic tetany at the end of the first week or beginning of the second week of life. Modified cow's milk formulas having significantly less phosphorus than unmodified cow's milk are widely used throughout the United States, and their use is rarely associated with this type of hypocalcemia. Some modified cow's milk formulas, such as Similac PM60:40 and SMA26, contain calcium and phosphorus concentrations similar to those found in breast milk.

Other factors that may predispose the newborn infant to hypocalcemia are delayed oral feedings and rapid correction of a metabolic acidosis with IV infusion of alkali. While the total calcium concentration does not decrease, the concentration of ionized calcium decreases as the pH of the blood rises. This problem may occur when correcting the acidemia associated with RDS.

Exchange transfusion with citrated blood is another cause of hypocalcemia associated with normal total serum calcium concentrations. Citrate, an anticoagulant, temporarily binds ionized calcium and leads to a functional hypocalcemia (34). Intravenous injection of 10% calcium gluconate solution at regular intervals during this procedure does little to raise the concentration of ionized calcium.

Clinical Manifestations

Hypocalcemia manifests in many ways and may easily be confused with such other neonatal disorders as hypoglycemia, sepsis, meningitis, CNS anoxia, intracranial bleeding and narcotic withdrawal. The most common clinical signs are tremulousness, apnea, cyanosis, vomiting and abdominal distension. Carpopedal spasm and laryngospasm are rare. Frank convulsions are more commonly seen with seventh-day hypocalcemia than in the early variety. Chvostek's sign occurs among normal newborn infants and hence is not of diagnostic value at this age.

A presumptive diagnosis of hypocalcemia may be made if the serum calcium concentration is below 8.0 mg/100 ml. Since the signs of hypocalcemia in the neonate are related to a decrease in ionized calcium rather than to the total calcium concentration, measurements of ionized calcium are preferable. About 50% of serum calcium exists in an ionized form, 40% is protein bound, and 10% is in a nonionized form but unbound to proteins. While electrodes capable of measuring ionized calcium are available, they have often proved unreliable in clinical usage.

When measuring total serum calcium concentrations, it is important to also measure the blood pH and total protein concentration. The concentration of ionized calcium decreases with a rising pH, and tetany may accompany alkalosis even in the presence of a borderline or normal total serum calcium concentration. At any given serum calcium concentration, the lower the total protein concentration, the greater the concentration of ionized calcium.

Measurements of serum phosphorus should be made concurrently with calcium determinations. These are elevated in both early and seventh-day hypocalcemia. Tsang et al (40) found mean phosphorus concentrations of 7.6 mg/100 ml at 8 hours and 8.1 mg/100 ml at 29 hours in infants with early hypocalcemia; phosphorus concentrations in seventh-day hypocalcemia may be even higher.

The signs of hypomagnesemia are similar to those of hypocalcemia, and magnesium concentrations should be measured at the same time as calcium concentrations. The reported coexistence of both conditions is another reason for determining the magnesium concentration (38).

Since a prolongation of the $Q-_oT_c$ interval (33) may be a feature of hypocalcemia, an ECG aids in the diagnosis, especially before the serum calcium concentration is known. With adequate therapy, this interval returns to normal.

In congenital absence of the thymus and parathyroid glands, a chest x ray is of value in confirming the diagnosis.

Treatment

The treatment of hypocalcemic seizures is discussed in the section Neonatal Seizures, Ch. 9.

If hypocalcemia is present, but signs are absent, 10% calcium gluconate, 1 to 2 ml/kg/day may be given, either intravenously or by the oral route, until serum calcium concentrations have stabilized. Calcium chloride, in a 1% to 2% solution administered orally (but never intravenously because of its caustic nature) has also been used in the treatment of neonatal hypocalcemia.

Calcium gluconate should not be mixed with bicarbonate-containing solutions, since a precipitate of calcium carbonate will form. Calcium has a potentiating effect on digitalis and should be administered with great caution to infants receiving this drug.

In general, the prognosis is favorable for infants who have been treated for hypocalcemic seizures.

MAGNESIUM METABOLISM

Magnesium (Mg^{++}) is a bivalent ion involved in many metabolic processes. It is required for release of acetylcholine at neuromyal junctions and is involved in activation of ATPase, protein synthesis, DNA degradation and as a cofactor in oxidative phosphorylation. It is primarily an intracellular ion, present in bone, muscle and soft tissue, with the remainder present in extracellular fluid. About 25% of extracellular Mg^{++} is bound to protein.

FETAL LIFE

Mg^{++} crosses the placenta freely, and the fetus normally receives 4 to 5 mg/day from the maternal circulation. Since fetal concentrations reflect maternal concentrations, any

condition causing maternal hypomagnesemia will result in similar findings in the
fetus.

NEONATAL PERIOD

The normal serum Mg^{++} concentration in
the newborn infant is about 2.0 mEq/l. It is
lower in those who are small for gestational
age than in those who are appropriately
grown (51). Abnormally high concentrations have been reported in asphyxiated
newborn infants (48), presumably due to
transfer of Mg^{++} from the intracellular to
extracellular compartment. Hyperkalemia is
often an associated finding.

With advancing postnatal age, serum
Mg^{++} concentrations rise, probably because
of decreased urinary losses of Mg^{++} secondary to renal maturation.

Both increased and decreased Mg^{++} concentrations may result in serious neuromuscular disturbances. Therefore, biochemical
measurements of serum Mg^{++} concentrations are often necessary. This has been
greatly simplified by the availability of micromethods (primarily atomic absorbtion
spectrophotometry (49a) that require only
very small samples of blood.

Hypomagnesemia

Primary hypomagnesemic convulsions are
rare in the neonatal period (46, 47). They
may be due to either decreased GI absorbtion of Mg^{++} or increased urinary losses.

Hypocalcemia has been reported as a concomitant finding (38) and improves when
the primary condition is treated. Therapy
consists of IM administration of magnesium
sulfate followed by oral Mg^{++} salts, such as
magnesium citrate or sulfate. Decreased
concentrations of Mg^{++} ions accompany exchange transfusion when the blood used has
acid citrate dextrose (ACD) as its anticoagulant since the citrate chelates and forms a
nonionic complex with Mg^{++}.

Hypermagnesemia

While treatment of preeclamptic women
with magnesium sulfate usually has no adverse effects on the fetus, its prolonged or
excessive use may lead to fetal hypermagnesemia (49).

Neonatal manifestations begin to appear
when concentrations rise above 4 mEq/l.
These include low Apgar score, flaccidity,
absence of deep tendon reflexes (DTRs),
weak cry and apathy. At about 5 mEq/l,
conduction defect and a prolonged PR interval are noted on the ECG. At 10 mEq/l,
DTRs disappear, and at 15 mEq/l, respiratory arrest and coma occur. Further elevations are associated with cardiac arrest.

Treatment consists of assisted ventilation
(in the presence of respiratory failure), IV
fluid therapy and correction of the metabolic
acidosis that may ensue. While elevated
Mg^{++} concentrations may suppress parathyroid hormone secretion and thus lower
serum Ca^{++} concentrations, treatment with
IV Ca^{++} solutions is of little practical value.
Exchange transfusion with ACD blood has
been reported to be beneficial in treating
this disorder (45). The mechanism involved
here is chelation of Mg^{++} ions by the
citrate.

Since both hypomagnesemia and hypermagnesemia are examples of correctable
neonatal neurologic disorders, all hospitals
caring for sick newborn infants should have
laboratories capable of determining serum
Mg^{++} concentrations on an around the
clock basis.

HEAVY METAL POISONING

Increased environmental pollution with lead
and mercury has caused concern over fetal
poisoning with these two heavy metals, each
of which freely crosses the placenta and can
be stored in high concentrations in fetal tissues (e.g., lung, liver and brain).

LEAD

The effects of lead on the fetus are most
severe during the early stages of pregnancy;
abortion and fetal death following exposure
are extremely common. Liveborn infants
may show evidence of intrauterine growth
retardation, delayed postnatal growth and
dentition and CNS damage.

Unusually high fetal wastage among female mill workers and lead factory employees in nineteenth century England led to legislation banning women from working in lead industries. Since that time, there have been sporadic reports of maternal exposure to lead causing fetal damage. The use of "moonshine" whiskey, lead oxide, abortifacients and exposure to burning battery cases have all been implicated in fetal lead poisoning (52, 53).

Scanlon studied lead concentrations in newborn infants of mothers living in urban and suburban areas (55). His finding that urban infants had slightly increased umbilical cord blood lead concentrations suggests that atmospheric pollution from lead-containing gasoline fuel presents a potential danger to the developing fetus.

Rajegowda et al (54) established normal values for cord blood lead concentrations as 0.01 to 0.03 mg/100 ml. These values may be used as a guideline if lead poisoning is suspected in a newborn infant.

MERCURY

Fetal mercury poisoning is more likely to be due to maternal ingestion of organic mercury compounds than to exposure to elemental mercury. Snyder (56) reported the case of a woman consuming mercury-contaminated meat for three months, beginning in the third trimester of pregnancy. While the mother was unaffected, the infant developed myoclonic jerks, hypotonia, irritability and an abnormal EEG.

An epidemic of methylmercury poisoning in Iraq, caused by eating homemade bread prepared from wheat seed treated with a methylmercury fungicide, resulted in widespread brain damage in fetuses and suckling newborn infants (52a).

REFERENCES

RENAL DEVELOPMENT

1. Bernstein J: The morphogenesis of renal parenchymal maldevelopment (renal dysplasia). Pediatr Clin North Am 18:395, 1971
2. Crocker JFS, Brown DM, Vernier RL: Develop-

mental defects of the kidney. Pediatr Clin North Am 18:355, 1971
3. Vernier RL, Smith FG: Fetal and neonatal kidney. In: Biology of Gestation, Vol. II. Edited by NS Assali. New York, Academic Press, 1968

FLUIDS AND ELECTROLYTES

4. Benda GIM, Babson SG: Peripheral intravenous alimentation of the small premature infant. J Pediatr 79:494, 1971
5. Boeckman CR, Krill CE Jr: Bacterial and fungal infections complicating parenteral alimentation in infants and children. J Pediatr Surg 5:117, 1970
6. Bryan MH, Wei P, Hamilton JR, Chance GW, Swyer PR: Supplemental intravenous alimentation in low birthweight infants. J Pediatr 82:940, 1973
7. Cassady G: Bromide space studies in infants of low birthweight. Pediatr Res 4:14, 1970
8. Chan JCM, Asch MJ, Lin S, Hays DM: Hyperalimentation with amino acid and casein hydrolysate solutions. Mechanism of acidosis. JAMA 220:1700, 1972
9. Driscoll JM, Heird WC, Schullinger JN, Gongaware RD, Winters RW: Total intravenous alimentation in low birthweight infants: a preliminary report. J Pediatr 81:145, 1972
10. Dudrick SJ, Vars HM, Rawnsley HM, Rhoads JE: Total intravenous feeding and growth in puppies. Fed Proc 25:481, 1966
11. Edelmann CM Jr, Spitzer A: The maturing kidney. J Pediatr 75:509, 1969
12. Finberg L: Dangers to infants caused by changes in osmolal concentration. Pediatrics 40:1031, 1967
13. Ghadimi H, Abaci F, Kumar S, Rathi M: Biochemical aspects of intravenous alimentation. Pediatrics 48:955, 1971
14. Heird WC, Driscoll JM Jr, Schullinger JN, Grebin B, Winters RW: Intravenous alimentation in pediatric patients. J Pediatr 80:351, 1972
15. Olney JW, Oi LH, Rhee V: Brain damaging potential of protein hydrolysates. N Engl J Med 289:391, 1973
16. Pildes RS, Ramamurthy RS, Cordero GV, Wong PWK: Intravenous supplementation of L-amino acids and dextrose in low birthweight infants. J Pediatr 82:945, 1973
17. Shaw JCL: Parenteral nutrition in the management of sick low birthweight infants. Pediatr Clin North Am 20:333, 1973
18. Sinclair JC, Driscoll JM, Heird WC, Winters RW: Supportive management of the sick neonate. Pediatr Clin North Am 17:863, 1970
19. Travis SF, Sugerman HJ, Ruberg RL, Dudrick SJ, Delivoria-Papadapoulos M, Miller LD, Oski FA: Alterations of red-cell glycolytic intermediates and oxygen transport as a consequence of hypophosphatemia in patients receiving intravenous hyperalimentation. N Engl J Med 285:763, 1971

20. Wilmore DW, Groff DB, Bishop HC, Dudrick SJ: Total parenteral nutrition in infants with catastrophic gastrointestinal anomalies. J Pediatr Surg 4:181, 1969

20a. Winters RW: The Body Fluids in Pediatrics. Boston, Little, Brown, 1973

ACID-BASE BALANCE

21. Astrup P, Jorgensen K, Andersen OS, Engel, K: The acid-base metabolism: a new approach. Lancet 1:1035, 1960

22. Blechner JN: Fetal acid-base homeostasis. Clin Obstet Gynecol 13:621, 1970

23. James LS, Weisbrot IM, Prince CE, Holaday DA, Apgar V: The acid-base status of human infants in relation to birth asphyxia and the onset of respiration. J Pediatr 52:379, 1958

24. James LS: Fetal blood sampling. Clin Perinatol 1:141, 1974

25. Kildeberg P: Disturbances of hydrogen ion balance occurring in premature infants. I. Early types of acidosis. Acta Paediatr Scand 53:505, 1964

26. Kildeberg P: Disturbances of hydrogen ion balance occurring in premature infants. II. Late metabolic acidosis. Acta Paediatr Scand 53:517, 1964

27. Kildeberg P: Clinical Acid-Base Physiology. Baltimore, Williams & Wilkins, 1968

28. Koch G, Wendel H: Adjustments of arterial blood gases and acid-base balance in the normal newborn infant during the first week of life. Biol Neonate 12:136, 1968

29. Modanlou H, Yeh S-Y, Hon EH: Fetal and neonatal acid-base balance in normal and high-risk pregnancies. During labor and the first hour of life. Obstet Gynecol 43:347, 1974

30. Siggaard-Anderson O: The pH, log pCO_2 blood acid-base nomogram revised. Scand J Clin Lab Invest 14:598, 1962

31. Weisbrot IM, James LS, Prince CE, Holaday DA, Apgar V: Acid-base homeostasis of the newborn infant duing the first 24 hours of life. J Pediatr 52:395, 1958

CALCIUM AND PHOSPHOROUS METABOLISM

32. Bakwin H: Pathogenesis of tetany of newborn. Am J Dis Child 54:1211, 1937

33. Colletti RB, Pan MW, Smith EWP, Genel M: Detection of hypocalcemia in susceptible neonates: the Q-$_o$T$_c$ interval. N Engl J Med 290:931, 1974

34. Friedman Z, Hanley WB, Radde IC: Ionized calcium in exchange transfusion with THAM-buffered ACD blood. Can Med Assoc J 107:742, 1972

35. Gittleman IF, Pincus JB, Schmertzler E, Saito M: Hypocalcemia occurring in the first day of life in mature and premature infants. Pediatrics 18:721, 1956

36. Mizrahi A, Gold AP: Neonatal tetany secondary to maternal hyperparathyroidism. JAMA 90:155, 1964

37. Mizrahi A, London R, Gribetz D: Neonatal hypocalcemia. N Engl J Med 278:1163, 1968

38. Paunier L, Radde IC, Kooh SW, Conen PE, Fraser D: Primary hypomagnesemia with secondary hypocalcemia in an infant. Pediatrics 41:385, 1968

39. Taitz LS, Zarote-Salvador C, Schwartz E: Congenital absence of the parathyroid and thymus glands in an infant (III and IV pharyngeal pouch syndrome). Pediatrics 38:412, 1966

40. Tsang RC, Oh W: Neonatal hypocalcemia in low birth weight infants. Pediatrics 45:773, 1970

41. Tsang RC, Kleinman LI, Sutherland JM, Light IJ: Hypocalcemia in infants of diabetic mothers. J Pediatr 80:384, 1972

42. Tsang RC, Light IJ, Sutherland JM, Kleinman LI: Possible pathogenetic factors in neonatal hypocalcemia of prematurity. J Pediatr 82:423, 1973

43. Tsang RC, Chen IW, Friedman MA: Neonatal parathyroid functions: role of gestational age and postnatal age. J Pediatr 83:728, 1973

44. Tsang RC, Chen I, Hayes W, Atkinson W, Atherton H, Edwards N: Neonatal hypocalcemia in infants with birth asphyxia. J Pediatr 84:428, 1974

44a. Tsang R, Gigger M, Oh W, Brown DR: Studies in calcium metabolism in infants with intrauterine growth retardation. J Pediatr 86:936, 1975

MAGNESIUM

45. Brady J, Williams HC: Magnesium intoxication in a premature infant. Pediatrics 40:100, 1967

46. Davis JA, Harvey DR, Yu JS: Neonatal fits associated with hypomagnesaemia. Arch Dis Child 40:286, 1965

47. Dooling EC, Stern L: Hypomagnesemia with convulsions in a newborn infant. Can Med Assoc J 97:827, 1967

48. Eungel RR, Elin RJ: Hypermagnesemia from birth asphyxia. J Pediatr 77:63, 1970

49. Lipsitz PJ, English IC: Hypermagnesemia in the newborn infant. Pediatrics 40:856, 1967

49a. Sunderman WF Jr, Carrol JE: Measurements of serum calcium and magnesium by atomic absorption spectrophotometry. Amer J Clin Path 43:302, 1965

50. Tsang RC: Neonatal magnesium disturbances. Am J Dis Child 124:282, 1972

51. Tsang RC, Light IJ, Oh W: Serum magnesium levels in low birth weight infants. Am J Dis Child 120:44, 1970

HEAVY METAL POISONING

52. Angle CR, McIntire MS: Lead poisoning during pregnancy. Am J Dis Child 108:436, 1964

52a. Bakir F, Damluje SF, Amin-Zaki L, Murtadha M, Khalidi A, Al-Rawi NY, Tikriti S, Dhahir HI, Clarkson TW, Smith JC, Doherty RA: Methylmercury poisoning in Iraq. Science 181:230, 1973

53. Palmesano PA, Sneed RC, Cassady G: Untaxed whiskey and fetal lead exposure. J Pediatr 75:869, 1969

54. Rajegowda BK, Glass L, Evans HE: Lead concentrations in the newborn infant. J Pediatr 80:118, 1972

55. Scanlon J: Umbilical cord blood lead concentration. Am J Dis Child 121:271, 1971

56. Snyder RD: Congenital mercury poisoning. N Engl J Med 284:1014, 1971

11

Endocrine Disorders

ADRENAL CORTEX

Although the adrenal cortex and medulla are in anatomic proximity, they are unrelated in either embryonic origin or function. The cortex is derived from mesoderm, apparently originating from a cellular downgrowth of the coelomic epithelium. Medullary cells originate from the ectodermal chromaffin tissue located in primitive autonomic ganglia.

FETAL DEVELOPMENT AND FUNCTION

By the end of the second month of gestation, the fetal adrenal gland is organized into three components that are present until shortly after birth: 1) the medulla, 2) the so-called fetal zone and 3) the adult cortex. The fetal zone contributes to the extremely large mass of the fetal adrenal gland. The densely packed cells of this zone disappear rapidly after birth, and although their function remained a mystery for many years, it is now believed that they synthesize the precursor for placental estriol production (6). This zone seems to be under the control of the anterior pituitary gland during fetal life; anencephalic fetuses, who lack an anterior pituitary gland, have no fetal zone in their adrenals, and their mothers excrete little or no estriol in their urine.

Both corticosteroids and androgens are synthesized in the adrenal cortex by the third month of gestation. The presence in the adrenal at this time of cortisol, androgens and aldosterone, plus the enzymes necessary for their synthesis, is direct evidence of this. Indirect evidence of adrenal function at this time is the masculinization of female fetuses with adrenogenital syndrome. For this to occur, the fetal adrenal must be producing androgens by the third month of gestation (fusion of the labioscrotal folds under the influence of androgens derived from the testes occurs by this time).

By the fourth month of gestation, the fetal zone has grown so large that the adrenal is as large as or larger than the kidney. At this time the zona glomerulosa can be identified in the adult cortex, but the zona reticularis cannot be differentiated from the zona fasciculata. Adrenocortical growth rate decelerates after the fourth month of gestation so that by term the adrenal gland is one-third the size of the kidney.

The size of the fetal adrenal is greater, by an average of 20%, in infants with amniotic infection than in noninfected infants. This difference is due to both a greater mass of cellular cytoplasm in adult zone cells and a greater number of cortical cells in the infected infants (12). The incidence of RDS is lowest in those infants born with the largest adrenal glands, and the presence of infection appears to protect the infant to some degree from developing RDS. Experimental evidence indicates that corticosteroids enhance production of pulmonary surfactant in fetal rabbits (9) and that corticosteroids administered to mothers 24 to 48 hours prior to delivery significantly decreases the incidence of RDS in premature infants of less than 32 weeks' gestation (11). It is therefore likely that the adult cortex of the fetus responds to amniotic infection by cellular hypertrophy and hyperplasia and that the increased amount of corticosteroids produced as a result of the stress (infection) enhances surfactant production.

The adrenocortical-pituitary axis of the fetus seems to function autonomously and usually is little affected by deviations in maternal adrenocortical function. This is apparently due in large part to the fact that during pregnancy there is a marked increase in the level of maternal transcortin, a globulin that binds cortisol in the plasma. Although maternal cortisol is capable of crossing the placenta, it is likely that protein binding of cortisol limits the actual amount that crosses from the maternal to fetal circulation.

Although there is evidence that corticosteroids administered to pregnant animals cause cleft palate in the fetus, there is no indication that this is true in human neonates (3).

Nor is there evidence that administration of corticosteroids to pregnant women suppresses fetal adrenocortical function. This may be due to the fact that maternal serum concentrations are only intermittently elevated or that binding of corticosteroids to transcortin inhibits their transplacental passage.

Kreines and De Vaux (10) have described adrenal insufficiency in the infant of a mother with Cushing's disease secondary to an adrenal adenoma. In this case, the very high and consistently elevated maternal corticosteroid concentrations probably led to suppression of fetal adrenocorticotrophic hormone (ACTH) secretion.

Since conception is virtually impossible in women with untreated Addison's disease, the effect of maternal hypoadrenocorticism on the fetus is only a theoretic question. Fetuses of mothers with adequately treated Addison's disease suffer no apparent ill effects.

NEONATAL ASPECTS

Normal Physiology

The adrenal cortices are extremely large in relation to total body size at birth, having a combined weight of 6 to 8 g at term (this is about 0.2% of total body weight, compared to 0.01% in normal adults). The fetal zone involutes rapidly, so that by the end of the second week of life, weight of the adrenals has decreased by 50%.

Corticosteroid concentrations in the cord blood of infants born by vaginal delivery approximate those found in normal nonpregnant adults (5 to 20 μg/100 ml) but are considerably lower than maternal levels. With cesarean section in the absence of labor, both maternal and fetal corticosteroid concentrations are considerably lower than those found following vaginal delivery. A marked decrease in plasma corticosteroid concentrations occurs during the first days of life. Even in the presence of stress, these levels tend to remain low. Gutai et al (7) have demonstrated, however, that injections of ACTH cause a significant increase in cortisol secretion. These investigators have suggested that the reason for poor cortisol secretion in response to stress may be due to the fact that either the degree of stress is insufficient to stimulate a normally functioning pituitary adrenal axis or the hypothalamic pituitary system is unable to release sufficient ACTH in the presence of physical stress.

The concentration of androgens in cord blood is extremely high, being most marked in premature infants. These levels decline over the first days of life and thereafter remain low.

The half-life of cortisol in the neonate is about twice that of cortisol in the adult. This appears to be due to both a decreased rate of glucuronidation by the liver and a relatively slow rate of reduction of ring A of the cortisol molecule.

CLINICAL ASPECTS

Two major neonatal disease entities involve the adrenal gland: adrenal hemorrhage is relatively common, although an antemortem diagnosis is often difficult to make, congenital adrenal hyperplasia, although relatively uncommon, is of considerable clinical importance. Congenital hypoplasia of the adrenal gland is extremely rare in the presence of an intact pituitary.

Adrenal hemorrhage

The signs of adrenal hemorrhage in the newborn infant usually are so nonspecific that the correct diagnosis is difficult or impossible to make, and the condition is often confused with intracranial hemorrhage, sepsis or RDS:

I. Etiology
  A. Hemorrhagic diathesis
    1. DIC
    2. Hemorrhagic disease of the newborn
  B. Birth trauma: Difficult breech delivery
  C. Perinatal asphyxia
  D. Maternal diabetes mellitus
  E. Sepsis
    1. Endotoxemia
    2. DIC

II. Clinical Manifestations
  A. Shock
  B. Pallor
  C. Lethargy
  D. Cyanosis
  E. Respiratory distress
  F. Irritability and convulsion
  G. Flank mass

III. Diagnosis
  A. Suggestive history
  B. Falling hematocrit
  C. IVP
  D. Postmortem examination

IV. Therapy
  A. Blood transfusion
  B. Vitamin K
  C. Heparin (with proven DIC)
  D. Oxygen
  E. IV fluids and electrolytes
  F. Thermoneutral environment
  G. Antibiotics (if sepsis is present)

Manifestations appear very shortly after birth or sometime during the first week of life (5, 8).

With moderate or severe bleeding into the gland (Fig. 11–1), there is usually a shock-like picture. The infant appears limp and lethargic; cyanosis or pallor is present. Respirations are often labored, and the grunting and tachypnea may be mistaken for RDS. Hyperirritability and convulsions may occur in some infants, and many develop apneic episodes. A low or declining hematocrit is usually present. Rarely, a palpable flank mass that may be confused with renal vein thrombosis is present. An intravenous pyelogram (IVP) may confirm the diagnosis by revealing flattening and downward displacement of the calyceal system of the upper portion of the kidney lying below the involved gland. In infants who survive, follow-up abdominal x rays may show evidence of adrenal calcification. These calcifications have been noted occasionally in autopsies of infants who died of other causes. As yet, there is no proven relationship between neonatal adrenal hemorrhage and hypoadrenocorticism in later life.

Several etiologic factors may be responsible for bleeding into the adrenals. Hemorrhagic disease of the newborn, once a major cause, has now been all but eliminated by the prophylactic use of vitamin K. Obstetric trauma, especially with breech deliveries, seems to be involved in some cases. Peri-

FIG. 11–1. Bilateral adrenal hemorrhage following a difficult breech delivery. (Reprinted from Morison JE: Foetal and Neonatal Pathology; London: Butterworth, 1970)

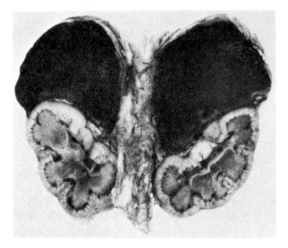

natal asphyxia has also been implicated. This may be related to disseminated intravascular coagulation (DIC) and the hemorrhagic diathesis that accompanies it. There also appears to be a relatively high incidence of adrenal hemorrhage in infants of diabetic mothers.

Therapy. Once the diagnosis is either strongly suspected or established, the treatment is symptomatic. Replacement of blood loss (with fresh whole blood if possible), administration of vitamin K, proper oxygenation, maintenance of fluid, electrolyte and acid-base balance and regulation of temperature are vitally important. If the diagnosis of DIC has been established, use of IV heparin may be of some value. When infection is suspected, the appropriate antibiotics should be administered. Use of corticosteroids has been suggested, but there is no clear-cut evidence that their administration plays any role in the treatment of this entity.

Congenital Adrenal Hyperplasia

Congenital adrenal hyperplasia is a syndrome associated with a group of enzymatic defects in the synthesis of glucocorticoids, mineralocorticoids and, rarely, androgens by the adrenal cortex (1, 2, 4, 13):

I. Etiology: Deficiency of
  A. 21-hydroxylase (95% of cases)
  B. 11β-hydroxylase
  C. 3β-hydroxycorticosteroid
  D. Desmolase

II. Clinical manifestations
  A. 21-hydroxylase deficiency (mild)
    1. Virilization of female fetus
    2. Mild enlargement of phallus in male
  B. 21-hydroxylase deficiency (severe, salt-wasting variety)
    1. Virilization of female fetus
    2. Mild enlargement of phallus in male
    3. Vomiting
    4. Diarrhea with shock and dehydration

    5. Hyponatremia and hypochloremia
    6. Hyperkalemia
    7. Metabolic acidosis
    8. Increased pigmentation
  C. 11β-hydroxylase
    1. Virilization of female fetus
    2. Hypertension
    3. No salt wasting
  D. 3β-hydroxysteroid dehydrogenase
    1. Mild virilization in females
    2. Incomplete masculinization in males
  E. Desmolase
    1. Severe salt wasting
    2. Universally fatal

III. Diagnosis
  A. Clinical manifestations
  B. Increased urinary 17-ketosteroids (21-hydroxylase and 11β-hydroxylase deficiencies) > 1 mg/24 hours after first week of life
  C. Increased urinary pregnanetriol excretion (in 21-hydroxylase deficiency)
  D. Decreased plasma cortisol concentrations
  E. Karyotype and buccal smear if sex is ambiguous
  F. X rays of female genitalia using contrast material

IV. Treatment
  A. Specific
    1. Cortisone acetate, 15 to 25 mg/day, to be increased as infant grows
    2. DOC, 1 to 2 mg/day IM, subcutaneous pellets when condition stabilizes (salt losers only)
    3. NaCl, 2 to 4 g/day dietary supplement (salt losers only)
  B. Nonspecific
    1. Treatment of fluid, electrolyte and acid-base imbalance
    2. Surgery for correction of ambiguous genitalia
    3. Genetic and psychologic counseling for families

These enzymatic defects, transmitted in an autosomal recessive manner, are associated with marked hypertrophy of the adrenal cortex, and with very rare exceptions, virilization of the female fetus. The incidence is about equal in both sexes. The affected male fetus usually appears normal at birth but may occasionally have slightly enlarged external genitalia.

In about 95% of all cases of congenital adrenal hyperplasia, the basic defect is a deficiency of the enzyme 21-hydroxylase. In its most severe form, there are defects in the production of both mineralocorticoids and glucocorticoids, and the infant presents with virilization and salt loss. In less severe forms, only glucocorticoid metabolism is impaired, and virilization is the only manifestation of the defect at birth. In its mildest forms, the disorder may not become apparent until early childhood.

The next most common defect is the absence of the enzyme 11β-hydroxylase, in which virilization and hypertension occur, but salt loss is not a problem. Other defects

that have been reported in rare instances are deficiencies in the enzymes desmolase and 3β-hydroxysteroid dehydrogenase.

21-Hydroxylase Deficiency

To understand the pathophysiology of congenital adrenal hyperplasia, reference should be made to Figure 11–2, which is a simplified form of the steps involved in the biosynthesis of androgens, mineralocorticoids and glucocorticoids in the adrenal cortex. As mentioned previously, this process begins during the second month of fetal life. Starting with cholesterol and pregnenolone as precursors, the cortex synthesizes sex hormones (primarily androgens), aldosterone and cortisol (or compound F).

The presence of 21-hydroxylase is necessary for the synthesis of both mineralocorticoids and glucocorticoids, but it is not required for the synthesis of sex hormones. With a marked deficiency of this enzyme,

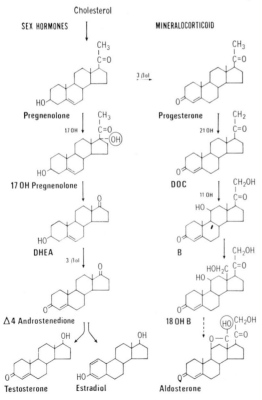

FIG. 11–2. A highly simplified scheme of the adrenocortical synthesis of cortisol. 3 β- ol, 3 β-hydroxysteroid dehydrogenase; 17 OH, 17-hydroxylase; 21 OH, 21-hydroxylase; 11 OH, 11 β-hydroxylase. (New MI: Pediatr Clin North Am 15:395, 1968)

the sequence of hormone synthesis will be blocked, so that there is an accumulation of both progesterone and 17-hydroxyprogesterone. Since cortisol cannot be synthesized, there is no negative feedback mechanism to the fetal pituitary gland; ACTH is continuously being secreted and stimulating the adrenal cortex. Formation of sex hormones continues unhindered in the absence of 21-hydroxylase, so their synthesis and secretion continues in an unchecked manner. The excessive circulating androgens (especially testosterone) that are formed tend to masculinize the female fetus. Aldosterone deficiency in utero does not affect the fetus since electrolyte balance is maintained by the placenta rather than the kidney. In the same manner, cortisol deficiency does not affect fetal carbohydrate metabolism since this is largely a placental function. If there is only a mild or moderate enzyme deficiency, aldosterone will be normally synthesized, and only cortisol metabolism will be impaired. Metabolic derangements associated with impaired or complete lack of secretion of cortisol and aldosterone do not manifest themselves until after birth when the infant can no longer rely on the placenta to regulate salt and carbohydrate metabolism.

11β-Hydroxylase Deficiency

Absence of 11β-hydroxylase, a less common defect, also involves the formation of aldosterone and cortisol. As with 21-hydroxylase deficiency, there is an increased secretion of androgens and virilization of the female fetus. Synthetic steps leading to the formation of cortisol proceed to compound S, with the defect occurring in the formation of cortisol from compound S. With regard to synthesis of mineralocorticoids, the process continues through the formation of desoxycorticosterone (DOC). Since this compound has the same salt-retaining effects as aldosterone, there is no salt wasting associated with a deficiency of 11β-hydroxylase. However, the increased secretion of DOC leads to the hypertension associated with this syndrome.

Desmolase Deficiency

In the absence of the enzyme desmolase, the conversion of cholesterol to pregnenolone cannot occur. There is complete impairment of adrenocortical function, and neonatal death has been universal.

3β-Hydroxysteroid Dehydrogenase

A deficiency of 3β-hydroxysteroid dehydrogenase blocks the conversion of pregnenolone to progesterone, thus causing impairment of both glucocorticoid and mineralocorticoid formation. The virilization that occurs in females is mild since this enzyme is required for the formation of testosterone from androgen precursors. In males, there is usually incomplete masculinization; perineal hypospadias and bifid scrotum may result.

Diagnosis

Clinical. Diagnosis of congenital adrenal hyperplasia in the neonatal period is usually made much more easily in the virilized female infant than in the male infant, in whom no external manifestations are apparent. The affected female will usually have clitoral hypertrophy (Fig. 11–3) ranging from mild enlargement to a phallus resembling a penis. There may be a common urogenital sinus, with the meatus at the base of the enlarged clitoris. In the most severe cases in females, there is fusion of the labioscrotal folds; thus, it may be extremely difficult to differentiate the severely affected newborn female from a male infant with perineal hypospadias and undescended testes. The male has normal external genitalia at birth, except in the very rare cases of 3β-hydroxysteroid and desmolase deficiency. In the case of mild to moderate 21-hydroxylase deficiency, untreated infants show no clinical symptomatology aside from progressive virilization. In the male, there is progressive enlargement of the external genitalia. There may be increased pigmentation of genitalia and areolae, probably due to increased circulating levels of ACTH and melanocyte-stimulating hormone.

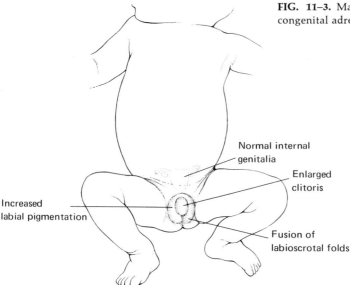

FIG. 11–3. Masculinization of female fetus with congenital adrenal hyperplasia.

Normal internal genitalia

Enlarged clitoris

Increased labial pigmentation

Fusion of labioscrotal folds

The salt-losing variety is more deadly in males than in females since in the latter there is usually some forewarning before the effects of the mineralocorticoid deficiency appear. The infant eats poorly and fails to gain weight; projectile vomiting may occur toward the end of the first week of life and may occasionally be confused with hypertrophic pyloric stenosis. Diarrhea and subsequent dehydration ensue, and the infant may go into shock quite rapidly. A metabolic acidosis with hyponatremia and hyperkalemia is present. This is a life-threatening condition, and immediate diagnosis and institution of therapy are mandatory.

Laboratory and Radiologic. There are several useful laboratory tests that help in establishing the diagnosis of congenital adrenal hyperplasia. In both the 21-hydroxylase and 11β-hydroxylase defect, there are marked elevations in excretion of urinary 17-ketosteroids. Since androgen excretion may be normally elevated during the first week of life, a 24-hour 17-ketosteroid excretion of more than 1 mg after the first week of life is tantamount to being diagnostic of the disorder. In the 21-hydroxylase deficiency, there is also increased urinary excretion of pregnanetriol, a metabolic product of 17-hydroxyprogesterone.

In the female infant with ambiguous genitalia, a buccal smear should be performed to confirm the presence of Barr bodies. A karyotype using peripheral lymphocytes is the most reliable way of determining genetic sex of the infant. X rays may also be helpful in outlining female genitalia, using contrast material inserted into the introitus.

Treatment

As soon as the diagnosis is made, replacement therapy with corticosteroids becomes mandatory. In the case of untreated mild 21-hydroxylase deficiency, further masculinization will occur, and although growth is rapid during the early years of life, short stature ultimately results because of early closure of epiphyses of long bones.

In the more severe 21-hydroxylase deficiency, failure to institute replacement therapy may lead to rapid demise, usually secondary to hyperkalemia. Even if a definitive diagnosis of congenital adrenal hyperplasia has not been made, treatment of this condition is a life-saving emergency. Treatment with sodium bicarbonate, insulin and ion exchange resins may effectively lower the serum potassium concentration. During the period of treatment, frequent biochemical studies must be performed. Measuring the amplitude of T waves on the ECG may be another means of monitoring the effectiveness of therapy in reducing the serum potassium concentration.

Cortisone acetate should be started in a dose of 15 to 25 mg daily and increased as the infant grows. In the case of salt losers, rehydration with parenteral fluids and electrolytes should be accompanied by an IM injection of 1 to 2 mg of DOC daily. Once the infant has stabilized, supplementary sodium chloride (2 to 4 g daily) should be included in the diet. The subcutaneous implantation of DOC pellets provides a sustained release mineralocorticoid preparation that should last for about a month. Hypertension associated with 11β-hydroxylase deficiency does not usually appear until the second year of life, so this is not a consideration in the neonatal period.

Genetic counseling of the involved family is extremely important; support of the family of an infant with ambiguous genitalia is also vital. Assignment of sex must be made at the earliest possible time, and psychologic counseling may be required for the entire family.

ADRENAL HYPOPLASIA

Hypoplasia, or absence of the adrenal cortex unassociated with a pituitary defect, is quite rare. Onset of clinical manifestations is apparently related to the amount of functioning tissue present; the signs usually present in the early neonatal period, but in less-severe cases they may not appear for weeks or months. Vomiting, diarrhea, dehydration, failure to gain weight and a shocklike collapse may all be signs of this disorder. Excessive pigmentation of the areolae of the nipples and scrotum may provide indications of the diagnosis. Both plasma cortisol levels and urinary 17-ketosteroid excretion are extremely low and cannot be increased by parenteral administration of ACTH.

THERAPEUTIC USE OF CORTICOSTEROIDS

Although corticosteroids have been frequently administered to neonates for a wide variety of illnesses, often as a desperate measure, their proven value is limited. Mineralocorticoids and glucocorticoids have their most important therapeutic use in the treatment of congenital adrenal hyperplasia and adrenal hypoplasia. Glucocorticoids also play a role (by inducing gluconeogenesis) in the treatment of resistant neonatal hypoglycemia. Their use in the treatment of infection, adrenal hemorrhage, perinatal asphyxia and sclerema has never been demonstrated.

Although the administration of corticosteroids to women just prior to the delivery of premature infants appears to decrease the incidence of RDS, their administration to the infant following delivery does not alter the course of the disease.

DISORDERS OF GONADAL DEVELOPMENT (see section Ambiguous Genitalia, Ch. 22)

EMBRYOLOGY

During early embryogenesis, the primitive gonad consisting of medullary and cortical portions is capable of developing into either ovaries or testes. Differentiation of this bipotential gonad begins at about the seventh week of fetal life. Development of the fetal testes depends on the presence of a Y chromosome, whereas ovarian development requires at least two X chromosomes. If there is no Y chromosome and only one X chromosome (as in Turner's syndrome), female genitalia will develop. Prior to differentiation of the gonad into testes or ovary, both the Wolffian and Müllerian ducts are present. Testicular growth stimulates the development of the Wolffian ducts, and an inhibitor substance secreted by the testes leads to a disappearance of the Müllerian ducts.

In the presence of androgens the labioscrotal folds fuse by the twelfth week of gestation, with formation of the scrotum and enlargement of the genital tubercle to form the penis. If androgens are not present, the labioscrotal folds remain unfused (forming the labia), and the genital tubercle develops into the clitoris.

PATHOGENESIS OF AMBIGUOUS GENITALIA

In congenital adrenal hyperplasia, a defect in the synthesis of cortisol leads to excessive secretion of ACTH through a feedback mechanism (Table 11–1). This in turn causes the adrenal cortex to secrete an excessive quantity of androgenic substances, and clitoral hypertrophy, often associated with fusion of the labioscrotal folds, occurs. The degree of masculinization depends on the severity of the enzymatic defect. In genetic males with this disorder the excessive secretion of androgens may lead to slight enlargement of the penis.

Progestins, used to maintain pregnancy in women with a history of habitual abortion, have an androgenic effect (16, 17). If administered prior to the 12th to 14th week of pregnancy, both clitoral hypertrophy and fusion of the labioscrotal folds occurs; if administered later, only clitoral hypertrophy occurs. Maternal ovarian and adrenal tumors that secrete androgenic substances

will in a similar manner lead to masculinization of the external genitalia of a female fetus.

In the case of the syndrome of complete testicular feminization (14), the testes of the male fetus secrete androgens in a normal manner, but there is an apparent end organ enzymatic defect, and masculinization of the external genitalia does not occur. These infants appear to be phenotypic females at birth, having a clitoris and a vagina that ends in a blind pouch. The testes remain in an intraabdominal position, and malignant change is common in later life. In incomplete variants of the disorder, varying degrees of feminization of the male fetus may be observed.

In males with 3 β-hydroxysteroid dehydrogenase deficiency, the enzymatic defect probably results in defective androgen synthesis by the testes, thus leading to ambiguous external genitalia.

The exact embryologic mechanism involved in the formation of gonads and genitalia in true hermaphroditism is poorly understood. Although peripheral lymphocytes usually show an XX sex chromosome pattern, other cell lines probably contain a Y chromosome. The pathogenesis of mixed gonadal dysgenesis, in which there is a testis on one side and an undifferentiated

TABLE 11–1. Ambiguous Genitalia in the Neonate

Condition	Pathogenesis	Clinical Manifestations
Congenital adrenal hyperplasia (21-hydroxylase deficiency)	Defect in synthesis of cortisol with excessive production of androgens	Virilization of external genitalia
Administration of progestins to habitual aborters during first trimester		Virilization of external genitalia
Androgen secreting maternal tumors		Virilization of external genitalia
Testicular feminization	End organ defect in response to androgenic stimulation in male fetus	Feminization of male fetus
3β-hydroxysteroid dehydrogenase deficiency	Defective androgen synthesis by testes	Ambiguous genitalia in males
True hermaphroditism	Poorly understood	External genitalia range from normal female to male with hypospadias
Mixed gonadal dysgenesis	Cytogenetic mosaicism(?)	Phallic enlargement, hypospadias, labioscrotal fusion

primitive streak on the other, is also poorly understood.

DIAGNOSTIC CRITERIA

Confronted with an infant having ambiguous genitalia, a careful family and maternal history is required. The diagnostic approach to the neonate with ambiguous genitalia is as follows:

I. History
   A. Previous history of infant with ambiguous genitalia
   B. Unexplained death of previous male infant (salt-losing form of congenital adrenal hyperplasia)
   C. Maternal ingestion of progestational agents

II. Physical examination
   A. Position of urethral meatus
   B. Presence or absence of vaginal orifice
   C. Size of phallus
   D. Fusion of labioscrotal folds
   E. Presence or absence of palpable gonad in inguinal canal or groin
   F. Abnormal dermatoglyphic patterns

III. Diagnostic investigations
   A. Buccal smear (Barr bodies)
   B. Urinary 17-ketosteroid and pregnanetriol concentrations
   C. Chromosomal analysis (if congenital adrenal hyperplasia has been eliminated)
   D. Contrast medium studies of GU tract
   E. Biopsy of palpable gonad
   F. Exploratory laparotomy (if diagnosis remains uncertain)

First, it must be ascertained whether siblings or other members of the family had similar findings at birth since congenital adrenal hyperplasia, the syndrome of testicular feminization and—occasionally—true hermaphroditism, may be familial. If the family history contains the unexplained death of a male in early infancy, congenital adrenal hyperplasia of the salt-losing type may be suspected. The mother should be questioned about ingestion of progestational substances early in pregnancy because of their association with virilization of the female fetus.

A careful examination of the genitalia must include observation of the position of the urethral meatus, presence or absence of a separate vaginal orifice, size of the phallus, degree of fusion of the labioscrotal folds and presence or absence of a palpable gonad in the inguinal canal or groin. Abnormal dermatoglyphic patterns may be observed in both XO/XX and XO/XY mosaicism.

Laboratory and Radiologic Studies

Various laboratory investigations help in establishing the diagnosis. A buccal smear must be done immediately. If Barr bodies (denoting the presence of more than one X chromosome) are seen, the diagnosis of female pseudohermaphroditism is likely, with true hermaphroditism or a form of sex chromosome mosaicism a less likely consideration. Since the most common form of female pseudohermaphroditism associated with the presence of Barr bodies is congenital adrenal hyperplasia, every effort must be made to rapidly identify this potentially life-threatening condition. Elevated levels of urinary 17-ketosteroids and pregnanetriol confirm this diagnosis, and appropriate medical therapy may then be undertaken. Abnormal serum electrolyte determinations may be the initial biochemical manifestation of this disorder. If the possibility of congenital adrenal hyperplasia is eliminated, or if the buccal smear shows an absence of Barr bodies, then an analysis of the chromosomal karyotype of peripheral lymphocytes should be performed. If the possibility of mosaicism is considered, the chromosomal composition of fibroblasts should also be studied.

Radiologic studies in which contrast media is introduced into the GU tract often delineate the presence of normal female organs of reproduction.

If a gonad is externally palpable, a biopsy aids in establishing the genetic sex of the infant. Occasionally, exploratory laparotomy may be required to establish a firm diagnosis.

MANAGEMENT

Although congenital adrenal hyperplasia represents the only situation in which ambiguous genitalia are present that requires immediate treatment, diagnostic procedures must nonetheless be carried out while the infant is in the neonatal nursery. Undue delay not only leads to an increased parental anxiety, it may also have an adverse effect on the psychosexual development of the infant.

Where female pseudohermaphroditism is associated with normal internal genitalia, plastic surgery can be performed to create a normal-sized clitoris and, if necessary, to reconstruct the introitus.

In male pseudohermaphroditism, true hermaphroditism or in conditions associated with sex chromosome mosaicism, the assigned sex should be determined by the appearance of the external genitalia. If the phallus is hypoplastic and there is little chance that it can eventually be used as a normal male penis, plastic construction of female genitalia is indicated. The decision to remove the gonads in these cases must be made on an individual basis.

In summary, the genitalia of all newborn infants must be carefully examined immediately after birth. Genital ambiguity must be investigated during the neonatal period, plastic surgery performed when indicated and phenotypic sex assigned as early in life as possible.

THYROID

FETAL DEVELOPMENT

Normal fetal growth and development, especially that of the brain, requires thyroid hormone. During the first half of pregnancy, the fetus depends largely on transplacental passage of maternal hormone (which is bound, to a large extent, to the plasma protein, thyroglobulin). After this, fetal thyroid function is, under normal circumstances, sufficiently developed to supply the needs of the fetus.

Although the fetal hypothalamic–pituitary–thyroid axis functions autonomously, maternal factors may have an adverse effect on the fetus. Since certain fetal thyroid disorders are preventable or treatable, the obstetrician must recognize these as early as possible to prevent the birth of a compromised infant.

By the third or fourth week of gestation, the cells that will form the thyroid gland have migrated from the base of the tongue to a position anterior to the trachea. At the end of the first trimester, follicles appear. At 14 weeks the concentration of iodide can be demonstrated, and at 19 weeks thyroxine can be detected. Thyrotropin also appears at about this time. Synthesis of the thyroglobulin molecule begins at about 11 weeks of gestation.

Before the 18th week of gestation, fetal levels of total thyroxine and free thyroxine are relatively low, but they increase progressively from 22 weeks' gestation to term (Fig. 11–4). The low levels of thyrotropin found prior to 18 weeks of gestation rise abruptly between the 18th and 22nd week, indicating rapid maturation of the fetal hypothalamic–pituitary–thyroid axis. Thyrotropin does not cross the placenta, and hence all that is measured is of fetal origin (20).

Thyroxine crosses the placental barrier slowly. Although an amino acid, it is transported in the blood primarily bound to thyroglobulin. Its concentration in maternal blood rises during the first trimester (to a level higher than that observed in nonpregnant women) and remains unchanged throughout the remainder of pregnancy. Fetal thyroxine concentrations continue to rise, so that at the end of the third trimester maternal and fetal concentrations are approximately equal (about 12 μg/100 ml). Thyroxine concentrations, however, are significantly lower in infants whose birth weights are below 1500 g. During the first trimester, free thyroxine levels in the mother are higher than those of the fetus (thus favoring diffusion of the hormone in the direction of the fetus). In the latter portion of pregnancy, a marked increase in maternal thyroglobulin production occurs secondary to stimulation by estrogen that

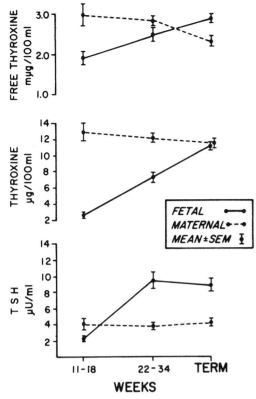

FIG. 11–4. Mean (± SEM) total thyroxine (T₄, µg/100 ml), free thyroxine (FT₄, µg/100 ml) and thyrotropin (TSH, µU/ml) concentrations from paired maternal and fetal serum specimens plotted for three periods of gestation: 11 to 18, 22 to 34 and 38 to 40 weeks. (Fisher DA et al: Pediatrics 46:208, 1970)

has been synthesized by the placenta. Therefore, by term, the normal fetal level of free thyroxine is higher than that of the mother (although total thyroxine levels are about the same). This favors diffusion of free thyroxine from fetus to mother during the latter part of pregnancy. By term, fetal thyrotropin levels have surpassed those of the mother. The high fetal free thyroxine concentration does not seem to suppress the hypothalamic pituitary axis in the same manner as in postnatal life. This may be due to the extremely low triiodothyronine (T₃) levels found in the fetus (19, 22, 24).

Maternal Influences

Although the fetal thyroid functions autonomously during the latter period of gestation, various maternal factors may modify its size and function. Both maternal hypothyroidism and hyperthyroidism and the ingestion of certain drugs can affect fetal thyroid function.

NEONATAL PERIOD

A marked increase in thyrotropin secretion occurs within the first hour after birth. This is followed by an elevation of thyroxine concentrations, which reach their maximum levels at about 24 hours of age. Triiodothyronine concentrations also begin to rise rapidly during the first hour after birth, and by age 24 hours are about ten times greater than fetal levels (19, 24). The increased I¹³¹ uptake observed both in full-term and premature infants is consistent with increased thyroid function during the early neonatal period. Exposure to low environmental temperature is associated with an even greater state of hyperthyroidism (21).

After the first week of postnatal life, thyroid function begins to return to normal adult levels (25).

IODINE BALANCE

Iodine Deficiency

Historically, the most important cause of fetal hypothyroidism has been inadequate iodide in the maternal diet. With the widespread use of iodized salt, endemic cretinism (characterized by deafness, mental deficiency, diplegia and squinting) has largely disappeared as a cause of fetal hypothyroidism. This remains a serious problem in some underdeveloped countries, as demonstrated by Pharoah et al (26) who have noted a high incidence of cretinism among neonates in the Western Highlands of New Guinea due to dietary deficiency of iodides. This problem was alleviated, to a large degree, by providing IM injections of iodized oil to women of childbearing age.

Excessive Use of Iodides

Ingestion of excessive amounts of iodides during pregnancy also affects the fetal thyroid. Iodides, prescribed as expectorants in the treatment of bronchial asthma, easily cross the placenta and lead to fetal thyroid enlargement. This excessive iodide probably blocks the release of thyroid hormone that has been produced by a normally functioning gland. An increase in thyrotropin secretion ensues, causing further synthesis (but impaired release) of thyroid hormone. The resulting colloid goiter may become extremely large. Although affected fetuses usually remain euthyroid, major difficulties often ensue following delivery when the large thyroid, impinging on the trachea, causes respiratory embarrassment. Tracheostomy alone may be insufficient to alleviate the respiratory symptoms, and a subtotal thyroidectomy may be required. The goiter spontaneously subsides over several weeks, and no specific medical therapy is necessary.

MATERNAL THYROID FUNCTION

Maternal Hypothyroidism

There is a high correlation between maternal and fetal hypothyroidism. Several factors may be involved, other than lack of iodides in the maternal diet. A genetically determined enzymatic defect common to both mother and fetus may account for both disorders. Antithyroid antibody, present in the maternal circulation in Hashimoto's disease, may cross the placenta and destroy fetal thyroid tissue.

Preliminary evidence indicates that treatment of a hypothyroid mother with very large doses of thyroid extract may have a beneficial effect on the fetus who is also hypothyroid (18). However, more studies are necessary. The therapeutic use of triiodothyronine, which crosses the placenta more easily than thyroxine, must also be evaluated. Measurements of amniotic fluid protein-bound iodine (PBI), triiodothyronine or thyroxine may be useful as a guide to therapy.

Maternal Hyperthyroidism

Thyrotoxicosis (Graves' disease) is an autoimmune disorder associated with the formation of an abnormal IgG immunoglobulin

known as long-acting thyroid stimulator (LATS). It is thought that LATS acts on microsomes of follicular cells and stimulates excessive secretion of thyroid hormone. Its chemical structure differs from that of thyrotropin, and it has a significantly longer half-life. Its secretion into the blood is not suppressed by the normal feedback mechanism that suppresses thyrotropin secretion in the presence of high blood levels of thyroid hormone. It is also thought to be responsible for the exophthalmos accompanying Graves' disease.

Signs and symptoms of hyperthyroidism in patients with Graves' disease may be alleviated by either medical or surgical therapy. However, suppression of LATS secretion is impossible since therapy is directed toward the end organ (thyroid gland).

NEONATAL HYPERTHYROIDISM (Table 11–2)

Being an IgG molecule, LATS readily crosses the placenta and stimulates excessive thyroid hormone secretion in the fetus. Therefore, no matter how the mother is treated during pregnancy, LATS continues to act on the fetal thyroid gland.

If the mother is treated with an antithyroid drug such as propylthiouracil (PTU) during pregnancy, suppression of both maternal and fetal thyroid hormone secretion occurs. Propylthiouracil given to control maternal illness may be just enough to combat fetal hyperthyroidism, with establishment of a euthyroid state, or it may actually cause fetal hypothyroidism. In the latter case, permanent neurologic sequelae may ensue, with a clinical picture of cretinism noted in the offspring. Treatment of a pregnant woman with I^{131} may totally ablate the fetal thyroid.

Prenatal Diagnosis*

With a knowledge of the normal range of amniotic fluid PBI values, Hollingsworth and Austin (23) were able to monitor thyroid function in fetuses of mothers with

---

* See Appendix A, Addendum 2.

TABLE 11-2. Neonatal Thyrotoxicosis

I. Etiology
  Maternal hyperthyroidism with transplacental
    passage of LATS
II. Clinical Manifestations
  Restlessness
  Tachycardia with occasional congestive heart
    failure
  Exophthalmos
  Goiter
  Irritability
  Fever
  Sweating
III. Laboratory and Radiologic Fndings
  Elevated thyroid function tests
  Presence of LATS in infant's serum
  Increased oxygen consumption
  Advanced bone age
IV. Therapy
  Maternal
    Antithyroid drugs (propylthiouracil)
  Neonatal
    Reserpine
    Propanolol
    Phenobarbital
    Propylthiouracil
    Digitalis (in presence of congestive heart
      failure)
    Oxygen (in presence of congestive heart
      failure)
    IV fluids (if dehydration is present)

Graves' disease. A very low amniotic PBI value was noted when the mother was treated with I^{131} and PTU; on the other hand, markedly elevated levels were found in another case in which the infant developed hyperthyroidism ten days after birth. Monitoring of both maternal and fetal thyroid function appears to be indicated in managing a pregnancy complicated by thyrotoxicosis.

Signs of Neonatal Thyrotoxicosis

If the mother is treated with only partial thyroidectomy, or receives no therapy at all, it is likely that the infant will be born in a hyperthyroid state and will exhibit such signs as tachycardia with congestive heart failure (which may be confused with congenital heart disease), restlessness, exophthalmos, irritability, fever, sweating, goiter, diarrhea and increased metabolic rate. Thrombocytopenia, hepatosplenomegaly and elevated levels of serum IgA and IgM may

occasionally be seen and can lead to a mistaken impression of generalized infection. Bilirubin levels are decreased, and RDS is rare in neonatal thyrotoxicosis.

These signs may vary in intensity from very mild to that of a life-threatening thyroid storm. They may appear at any time from birth to the second day of life. Cardiomegaly and advanced bone age may be apparent on x ray.

Therapy

Since the half-life of LATS is 7 to 18 days, therapy (which may be lifesaving) is only necessary for a relatively short period (29). In mild cases, spontaneous recovery may occur without treatment.

In severe cases, reserpine usually relieves many of the clinical signs. The mechanism of action of this drug is unknown, but it may be related to depletion of catecholamine stores. Propanolol hydrochloride, a β-adrenergic blockading agent has been used successfully in this disorder (28). A thyroidal blockading agent, such as PTU or an iodide, may also be of therapeutic value. However, this type of drug may require several days to take effect. Phenobarbital may be of value in sedating the infant. If dehydration is present, correction with IV fluids is necessary. If congestive heart failure is present, digitalization and oxygen administration are necessary. The infant's status may be followed by his clinical condition, by a fall in serum PBI or thyroxine (provided iodides have not been administered) and by the return of his resting oxygen consumption to a normal level.

If treatment of the mother with PTU has led to fetal hypothyroidism, the newborn infant continues to show signs of thyroid ablation for several days postnatally. However, once the effect of the transplacentally transmitted PTU wears off, the infant usually shows signs of hyperthyroidism and may require treatment. Those infants who show permanent signs of hypothyroidism because of maternal treatment during pregnancy require long-term replacement therapy.

NEONATAL HYPOTHYROIDISM (Cretinism)

Hypothyroidism is often difficult to diagnose in the early neonatal period. Although the fetus may be hypothyroid, enough maternal thyroxine usually crosses the placenta to mask the frank signs of hypothyroidism. A history of maternal hypothyroidism or the delivery of a cretin following a previous pregnancy should alert the physician to the possibility of a hypothyroid infant. During the pregnancy abnormally low levels of amniotic fluid PBI or thyroxine may raise the suspicion of fetal hypothyroidism (23). The presence of antithyroid antibodies in the blood of women who have previously delivered cretins (these antibodies presumably cross the placenta and attack the fetal thyroid) should also raise the suspicion of hypothyroidism.

In addition to the obstetric history, there are many neonatal signs that should arouse the suspicion of congenital hypothyroidism

FIG. 11–5. Signs of neonatal hypothyroidism.

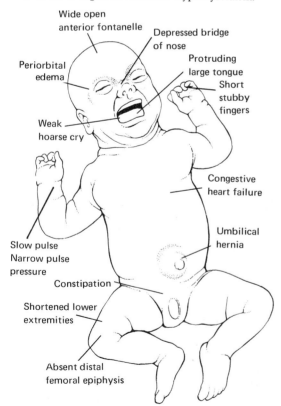

Wide open
anterior fontanelle
Depressed bridge
of nose
Periorbital
edema
Protruding
large tongue
Short
stubby
fingers
Weak
hoarse cry
Congestive
heart failure
Umbilical
hernia
Slow pulse
Narrow pulse
pressure
Constipation
Shortened lower
extremities
Absent distal
femoral epiphysis

(Fig. 11–5). The classic picture is one of a sluggish and lethargic infant with a hoarse and weak cry. An umbilical hernia and large, protruding tongue may be present. Constipation, an unusually slow pulse and unexplained jaundice are frequent signs. The lower extremities are shortened, and the hands may appear spadelike with short stubby fingers. Myxedema is occasionally seen. There may be cyanosis, respiratory distress and an unexplained heart murmur. The anterior fontanelle may be wide open. On radiologic examination, the distal femoral epiphyses, which normally appear at about 38 weeks of gestation, may be absent after this time. The resting oxygen consumption is abnormally low. Abnormalities in thyroid function tests depend on the type of defect causing the hypothyroidism. It is unusual for a clear-cut case of cretinism to become apparent in the neonatal period. Since the ultimate prognosis is best in those infants who have had the benefit of exposure to thyroid hormone in utero (and therefore would be expected to have the least brain damage), the presence of any signs or symptoms even remotely resembling hypothyroidism should be enough to warrant a diagnostic evaluation for this disorder.

Athyrotic Cretinism

The most common type of hypothyroidism is athyrotic cretinism. The etiology of this is obscure. The occasional familial incidence of this may indicate a failure of the normal migration of the thyroid from the base of the tongue to its normal position anterior to the trachea or the presence of maternal antithyroid antibodies directed against the fetal thyroid. Diagnosis of this disorder depends on markedly decreased levels of serum PBI, triiodothyronine and thyroxine and elevated levels of TSH. Serum cholesterol levels are usually elevated, but this is a less consistent finding. The diagnosis of athyrotic (or hypothyrotic) cretinism is confirmed by zero or minimal (less than 10%) radioactive iodine (I^{131}) uptake in 24 hours.

Once the diagnosis is established, it is

imperative that adequate treatment be started at once in order to minimize CNS damage. Either dessicated thyroid, purified thyroxine or triiodothyronine (Cytomel) may be used to institute treatment. Although triiodothyronine has the most rapid onset of action of the three, there is probably no particular advantage to using it instead of dessicated thyroid. The latter drug has the advantage of low cost, and its effectiveness will be reflected by serum PBI or thyroxine levels. (When triiodothyronine is used therapeutically, the infant may be euthyroid in the presence of a very low serum PBI or thyroxine concentration, however, measurements of triiodothyronine by radioimmunoassay may reflect the infant's euthyroid state.)

The initial daily dosage of thyroid extract in the neonatal period is usually 16 mg. This dosage may be raised weekly until an average intake of 64 mg/day is attained. The range may vary from 45 mg to 75 mg/day. Acceleration of growth to normal rates is probably the most sensitive indicator of adequacy of therapy. The persistence of symptoms of hypothyroidism usually indicates inadequacy of therapy, and an increment in dosage is indicated. With overtreatment, such signs of hyperthyroidism as tachycardia, restlessness, diarrhea and sweating may appear. With these findings, the dosage should be decreased. Although early treatment does not guarantee achievement of an optimal level of intelligence, the longer treatment is delayed, the worse will be the eventual outcome (27).

Dussault et al (19a) have developed an immunoassay which can rapidly measure thyroxine concentrations in the eluate of blood spotted on filter paper. Using this method, they have screened 47,000 newborn infants on the fifth day of life, and detected 7 cases of congenital hypothyroidism.

Inborn Errors of Thyroid Metabolism

A group of inborn errors of thyroid gland metabolism may also cause neonatal hypothyroidism. These may be associated with goitrous enlargement of the thyroid gland.

Goiter, however, is rare in the neonatal period in this group and may not appear for several years.

In Pendred's syndrome, there is an association between familial goitrous hypothyroidism and deafness. The primary defect is a deficiency of peroxidase enzymes, which normally oxidize iodide to iodine in the thyroid. As opposed to athyrotic cretinism, in which radioactive iodide levels are zero or markedly diminished, there is an increased I^{131} uptake in this condition. Administration of perchlorate or thiocyanate causes rapid discharge of iodine from the gland. As in athyrotic cretinism, these infants must be treated with full replacement therapy.

There are, in addition, other very rare inborn errors of thyroid hormone synthesis and metabolism. These include defects of iodide trapping and organification, coupling defects of iodotyrosines and deiodination defects. Congenital absence of thyroglobulin has also been observed.

REFERENCES

ADRENAL CORTEX

1. Bongiovanni AM, Eberlein WR, Goldman AS, New M: Disorders of adrenal steroid biogenesis. Recent Prog Horm Res 23:375, 1967

2. Childs B, Grumbach MM, Van Wyk JJ: Virilizing adrenal hyperplasia: a genetic and hormonal study. J Clin Invest 35:213, 1956

3. Cleveland WW: Maternal fetal hormone relationships. Pediatr Clin North Am 17:273, 1970

4. Eberlein WR: The salt-losing form of congenital adrenal hyperplasia. Pediatrics 21:667, 1958

5. Gross M, Kottmeier PK, Waterhouse K: Diagnosis and treatment of neonatal adrenal hemorrhage. J Pediatr Surg 2:308, 1967

6. Frandsen VA, Stakemann G: The site of production of oestrogenic hormones in human pregnancy. II. Experimental investigations on the role of the foetal adrenal. Acta Endocrinol (Kbh) 43:184, 1963

7. Gutai J, George R, Koeff S, Bacon GE: Adrenal response to physical stress in the affect of adrenocorticotrophic hormone in newborn infants. J Pediatr 81:719, 1972

8. Klingenberg A: Massive adrenal hemorrhage in newborn infants. Schweiz Med Wochenschr 100:417, 1970

9. Kotas R, Avery ME: Accelerated appearance of

pulmonary surfactant in the fetal rabbit. J Appl Physiol 30: 358, 1971

10. Kreines K, De Vaux WD: Neonatal adrenal insufficiency associated with maternal Cushings syndrome. Pediatrics 47:516, 1971

11. Liggins GC, Howie RN: A controlled trial of antepartum glucocorticoid treatment for prevention of the respiratory distress syndrome in premature infants. Pediatrics 50:515, 1972

12. Naeye RL, Harcke H, Blanc W: Adrenal gland structure and the development of hyaline membrane disease. Pediatrics 47:650, 1971

13. New MI: Congenital adrenal hyperplasia. Pediatr Clin North Am 15:395, 1968

DISORDERS OF GONADAL DEVELOPMENT

14. Perez-Palacios G, Jaffe RB: The syndrome of testicular feminization. Pediatr Clin North Am 19:653, 1972

15. Sohval AR: Hermaphroditism with atypical or mixed gonadal dysgenesis. Am J Med 36:281, 1964

16. Voorhess ML: Masculinization of the female fetus associated with norethindrone-mestranol therapy during pregnancy. J Pediatr 71:128, 1967

17. Wilkins L: Masculinization of female fetus due to orally given progestins. JAMA 172:1028, 1960

THYROID

18. Bacon GE, Lowrey GH, Carr EA: Prenatal treatment of cretinism: preliminary studies of its value in postnatal development. J Pediatr 71:654, 1967

19. Czernichow P, Greenberg AH, Tyson J, Blizzard RM: Thyroid function studied in paired maternal-cord sera and sequential observations of thyrotropic hormone release during the first 72 hours of life. Pediatr Res 5:53, 1971

19a. Dussault JH, Coulombe P, Laberge C, Letarte J, Guyda H, Khoury, K. Preliminary report on a mass screening program for neonatal hypothyroidism. J Pediatr 86:670, 1975

20. Fisher DA, Hobel CJ, Garza R, Pierce CA: Thyroid function in the preterm fetus. Pediatrics 46:208, 1970

21. Fisher DA, Oddie TH, Makoski EJ: The influence of environmental temperature on thyroid, adrenal and water metabolism in the newborn human infant. Pediatrics 37:583, 1966

22. Fisher DA, Odell WD, Hobel CJ, Garza R: Thyroid function in the term fetus. Pediatrics 44:526, 1969

23. Hollingsworth DR, Austin E: Thyroxine derivatives in amniotic fluid. J Pediatr 79:923, 1971

24. Lieblich JM, Utiger RD: Triiodothyronine in cord serum. J Pediatr 82:290, 1973

25. O'Halloran MT, Webster HL: Thyroid function assays in infants. J Pediatr 81:916, 1972

26. Pharoah POD, Buttfield IH, Hetzel BS: Neurological damage to the fetus resulting from severe iodine deficiency during pregnancy. Lancet 1:308, 1971

27. Raiti S, News GH: Cretinism: early diagnosis and its relation to mental prognosis. Arch Dis Child 46:692, 1971

28. Smith CS, Howard NJ: Propanolol in treatment of neonatal thyrotoxicosis. J Pediatr 83:1046, 1973

29. Sunshine P, Kusumoto H, Kriss JP: Survival time of LATS in neonatal thyrotoxicosis: implications for diagnosis and therapy of the disorder. Pediatrics 38:869, 1965

12

The Gastrointestinal Tract and Perinatal Metabolism

ANATOMIC DEVELOPMENT OF THE GI TRACT

Abnormal embryogenesis of the gastrointestinal (GI) tract leads to a variety of congenital anomalies, ranging from minor to severe, life-threatening conditions, many of which are discussed in Chapter 23, Surgical Problems.

The fetal GI tract develops in two portions: 1) the endoderm-lined primitive gut (located within the embryo) and 2) extraembryonic structures (the yolk sac and allantois). The primitive, tubelike gut has two blind ends (foregut and hindgut) and is connected in its midportion (midgut) to the yolk sac by the vitelline duct.

FOREGUT

Pharyngeal Arches

At the cephalic end of the tract the pharyngeal gut develops as five pharyngeal arches separated by clefts, during the fourth and fifth weeks of gestation. The first two arches give rise to the bones of the middle ear, a portion of the temporal bone and several muscles and nerves. The hyoid bone and associated muscles and nerves are derived from the third arch, whereas the fourth and fifth fuse to form the thyroid, cricoid and arytenoid cartilages and their associated muscles and nerves.

Of the five pairs of pharyngeal pouches that are formed, the first gives rise to the middle ear, eustachian tube and tympanic membrane. The second gives rise to the palatine tonsils; the thymus and parathyroid glands are derived from the third, with the fourth forming the superior parathyroid gland and the fifth a portion of the thyroid gland.

Several congenital anomalies result from abnormal differentiation of the pharyngeal arches and pouches during the embryologic period. For example, midline branchial cysts form when the second pharyngeal arch fails to fuse with the third and fourth arches. Failure of differentiation of the thymus and parathyroid glands from third and fourth pouches (DiGeorge's syndrome) leads to severe, unremitting hypocalcemia, immunologic deficit regarding the thymic-dependent lymphocytes (delayed hypersensitivity) and early death.

Failure of the arches to fuse results in persistent spaces (clefts) between them. Persistence of the first pharyngeal cleft leads to preauricular sinus formation, whereas remnants of the second, third and fourth clefts that remain open form a cervical sinus, located on the lateral aspect of the neck, just anterior to the sternocleidomastoid muscle.

Thyroglossal Cysts and Aberrant Thyroid Tissue

Thyroglossal cysts are midline remnants of the thyroglossal duct, a structure that, in the embryo, connects the thyroid gland to the floor of the pharynx. The cysts are located in the midline of the neck, with about half of them in the area of the hyoid bone. They may also be found at the base of the tongue or close to the thyroid cartilage. Aberrant thyroid tissue may be found anywhere along the path of descent of the thyroid gland from the base of the tongue to the neck.

Esophageal Atresia and Tracheoesophageal Fistula

The mechanisms of formation of esophageal atresia and tracheoesophageal fistulas are unknown. Several anatomic variants exist, most of which are life-threatening and require operative intervention immediately after birth. They are discussed in detail in Chapter 23, Surgical Problems.

Lungs, Esophagus and Stomach

The lungs form from respiratory buds, which are an outbranching of the foregut. Abnormal budding leads to the formation of ectopic lobes that develop independently of the respiratory system. Congenital lung cysts, which may become chronically infected, are derived from these lobes.

The remainder of the foregut forms the esophagus, stomach, liver, gall bladder and pancreas. The stomach develops as a dilatation of the foregut during the fifth week of gestation. After undergoing a variety of positional changes, the greater and lesser curvatures are formed, and the pyloric portion moves to the right while the cardiac portion moves to the left. If there is hypertrophy of the circular or longitudinal musculature in the pyloric region, pyloric stenosis will result. During the period of

rotation of the stomach, the duodenum forms as a U-shaped loop that will eventually lie in the retroperitoneal space.

Liver, Gall Bladder and Pancreas

Liver development begins during the third week of gestation with an outgrowth of the endodermal epithelium (hepatic diverticulum) at the distal end of the foregut. By the tenth week of gestation the liver comprises about 10% of total body weight. After this time growth of the liver decelerates in relation to that of the rest of the body so that at term the liver comprises about 5% of body weight. The hepatic diverticulum gives rise to the bile ducts and gall bladder. Failure to establish a lumen in these structures may lead to either a partial or total atresia.

The pancreas develops from two buds derived from the endodermal epithelium of the duodenum. If the ventral bud fails to undergo its usual rotation, annular pancreas (with encirclement of the duodenum) and intestinal obstruction occur.

MIDGUT AND HINDGUT

The midgut comprises the entire intestinal tract from the distal portion of the duodenum to the proximal two-thirds of the transverse colon. Initially, it is connected to the yolk sac by means of the vitelline, or omphalomesenteric duct. Persistence of a vestige of this structure, Meckel's diverticulum (with ectopic gastric mucosa) may lead to ulceration, bleeding or perforation during postnatal life.

Because of the rapid growth of this portion of midgut, it is extended from the abdominal cavity during the sixth week of fetal life, during which time growth and rotation 270° counterclockwise around the axis of the superior mesenteric artery occur. Developmental abnormalities during this period may lead to malrotation or volvulus. Intestinal contents return to the abdominal cavity by the end of the third month of gestation. If this does not occur, an omphalocele will result.

The hindgut begins at the distal third of

the transverse colon and ends at the upper portion of the anal canal. Because of its communication with the cloaca early in gestation, fistulas may persist between the rectum and genitourinary (GU) tract, usually in conjunction with imperforate anus. The distal portion of the anal canal arises from an ectodermal depression (proctodeum). Failure of the hindgut to communicate with the proctodeum leads to imperforate anus.

PHYSIOLOGIC DEVELOPMENT OF THE GI TRACT

FETAL LIFE

The nutritional status of the fetus depends primarily on intact placental function. However, the newborn infant relies on his GI tract to provide nutrition for optimal growth and development.

The ability to suck and swallow develops during fetal life. By the 33rd or 34th week of gestation, there is efficient coordination between these functions, and the fetus swallows amniotic fluid. In an upper GI tract obstruction, hydramnios is likely to develop (this may also accompany anencephaly or diabetes mellitus).

NEONATAL PERIOD

At term the GI tract is about 250 cm long, sterile and airless. Bacterial colonization develops within 24 to 48 hours after birth, the time of appearance and nature of the organisms reflecting both the type and quantity of the milk received by the infant. Air normally enters the stomach following delivery and fills the small intestine by 12 hours and the large intestine by 24 hours. Meconium, which has accumulated during fetal life, is passed within 24 hours in the great majority of infants.

The normal full-term infant is capable of efficiently digesting, absorbing and assimilating breast milk and all commercially prepared infant formulas. Hydrochloric acid is produced by the stomach immediately after birth (1, 2). Although the pH of gastric fluid

is nearly neutral at birth (due to the amniotic fluid), there is a rapid drop over the first six hours of postnatal life. Many premature infants, however, have achlorhydria during the first day of life.

The ability to digest all dietary carbohydrates is established at term. Maltase and sucrase reach their maximum enzymic activity by the sixth or seventh month of gestation, whereas lactase activity reaches its peak at term (3). With the exception of infants with mucoviscidosis, pancreatic enzyme function is well established, even in premature infants. In the latter group, vegetable fats are more easily digested and absorbed than animal fats. Gastrointestinal function is extremely sensitive to a variety of insults that may affect the neonate. Hypoxia, sepsis and hypoglycemia are some of the more commonly encountered nonsurgical conditions that lead to neonatal paralytic ileus.

CARBOHYDRATE METABOLISM

FETAL PHYSIOLOGY

Glucose is the principal nutrient available to the fetus for energy metabolism and, like other monosaccharides, it probably crosses the placenta by facilitated active transport rather than by simple diffusion. Disaccharides, such as sucrose and lactose, cannot cross the placental barrier and are therefore unavailable to the fetus.

Stored as glycogen in both placenta and fetus, glucose has been demonstrated in the germinal disc of a 13-day-old fetus. By 8 weeks it is present in the placenta, but it does not appear in the liver until the 12th to 15th week of gestation. Until the 20th to 24th week of gestation, liver glycogen is not present in sufficient quantities to maintain adequate blood glucose levels. Up to this time, the placenta participates in the regulation of blood glucose by releasing glycogen; afterwards, placental glycogen stores gradually decrease until term. In diabetic pregnancies, glycogen stores in the placenta are increased.

Liver glycogen stores increase markedly during the last weeks of pregnancy, so that by term, the liver glycogen content is 80 to 120 mg/g of wet tissue, about twice the normal adult value. Cardiac glycogen is extremely high, reaching about ten times the adult level by term. Skeletal muscle glycogen is also increased throughout gestation and is about three to five times the adult level at term. The amount of glycogen stored in the lungs reaches maximum concentrations during the middle of pregnancy, but decreases to adult levels by term.

In malnourished fetuses with retarded intrauterine growth, glycogen stores are usually depleted. This depletion also occurs in undergrown fetuses of diabetic mothers with toxemia and vascular insufficiency.

The fetal blood glucose concentration is about 60% to 75% of that of the mother's (25, 31). The rate of umbilical uptake of glucose from the maternal circulation is unknown, but measurements have been made of concurrent glucose concentrations in umbilical arterial and venous blood. In several series (both in humans and experimental animals) the differences have ranged from 3 to 11 mg/100 ml, with an average difference of about 5 or 6 mg/100 ml (17, 25, 29).

During fetal life, blood glucose levels normally remain within a relatively narrow range, reflecting maternal levels. The fetal endocrine pancreas (beta cells of the islets of Langerhans), which begins to secrete insulin between the 14th and 20th week of gestation, does not seem to play a major role in fetal glucose homeostasis. (The fact that the fetal pancreatic insulin secretion is more responsive to increased blood concentrations of arginine than to glucose (18) suggests that the fetal endocrine pancreas plays a role in intrauterine protein metabolism.) Insulin secreted by the maternal pancreas does not cross the placenta and therefore has no effect on the fetus. At the time of delivery, the islet cells secrete insulin sluggishly and respond poorly to an increased blood glucose concentration. This lack of responsiveness is even more apparent in infants of very low gestational age (12, 14, 23). Only after postnatal feedings

have been established does insulin play its full role in the regulation of glucose metabolism.

Maternal Diabetes Mellitus

Diabetes mellitus in the mother has a profound influence on fetal pancreatic function, carbohydrate and fat metabolism and growth (16, 26). The wide fluctuations of blood glucose in the mother are reflected in the fetus, but this is usually more of a problem when the onset of the diabetes has preceded the pregnancy and when it is under poor control. These fluctuations result in elevated fetal blood glucose levels and cause hyperplasia and hypertrophy of fetal islet cells with a resulting hyperinsulinemia that leads to accelerated fetal growth, due probably both to the lipogenic effect of insulin and its positive effect on fetal protein anabolism. The greater the weight of the fetus, the more marked the degree of beta-cell hyperplasia.

The abnormal intrauterine environment brought about by maternal diabetes is not conducive to a normal gestation. Fetal morbidity and mortality are increased, and there is a higher than normal incidence of congenital anomalies. Aberrations of maternal acid-base metabolism (ketoacidosis) may also adversely affect fetal oxygenation by decreasing the erythrocyte concentration of 2,3-diphosphoglycerate (24).

Erythroblastosis Fetalis and Endocrine Influences

The fetal endocrine pancreas is also affected by erythroblastosis fetalis (7). Islet cell hyperplasia with increased insulin secretion and subsequent neonatal hypoglycemia may occur. Though the reason for this remains unclear, it may represent a compensatory mechanism for the binding and destruction of insulin by antibodies that are present in this disorder.

The fetal endocrine system (other than pancreatic beta cells) appears to play a role in the regulation of glucose metabolism. Fetal pituitary hormones and corticosteroids seem to be required for glycogen accumulation. Glucagon and epinephrine are probably necessary for the conversion of glycogen to glucose. The inability of some hypoglycemic infants, e.g., the infants of diabetic mothers (19) and small-for-gestational-age infants with a history of fetal malnutrition (30), to secrete epinephrine postnatally may indicate that this mechanism is exhausted attempting to maintain normal blood glucose levels in the fetus.

INTRAPARTUM

Nature normally endows the fetus at term with ample supplies of glycogen to provide enough fuel for energy metabolism during the hours immediately prior to delivery, when stress is present and the oxygen supply often low. Glycogen is also necessary for the period following delivery when the infant's caloric intake is either low or non-existent. Because of the high utilization of glycogen during this critical period, liver glycogen decreases to 10% of its original value in two to three hours after birth and does not reach adult levels until age two to three weeks. Skeletal muscle and cardiac glycogen decrease at a slower rate. The decrease in cardiac glycogen content is, however, accelerated in the presence of asphyxia.

Together with the rapid decrease in glycogen following delivery, the respiratory quotient (CO_2 production/O_2 consumption) decreases from about 1.0 at birth to 0.70 to 0.75 (in starved infants) by the second day and does not rise to levels of 0.80 to 0.85 until adequate feeding is established. This indicates that energy metabolism is primarily dependent on fat rather than glucose. Glycogen reserves, which can be depleted very rapidly, are therefore preserved, and the source of glucose necessary for brain and RBC metabolism remains largely intact.

POSTNATAL

Following delivery, blood glucose concentrations in the infant vary from 40 to 90 mg/100 ml, but these may be considerably elevated if the mother has received glucose intravenously. In the hours after delivery, blood glucose levels decline, generally becoming stabilized at levels of 45 to 60 mg/100 ml by age four to six hours. The limits of blood glucose levels in the newborn infant are set by a balance between glucose entry into the blood (from glycogen stores, via the GI route, or by IV infusion) and tissue utilization. The concentration of glucose in the circulation depends on the magnitude of glycogen stores, the amount of glucose that enters the blood following feedings, the glycogenolytic effects of glucagon and epinephrine and the gluconeogenic effect of 17-hydroxycorticosteroids. Glucose utilization depends on muscular activity, the mass of metabolically active tissue, available oxygen and oxygen consumption, pH and insulin secretion. As noted previously, insulin secretion may be "sluggish" during the first days of life. Any aberrations may lead to hypoglycemia or hyperglycemia.

Once oral feedings have started, the glucose levels in normal neonates begin to rise, with a wide degree of fluctuation noted. The normal blood glucose level during the first week of life is about 55 to 70 mg/100 ml, with most infants having levels greater than 50 mg/100 ml after 72 hours of age. In normally grown full-term infants, blood glucose levels of less than 30 mg/100 ml may be interpreted as abnormal during the first three days of life, and 40 mg/100 ml thereafter.

Hypoglycemia and Low Birth Weight

Low-birth-weight infants tend to have lower blood glucose concentrations both in the immediate neonatal period and during the first month of life than do normal full-term infants (Table 12–1). Baens et al (6) show that 15% to 20% of low-birth-weight infants have blood glucose levels of less than 30 mg/100 ml (considered hypoglycemic for normal full-term infants). Cornblath (11) considers a blood glucose level of less than 20 mg/100 ml indicative of hypoglycemia in low-birth-weight infants.

Low-birth-weight infants are, however, a heterogenous group. In infants who are small for gestational age because of fetal

TABLE 12–1. Neonatal Hypoglycemia

Causes	Mechanism
Maternal diabetes mellitus* Frank (up to 50% of offspring) or Gestational (up to 20% of offspring)	Increased insulin secretion, decreased epinephrine secretion
Intrauterine growth failure due to 1) maternal malnutrition, 2) toxemia of pregnancy or 3) in smaller of twins	Decreased liver glycogen stores secondary to placental dysfunction, increased utilization by the brain, decreased epinephrine secretion, inappropriate insulin secretion (uncertain)
Hypoxia	Depletion of glycogen stores during intrapartum period
Cold Stress	Increased glucose utilization secondary to increased oxygen consumption

Miscellaneous:
  Galactosemia
  Type I glycogen storage disease
  Maple syrup urine disease
  Beckwith's syndrome
  Erythroblastosis fetalis
  Insulinoma
  Leucine sensitivity	

* Onset of signs usually within a few hours after birth.

malnutrition, the finding of low blood glucose levels is relatively common, and this is consistent with the autopsy findings of Shelly (28) that these infants have a very diminished liver glycogen content. Melichar et al (21) found no umbilical arteriovenous difference in blood glucose concentrations in these infants, their umbilical venous glucose levels being approximately 50% less than those found in normal full-term infants. This suggests that the reason for the low liver glycogen content in these infants is inadequate glucose transfer across the placenta to the fetus.

In addition to depleted hepatic glycogen stores, the rapid uptake and utilization of glucose by the metabolically active brain is probably another factor contributing to low blood glucose levels.*

In normally grown infants of low gestational age, abnormally low blood glucose concentrations present less of a problem. These infants usually have better liver glycogen stores than undergrown infants of similar weight but of higher gestational age. A diabetic-like glucose tolerance curve is usually present and is apparently due to the unresponsiveness of the infant's immature

* See Appendix A, Addendum 3.

beta cells to a glucose stimulus. Hyperglycemia may also be encountered if the infant is receiving an infusion of glucose, especially if the glucose concentration of the fluid is 10% or greater (14).

Hypoxia and Chilling. Both perinatal hypoxia and postnatal chilling tend to lower blood glucose levels. The inefficient anabolic utilization of glucose for energy metabolism via the tricarboxylic acid cycle during period of oxygen deprivation greatly decreases glycogen stores and hence leads to hypoglycemia. In the presence of cold stress, nonshivering thermogenesis is dependent on adequate glucose reserves necessary for the resynthesis of fat in brown adipose tissue, which is necessary for the maintenance of normal body temperature.

Discordant Twins. Hypoglycemia is very common in the smaller of discordant twins, especially if the smaller twin weighs less than 2000 g and is 25% or more lighter than the larger twin (27). This is most likely due to the decreased in utero blood supply to the undergrown twin.

Infants of Diabetic Mothers. Infants of diabetic mothers have an unusually high incidence of hypoglycemia during the immediate postnatal period. The incidence varies with individual observers and depends largely on the frequency of observations. Cornblath (13) found that 50% of infants of mothers with frank diabetes developed hypoglycemia, while 20% of infants of mothers with gestational diabetes were hypoglycemic.

It is likely that the hypoglycemia noted in this group of infants (the more severe the maternal diabetes, the greater the likelihood of significant hypoglycemia) is related to hyperinsulinism. The rate of fall of blood glucose in affected infants varies directly with the concentration in maternal blood at the time of delivery. The level at which the blood glucose finally stabilizes does not correlate with the cord blood level noted following delivery. Increased plasma insulin levels have been demonstrated in infants of both frank and gestational diabetic mothers (8, 22, 26). The beta-cell hypertrophy and hyperplasia present at postmortem examinations of infants with diabetic mothers who have died correlates with biochemical findings. The increased growth in these infants is probably due to both the lipogenic effects of insulin and its anabolic effect in protein metabolism. The higher the weight of the infant, the greater is the degree of beta-cell hyperplasia.

Another factor that may predispose infants of insulin-dependent diabetic mothers to hypoglycemia is their inability to secrete epinephrine in response to the hypoglycemic stimulus (25), which thus results in a failure to mobilize plentiful glycogen stores. The hypoglycemia in these infants is usually of relatively short duration, and blood glucose levels usually revert to normal by the second day of life.

The inability of the hypoglycemic neonate to maintain adequate blood glucose levels is of considerable clinical significance. Since glucose is the principal source of energy for brain metabolism, decreased blood levels may lead to the appearance of abnormal signs. If immediate therapy is not started, permanent neurologic sequelae may ensue (5, 9, 15).

Signs of Hypoglycemia

The signs of neonatal hypoglycemia are related to a malfunctioning CNS and include excessive jitteriness, tremors, lethary, high-pitched cry, poor suck and difficulty in feeding, cyanosis, limpness and generalized seizure activity. Cardiomegaly has also been reported in neonatal hypoglycemia (4). Upon biochemical correction, the heart size returns to normal. Many of these signs are also manifestations of such other disorders (Table 12–2) as hypocalcemia, CNS bleeding, infection or anoxia and the narcotic withdrawal syndrome. Often, hypoglycemia may coexist with one of these other conditions. One way of determining if a specific sign is due to hypoglycemia is by observing the clinical (and possibly electroencephalographic) response to an adequate IV injection of glucose. A rapid clearance of glucose from the blood is associated with these signs (in hypoglycemia) and tends to confirm the diagnosis.

Biochemical Diagnosis

Blood glucose determinations should be performed on all infants with the previously noted signs. In addition, all infants who are inappropriately grown for gestational age, all low-birth-weight infants and all infants of diabetic mothers should undergo at least one screening test for the determination of

TABLE 12–2. Differential Diagnosis of Neonatal Hypoglycemia

I. Infectious causes
  Sepsis
  Meningitis
  Encephalitis
II. Metabolic disorders
  Hypocalcemia
  Hypomagnesemia
  Hyponatremia or hypernatremia
  Pyridoxine dependency
  Withdrawal from addictive drug
III. Bleeding
  Intraventricular hemorrhage
  Subdural hematoma
  Adrenal hemorrhage
IV. Congenital anomalies of the CNS

blood glucose levels. In small-for-gestational-age infants, this should be repeated daily for three days since the hypoglycemia may not be apparent immediately after birth.

The use of Ames Dextrostix* has greatly simplified the process of screening for neonatal hypoglycemia. A drop of freely flowing blood is allowed to cover the end of this glucose oxidase reagent strip for exactly one minute, after which it is washed off and the resultant color compared with a prepared chart. With this method false negative results are rare. Dextrostix Reflectance Meters (small photoelectric units that can "read" the Dextrostix values) have a fairly good degree of accuracy, but in the presence of a high hematocrit, the reflectance meter readings may be falsely low.

If there is any question about the presence of hypoglycemia, a biochemical determination, such as the glucose oxidase method (20), should be performed. Processing the sample is of great importance in obtaining an accurate result for if the serum is allowed to remain in contact with the red blood cells for a prolonged period, glycolysis occurs, causing a decrease in the serum

* Ames Co., Elkhart, Indiana 46514

FIG. 12–1. Typical appearance of an infant of a diabetic mother.

glucose concentration. The addition of sodium fluoride to the specimen halts this process.

Because of the wide overlap of signs of hypoglycemia with other potentially treatable disorders, further investigations for such conditions as neonatal sepsis, hypocalcemia, hypomagnesemia, hyponatremia, hypernatremia, polycythemia, drug withdrawal, intracranial bleeding and pyridoxine dependency are warranted if the clinical manifestations attributed to hypoglycemia do not subside with the IV administration of glucose.

The diagnosis of hypoglycemia must be based on two abnormal sequential readings (below 20 mg/100 ml for infants weighing less than 2500g, below 30 mg/100 ml for fully grown infants less than 72 hours of age or below 40 mg/100 ml after that time). Once the diagnosis is established, an etiology should be determined. Infants of diabetic mothers are usually easy to recognize, both from their characteristic general appearance and maternal history (Fig. 12–1). Undergrown infants are also usually easy to recognize. This is especially true for the smaller of discordant twins.

Other relatively common conditions associated with hypoglycemia (e.g., anoxia, chilling, intracranial bleeding infection and adre-

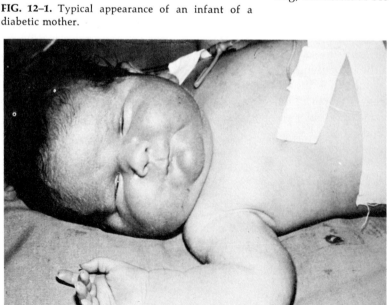

nal hemorrhage) should be suspected if no obvious cause is found. In prolonged and persistent hypoglycemia less common entities, such as glycogen storage disease, galactosemia, maple syrup urine disease, insulinoma or leucine-sensitive hypoglycemia, congenital fructose intolerance or Beckwith's syndrome may be suspected.

Therapy

Infants with symptomatic hypoglycemia (Table 12–3) must always be treated; although the necessity for treating asymptomatic infants is still controversial, most observers recommend treating them as well (8). In small-for-gestational-age hypoglycemic infants a solution of 1 to 2 ml/kg of 50% glucose or 2 to 4 ml/kg of 25% glucose is infused over a five-minute period into a peripheral vein. This is followed by an infusion of 10% or 15% glucose solution (approximately 75 ml/kg/day during the first two days of life). Oral feedings may be instituted if the infant is asymptomatic. After 48 hours the concentration of the solution may be lowered gradually and discontinued after the infant has normal blood glucose levels for 24 to 48 hours. These infants should never be treated solely by oral administration of glucose. However, the early institution of feedings (prior to four hours of age) in low-birth-weight infants is associated with a decreased incidence of hypoglycemia. Glucagon or epinephrine

TABLE 12–3. Therapy of Neonatal Hypoglycemia

II. Diabetes Mellitus
    A. Glucagon, 0.3 mg/kg (up to 1.0 mg or epinephrine 0.01 mg/kg, IM, if infant is asymptomatic)
    B. If infant is symptomatic, 1 to 2 ml/kg of 50% glucose or 2 to 4 ml/kg 25% glucose IV over a 5-minute period, followed by infusion of 10 or 15% glucose solution for 48 hours, to be followed by 5% glucose solution for 24 hours.
    C. If hypoglycemia is unresponsive to above, hydrocortisone 5 mg/kg/day IM in two divided doses.
II. Fetal Malnutrition
    A. Early feedings, if tolerated
    B. Follow guidelines of I., B. and I., C.

should not be used in these infants since glycogen stores are very low. Blood glucose levels, which must be carefully monitored during the course of therapy, should return to normal fairly rapidly following institution of therapy. If no response occurs after 6 to 12 hours, hydrocortisone, 5 mg/kg/day, may be given IM in two divided doses in an attempt to promote gluconeogenesis.

Although hypoglycemia associated with fetal malnutrition may not become apparent until after the first day of life, the onset of hypoglycemia in infants of diabetic mothers is usually early. If the latter infant is asymptomatic, oral feedings may be initiated and either glucagon (0.3 mg/kg, up to 1.0 mg) or epinephrine (0.01 mg/kg) given IM since glycogen stores are usually ample. Pharmacologic action of both of these preparations is moderately short; however, glucagon may have an additional adverse effect of stimulating insulin release, thus causing a rebound hypoglycemia.

Prognosis

The ultimate outcome for untreated infants with symptomatic hypoglycemia is poor, with a high incidence of convulsive disorders and brain damage. However, prompt treatment is associated with a more favorable prognosis.

Infants of diabetic mothers with hypoglycemia seem to have a better overall prognosis than hypoglycemic infants who are small for gestational age. This may be due to the fact that the latter group has suffered either hypoglycemic or hypoxic brain damage for a variable length of time prior to delivery.

UNCOMMON DISORDERS

Galactosemia

Galactosemia is a rare inborn error of galactose metabolism, which if undetected and untreated leads either to death or to severe brain and liver damage and cataract formation (39). This disorder, which has an autosomal recessive mode of inheritance, is due to the absence of the enzyme galactose-1-

phosphate uridyl transferase, necessary for the conversion of galactose-1-phosphate to glucose-1-phosphate. Absence of the enzyme galactokinase, the catalyst for the conversion of galactose to galactose-1-phosphate, has also been demonstrated as a cause of a less serious form of galactosemia that is detected only occasionally in the neonate, having as its principal toxic effect cataract formation.

The incidence of galactosemia is reported to be as high as 1:18,000 (38). However, Shih et al (43) discovered only 2 cases among over 374,000 infants who were screened in Massachusetts in 4½ years. Kelly et al (40) found 4 homozygotes among approximately 141,000 infants whom they screened.

Etiology and Clinical Manifestations. The symptoms seem to be related to the accumulation of galactose-1-phosphate rather than to the increased blood levels of galactose and the hypoglycemia that are usually present. Manifestations of the disorder only follow the ingestion of galactose (in the form of lactose in the milk-drinking neonate), and the fetus remains unharmed in utero since the mother is usually capable of metabolizing excessive galactose. Some heterozygous mothers, with a partial deficiency of uridyl transferase may have difficulty in metabolizing a large galactose load. Whether this has a deleterious effect on the homozygous fetus has not yet been determined.

Neonatal clinical signs may begin several days after the institution of milk feedings and include vomiting, diarrhea, failure to gain weight, persistent jaundice, hepatosplenomegaly and ascites. The mechanisms of toxicity are poorly understood. The fact that increased concentrations of galactose-1-phosphate within the erythrocyte impair oxygen uptake may be related to the pathologic changes of this disorder. Many of the infants appear to be susceptible to fulminating infection, especially *E. coli* septicemia. It is likely that the high incidence of infection secondary to lactose-fermenting organisms is related to the high concentrations of milk

sugars that accumulate in body fluids. The usual aminoaciduria and proteinuria are probably secondary to the toxic effects of abnormal metabolites on the renal tubules.

If the disorder remains unrecognized and milk feedings are continued, the clinical condition deteriorates. Malnutrition becomes severe, and hepatic enlargement leads to eventual cirrhosis. Cataracts may appear by the end of the first month of life, and psychomotor retardation becomes evident within several months after birth.

Treatment. The signs quickly disappear when lactose is completely removed from the diet. Appetite improves; hepatomegaly, jaundice, vomiting and diarrhea subside; and weight is gained. It is relatively easy to maintain a lactose-free diet during early infancy by using a non-carbohydrate-containing formula (such as Cho-Free) or one like Nutramigen, which contains sucrose as its carbohydrate. Maintaining this regimen becomes much more difficult, however, as the infant grows and more foods are added to the diet.

Since galactosemia is a treatable disorder, it must be suspected whenever suggestive signs are present. A test for reducing substances (such as with Clinitest) is positive in the presence of galactosuria. However, when the same urine specimen is tested specifically for glucose with a glucose oxidase reagent, none is detected. A definitive diagnosis is based on the finding of an abnormal galactose tolerance test and the complete absence of the enzyme galactose-1-phosphate uridyl transferase from the patient's red blood cells.

Screening. In 1974, testing of all newborn infants for galactosemia became mandatory in New York state, with blood samples being taken prior to discharge from the nursery.

Routine screening for RBC uridyl transferase activity has a dual purpose. The primary one is to determine which infants are homozygous for the disorder and therefore require immediate treatment. Since asymptomatic, heterozygous carriers usually have decreased levels of red blood cell uridyl transferase, these individuals may also be discovered, and the knowledge of being a heterozygous carrier is of potential importance in family planning.

Glycogen Storage Disease

Both type I (von Gierke's) and type II (Pompe's) glycogen storage disease may occasionally produce clinical signs during the neonatal period (33, 36). Although the primary manifestations of von Gierke's disease are hypoglycemia and acidosis, there are no apparent derangements of carbohydrate metabolism in Pompe's disease.

Von Gierke's disease is a disorder with an autosomal recessive mode of inheritance, characterized by absence of the hepatic enzyme G-6-phosphatase. Since this enzyme is necessary for the normal breakdown of hepatic glycogen to glucose, the affected infant may become profoundly hypoglycemic and acidotic unless fed at frequent intervals. Ketosis, rarely observed in the neonatal period, may be present in this disorder.

The diagnosis may be suspected when there is hepatomegaly associated with unresponsive hypoglycemia and an inability of the blood glucose concentration to rise following an injection of epinephrine or glucagon. The definitive diagnosis can be made following a liver biopsy, when abnormally large amounts of glycogen and absence of G-6-phosphatase are demonstrated.

In *Pompe's disease*, which is also inherited by an autosomal recessive gene, there is an absence of the enzyme α-1,4 glucosidase. It is characterized by accumulation of glycogen in cardiac and muscle tissue, but the liver generally is spared. Hypoglycemia is never present, and the primary manifestations in the neonatal period are those of cardiac failure, muscular weakness and respiratory insufficiency. Diagnosis is made by muscle biopsy, in which increased glycogen stores and absence of the involved enzyme are noted. While little can be done therapeutically for the affected infant, a prenatal diagnosis can be made (when there have been previous cases in the family) by the absence of α-1,4 glucosidase from amniotic fluid (see Ch. 14, Genetic Disorders).

Beckwith's Syndrome

In Beckwith's syndrome, hypoglycemia is associated with microcephaly, macroglossia, omphalocele or umbilical hernia, visceromegaly and pancreatic beta-cell hyperplasia (34). Since a recurrence among siblings is reported, the disorder is probably hereditary.

Leucine Sensitivity

Leucine-induced hypoglycemia may occasionally be seen during the neonatal period (35), and severe, symptomatic hypoglycemia may occur following a feeding that is relatively high in protein. A decline in blood glucose to 50% of the fasting level within 20 to 45 minutes following a leucine tolerance test is diagnostic.

Insulinoma

Islet cell adenomas, although rare in the neonatal period, have been reported to cause severe and persistent hypoglycemia (41). The definitive diagnosis can only be made following surgical exploration.

Transient Neonatal Diabetes

Transient neonatal diabetes mellitus is a very uncommon disorder of carbohydrate metabolism, that usually appears before three weeks of age and is most common in infants who are undergrown for gestational age. Spontaneous remission is usually noted within three or four months.

The presenting signs are glycosuria, hyperglycemia, dehydration, acidosis in the absence of ketosis. The etiology is poorly understood, but Shiff et al (42) speculate that fetal malnutrition may influence the maturational process of insulin-secreting cells well into postnatal life and that an exogenous source of insulin is required until the infant's endocrine pancreas begins to function normally.

Therapy consists of rehydration of the infant, reestablishment of normal acid-base and electrolyte balance, and control of the hyperglycemia by the administration of one to three units of crystalline insulin per kilogram per day. Although it is rare for true diabetes mellitus to manifest itself during the neonatal period, its appearance has been reported as early as the ninth day of life.

Hereditary Fructose Intolerance

Hereditary fructose intolerance (32), secondary to a marked deficiency of hepatic fructose-1-phosphate aldolase, is rarely diagnosed in the neonatal period. If fructose or a fructose-containing disaccharide, e.g., sucrose, is included in the diet, such signs as persistent jaundice, vomiting and failure to thrive may be observed. Definitive diagnosis is made by demonstrating decreased enzyme activity in fresh or deep frozen liver tissue specimens.

PROTEIN METABOLISM

FETAL PHYSIOLOGY

The anabolic state of the fetus depends on the optimal placental transfer of maternal amino acids. Evidence indicates that amino acids cross the placenta by an active transport mechanism against a concentration gradient and that this transport mechanism favors L-amino acids over D-amino acids. Curet (44) postulates their storage in uteroplacental tissue after they leave the maternal circulation and their subsequent release to the fetus as required by a process of simple diffusion.

Even though this active transport process favors accumulation of amino acids on the fetal side of the placenta, severe maternal protein malnutrition may nonetheless limit the amount that the fetus receives. Functional disorders of the placenta, such as toxemia of pregnancy, can also significantly decrease amino acid flow to the fetus, with subsequent impairment of fetal growth.

Most of the amino acids transferred from the mother to the fetus are utilized in tissue formation following their conversion to proteins by the fetal liver. As gestation progresses, more and more protein is utilized by the growing fetus, so that by the last months of pregnancy, the fetus is retaining about 2 g of protein per kilogram of body weight per day.

Prior to term, the fetal liver is deficient in certain enzymes involved in amino acid metabolism which are present in the full-term infant and older individuals. The absence of cystathionase, for example, prevents conversion of methionine to cysteine and cystine. The fetus is therefore dependent on a normal maternal dietary intake of these amino acids for optimal protein metabolism.

During the third month of fetal life, the total plasma protein concentration is about 1.6 g/100 ml, with about 90% of it albumin. By term, the concentration is almost 6 g/100 ml, with an albumin-globulin ratio of approximately 3:2.

There is evidence that protein and amino acids also serve as a significant substrate for energy metabolism in the fetus. Breakdown products of protein metabolism (e.g., urea, uric acid and ammonia N) have been found by Rubaltelli and Formentin (46) to be higher in umbilical arterial than in umbilical venous blood. Gresham et al (45) have found that at parturition urea concentrations are significantly higher in fetal umbilical arterial blood than in maternal venous blood. Just how much protein is utilized by the fetus to meet his growth requirements and how much is diverted towards energy expenditure remains to be determined.

NEONATAL PERIOD

Postnatal problems in protein metabolism arise primarily in premature infants. Deprived of a maternal source of amino acids, they must continue to receive enough protein to meet the requirements of a rapidly growing brain.

Two types of difficulties arise here, the first of which is providing protein in sufficient quantity to meet the infant's growth needs. Since oral intake is limited by both a poor sucking reflex and a reduced gastric capacity during the first week of life, the premature infant usually receives a suboptimal protein intake by the oral route during this period.

The second type of problem involves the composition of the protein that the infant receives. Because of hepatic enzyme immaturity (47), protein containing a low content of cystine and a high quantity of methionine may not be ideal for optimal growth. Enzymes that metabolize phenylalanine and tyrosine also function poorly in the preterm infant. Since excessive blood concentrations of these two amino acids may lead to intellectual impairment, care must be taken to limit their intake.

The optimal protein intake for premature infants, both by the oral and parenteral routes, is discussed in the section Feeding the Low-Birth-Weight Infant and in the section Total Parenteral Alimentation, Chapter 10.

Several disorders of protein metabolism may affect the newborn infant, several of which are treatable.

PHENYLKETONURIA

Phenylketonuria (PKU), an inborn error of the amino acid phenylalanine, has a deleterious effect on the CNS that is amenable to preventative therapy. Transmitted by an autosomal recessive gene, it affects about 1:10,000 infants born in the United States. Its incidence is highest among fair-skinned people of northern European descent; it is found very infrequently in dark-skinned races.

ETIOLOGY

In the absence of the enzyme phenylalanine hydroxylase (Fig. 12–2), which converts phenylalanine to tyrosine, phenylalanine accumulates in the blood (48). By the alternate pathway of transamination, phenylpyruvic acid forms and is subsequently either reduced to phenyllactic acid or decar-

boxylated to form phenylacetic acid. The latter compound may be conjugated to form phenylacetyl glutamine. The accumulation of these metabolites in unusually large quantities is responsible for severe brain damage, and mental retardation occurs in most children affected by this disorder. Experimental evidence suggests that CNS toxicity may be caused by the abnormal metabolite accumulation (such as phenylpyruvate) rather than by the excessively high phenylalanine level per se. Perry et al (57) suggest that that the mental retardation in PKU may be associated with decreased levels of the amino acid glutamine, which is sometimes observed in this disorder.

FETAL PHYSIOLOGY

Although the enzymatic defect is present, the growing homozygous fetus appears to be protected in utero from the deleterious effects of PKU. It is speculated that when levels of phenylalanine rise in the affected fetus, the active transport mechanism of amino acids across the placenta prevents further transfer from mother to fetus. The toxic effects of this disorder begin to appear only after birth.

Studies conducted on the offspring of phenylketonuric mothers have shown that they are usually heterozygotes. Widespread evidence indicates that the vast majority of these fetuses have severe intrauterine growth retardation, an extremely high incidence of birth defects, microcephaly, subsequent mental retardation and convulsions (52, 56, 58). The very high maternal phenylalanine levels in women on an unrestricted diet cause marked elevations in fetal concentrations of this amino acid, which are reflected by marked increases in amniotic fluid phenylalanine concentrations. As a normal pregnancy progresses, the amniotic fluid concentrations of all amino acids decline steadily, but the opposite appears to be true in pregnant women with PKU (59).

Because of recent advances in the treatment of this disorder, more and more women with PKU will become potential

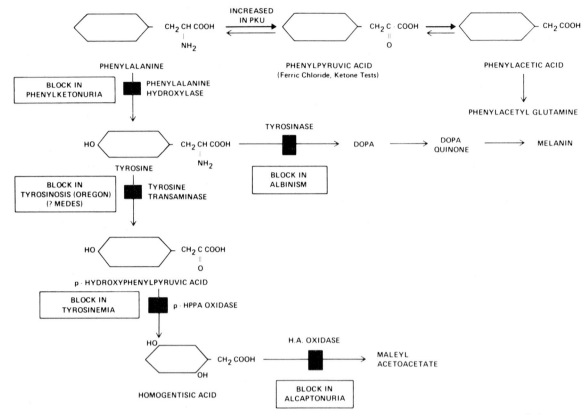

FIG. 12–2. Phenylalanine and tyrosine metabolism. (Frimpter GW: N Engl J Med 289:835, 1973. Reprinted by permission.)

bearers of children. Two options are open to these women: 1) they may practice complete contraception and refrain from having any children or 2) they may maintain a low-phenylalanine diet during pregnancy. Arthur and Hulme (49) report the birth of an infant of normal intelligence to a phenylketonuric mother whose blood phenylalanine concentration was maintained between 2 and 6 mg/100 ml during pregnancy by means of a synthetic low-phenylalanine diet.

NEONATAL DIAGNOSIS

Since the brain is undamaged at birth and the harmful effects of the disorder take weeks or months to appear, immediate diagnosis on a biochemical rather than clinical basis is necessary. A therapeutic regimen can prevent many of the ravages of this disorder and allow most phenylketonuric infants to lead a normal, or near normal, life. Because of this, testing for PKU has

become a routine nursery practice, and most states now mandate this testing by law.

The most effective and inexpensive available means of detecting PKU in large numbers of very young infants is by the bacterial inhibition method introduced by Guthrie in 1960 (53), with which blood phenylalanine levels of over 6 mg/100 ml may be detected. A drop of the infant's blood is allowed to fill a circle on a piece of filter paper. After the blood has dried, these filter papers are usually forwarded to a central health department laboratory where large-scale testing is performed. The filter paper with blood is incubated with *B. subtilis* and β-2-thienylalanine, a phenylalanine analogue that inhibits the growth of the bacteria. If phenylalanine is present in the blood in significant concentrations, the growth inhibition is overcome and the microorganism grows. There may, however, be false positive and negative results. Elevated levels may be detected in premature infants who are on a relatively high protein and low ascorbic acid intake, this elevation usually being associated with increased tyrosine concentrations (see section, Tyrosine Metabolism). False negative findings may occur in an affected infant who has not yet received any milk feedings or in those whose blood samples were taken before phenylalanine concentrations had a chance to become elevated. Therefore, the test should not be performed unless the infant has been on milk feedings for at least two or three days.

If this screening test reveals a phenylalanine concentration of more than 6 mg/100 ml, further testing for phenylalanine by biochemical methods is indicated. Serum phenylalanine concentrations greater than 30 mg/100 ml are presumptive evidence of PKU and are usually associated with tyrosine concentrations of less than 5 mg/100 ml.

Urinary screening for the detection of PKU in the neonatal period is contraindicated. Positive Phenistix or ferric chloride tests, which depend on the presence of phenylpyruvic acid in the urine, usually do not occur unless the serum phenylalanine concentration exceeds 20 mg/100 ml.

CLINICAL MANIFESTATIONS

Signs of PKU do not appear in the neonatal period unless the infants have been exposed in utero to maternal disease. The first sign to appear is usually vomiting, which is often present by the end of the first month of life. Irritability may also appear at about this time. Eczema, which is secondary to abnormal tyrosine metabolism, appears in about 25% of affected infants but is rarely seen before the third or fourth month. The peculiar, "mousy" smell of urine of phenylketonuric infants is another relatively early finding, but this is almost never encountered in the neonatal period. Convulsions, frank neurologic and EEG abnormalities and cortical atrophy are later findings.

TREATMENT AND PROGNOSIS

The prognosis of PKU depends to a large extent, but not completely, on when a special low-phenylalanine diet is started (54, 55). For each ten weeks that treatment is delayed, there is an estimated five-point decrease in the potential intelligence quotient.

The use of specially prepared low-phenylalanine formulas such as Lofenolac rapidly lowers the blood phenylalanine concentration, often below the normal level of 2 to 6 mg/100 ml. Since the excessive restriction of phenylalanine may be associated with hematologic and osseous abnormalities, hypoglycemia and growth retardation, infants receiving this diet must have their blood phenylalanine concentrations determined at frequent intervals. By age three or four years, significant brain growth has ceased, and dietary phenylalanine restriction may be lessened without any adverse neurologic effects.

Although most observers accept the fact that a low-phenylalanine diet started early in infancy largely prevents or at least mitigates intellectual and neurologic deterioration, some investigators question the efficacy of this diet in preventing mental retardation in affected infants (50, 51).

The low-phenylalanine diet must of course be reinstituted in any woman who is either pregnant or contemplating pregnancy.

TYROSINE METABOLISM

Levine et al (61) first described a transient defect in the metabolism of the amino acid tyrosine that most commonly occurs in low-birth-weight infants receiving a high-protein intake. The enzymes responsible for tyrosine metabolism (tyrosine transaminase and p-hydroxyphenylpyruvic oxidase), whose activity is normally sluggish in infants of low gestational age, are further inhibited by high dietary protein ingestion. This causes a temporary elevation of blood tyrosine concentrations; phenylalanine concentrations are sometimes elevated as well.

Avery et al (60) investigated 15,000 infants and found that 10% of full-term infants had mild tyrosinemia during the first week of life, whereas 30% of premature infants were severely affected. Tyrosine levels declined with increasing gestational age. In those infants of lowest gestational age, tyrosine levels were most elevated in the presence of a high-protein intake (6 g/kg/day). Ascorbic acid, which protects the involved enzyme against inactivation by its substrate, was only partially successful (at a dose of 60 mg/day) in lowering tyrosine levels in infants on high-protein diets. Although some lethargy was noted in infants with the highest tyrosine levels, no permanent neurologic sequelae could be related to them by this group.

Partington (64) also detected high levels of blood tyrosine (greater than 10 mg/100 ml) in infants of low birth weight and gestational age, but could not detect any signs in those infants with elevated levels.

Watkins et al (65) found that one or two injections of 100 mg of ascorbic acid significantly lowered blood tyrosine levels even in those premature infants receiving high-protein intakes.

The harmlessness of elevated blood tyrosine levels in low birth weight infants was questioned by Menkes et al (63). Psychologic testing performed on seven and eight-year-old, ex-premature infants whose blood tyrosine levels had been monitored during their stay in the nursery associated elevated tyrosine levels in infants whose birth weight was more than 2000 g with significantly decreased intellectual performance, especially in the area of visual perceptions.

Mamunes et al (62) followed 36 full-term infants with severe tyrosinemia. At age three to five years, these children demonstrated impaired visual discrimination, verbal fluency, conceptualization and auditory discrimination.

While further studies are needed, it would appear that high-protein diets should be avoided in newborn infants unless blood tyrosine concentrations can be carefully monitored.

UNCOMMON DISORDERS OF AMINO ACID AND PROTEIN METABOLISM

There is an ever-increasing list of inborn errors of amino acid and protein metabolism that are known to affect man (68, 74), but which are rarely encountered as clinical entities during the neonatal period.

MAPLE SYRUP URINE DISEASE

Like PKU, maple syrup urine disease is a genetically transmitted (autosomal recessive) disorder of amino acid metabolism that causes severe cerebral damage. Unlike PKU, however, it manifests itself during the first week of life, with death often ensuing by the end of the first month of life if no therapy is instituted. In this disorder, there is an accumulation of the branched chain amino acids (leucine, isoleucine and valine) in the blood; there is also an excessive excretion of these amino acids plus their keto acid analogs in the urine. The enzymatic defect may be in the oxidative decarboxylation of these keto acids.

The diagnosis is suspected in infants who have been apparently well for the first few days of life, but who subsequently develop lethargy, poor suck, dyspnea, sluggish Moro reflex, muscular rigidity and often convulsions and whose urine has a smell reminiscent of maple syrup. The diagnosis can be confirmed by chromatographic examination of the blood and urine. Dancis et al (67) demonstrated that the enzymatic defect can be identified in white blood cells and cultures of skin fibroblasts.

If left untreated, the disease is progressively fatal, with pathologic examination of the brain revealing evidence of cerebral degeneration.

Treatment consists of a diet low in leucine, isoleucine and valine. This is accomplished with a synthetic amino acid formula that has a low concentration of the involved branched chain amino acids. Success with this mode of therapy leads to normal neurologic development (87).

ISOVALERICACIDEMIA

Isovalericacidemia is a rare disorder that leads to severe, resistant metabolic acidosis, convulsions and death in the neonatal period. The urine and sweat have a characteristic odor of sweaty feet. Serum concentrations of isovaleric acid 1500 times the normal value have been reported (73). The disorder is caused by the absence of an enzyme responsible for the dehydrogenation of isovalerylcoenzyme A.

METHYLMALONIC ACIDEMIA

Methylmalonic acidemia is an inborn error of amino acid metabolism related to the branched chain aminoacidurias which leads to acidosis and failure to thrive in infancy (65a, 68). In one form of the disorder, serum concentrations of methylmalonic acid can be decreased by administration of extremely high doses of vitamin B_{12}. In one instance where a previous child died with this disorder, a large dose of vitamin B_{12} given to the mother during a successive pregnancy brought about decreased serum concentrations of methylmalonic acid in an affected fetus.

ALBINISM

Albinism is a genetically transmitted (autosomal recessive) defect in the conversion of tyrosine to melanin, caused by the absence of the enzyme tyrosinase, so that melanin cannot be produced by the melanocyte. This disorder may affect all areas of the body (universal albinism) or localized portions of the body.

The incidence of albinism varies from about 1:5,000 to 1:25,000 deliveries. It is of little clinical importance in the neonatal period and may not be easily recognized in light-skinned races. With advancing years, however, albinos develop photophobia, decreased visual acuity and increased sensitivity of the skin to sunlight with an excessively high degree of susceptibility to skin cancer.

HOMOCYSTINURIA

Homocystinuria is an autosomal recessive defect of amino acid metabolism marked by the absence or decrease in activity of the enzyme cystathionine synthetase. This results in a progressive accumulation of homocystine and methionine in the blood and urine, with clinical manifestations such as intellectual impairment and dislocated lens evident by the second or third year of life.

Although clinical manifestations do not appear in the neonatal period, if dietary restriction of methionine and supplementation with cystine is begun very early in life (69), normal development may ensue.

LESCH-NYHAN SYNDROME

The Lesch-Nyhan syndrome is a sex-linked recessive disorder of amino acid metabolism caused by an absence of the enzyme hypoxanthine-guanine phosphoribosyl transferase, which leads to severe mental retardation, spasticity and self-mutilation (70).

The diagnosis can be made antenatally by demonstration of absence of the enzyme in cells cultured from amniotic fluid. Although clinical signs are not apparent in affected neonates, extremely high serum uric acid concentrations are seen. Treatment with allopuranol (a xanthine oxidase inhibitor) in the neonatal period is successful in reducing uric acid levels but not in preventing later manifestations of the disease (71).

HYPERAMMONEMIA

Hyperammonemia is an inborn error of ammonia metabolism associated with the absence of the enzyme ornithine transcarbamylase (OTC) and reported to be a cause of neonatal death (66). Partial absence of this enzyme is associated with elevated blood ammonia levels, failure to thrive and mental retardation in female infants after the neonatal period, but total absence of the enzyme, which is associated with extraordinarily high ammonia levels, coma and death, is observed only in males, suggesting that the defect may be transmitted as a sex-linked trait. Although reduction in protein intake has been partially successful in the treatment of affected females, it was of no benefit in the newborn male infant, who expired (66).

TABLE 12–4. Total Fetal Lipid Content at Various Stages of Gestation

Fetal age (weeks)	Fetal weight (grams)	Fetal lipids (grams)	Percent of lipids
12–14	20	0.102	0.5
18–20	200	1.0	0.5
24–25	635	16.9	2.6
36–37	2240	156.8	7.0
40–42	3240	295.8	9.0

(Harding: Clin Obstet Gynecol 14:685, 1971)

LIPID METABOLISM

Lipids play an essential biologic role in both the fetal and neonatal periods (78, 83). Triglycerides, or neutral fats, must be stored during gestation to provide a concentrated source of calories for the newborn infant. Fat also serves as a thermal insulator and mechanical cushion for the neonate.

Other lipids, such as phospholipids and sterols, are essential for both histologic and physiologic development in the perinatal period.

FETAL DEVELOPMENT

The lipid content of the embryo during the early weeks of gestation is minimal. Between the first and ninth months of pregnancy, however, fetal lipid increases 300-fold, so that at term it comprises 9% to 16% of the total body weight (Table 12–4).

Adipose tissue becomes grossly apparent at about the 24th week of gestation, but it is not until about the 34th week that marked fat deposition (5 to 10 g/day) occurs. This development coincides with increased pancreatic islet cell function, and presumably the lipogenic activity of insulin is associated with the increased rate of fat deposition.

Triglycerides are synthesized within the fat cell from free fatty acids and glycerol. During the first two trimesters the fetus is essentially incapable of synthesizing free fatty acids, which are primarily derived from the maternal circulation. During the third trimester free fatty acids are largely of fetal origin, being synthesized from glucose and acetate precursors.

Ordinarily fat is not utilized for energy metabolism during gestation, the fetus being primarily dependent on glucose as a source of calories. Under certain abnormal circumstances, however, such as hypoxia, the fetus is capable of utilizing fat.

Fat is mainly stored in adipose tissue, although it is found in such other organs as the heart, liver, kidneys and skeletal muscle. Two types of adipose tissue develop during fetal life: 1) white adipose tissue and 2) brown adipose tissue. The major function of white adipose tissue is to provide an energy reserve (each gram of fat yields 9 calories) in the face of starvation or semistarvation during the neonatal period, whereas brown adipose tissue is mainly concerned with heat production during exposure to subthermoneutral environmental temperatures.

Composed of adipocytes containing a single lipid vacuole, white adipose tissue is widely distributed throughout the body. In addition to being a storehouse of energy reserves, it acts as an insulator against heat loss and serves as a mechanical cushion against trauma to the deep organs of the body.

Primarily located in the intrascapular space and mediastinum, brown adipose tissue (see Ch. 13, Thermoregulation) reaches maximal anatomic and physiologic development at term and begins to regress several weeks postpartum. Histologically it is differentiated from white adipose tissue in that each cell has many lipid-containing vacuoles, together with a high concentration of cytochrome-containing oxidative enzymes in the mitochondria (Fig. 12–3). Depletion of fat from these cells imparts a

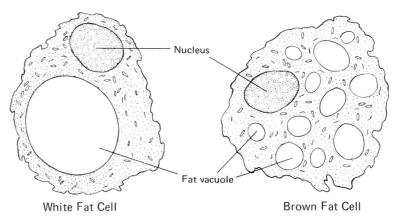

White Fat Cell   Brown Fat Cell

FIG. 12–3. Comparative structure of brown and white fat cells.

yellowish brown cast to the tissue, thus the name.

In infants who are small for gestational age because of malnutrition in utero, the amount of fat (brown and white adipose tissue) accumulated during gestation is diminished. This condition may be due both to an inadequate supply of glucose reaching the fetus from the maternal circulation and to an enzymatic defect interfering with the deposition of fat in adipose tissue. The low total body fat content of premature infants is due to shortened gestation rather than to a defect in the deposition of fat.

Dysmature and postmature infants, whose growth is normal until late in gestation, also show a decrease in the amount of fat in subcutaneous tissue. In this set of circumstances fat deposition proceeds normally until the fetus is faced with a decrease in its supply of glucose and oxygen, at which time fat stores (together with glycogen) are depleted to meet the energy requirements of the compromised fetus.

An excessive deposition of fat is observed in the fetuses of diabetic mothers presumably owing to the lipogenic activity of insulin, excessive quantities of which are secreted by the endocrine pancreas of these fetuses.

NEONATAL PERIOD

At parturition, carbohydrate is the major source of energy for the infant. Very shortly thereafter plasma concentrations of glycerol and free fatty acids increase sharply (82, 85), accompanied by a decline in the RQ. It is not until feedings are well established that the phenomenon is reversed (see section Carbohydrate Metabolism). Severely hypoxemic infants, however, are unable to mobilize fatty acids to meet their energy requirements (79).

Premature infants and those who are small for gestational age, because they enter extrauterine life with grossly inadequate fat stores, face an acute energy deficit (see section Feeding the Low-Birth-Weight Infant). Their survival is threatened unless adequate caloric intake—which can both meet ongoing energy requirements and provide a substrate for growth of the infants (including deposition of fat in adipose tissue—is assured.

Maintaining a thermoneutral environment in low-birth-weight infants during the early neonatal period supports survival, presumably through the preservation of limited fat stores (77). The lipolysis that occurs in brown adipose tissue secondary to chemical thermogenesis depletes this tissue of its triglyceride stores. There is some evidence that the triglyceride of brown adipose tissue can be replenished by transfer of fatty acids from white adipose tissue, the procedure ultimately depleting the latter organ of its fat reserves (78).

Adequate storage of fat during the latter stage of gestation is vital if the newborn infant is to adapt successfully to the extra-uterine environment.

The number, rather than the size, of fat cells in infants determines the likelihood of obesity (80). For infants with a normal cell count, subsequent obesity is easier to treat.

HYPERLIPOPROTEINEMIA

Of several biochemically distinct forms of genetically determined hyperlipidemia, familial hypercholesterolemia (type II hyperlipidemia), a relatively common condition associated with premature onset of arteriosclerotic heart disease, may be detectable in the neonatal period.

Although abnormal physical findings are absent at this time, several investigators suggest that elevations of umbilical cord blood levels of low density lipoproteins and total cholesterol are diagnostic of the disorder (76, 81). Other investigators are unable to confirm this finding (77).

Since early diagnosis may lead to preventive treatment, routine screening of cord blood for lipids and cholesterol would become part of the nursery routine if further studies confirmed the correlation between elevated levels and development of hyperlipoproteinemia.

FEEDING THE LOW-BIRTH-WEIGHT INFANT

The optimal approach to the feeding of low-birth-weight infants is a matter of long-standing controversy. Early alimentation has been associated with increased rates of survival (93, 102), but while several types of early feeding regimens have been advocated, none has yet been proven superior to any other. In addition to the effect on overall survival in these infants, concern also exists about the long-term effects of inadequate nutrition (including both total calories and protein intake) in a rapidly growing CNS (100). Intrauterine malnutrition that has resulted in impaired growth of the CNS (104) may compound this problem in certain infants. Caloric stores are minimal in low-birth-weight infants, and since their nutritional requirements are high, a means of meeting these needs must be found.

The question of when to begin feeding low-birth-weight infants was raised during the 1920s, when Hess and Lundeen (97) advocated early feeding of breast milk to premature infants. Fasting and thirsting of low-birth-weight infants for 36 to 96 hours became customary in the 1940s and 1950s, partly because of the danger of aspiration of feedings and partly because of the belief that edematous premature infants excreted water and solutes more efficiently when they were not fed during the first few days of life (103). Smallpiece and Davies (102) found that premature infants who received early feedings of breast milk had a prolonged survival. Cornblath et al (93) showed that early IV infusions of glucose and water were responsible for increased survival when compared to a regimen of either total starvation or enteral glucose and water during the first three days of life. Early parenteral feedings reverse some of the catabolic processes accompanying starvation and protect against the development of hypoglycemia (89, 90).

Davies and Davis (95) suggest in a retrospective study that low caloric intake during the early neonatal period is associated with a relatively small head circumference (implying retarded brain growth), which continues into childhood.

Early parenteral feedings have also been shown to decrease serum bilirubin concentrations in both low-birth-weight infants and infants of diabetic mothers (98, 105). All of these findings justify early administration of adequate amounts of nutrients to low-birth-weight infants. It would be ideal if an intake of 60 to 80 calories/kg/day could be achieved with breast milk or formula feedings by the second day of life and advanced in rapid increments to about 120 calories/kg/day, the amount required for normal growth, but for several reasons the quantity of milk feedings that the infant receives must be increased at a much slower rate.

Premature infants have a limited gastric capacity (Table 12–5) and feedings must be introduced with great care since excessive

TABLE 12–5. Average Physiologic Capacity of the Stomach in the First Ten Days of Life

Day of life	Stomach capacity (ml/kg birth wt)
1	2
2	4
3	10
4	16
5	19
6	19
7	21
8	23
9	25
10	27

(Silverman WA: Dunham's Premature Infants, 3rd ed. New York: Harper & Row, 1961)

gastric distension may rupture the stomach. In addition, the danger of regurgitation with subsequent aspiration into the lungs and the high incidence of respiratory distress limit the volume of enteral feedings tolerated by premature infants during the early days of life.

Infants who are small for gestational age have a lower incidence of respiratory distress, greater gastric capacities and a better ability to suck than those of similar birth weight, but lower gestational age. However, they also have greater caloric requirements and a higher incidence of hypoglycemia, and their total nutritional requirements often cannot be met by enteral feedings during the early days of life.

Several techniques have improved the enteral feeding of low-birth-weight infants. Because infants with gestational ages of less than 32 to 34 weeks cannot coordinate nutritive sucking and swallowing, methods have been developed that permit the introduction of either formula or breast milk into their stomachs. With intermittent gavage feedings, a soft rubber No. 8 French catheter is introduced into the stomach through the mouth before each feeding and removed after its conclusion. A second method, which we have employed and found satisfactory, is the use of the indwelling polyvinyl nasogastric feeding tube (either No. 3½ or No. 5 French). These tubes are chemically inert and may be left in place for at least a week without causing irritation.

Bradycardia, secondary to vagal stimulation, may occasionally be encountered during insertion of a tube via the esophagus into the stomach (92).

NUTRITIONAL REQUIREMENTS AND FEEDING REGIMENS

Although there is no clear-cut definition of optimal weight gain in low-birth-weight infants, the figure of 15 g/kg/day is usually used (96). This can be accomplished with an average caloric intake of 120 calories/kg/day (with a range of 110 to 140 calories/kg/day), under thermoneutral conditions. Requirements may be somewhat higher in infants who are small for gestational age and have high resting metabolic rates. Accelerated rates of weight gain can be achieved by increasing caloric intake, but there is no biologic evidence that this is advantageous to the infant.

Both human breast milk and many commercially available formulas have a caloric content of 20 calories/oz (0.67 cal/ml). In order to achieve a caloric intake of 120 calories/kg/day, a fluid intake of 180 ml/kg/day is therefore required, and this quantity usually exceeds gastric capacity during the first seven to ten days of life. To avoid this problem, several more highly concentrated formulas have been developed containing 24 and 27 calories/oz (0.8 and 0.9 calories/ml, respectively). The electrolyte content of these formulas is adequate to meet growth needs without exceeding the limited renal concentrating ability of 600 to 800 mOsm/l during the early days of life.

Protein

The optimal protein requirement for premature infants is not known. Full-term infants grow at a normal rate with the protein provided by human breast milk (about 2 g/kg/day) in the usual daily volume of about 200 ml/kg/day. The premature infant requires at least 3 to 4 g protein/kg/day contained in a modified cow's milk formula in order to grow at an optimal rate (94).

Räihä (100) points out that cow's milk protein, which is predominantly casein, contains a low concentration of cystine, an essential amino acid for premature infants, and relatively high concentrations of phenylalanine and tyrosine, which may have adverse effects on the CNS. Human milk, on the other hand with a 3:2 lactalbumin-casein ratio, has a relatively high cystine content and low concentrations of phenylalanine and tyrosine. Räihä then speculates that the quality as well as the quantity of protein that a premature infant receives in his diet is important in providing for optimal growth.

A variety of commercially prepared formulas (Table 12–6) are available for use in low-birth-weight infants, varying in their caloric and protein content and in the qualitative composition of the protein (SMA and Similac PM 60:40 have lactalbumin-casein ratios of 3:2, whereas most of the other prepared formulas have ratios similar to that of cow's milk).

Further prospective clinical trials are necessary before a judgment can be made concerning optimal protein requirements in this group of infants.

Carbohydrates

Carbohydrates serve primarily as a source of calories for energy metabolism. Except for rare instances of specific intolerance states, all of the commonly used carbohydrates are easily absorbed from the GI tract and metabolized by low-birth-weight infants.

Fats

Although fats comprise a major source of dietary calories, normal growth is possible even when they are absent from the diet, e.g., in infants who are receiving total parenteral alimentation. Because of relatively poor intestinal fat absorption in low-birth-weight infants, most artificial formulas use unsaturated vegetable oils which are more easily absorbed than animal fats. Medium-chained triglycerides have been used experimentally as a source of dietary fat in low-birth-weight infants, with improvement in weight gaining and a decrease in stool fat loss (101a).

Vitamins

Vitamins are added to all proprietary formulas, but the small volumes that are initially given to low-birth-weight infants necessitate a supplementary source. Most of the commercially available vitamin supplements contain sufficient vitamins A, B_{12}, C, D and E, pyridoxine, niacin, pantothenic acid, folic acid and riboflavin.

TABLE 12–6. Composition of Human Milk, Cow's Milk and Commercial Formulas (per 100 ml)

Formula	Protein (g)	Carbo-hydrate (g)	Fat (g)	Calories	Comments
Cow's Milk	3.3	4.8	3.7	67	
Enfamil 20	1.5	7.0	3.7	67	
Enfamil 24	1.8	8.3	4.5	81	
Human Milk	0.9–1.2	7.0	3.5	67	
Nutramigen	2.2	8.6	2.6	67	Protein hydrolysate, carbohydrate is sucrose
Prosobee	2.6	3.8	5.7	67	Protein derived from soy beans
Similac 20	1.8	7.0	3.6	67	
Similac 24	2.2	8.4	4.3	81	
Similac 27	2.5	9.4	4.9	91	
Similac PM 60:40	1.6	7.6	3.5	67	Lactalbumin-casein ratio 3:2 low solute content
SMA 20	1.5	7.2	3.6	67	Lactalbumin-casein ratio 3:2 low solute content
SMA 24	1.8	8.64	4.32	81	Lactalbumin-casein ratio 3:2 low solute content

Iron

Although dietary iron usually cannot be utilized in hematopoiesis during the first four to six weeks of life, it is nonetheless absorbed in the GI tract and stored within the reticuloendothelial system for future use. Low-birth-weight infants, whose iron reserves are lower than those of normal full-term infants, should be fed formulas containing iron in order to prevent iron deficiency anemia during infancy.

Feeding Regimens

The feeding regimen must be individualized for each low-birth-weight infant, taking into account the birth weight, gestational age and general clinical condition, e.g., respiratory distress, vomiting and abdominal distension. Enteral feedings that do not fully meet the infant's nutritional requirements are supplemented with an IV infusion of glucose and water until the infant can tolerate about 100 ml/kg/day of fluids by the enteral route.

Several new methods that bypass the stomach as the portal of entry for nutrients have been described in the late 1960s and early 1970s and will be discussed later in this section. The following are examples of feeding regimens for various categories of low-birth-weight infants.

Small Premature Infants. Small premature infants (birth weights below 1500 g and gestational ages below 30 to 32 weeks) usually require an IV infusion of 10% glucose solution, which should be started within the first four hours of life. In the absence of any evidence of serious illness, e.g., respiratory distress or abdominal distension, enteral feedings can also be instituted at this time, either by indwelling feeding tube or intermittent gavage. Total fluid intake should be limited to 70 to 80 ml/kg during the first 24 hours of life and increased by 10 ml/kg/day until a daily fluid intake of about 150 ml/kg is attained. The volume given by the enteral route should be subtracted from the fluid infused intravenously. The first two enteral feedings should consist of 2 ml of 10% glucose solution per kg of body weight. If these are tolerated, formula can be introduced at the third feeding. Although some clinicians prefer one-half strength formula during the first 48 hours of life, we have encountered no difficulty using full-strength formula.

A feeding schedule every three hours is usually well tolerated. Prior to each feeding, gastric contents should be aspirated, measured and placed back into the stomach, and the volume subtracted from the volume of the feeding. With each successive day small increments may be made in the volume of each feeding (Fig. 12–3) until the caloric intake reaches 120 calories/kg/day. The IV infusion may be discontinued when the infant is receiving about 100 ml (80 to 90 calories/kg/day) by the enteral route. Enteral feedings should be immediately discontinued if there is evidence of respiratory distress, vomiting, diarrhea, abdominal distension or any other debilitating condition, and reinstitution deferred until abnormal signs have subsided. Bottle feedings, using a premature nipple, can generally be started when the infant reaches a postconceptional age of 32 to 34 weeks. Until the time when stable body temperature can be maintained in a room air environment, these infants are fed while in the incubator. There should be

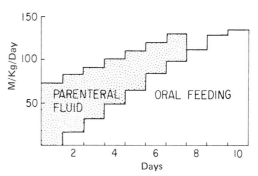

FIG. 12–4. Combined parental and oral feeding in ml/kg/day for a newborn infant weighing less than 1500 g at birth who is unable to suck. The proportion of oral and parenteral fluids will vary with the ability of the individual infant to tolerate oral fluids. (Babson SG: J Pediatr 79:694, 1971)

no time pressure placed on the nurse, since a protracted period of time may be required to complete feedings.

Larger Premature Infants. Larger and more-mature preterm infants usually pose less difficulty. In the absence of serious medical problems, they suck well and can often be maintained on oral feedings alone, without a supplementary IV infusion. Feedings should be instituted within the first four to six hours of life. The first two should consist of 5 to 15 ml of 10% glucose water solution, depending on the infant's size and sucking ability. Following this, full strength formula (usually 24 calories/oz), can be started with daily increments of 5 to 10 ml/feedings. Either a three or four hourly feeding schedule may be maintained.

Small-For-Gestational-Age Infants. Infants who are small for gestational age (under the tenth percentile for birth weight) present special problems because of intrauterine malnutrition. Since they develop hypoglycemia easily and have poor fat stores and high resting metabolic rates, enteral feedings should be started, if possible, within the first two to four hours of life, with the caloric intake being advanced rapidly. In addition to oral feedings, an infusion of 10% or 15% glucose solution can be started in addition to the liberal oral feedings. As is the case with other small infants, the first two feedings should be glucose and water, followed by full-strength formula (see section Intrauterine Growth Retardation, Ch. 4).

Alimentation of sick infants who are unable to tolerate enteral feedings is discussed in the section Fluids and Electrolytes, Chapter 10.

Some basic principles apply to the feeding of all low-birth-weight infants. A thermoneutral environment should be maintained when caloric intake is low in order to minimize the expenditure of energy for maintenance of body temperature. Infants should be weighed at least three times a week (daily when receiving IV supplementation). A record should be maintained of intake and output, including regurgitated food and urinary and fecal losses.

Newer Feeding Methods

These conventional feeding methods do not provide an adequate protein intake until at least one week of age. The long-term effects of limited protein intake on a growing CNS are not known. Acceleration of enteral feedings to provide protein is often futile, especially when the infant is physiologically incapable of tolerating the relatively large volumes of fluid placed in his stomach. Several new methods of nonoral feeding for low-birth-weight infants, which were introduced in the 1970s, thus have the advantage of being able to provide a relatively large protein and caloric intake during the first days of life.

Total Parenteral Alimentation. There have been several reports concerning total parenteral alimentation for feeding very small infants (see section Fluids and Electrolytes, Ch. 10). Although infants treated with this regimen grew rapidly, potential complications countermand its routine clinical use except in those cases where the GI tract remains nonfunctional for a prolonged period of time.

Peripheral Alimentation. Several investigators have successfully supplemented oral feedings with IV infusions containing either a protein hydrolysate or L-amino acids (see section Fluids and Electrolytes, Ch. 10). Since the osmolarity of these solutions is considerably less than the osmolarity of solutions used for total parenteral alimentation, they can be successfully administered by a peripheral vein. In all of the series weight gain in the treated groups was superior to weight gain among infants who received enteral feedings supplemented by an IV infusion of 10% glucose. No differences in mortality were noted between study and control groups. Although this type of feeding regimen avoids many of the pitfalls of total parenteral alimentation, further evaluation, including long-term follow-up of infants is necessary.

Enteric Techniques. Two methods utilizing the GI tract to deliver a high-caloric input have been described. Landwirth et al (99) have continuously infused formula into the stomach using an indwelling nasogastric tube, while Cheek and Staub (91) and Rhea et al (101) have introduced formula directly into the jejunum by an indwelling nasojejunal tube. In the latter method the feedings enter the GI tract distal to the pyloric sphincter, eliminating the possibility of regurgitation and aspiration. Both methods must undergo further evaluation and be compared to techniques employing IV alimentation.*

Improved feeding techniques have contributed to a decrease both in morbidity and in mortality among low-birth-weight infants. Refinements must provide for optimal development of a rapidly growing CNS.

REFERENCES

1. Harries JT, Fraser AJ: Acidity of gastric contents of premature babies during the first 14 days of life. Biol Neonate 12:186, 1968
2. Khan AJ, Mehta S, Walia BSN: Basal gastric acid secretion in the newborn. Indian J Pediatri 6:608, 1969
3. Sheehy TW: Fetal disaccharidases. Am J Dis Child 121:464, 1971

CARBOHYDRATE METABOLISM

4. Amatayakul O, Cumming GR, Haworth JC: Association of hypoglycemia with cardiac enlargement and heart failure in newborn infants. Arch Dis Child 45:717, 1970
5. Anderson JM, Milner RDG, Stritch SJ: Pathological changes in the nervous system in severe neonatal hypoglycemia. Lancet 2:372, 1966
6. Baens GS, Lundeen E, Cornblath M: Studies of carbohydrate metabolism in the newborn infant. VI. Levels of glucose in blood in premature infants. Pediatrics 31:580, 1963
7. Barrett CT, Oliver TK Jr: Hypoglycemia and hyperinsulinism in infants with erythroblastosis fetalis. N Engl J Med 278:1260, 1968

* See Appendix A, Addendum 4.

8. Beard A, Cornblath M, Gentz J, Kellum M, Persson B, Zetterstrom R, Haworth JR: Neonatal hypoglycemia: a discussion. J Pediatr 79:314, 1971
9. Chase HP, Marlow RA, Dabiere CS, Welch NN: Hypoglycemia and brain development. Pediatrics 27:378, 1961
10. Cornblath M, Ganzon AF, Nicolopoulos D, Baens GS, Hollander RS, Gordon MW, Gordon HH: Studies of carbohydrate metabolism in the newborn infant. III. Some factors influencing the capillary blood sugar and the response to glucagon during the first hours of life. Pediatrics 27:378, 1961
11. Cornblath M, Schwartz R: Disorders of Carbohydrate Metabolism in Infancy. Philadelphia, Saunders, 1966
12. Cornblath M, Wybregt SH, Baens GS: Studies of carbohydrate metabolism in the newborn infant. VIII. Tests of carbohydrate tolerance in premature infants. Pediatrics 32:1007, 1963
13. Crenshaw C: Fetal glucose metabolism. Clin Obstet Gynecol 13:579, 1970
14. Dweck H, Cassady, G: Glucose intolerance in infants of very low birth weight. I. Incidence of hypoglycemia in infants of birth weights 1100 grams or less. Pediatrics 53:189, 1974
15. Haworth JC, McRae KN: The neurological and developmental effects of neonatal hypoglycemia. Can Med Assoc J 92:861, 1965
16. Hoet JJ: Normal and abnormal foetal weight gain. In: Foetal Autonomy. Edited by GEW Wolstenholme, M O'Connor. London, J & A Churchill, 1969
17. Jarrett IG, Jones GB, Potter BJ: Changes in glucose utilization during development of the lamb. Biochem J 90: 189, 1964
18. King KC, Butt J, Raivo K, Räihä N, Roux J, Teramo K, Wamaguchi K, Schwartz R: Human maternal and fetal insulin response to arginine. N Engl J Med 285:607, 1971
19. Light IJ, Sutherland JM, Loggie JM: Impaired epinephrine release in hypoglycemic infants of diabetic mothers. N Engl J Med 277:94, 1967
20. Marks V: An improved glucose oxidase method for determining blood, CSF and urine glucose levels. Clin Chim Acta 4:395, 1959
21. Melichar V, Novak M, Hahn P: Peculiarities in carbohydrate and lipid metabolism in hypotrophic infants. In: Intra-Uterine Dangers to Foetus. Edited by J Horsky, ZK Stembera. New York, Excerpta Medica Foundation, 1967
22. Obenshain SS, Adam PAJ, King KC, Teramo K, Raivio KO, Räihä N, Schwartz R: Human fetal insulin response to sustained maternal hyperglycemia. N Engl J Med 283:566, 1970
23. Pagliara AS, Karl IE, Haymond M, Kipnis DM: Hypoglycemia in infancy and childhood. Parts I and II. J Pediatr 82:365, 558, 1973
24. Pang SJ, Bleicher SJ: Pregnancy, diabetes and RBC 2,3-diphosphoglycerate (DPG) levels, (abstr). Diabetes 22:298, 1973
25. Patterson P, Phillips L, Wood C: Relationship

between maternal and fetal glucose during labor. Am J Obstet Gynecol 98:938, 1967

26. Pildes RS: Infants of diabetic mothers. N Engl J Med 289:902, 1973

27. Pildes RS, Forbes AE, Cornblath M: Studies of carbohydrate metabolism in the newborn infant. IX. Blood glucose levels and hypoglycemia in twins. Pediatrics 40:69, 1967

28. Shelly HJ: Carbohydrate metabolism in the foetus and newly-born. Proc Nutr Soc 28:42, 1969

29. Stenger V, Henry J, Cestaric E: Movements of glucose in the human pregnant uterus. Am J Obstet Gynecol 94:261, 1966

30. Stern L, Sorenkes TL, Räihä N: The role of the adrenal medulla in the hypoglycemia of fetal malnutrition. Biol Neonate 11:129, 1967

31. Zuspan FP, Whalley WH, Nelson GH: Placental transfer of epinephrine. I. Maternal-fetal metabolic alterations of glucose and non-esterified fatty acids. Am J Obstet Gynecol 95:284, 1966

UNCOMMON DISORDERS

32. Black, JA, Simpson K: Fructose intolerance. Br Med J 4:138, 1967

33. Brown BI, Brown, DH: The glycogen storage diseases, types I, II, IV, V, VII and unclassified glycogenosis. In: Carbohydrate Metabolism and Its Disorders. Edited by F Dickens, PJ Randles, WS Whalen. New York, Academic Press, 1968

34. Combs JT, Grunt JA, Brandt IC: New syndrome of neonatal hypoglycemia. Association with visceromegaly, macroglossa, microcephaly, and abnormal umbilicus. N Engl J Med 275:236, 1966

35. DiGeorge AM, Auerbach VH: Leucine-induced hypoglycemia: A review and speculations. Am J Med Sci 240:792, 1960

36. Field RA: Glycogen deposition diseases. In: The Metabolic Basis of Inherited Disease. Edited by JB Stanbury, JG Wyngaarden, DA Frederickson. New York, McGraw-Hill, 1960

37. Gitzelmann R: Hereditary galactokinase deficiency. a newly recognized cause of juvenile cataracts. Pediatr Res 1:14, 1967

38. Hansen RG, Bretthauer RK, Mayes J, Nordin JH: Estimation of frequency of occurrence of galactosemia in the population. Proc Soc Exp Biol Med 115:560, 1964

39. Isselbacher KJ: Galactosemia. In: The Metabolic Basis of Inherited Disease, 2nd ed. Edited by JB Stanbury, JB Wyngaarden, DS Fredrickson. New York, McGraw-Hill, 1966, p. 178

40. Kelly S, Katz S, Burns J: Screening for galactosemia in New York state. Public Health Rep 85:575, 1970

41. Salinas ED, Mangurten HH, Robert SS, Simon WH, Cornblath M: Functioning islet cell adenoma in the newborn. Pediatrics 41:646, 1968

42. Schiff, D, Colle E, Stern L: Metabolic and growth patterns in transient neonatal diabetes. N Engl J Med 287:119, 1972

43. Shih VE, Levy HI, Karolkewicz V: Galactosemia screening of newborns in Massachusetts. N Engl J Med 284:753, 1971

PROTEIN METABOLISM

44. Curet LB: Physiological aspects of amino acid transport across the placenta. Clin Obstet Gynecol 13:586, 1970

45. Greshan EL, Simons PS, Battaglia FC: Maternal-fetal urea concentration difference in man: metabolic significance. J Pediatr 79:809, 1971

46. Rubaltelli FF, Formentin PA: Ammonia nitrogen, urea and uric acid blood levels in mother and umbilical vessels at delivery. Biol Neonate 13:147, 1968

47. Sturman JA, Gaull G, Räihä NCR: Absence of cystathionase in human fetal liver. Science 169:74, 1970

PKU

48. Allen RJ, Heffelfinger JC, Masotti RE. Tsau MV: Phenylalanine hydroxylase activity in newborn infants. I. Relation to the appearance of metabolites in blood and urine in normal and enzyme deficient states. II. Relations to the clinical diagnosis of phenylketonuria. Pediatrics 33:512, 1964

49. Arthur LJH, Hulme JD: Intelligent, small for dates baby born to oligophrenic phenylketonuric mother after low phenylalanine diet during pregnancy. Pediatrics 46:235, 1970

50. Bessman SP: Legislation and advances in medical knowledge acceleration or inhibition? J Pediatr 69:334, 1966

51. Birch HG, Tizard J: The dietary treatment of phenylketonuria: not proven? Dev Med Child Neurol 9:9, 1967

52. Brown ES, Waisman HA: Mental retardation in four offspring of a hyperphenylalaninemic mother. Pediatrics 48:401, 1971

53. Guthrie R, Susi A: A simple phenylalanine method for detecting phenylketonuria in large populations of newborn infants. Pediatrics 32:338, 1963

54. Kany ES, Sollee ND, Gerald PS: Results of treatment and termination of the diet in PKU. Pediatrics 46:881, 1970

55. Knox WE: An evaluation of the treatment of phenylketonuria with diets low in phenylalanine. Pediatrics 26:1, 1960

56. Mabry CC, Denniston JC, Coldwell JG: Mental retardation in children of phenylketonuric mothers. N Engl J Med 275:1331, 1966

57. Perry TL, Hansen S, Tischler B: Glutamine depletion in phenylketonuria: a possible cause

of the mental defect. N Engl J Med 282:761, 1970

58. Stevenson RE, Huntley CC: Congenital malformations in offspring of phenlyketonuric mothers. Pediatrics 40:33, 1967

59. Thomas GH, Parmley TH, Stevenson RE, Howell RR: Developmental changes in amino acid concentrations in human amniotic fluid: abnormal findings in maternal phenylketonuria. Am J Obstet Gynecol 111:38, 1971

TYROSINE METABOLISM

60. Avery ME, Clow CL, Menkes JH, Ramos A, Scriver CR, Stern L, Wasserman BP: Transient tyrosinemia of the newborn: dietary and clinical aspects. Pediatrics 39:378, 1967

61. Levine S, Marples E, Gordon H: A defect in the metabolism of tyrosine and phenylalanine in premature infants: identification and assay of intermediary products. J Clin Invest 20:199, 1941

62. Mamunes P, Prince PE, Hunt PA, Hitchcock ES, Hoffman DE: Adverse sequelae in transient tyrosinemia of the term neonate, (abstr). Pediatr Res 7:193, 1973

63. Menkes JH, Chernick V, Ringel B: Effect of elevated blood tyrosine on subsequent intellectual development of premature infants. J Pediatr 69: 583, 1966

64. Partington MW: Neonatal tyrosinemia. Biol Neonate 12:316, 1968

65. Watkins ML, Crump EP, Hara S: Management of transient hyperphenylalaninemia and tyrosinemia in low-birth-weight Negro infants fed high-protein diets. J Natl Med Assoc 65:241, 1971

UNCOMMON DISORDERS OF AMINO ACID AND PROTEIN METABOLISM

65. Ampola MG, Mahoney MJ, Nakamura E, Tanaka K: In utero treatment of methylmalonic acidemia (MMA-emia) with vitamin B_{12}. Ped Research 8:387, 1974

66. Campbell AGM, Rosenberg LE, Snodgrass PJ, Nuzum CT: Ornithine transcarbamylase deficiency: a cause of lethal neonatal hyperammonemia in males. N Engl J Med 288:1, 1973

67. Dancis J, Hutzler J, Snyderman SE, Cox RP: Enzyme activity in classical and variant forms of maple syrup urine disease. J Pediatr 81:312, 1972

68. Frimpter GW: Aminoacidureas due to inherited disorders of metabolism. Parts I and II. N Engl J Med 289:835, 895, 1973

69. Komrower GM, Lambert AM, Cusworth DC, Westall RG: Dietary treatment of homocystinuria. Arch Dis Child 41:666, 1966

70. Lesch M, Nyhan WL. A familial disorder of uric acid metabolism and central nervous system function. Am J Med 36:561, 1964

71. Marks JF, Baum J, Keele DK, Kay JL: Lesch-Nyhan syndrome treated from early neonatal period. Pediatrics 42:357, 1968

72. Newman CGH, Wilson BDR, Callaghan P, Young L: Neonatal death associated with isolvaleric acidemia. Lancet 2:439, 1967

73. Synderman SE: Maple syrup urine disease. In: Amino Acid Metabolism and Genetic Variation. Edited by WL Nyhan. New York, McGraw-Hill, 1967, p 171

74. Stanbury JB, Wyngaarden JB, Frederickson DS: The Metabolic Basis of Inherited Disease, 3rd ed. New York, McGraw-Hill, 1972

LIPID METABOLISM

75. Darmady JM, Fosbrooke AS, Lloyd JK: Prospective study of serum cholesterol levels during first year of life. Br Med J 2:685, 1972

76. Glueck CJ, Heckman F, Schoenfeld M, Steiner P, Pearce W: Neonatal familial type II hyperlipoproteinemia: cord blood cholesterol in 1800 births. Metabolism 20:597, 1971

77. Hull D: Nutrition and temperature control in the newborn baby. Proc Nutr Soc 28:56, 1969

78. Harding PGR: The metabolism of brown and white adipose tissue in the fetus and newborn. Clin Obstet Gynecol 14:685, 1971

79. Harris RJ: Plasma nonesterified fatty acid and blood glucose levels in healthy and hypoxemic newborn infants. J Pediatr 84:578, 1974

80. Hirsh J, Knittle JL: Cellularity of obese and nonobese human adipose tissue. Fed Proc 29:1516, 1970

81. Kwiterovich PO, Levy RI, Frederickson DS: Neonatal diagnosis of familial type II hyperlipoproteinemia. Lancet 1:118, 1973

82. Novak M, Melichar V, Hahn P: Postnatal changes in the blood serum content of glycerol and FFA in human infants. Biol Neonate 7:179, 1964

83. Roux JF, Yoshioka T: Lipid metabolism in the fetus during development. Clin Obstet Gynecol 13:595, 1970

84. Sabata V, Stembera ZKS, Novak M: Levels of unesterified and esterified fatty acids in umbilical blood of hyposic fetuses. Biol Neonate 12:194, 1968

85. Zee P: Lipid metabolism in the newborn. II. Neutral lipids. Pediatrics 41:640, 1968

FEEDING THE LOW-BIRTH-WEIGHT INFANT

86. Auld PAM, Bhangananda P, Mehta S: The influence of an early caloric intake with I-V glucose on catabolism of premature infants. Pediatrics 37:592, 1966

87. Babson SG: Feeding the low-birth weight infant. J Pediatr 79:694, 1971

88. Beard AG, Panos TC, Marasigan BV,

Eminians J, Kennedy HF, Lamb J: Perinatal stress and the premature neonate. 2. Effect of fluid and calorie deprivation on blood glucose. Pediatrics 68:329, 1966

89. Cheek JA, Staub GF: Nasojejunal alimentation for premature and full term newborn infants. J Pediatr 82:955, 1973

90. Cordero L, Hon EH: Neonatal bradycardia following nasopharyngeal stimulation. J Pediatr 78:441, 1971

91. Cornblath M, Forbes AE, Pildes RS, Luebben G, Greengard J: A controlled study of fluid administration on survival of low birth weight infants. Pediatrics 38:547, 1966

92. Davidson M: Formula feeding of normal term and low birth weight infants. Pediatr Clin North Am 17:913, 1970

93. Davidson M, Levine SZ, Bauer CH, Dann M: Feeding studies in low-birth-weight infants. I. Relationships of dietary protein, fat and electrolyte to rates of weight gain, clinical courses, and serum chemical concentrations. J Pediatr 70:695, 1967

94. Davies PA, Davis JP: Very low birth weight and subsequent head growth. Lancet 2:1216, 1970

95. Gordon HH, Levine SZ: Respiratory metabolism in infancy and childhood. XVIII. Daily energy requirement of premature infants. Am J Dis Child 59:1185, 1940

96. Hess JH, Lundeen EC: The Premature Infant: Its Medical and Nursing Care. Philadelphia, Lippincott, 1941, p 309

97. Holt LE, Snyderman SE: The feeding of premature and newborn infants. Pediatr Clin North Am 13:1103, 1966

98. Hubbell JP, Drorbaugh JE, Rudolph AJ, Auld PAM, Cherry RB, Smith CA: "Early" versus "late" feeding of infants of diabetic mothers. N Engl J Med 265:835, 1961

99. Landwirth J: Continuous nasogastric infusion versus total intravenous alimentation (letter). J Pediatr 81:1037, 1972

100. Räihä NCR: Biochemical basis for nutritional management of preterm infants. Pediatrics 53:147, 1974

101. Rhea JW, Ghazzowi O, Weidman W: Nasojejunal feeding: an improved device and intubation technique. J Pediatr 82:951, 1973

101a. Roy CC, Ste-Marie M, Weber A, Bard H, Doray B: Correction of the "physiologic" malabsorption of the premature by a medium chain triglyceride (MCT) formula (abstr). Ped Research 8:385, 1974

102. Smallpiece V, Davies PA: Immediate feeding of premature infants with undiluted breast milk. Lancet 2:1349, 1964

103. Smith CA: Reasons for delaying the feeding of premature infants. Ann Paediatr Fenniae 3:261, 1957

104. Winick M: Cellular growth in intrauterine malnutrition. Pediatr Clin North Am. 17:69, 1970

105. Wu PYK, Teilmann P, Cabler M, Yaugn M, Metcalf J: "Early" versus "late" feeding of low birth weight neonates. Pediatrics 39:733, 1967

13

Thermoregulation

The importance of thermal environment in the care of low-birth-weight infants has been recognized since the latter part of the nineteenth century, when Budin was able to improve the survival rates of these infants by rearing them in incubators (7). However, a detailed understanding of thermoregulatory mechanisms in newborn infants did not evolve until the 1960s.

FETAL THERMOREGULATION

The growing fetus produces heat. To maintain a thermal steady state, mechanisms must be available for the dissipation of this heat, and a temperature differential between mother and fetus must thus exist.

During a cesarean section, it is obvious to the obstetrician that the gravid uterus and adnexa feel warmer than the surrounding tissues. There is also experimental evidence that the brain of the fetal lamb is 0.4° to 0.8° C warmer than maternal aortic blood and that umbilical arterial blood is warmer than umbilical venous blood (1).

Little is known about the mechanisms of fetal heat loss. The placenta is generally considered to be the major organ for heat exchange between fetal and maternal blood, although there is probably some loss by conduction to amniotic fluid and maternal tissues. In cases of fetal death, the temperature differential between mother and fetus disappears.

Following delivery, the homeothermic newborn infant still is faced with the problem of maintaining a constant body temperature, but at this point the problem becomes one of preserving (rather than dissipating) heat in the "cool" world outside of the uterus.

HEAT DISSIPATION

The newborn infant produces heat primarily through chemical means and dissipates heat through physical means. The balance of body temperature in the neonate probably is regulated by the hypothalamus (the central "thermostat"), which attempts to maintain a constant "set point" core temperature. This is the temperature at which the organism optimally functions at a minimal metabolic rate. In larger premature and full-term infants, this set point is approximately 37.0° C. Brück et al (6), however, have found that this may be somewhat lower in very small premature infants.

The thermosensitive cells of the CNS are responsive to changes both in blood temperature and afferent stimuli from peripheral thermoreceptors. Through a complex mechanism, the central integraters of temperature regulation attempt to strike a balance between heat production and heat loss (Figs. 13–1 and 13–2). When this mechanism is overwhelmed, usually by heat loss exceeding heat production in low-birth-weight infants, the physician caring for the infant must intervene to establish thermal balance.

The human infant readily loses heat to the environment because its surface area is relatively large in relationship to body weight. The full-term infant has 5% of the mass of an adult, but 15% of the surface area; in a low-birth-weight infant, this situation is exaggerated. Heat is lost by radiation, evaporation, conduction and con-

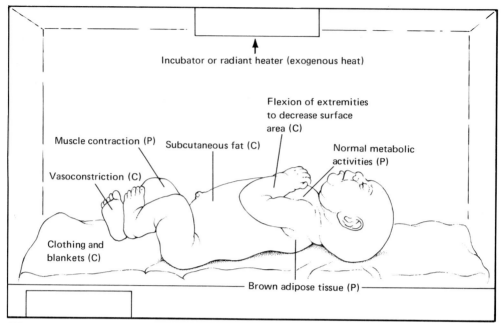

FIG. 13–1. Mechanisms of heat production (P) and conservation (C) in newborn infants.

FIG. 13–2. Mechanisms of heat loss in newborn infants.

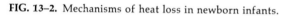

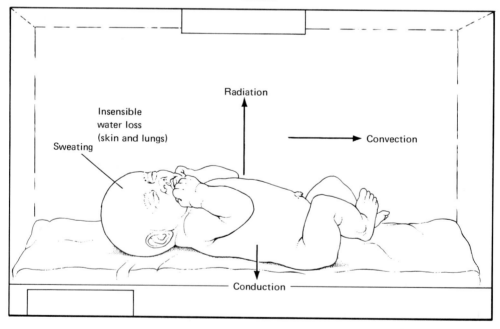

vection. Factors influencing heat loss are: surface area to body mass ratio, passage of moving air over the surface of the infant, surface conductivity of heat (dependent on effective tissue insulation, including clothing), effective air temperature,* relative humidity and physical characteristics of surrounding objects.

Tissue Insulation

The full-term infant is better adapted to protect himself against heat loss than is the low-birth-weight infant. The thick layer of subcutaneous tissue in the normally grown full-term infant provides insulation against loss of body heat to the environment. This layer is poorly developed both in premature infants and in those with intrauterine growth retardation, even when the gestational age is well advanced.

However, both normally grown full-term infants and those with intrauterine growth retardation can reduce body surface area by assuming a flexed posture, thus limiting loss of heat by radiation. The premature infant is unable to do this.

Heat loss is limited by peripheral vasoconstriction, which increases effective tissue insulation. This function is present even in infants of very low gestational age provided the CNS is intact.

In a warm environment peripheral blood vessels dilate, decreasing tissue insulation and enhancing dissemination of heat to the environment.

Radiant Heat Loss

Radiant heat loss accounts for much of the heat dissipated by the newborn infant to the environment. This can be decreased effec-

---

* Since the room air outside of the incubator is cooler than the air within the incubator, the inner wall temperature of the incubator will be lower than the incubator air temperature. The infant will therefore lose more heat by radiation to the incubator wall that it would if the incubator wall temperature were the same as the air temperature. For approximately each 7° C that the room air temperature falls below the incubator air temperature, 1° C must be subtracted from the latter to determine the effective air temperature of the incubator.

tively by insulating the infant with clothes and blankets, or in the case of a small premature infant, by placing him in a warm incubator.

Conduction and Convection

Heat loss by conduction occurs through direct contact of the skin with the immediate environment. Air is a relatively poor conductor of heat. If the unclothed infant is inadvertently placed on a metal or other highly conductive surface, this type of heat loss becomes a major factor.

Convective heat loss only occurs when a portion of the infant's skin is exposed to a stream of moving air.

Insensible Water Loss and Sweating

About one-fourth of the normal heat loss under basal conditions occurs by insensible water loss, which is evaporation of water through the skin and lungs. Fanaroff et al (14) have found, however, that in small premature infants (less than 1250 g), insensible water loss may be unusually large, especially during the first ten days of life. This may be due to thin skin that is extremely permeable and has an increased water content. Under usual thermal conditions, heat loss through sweating does not occur. In the presence of excessively high environmental temperatures, usually associated with deep body temperatures greater than 37.2° C, the full-term and larger premature infant can dissipate heat by sweating. In infants of less than 37 weeks' gestation, the ability to sweat is either absent or markedly impaired (22).

Because of the immaturity of the sweating apparatus in most premature infants, hyperthermia will usually ensue if they are placed in overheated incubators.

The ability to dissipate heat through either insensible water loss or sweating is decreased as the relative humidity increases. Increasing the relative humidity of incubators has, in fact, been one way of decreasing the heat loss in small premature infants (28). This method is, however, comparatively inefficient (25).

HEAT PRODUCTION

Since the newborn human infant loses heat rapidly, nature has provided an efficient method for increasing heat production. This process, called nonshivering or chemical thermogenesis, far surpasses the adult method of increasing heat production, i.e., shivering when exposed to cool environmental temperatures. Chemical thermogenesis occurs when the infant is exposed to environmental temperatures below the thermoneutral zone, i.e., the temperature range in which a resting infant maintains normal body temperature (both superficial and deep), along with a minimal rate of oxygen consumption (6, 20, 23, 33, 34). The thermoneutral zone varies with the size and body composition of the infant, postnatal age and the amount of clothing (if any) he is wearing (Fig. 13–3). In the clothed infant, this zone is lowered by several degrees, depending on the physical properties of the

FIG. 13–3. Thermoneutral zone range for naked and clothed newborn infants. (Hey EN: Physiological principles involved in the care of the preterm human infant. In: The Mammalian Fetus in Vitro. Edited by CR Austin. London, Chapman and Hall, 1973)

clothes and blankets. In the nude infant, the lower limit of the thermoneutral zone is surpassed when the gradient between skin and environmental air temperature exceeds 1.5° C. Because of the greater ratio of surface area to mass and the higher thermal conductance of low-birth-weight infants, these infants require higher environmental temperatures than those needed by full-term infants to maintain thermoneutrality.

Resting oxygen consumption, or minimal metabolic rate, is lowest immediately after birth; it rises with increasing postnatal age throughout the neonatal period (Table 13–1). During the early neonatal period, the rate of oxygen consumption of full-term infants is significantly higher than that of premature infants. The resting oxygen consumption of infants who are small for gestational age is usually higher than that of preterm infants of similar weight but lower gestational age. This may be due to the higher proportion of metabolically active tissue, including the brain, found in this former group of infants (37).

When exposed to a relatively cool or sub-thermoneutral environmental temperature, the full-term infant has the capacity to more

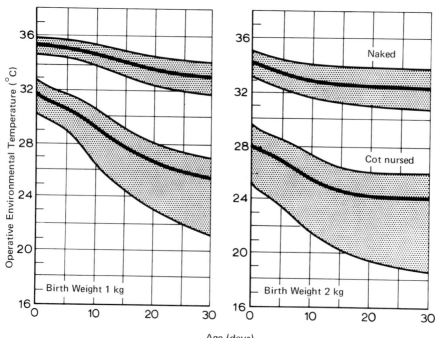

Age (days)

TABLE 13–1. Typical Minimal Metabolic Rates During the Neonatal Period

		Minimal Metabolic Rate	
	Postnatal Age	calorie/kg/24 hr	calorie/m²/24 hr*
Full-term			
(3500 g)	Birth to 6 hours	32	470
	Latter half of first day	37	550
	Second or third day	43	630
Preterm			
(1500 g)	First day	34	380
	Sixth day	42	470
	2 to 4 weeks	50	590
	4 to 6 weeks	59	760

* Surface area calculated as $A = kW^{2/3}$, using Lissauer's constant, $k = 10.3$.
(Sinclair: Pediatr Clin North Am 17:147, 1970)

than double his heat production as early as 15 minutes after birth (6). Both premature infants and those with intrauterine growth retardation can increase heat production under these conditions, but not to the extent seen in the full-term infant. As environmental temperature falls, heat production increases in a linear manner. Since the infant's primary thermoreceptors are located superficially in facial skin and tracheal mucosa (27, 32), a drop in the environmental temperature rapidly initiates mechanisms to increase heat production. When enough heat is being produced to equal heat loss, the infant's core or rectal temperature remains stable. When heat loss exceeds heat production, the core temperature begins to fall.

CHEMICAL THERMOGENESIS

The cold-induced increase in heat production in newborn infants is rarely accompanied by shivering. The site of this heat production is thought to be brown adipose tissue (12, 18), which appears as a thin sheet of fat in the interscapular area and neck and to a lesser extent around the kidney and adrenal glands (Fig. 13–4). With a full fat content, brown adipose tissue has a yellowish appearance, but it turns darker with fat depletion. Its cells, which begin to differentiate at 26 to 30 weeks of gestation, contain multilocular lipid cytoplasmic inclusions. White adipose tissue cells, on the other hand, have a single lipid cytoplasmic

inclusion. Although white adipose tissue has a relatively poor blood supply, brown adipose tissue is highly vascularized.

White adipose tissue serves as a source of nutrient for energy metabolism in the presence of total or partial starvation under thermoneutral conditions. The fat of brown adipose tissue is utilized as a source of energy only under conditions of cold stress. In cases of intrauterine malnutrition, there is usually a marked depletion of fat in white (but not brown) adipose tissue. In infants who have been exposed to low environmental temperatures and have received a subnormal caloric intake for at least 36 to 48 hours, a depletion of fat in brown adipose tissue has been noted at autopsy (3).

Following exposure to an acute cold stress, afferent nerve fibers ending in the cervical cord transmit the stimulus to efferent sympathetic fibers, which mediate the release of norepinephrine. An increase in 3':5'-cyclic adenosine monophosphate

FIG. 13–4. Distribution of brown adipose tissue in the human neonate. (Modified from Dawkins MR, Hull D: The production of heat by fat. Scient Am 213:62, 1965)

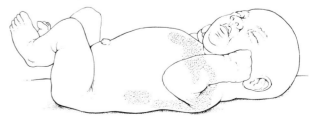

(cAMP) is followed by activation of a lipase, which hydrolyzes the fat in brown adipose tissue to glycerol and fatty acids. The fatty acids are oxidized in the brown adipose cells in a highly exothermic reaction. The heat of this reaction warms the venous blood returning from the brown adipose organ into the mediastinum, with a subsequent elevation of the infant's core temperature.

Nonshivering (or chemical) thermogenesis remains the primary mechanism for cold-induced heat production in the newborn infant for several weeks after birth. With the disappearance of the brown adipose organ, the infant's primary method of heat production in the presence of cold stress changes to shivering.

CLINICAL CONSIDERATIONS

THE DELIVERY ROOM

The newborn infant experiences his first thermal challenge in the moments after delivery. He emerges wet into an environment at least 10° C cooler than that of the amniotic cavity and immediately begins to lose heat by radiation, evaporation and convection. Although he responds to this stress by heat production via nonshivering thermogenesis, heat loss exceeds heat production, and there is rapid decline in core temperature. Those infants who have become hypoxic in utero may have an impaired ability to respond to cold stress, and an even greater decrease in body temperature may occur (9).

Dahm and James (10) have measured the heat loss of vigorous infants in the delivery room at an average air temperature of 25° C (Fig. 13–5). In infants who remained wet in room air, the heat loss was 100.5 calories/kg/min. When the infant was dried but left unwrapped, heat loss was reduced to 81.4 calories/kg/min. Drying and wrapping the infant in a blanket further reduced the heat loss to 39.0 calories/kg/min, while with drying and placing the infant under a radiant heater, the heat loss was 22.5 calories/kg/min.

The vigorous full-term infant tolerates the cold stress of the delivery room (this may actually play some role in the initiation of respiration), and hence drying and wrapping the infant in a blanket after delivery are alone adequate measures. The management of low-birth-weight and asphyxiated infants, however, is another matter. Infants whose capacity to produce heat and limit heat loss may be impaired are in particular jeopardy. The acidosis and hypoxia already present may be worsened by exposure to the cool environment. This may be related to the vasoconstricting effect of nonrepinephrine on pulmonary arterioles, with subsequent pulmonary hypoperfusion and right-to-left shunting of blood within the lungs.

Heat loss may be minimized in these high-risk infants by drying and placing them under radiant heaters immediately after delivery, especially if resuscitation is required. Body wraps made of aluminum foil or a transparent material (plastic food wrap) have been used to limit heat loss in the delivery room, but have not gained widespread clinical acceptance (4).

The transfer of low-birth-weight infants

FIG. 13–5. Mean deep body temperatures (T_R) of each group during the first 30 minutes of life. ■ wet infants in room air; □ dry infants in room air; ● wet infants under the radiant heater; △ dry infants wrapped in a blanket; ○ dry infants under the radiant heater. (Dahm LS, James LS: Pediatrics 49:504, 1972)

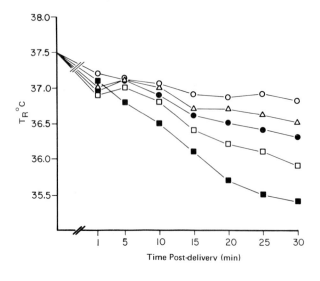

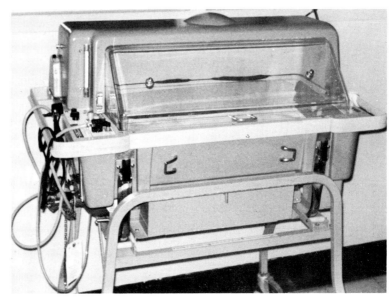

FIG. 13–6. Air-Shields portable transport incubator. (Air-Shields Co., Hatboro, Pa.)

from the delivery room to the nursery has long been associated with excessive heat loss and decrease in body temperature. The introduction of battery-powered transport incubators (Fig. 13–6) now allows the smallest infants to be transported long distances in a thermoneutral environment.

EARLY NEONATAL PERIOD

To determine the optimal thermal environment for low-birth-weight infants, Silverman et al (35) studied the effect of incubator air temperatures on survival rates of these infants. They were able to demonstrate that small infants raised with average incubator air temperatures of 29° C during the early neonatal period had significantly higher mortality rates than those infants whose incubator air temperatures averaged 32° C.

In simultaneously published studies (8, 13), it was shown that infants with birth weight of less than 1600 g raised under thermoneutral conditions had significantly lower mortality rates during the first three days of life than infants reared in a slightly cool environment (incubator air temperatures about 32° C). The reason for increased mortality rates in infants reared under cooler environmental temperatures could not be determined, but it has been specu-

lated that this was related to the diversion of calories to heat production and the depletion of fat depots in the cooler infants.

Premature Infants

On the basis of this information, it is recommended that small and sick premature infants, who have little caloric reserve and limited food intake, be reared under thermoneutral conditions during the early neonatal period.

The recognition that in premature infants abdominal skin temperatures of 36.3° to 36.5° C are associated with minimal rates of oxygen consumption led to the development of servocontrolled incubators that can maintain the desired skin temperature. A thermistor probe that is taped to the infant's skin causes the incubator heating unit to be turned on when the skin temperature falls below the desired level and evokes discontinuation of heat input when the skin temperature exceeds this level.

The more recent development of radiant heaters has allowed premature infants to be raised in thermoneutral environments outside of the confines of incubators (Fig. 13–7). These have the advantage of providing ready accessibility to the infant. However, a possible disadvantage is exposure of infants to environmental microorganisms. Vertical air columns around the radiant heater may decrease the amount of dust and microorganisms in the air surrounding the infant (29).

If only standard incubators are available, care should be taken to prevent inadvertent cooling or overheating of the nude infant. Axillary temperatures should be measured at least every four hours. Every attempt must be made to maintain these temperatures within a range of 36.8° to 37.0° C.

In premature infants of very low birth weight, care must be taken to avoid rapidly rising environmental temperatures and abdominal skin temperatures of over 36.5° since both of these conditions are associated with increased numbers of apneic episodes (11, 31). The explanation of this phenomenon is unknown.

In low-birth-weight infants who are otherwise free of illness, a thermoneutral state may be achieved outside of incubators by dressing the infant in a diaper and long-sleeved shirt, covering him with a blanket and maintaining room temperature at about 30° C (26). The use of clothing and blankets simplifies thermal control, but has disadvantages since the infant is not so easily observed and is deprived of beneficial photo-oxygenation effects of normal room lighting on unconjugated bilirubin. In the presence

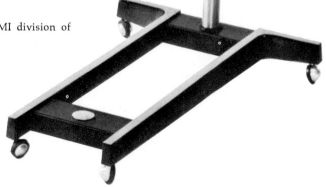

FIG. 13–7. IMI Radiant Warmer. (IMI division of BD Electrodyne, Sharon, Mass.)

of minimal cooling, the core or axillary temperatures may not decline. This is due to the fact that increased heat production compensates for heat loss. Under this circumstance, the skin temperature will begin to fall, and the core to skin temperature gradient (which is about 0.5° C under thermoneutral conditions) will begin to increase. The core temperature will start to fall when heat loss exceeds heat production.

Full-Term Infants

Full-term infants who are critically ill should be reared under thermoneutral conditions, whether in incubators or under radiant heaters. These infants have a poor capacity to produce heat and will become hypothermic if no supplementary heat is provided. For this group of infants abdominal skin temperatures of 36.1° to 36.2° C are associated with a thermoneutral state.

Care must be taken to minimize inadvertent chilling in infants raised in incubators. Opening of the incubator portholes can pose a thermal stress. Of greater consequence is lifting the incubator hood to perform a procedure. If complete access to the infant is necessary, e.g., in umbilical artery catheterization, the procedure should be performed in a thermoneutral environment under a radiant heater. The use of chilled blood during an exchange transfusion can cause a significant decrease in the infant's core temperature (24); blood must be warmed to body temperature before it is given to an infant.

LATE NEONATAL PERIOD

It is universally agreed that small and sick newborn infants who are receiving a suboptimal caloric intake should be raised under thermoneutral conditions to prevent excessive caloric expenditures; however, the ideal thermal conditions for low-birth-weight infants after the critical first days of life have not been fully defined.

The role of the thermal environment in the late neonatal period was studied by Glass et al (16). It was demonstrated that the rearing of unclothed infants in thermoneutral environments after the first week of life (median incubator air temperatures of 34.5° C) was associated with a growth rate significantly greater than that of an isocalorically fed group of infants reared under cooler ambient conditions (median incubator air temperatures of 32.0° C). The growth rates of the latter group improved, however, when those infants were given a small caloric supplement (24). Infants raised under the cooler conditions had significantly elevated resting metabolic rates, and it was speculated that decreased rates of growth were due to diversion of calories from storage to heat expenditure. The ability to resist an acute cold stress was diminished in those infants raised nude under thermoneutral conditions, with indirect evidence pointing to decreased physiologic competence of the brown adipose organ under these conditions. It also has been suggested that the clothing and blanketing of low-birth-weight infants after the first week of life, with faces exposed to air temperatures of 29° to 30° C, is associated with optimal growth and enhanced ability to resist an acute cold stress, when compared to a similar group of infants raised nude under thermoneutral conditions (17).

Clinical Implications

The clinical implications of these findings are that once low-birth-weight infants are free of illness and receiving adequate oral feedings, slightly decreased environmental temperatures do not affect survival but may slow the rate of growth. The physician caring for these infants should provide extra calories if environmental temperatures are below the thermoneutral range (17a). The increased resistance to cold stress noted in infants raised under subthermoneutral conditions may be of clinical importance if they are inadvertently discharged to homes having inadequate heating.

Low-birth-weight infants may be transferred safely from incubators to open bassinets at a time when they are able to maintain a stable core temperature without supplementary heat input. This usually occurs when they are between 1800 and 2000 g and are taking feedings well.

Hey and O'Connell (26) have shown that healthy full-term infants who were clothed and blanketed had minimal rates of oxygen consumption when nursery air temperatures were about 25° C. This would be the most desirable year round air temperature for normal nurseries. During very warm days, air temperatures rise considerably above this level in nurseries without air conditioning, and the infants may become hyperthermic. Removal of clothing and blankets would then allow excessive heat to be lost through evaporation of sweat from the skin.

Upon discharge from the hospital nursery, the infant is best kept in a bedroom where air temperature is about 25° to 26° C (77° to 79° F). Although cold injury to newborn infants is unusual in the United States today, it is nonetheless occasionally encountered. Signs of cold injury are lethargy, poor suck, hypothermia and sclerema. Treatment is gradual rewarming in a thermoneutral environment.

REFERENCES

1. Abrams R, Caton D, Curet LB, Crenshaw C, Mann L, Barron DH: Fetal brain-maternal aorta temperature differences in sheep. Am J Physiol 217:1619, 1969

2. Adamsons K Jr: The role of thermal factors in fetal and neonatal life. Pediatr Clin North Am 13:599, 1966

3. Aherne W, Hull D: Brown adipose tissue and heat production in the newborn infant. J Pathol 91:223, 1966

4. Besch NJ, Perlstein PH, Edwards NK, Keenan WJ, Sutherland JM: The transparent baby gag: a shield against heat loss. N Engl J Med 284:121, 1971

5. Brück K: Temperature regulation in the newborn infant. Biol Neonate 3:65, 1961

6. Brück K, Parmelee AH, Brück M: Neutral temperature range and range of "thermal comfort" in premature infants. Biol Neonate 4:32, 1962

7. Budin P: Le Nourrisson. Paris, O Doin, 1900. Translation by W Maloney: The Nursling. London, Caxton, 1907

8. Buetow KC, Klein SW: Effect of maintenance of 'normal' skin temperature on survival of infants of low birth weight. Pediatrics 34:163, 1964

9. Burnard ED, Cross KW: Rectal temperature in the newborn after birth asphyxia. Br Med J 2:1197, 1958

10. Dahm LS, James LS: Newborn temperature and calculated heat loss in the delivery room. Pediatrics 49:504, 1972

11. Daily WJR, Klaus M, Meyer HBP: Apnea in premature infants: monitoring, incidence, heart rate changes, and an effect of environmental temperature. Pediatrics 43:510, 1969

12. Dawkins MJR, Scopes J: Non-shivering thermogenesis and brown adipose tissue in the human newborn infant. Nature 206:201, 1965

13. Day RL, Caliguiri L, Kamenski C, Ehrlich F: Body temperature and survival of premature infants. Pediatrics 34:171, 1964

14. Fanaroff AA, Rand MB, Wald M. Gruber HS, Klaus MH: Insensible water loss in low birth weight infants. Pediatrics 50:236, 1972

15. Glass L, Silverman WA, Sinalcir JC: Effect of the thermal environment on cold resistance and growth of small infants after the first week of life. Pediatrics 41:1033, 1968

16. Glass L, Silverman WA, Sinclair JC: Relationship of thermal environment and caloric intake to growth and resting metabolism in the late neonatal period. Biol Neonate 14:324, 1969

17. Glass L, Sinclair JC, Floyd MV: Effect of differential cooling on cold resistance and growth in low birth weight infants. Soc Ped Res Program and Abstracts, Atlantic City, 1971, p 258

17a. Glass L, Lala RV, Jaiswal V, Nigam SK: Effect of thermal environment and caloric intake on head growth of low birth weight infants during the late neonatal period. Arch Dis Child 50:571, 1975

18. Harding PGR: The metabolism of brown and white adipose tissue in the fetus and newborn. Clin Obstet Gynecol 14:685, 1971

19. Heim T: Thermogenesis in the newborn infant. Clin Obstet Gynecol 14:790, 1971

20. Hey E: The relation between environmental temperature and oxygen consumption in the newborn baby. J Physiol 200:589, 1969

21. Hey EN: Thermal regulation in the newborn. Br J Hosp Med July 1972, p 51

22. Hey E, Katz, G: Evaporative water loss in the newborn baby. J Physiol 200:605, 1969

23. Hey EN, Katz G: Optimum thermal environment for naked babies. Arch Dis Child 45:328, 1970

24. Hey EN, Kohlinsky S, O'Connell B: Heatlosses from babies during exchange transfusion. Lancet 1:335, 1969

25. Hey EN, Maurice NP: Effect of humidity on production and loss of heat in the newborn baby. Arch Dis Child 43:166, 1968

26. Hey EN, O'Connell B: Oxygen consumption and heat balance in the cot-nursed baby. Arch Dis Child 45:335, 1970

27. Mestyán J, Jarái I, Bata G, Fekete M: The significance of facial skin temperature in the chemical heat regulation of premature infants. Biol Neonate 7:243, 1964

28. Miller JC, Behrle FC, Hagar DL, Denison TR: The effect of high humidity on body temperature and O_2 consumption of newborn premature infants. Pediatrics 27:740, 1961

29. Musch B, Adams ST, Sunshine P: An air incubator for use in an intensive care nrusery. J Pediatr 79: 1024, 1971

30. Oliver TK Jr: Temperature regulation and heat production in the newborn. Pediatr Clin North Am 12:765, 1965

31. Perlstein PH, Edwards NK, Sutherland JM: Apnea in premature infants and incubator air temperature changes. N Engl J Med 282:461, 1970

32. Pribylová H: The importance of thermoreceptive regions for the chemical thermoregulation of the newborn. Biol Neonate 12:13, 1968

33. Scopes JW, Ahmed I: Minimal rates of oxygen consumption in sick and premature newborn infants. Arch Dis Child 41:407, 1966

34. Scopes J, Ahmed I: Range of critical temperature in sick and premature newborn babies. Arch Dis Child 41:417, 1966

35. Silverman WA, Fertig JW, Berger AP: The influence of the thermal environment upon the survival of newly born premature infants. Pediatrics 22:876, 1958

36. Sinclair JC: Heat production and thermoregulation in the small for date infant. Pediatr Clin North Am 17:147, 1970

37. Sinclair JC, Silverman WA: Relative hypermetabolism in undergrown human neonates. Lancet 2:49, 1964

14

Genetic Disorders

MELVIN GERTNER

There is a wide variety of genetically transmitted disorders that affect the newborn infant. Some are associated with known chromosomal abnormalities; the majority are not. Advances made in the field of medical genetics have led to specific treatment of genetically transmitted disorders in a few conditions, such as phenylketonuria, hemophilia and the adrenogenital syndrome, and new diagnostic techniques together with an increased understanding of many of these disorders have made genetic counseling available to potentially high-risk parents. It has been speculated that at some time in the future "molecular engineering" may reverse the deleterious effects of many of these conditions.

CELL DIVISION AND CHROMOSOMAL ABNORMALITIES

Chromosomal abnormalities are associated with a variety of clinical disorders that are recognizable in the newborn infant. The normal chromosome complement consists of 44 autosomes and 2 sex chromosomes: an X and a Y chromosome in males and two X chromosomes in females. Chromosomes are arranged in groups according to size and morphology, and the resultant arrangement is known as the karyotype. A chromosome is composed of two strands called chromatids, which are attached at a point called the centromere or primary constriction. The location of the centromere determines the morphology of the chromosome. If the centromere is in the middle, the chromosome is metacentric; if the centromere is between the middle and the end of the chromosome, it is submetacentric; if the centromere is close to the end of the chromosome it is acrocentric (Fig. 14–1). Metacentric chromosomes, therefore, have arms of approximately equal length, whereas submetacentric chromosomes have short arms and long arms, and acrocentric chromosomes have minute short arms.

The autosomal chromosome pairs are divided into seven groups: group A, 1–3; group B, 4–5; group C, 6–12; group D, 13–15; group E, 16–18; group F, 19–20; group G, 21–22. The X chromosome most closely resembles a C group chromosome, and the Y chromosome most closely resembles a G group chromosome (Fig. 14–2). Two chromosomes that comprise a pair are known as homologues.

In order to understand the pathogenesis of conditions associated with chromosomal abnormalities, a knowledge of the physiology of cellular division (mitosis) and gametogenesis (meiosis) is necessary.

MITOSIS

The process by which somatic cells divide to produce two identical cells is known as

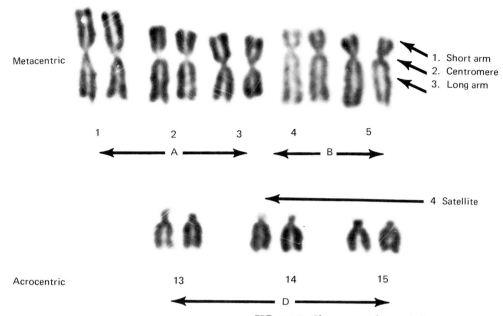

FIG. 14–1. Chromosomal morphology.

mitosis (Fig. 14–3). This occurs without any significant alteration of primary genetic material and is divided into four stages: 1) the prophase, 2) metaphase, 3) anaphase and 4) telophase.

Prophase

Two chromatids are formed from a single one. An accessory mitotic apparatus appears, consisting of 2 centrioles, each with an aster and a group of filaments called a spindle. The nuclear membrane and nucleoli that are present during the interphase disappear.

Metaphase

The formation of the spindle progresses, and the chromosomes arrange themselves with their centromeres on the equatorial plane. The two chromatids of each chromosome lie parallel to each other and are attached only at the centromere. Longitudinal splitting through the centromere then occurs.

Anaphase

At the onset of anaphase the daughter centromeres separate from one another and

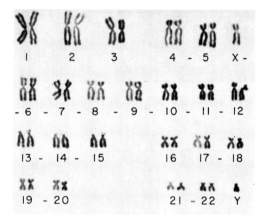

FIG. 14–2. Normal human male karyotype.

move up the spindle toward the poles, pulling the chromatids that are attached to them apart from one another. These are now called daughter chromosomes. As the centromeres are separating from one another, the equatorial region of the spindle elongates.

Telophase

Telophase begins when the polar migration of the chromosomes ends. At this time daughter nucleoli and, nuclear membranes

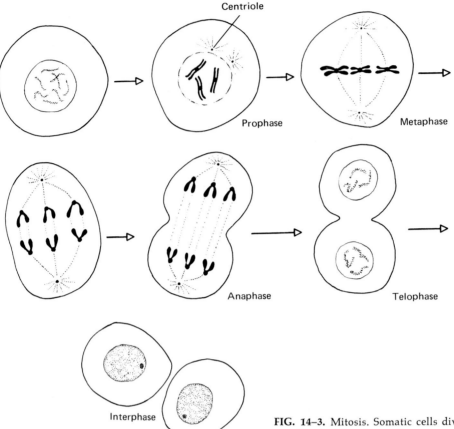

FIG. 14–3. Mitosis. Somatic cells divide to produce two identical daughter cells.

reappear, and the chromosomes become loosely coiled and elongated. The cytoplasm then segments and separates (a process known as cytokinesis), and two individual cells are formed.

MEIOSIS

The process of chromosome reduction by which mature germ cells (with half the number of chromosomes) are formed is called meiosis (Fig. 14–4). This process involves two cell divisions with only one chromosome duplication and results in mature haploid cells arising from the precursor diploid cells.

In the first stage of meiosis, each pair of homologous chromosomes is represented by two pairs of chromatids. The two pairs of homologous chromatids line up side-by-side on a single spindle fiber in this metaphase,

with each chromatid pair held together by a centromere (one maternal and one paternal). The centromeres, along with the two chromatids, move to opposite poles, and the two daughter cells that are formed immediately redivide.

During the second meiotic division the centromeres with the two chromatids assemble on the spindles of the newly formed cells. The centromeres now divide, as in mitosis, and the daughter centromeres are joined to one chromatid. The daughter centromeres along with the single chromosome strand (chromatid) then move to the opposite poles, and two new cells are formed.

Each premeiotic germ cell with two sets of chromosomes thus produces four germ cells, each of which has a single set of chromosomes. The meiotic divisions are therefore known as reduction divisions. During the first meiotic division the number of centro-

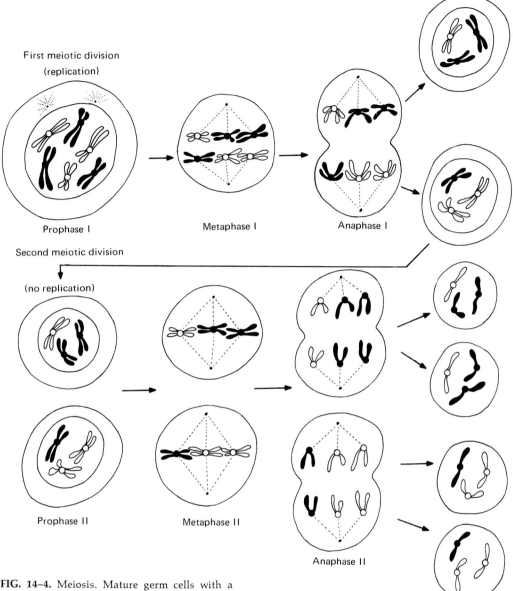

First meiotic division
(replication)

Prophase I　　　Metaphase I　　　Anaphase I

Second meiotic division

(no replication)

Prophase II　　　Metaphase II

Anaphase II

FIG. 14–4. Meiosis. Mature germ cells with a haploid number of chromosomes are formed.

meres is reduced by half, and during the second division the number of chromatids (chromosome strands) is reduced to half. In the male, meiosis in the spermatocyte leads to the formation of four mature sperm cells. In the female, however, meiosis in the oocyte leads to the formation of one mature egg cell and three polar bodies. This occurs because of unequal distribution of the cytoplasm with each division. Thus, during the first division a small bud of the oocyte be-

comes the first polar body and the larger daughter cell then divides unequally again to form the mature egg and another polar body (the first polar body also divides at this time to produce two polar bodies).

BREAKAGE AND RECOMBINATIONS

Chromosome breakage and recombinations result in a variety of abnormal chromosomes. When two acrocentric chromosomes

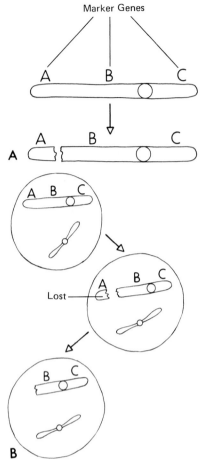

Marker Genes

A

B

FIG. 14–5. A. Chromosomal breakage results in the formation of 2 fragments; the fragment containing marker genes B and C contains the centromere, while that containing marker gene A does not. **B.** The fragment containing marker gene A is lost, while the one containing marker genes B and C, although deficient in genetic material, may then behave like a normal chromosome.

lose their small short arms and fuse at the centromeres, the new chromosome is relatively stable. This translocation chromosome produces no phenotypic abnormalities because there is an insignificant loss of chromosome material. However, during meiosis and subsequent fertilization, cells with extra chromosomal material (usually lethal) or new cells with the same balanced translocation may be formed.

Chromosomes may break at one or more locations. A break at any one location results in two fragments, only one of which contains the centromere (Fig. 14–5A). The fragment without the centromere is lost during mitosis (Fig. 14–5B) and the new cells are deficient in the genetic material carried by that fragment. Since only the centromere can attach to the mitotic spindle, only the centromere-bearing fragment can be transmitted to an entire line of subsequent cells.

The fragment with the centromere may then behave like a normal chromosome and continue to divide normally, producing daughter cells that contain the new chromosome, which is stable although deficient in genetic material. This fragment may, however, reduplicate to form two new fragments with broken ends that unite to form a new long unstable chromosome with two centromeres. During the subsequent division, the centromeres migrate to opposite spindle poles, stretching the chromo-

FIG. 14–6. "Break-fusion-bridge-breakage cycle," following division of fragmented chromosome.

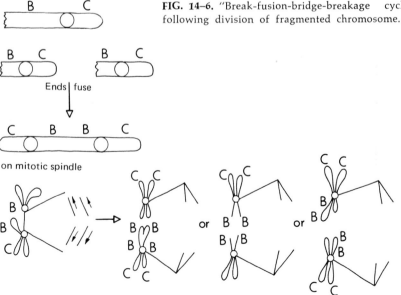

some and eventually breaking it at an unpredictable point. This leads to the formation of two daughter cells, one with a doubled chromosome portion and one completely lacking in that chromosome portion. The "break-fusion-bridge-breakage" cycle is then repeated in the next cell cycle, leading to cells with a variety of genotypes (Fig. 14–6).

Inversions and Ring Chromosomes

Another consequence of chromosomal breakage is the formation of inversions and ring chromosomes. When a chromosome breaks at two points, several possibilities for reunion occur. The first is union of the two pieces in the same order in which they were broken, but they may reunite with the middle piece inverted, giving rise to an inversion chromosome. If the two breaks are on the same side of the centromere, the two end fragments of the chromosome may be lost immediately; if the fragment bearing the centromere is lost, it may form a ring chromosome by fusion of its two ends before being lost.

Inversions may further be divided into paracentric inversions, in which the breakage points are on the same arm of the chromosome (so that the rearrangement is not apparent because it does not alter the relative arm lengths), or pericentric inversions, in which the two breaks occur in different arms. A chromosome that has undergone pericentric inversion is usually quite apparent because there is a change in relative arm lengths (Fig. 14–7).

Mitosis can proceed normally in inversion chromosomes. During meiosis, however, crossing over (exchange of genetic material between two chromosomes) may occur, resulting in the formation of many abnormal chromosomes. Some of these are deficient in genetic material, whereas others contain duplicated genetic material. Cells that contain both new chromosomes have the normal amount of genetic material, but when the two chromosomes segregate into different gametes during meiosis a deficiency of material occurs in one gamete and

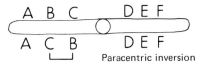

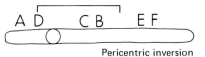

FIG. 14–7. Chromosomal paracentric and pericentric inversions.

a duplication occurs in the other (Fig. 14–8).

The same mechanism for the production of "duplication deficiency" chromosomal defects occurs in carriers of "balanced reciprocal translocations." Here, breaks have occurred in two homologous chromosomes. The carrier of such a translocation is normal because the cells contain the normal total amount of genetic material. During the meiosis, however, the two translocation chromosomes may go to the opposite pole from the two normal homologues, or one normal chromosome and one translocated chromosome may go to one pole, while the other normal chromosome and translocated chromosome go to the other pole. In the first case two balanced gametes are formed; in the second case, two unbalanced ones are formed (Fig. 14–9).

ABNORMAL HUMAN KARYOTYPES

Changes in the number or structure of chromosomes result in abnormal karyotypes that may be related to pathologic states. The normal number of chromosomes in a somatic cell is termed diploid. The sperm and ova contain half the number of chromosomes (haploid). Multiples of the haploid number of chromosomes are known as polyploidy, i.e., triploid (3 × haploid, or 69 chromosomes in man) or tetraploid (4 × haploid). Euploidy refers to the normal number, i.e., 46, and aneuploidy to any abnormal number, e.g., 45, 47, 48.

The presence of three homologues of a given autosome instead of the usual two is

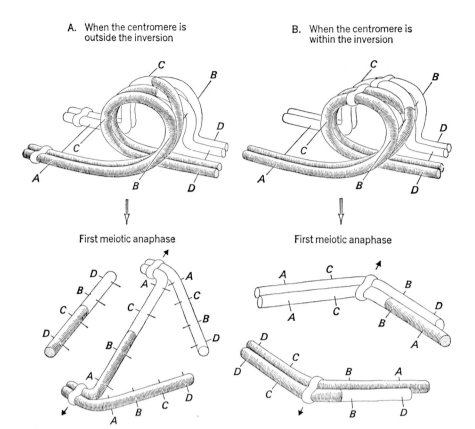

A. When the centromere is outside the inversion

B. When the centromere is within the inversion

First meiotic anaphase

First meiotic anaphase

FIG. 14–8. Crossing over within the inversion loop of an inversion heterozygote results in aberrant chromatids with duplications or deficiencies. **A.** Centromere outside the inversion **B.** Centromere within the inversion. (Srb AM, Owen RD, Edgar RS. General Genetics, 2nd ed. San Francisco, Freeman, 1965)

referred to as trisomy; the absence of one of a pair of homologues is known as monosomy.

A deletion is a loss of chromosome material resulting after breaks of a chromosome arm. A translocation is the transfer of a segment of one chromosome to another chromosome or to a different position on the same chromosome. Isochromosomes are two identical arms united by a centromere. Mosaicism refers to the existence of two or more cell lines with different karyotypes occurring in a single individual.

AUTOSOMAL TRISOMY SYNDROMES

Down's Syndrome (Trisomy 21)

Down's syndrome, or trisomy 21 (also known as monogolism) is the most common

autosomal trisomy, occurring in approximately 1:600 live births (9). The clinical manifestations of Down's syndrome are numerous, but none of the features other than the mongoloid facies (Fig. 14–10) are consistently present (8, 11). At birth the infant is often hypotonic. The head is typically brachycephalic, and there is an upward and outward slant of the eyes, which have prominent internal epicanthal folds. Small whitish dots at the periphery of the iris known as Brushfield spots may be present. The nasal bridge is flattened, and there may be a high-arched palate and large tongue. At birth there is often an absence of the breast tissue that is normally present in infants secondary to maternal hormonal stimulation. The hands are often short, and there is frequently a short incurved fifth finger, secondary to the absence or dysplasia of the middle phalanx. Dermatoglyphic patterns are abnormal (3) (Fig. 14–11). There is often a single palmar crease known as a simian line and a distally displaced triradius. A spacing between the first and second toes

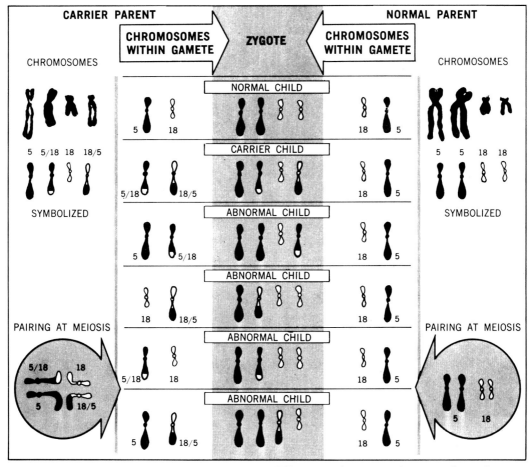

FIG. 14–9. Inheritance of reciprocal translocation. (Redding BA, Hirschhorn K: Guide to Human Chromosome Defects. In: Birth Defects, Original Article Series. White Plains, The National Foundation, September 1968)

with a deep plantar crease is usually noted. Umbilical hernias are frequently present, and these infants have an increased incidence of duodenal stenosis or atresia. Congenital cardiac defects are common; defects of the atrioventricular canal occur with unusual frequency. Cryptorchidism is common in males. Although both male and female patients with trisomy 21 undergo puberty, the males are presumably sterile. Roentgenographically, there is flattening of the lower edge of the ilium and flaring of the iliac wings. Mental development is retarded, and even those infants whose psychomotor development appears normal often slow down in mental development as they grow older. Patients with Down's syndrome experience a relatively high incidence of respiratory infections. Shortness of stature and premature aging are common. There is a marked increase of leukemia among children with Down's syndrome (13).

Genetics. The overall incidence of trisomy 21 is approximately 1:600 live births. The incidence, however, increases significantly with advancing maternal age. In women under 30, the incidence is about 0.6:1000 births; this increases to approximately 20:1000 for mothers aged 45 and over (6).

Several mechanisms are responsible for the production of the chromosomal aberration. Since most cases of nonmosaic Down's

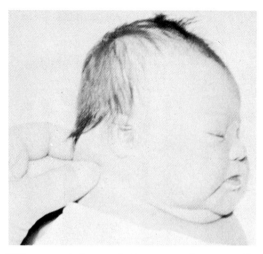

FIG. 14–10. Infant with Down's syndrome. (Gellis S, Feingold M: Syndromes in Pediatrics. New York, Medcom, 1969)

syndrome occur spontaneously in parents with normal karyotypes, it is presumed that primary meiotic nondisjunction of a normal germinal cell gives rise to an abnormal gamete containing the extra 21 chromosome. Since the maternal age effect is so striking, it is presumed that the nondisjunction usually occurs during oogenesis in most cases.

FIG. 14–11. Palmar dermatoglyphics in monozygotic twins with Down's syndrome. There are 10 ulnar loops on digits, distal axial triradii on both palms and bilaterial third interdigital loops. There are normal flexion creases on the left and a flexion crease on the right. (Uchida IA, Soltan HC: Evaluation of dermatoglyphics in medical genetics. Pediatr Clin North Am 10:409, 1963)

Approximately 3% of patients with Down's syndrome are translocation-trisomics (10). In these patients a G group chromosome is translocated to a D group or to another G group chromosome. Parents of translocation-trisomics may have normal karyotypes, in which case the aberration is said to be sporadic, or one of the parents may be a translocation carrier, in which case the aberration is inherited. In the latter case, the translocation carrier parent is phenotypically normal and has 45 chromosomes, one of which is a product of the translocation between a chromosome 21 and either a D or G group chromosome. Because the translocation carrier has a normal chromosome complement, the carrier is called a balanced translocation carrier. The balanced translocation carrier, however, has a greater risk of producing an affected offspring, and this tendency is independent of maternal age (4).

Approximately 1% of patients with Down's syndrome are mosaics with two cell lines, one with 47 chromosomes and one with 46 chromosomes (7). Occasionally, phenotypically normal parents of patients with Down's syndrome have been found to be mosaics (12).

The risk of recurrence of Down's syndrome in subsequent pregnancies is considerably higher than the random risk in women under age 30 (5). Translocation carriers, of course, have a high risk of producing offspring with Down's syndrome (10).

Modern techniques of prenatal genetic

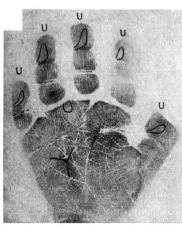

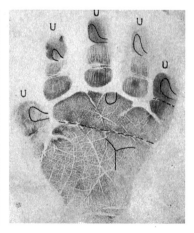

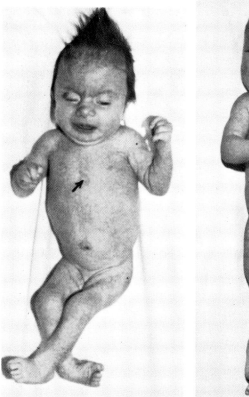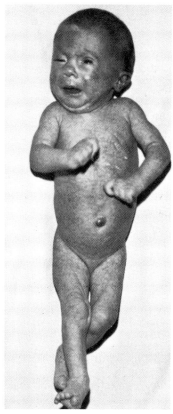

FIG. 14–12. Trisomy 18 syndrome. Arrow indicates lower end of short sternum. (Smith DW: Autosomal abnormalities. Am J Obstet Gynecol 910:1055, 1964)

diagnosis make it possible to determine the fetal karyotype antenatally in high-risk pregnancies.

Trisomy 18

The incidence of trisomy 18 has been estimated to be 0.3:1000 live births (17). Females are affected three times as often as males. The infants are generally small for gestational age. Prenatal history often reveals weak fetal movements and polyhydramnios. Multiple abnormalities in all organ systems have been noted in infants with this syndrome, but no one malformation has been found in all the infants studied. Only the more common anomalies are listed in this section. Infants trisomic for chromosome 18 (Fig. 14–12) usually have a prominent occiput, short sternum and small pelvis. Flexion deformities of the fingers with the index finger overriding the third finger are common. Dermatoglyphics reveal distal palmar triradii and a low arch dermal ridge pattern on six or more digits. Low-set malformed ears, micrognathia, ventricular septal defects and cryptorchidism are frequently observed in males. These infants generally fail to thrive, and most succumb during the first few months of life. Trisomy 18 occurs more frequently with advanced maternal age (11, 15).

Trisomy 13

As in the trisomy 18 syndrome, all organ systems may be involved, but no single defect has been detected in all infants with the syndrome. The more common anomalies include cleft lip, cleft palate, microphthalmos, hyperconvex narrow fingernails, midline scalp defects and cryptorchidism in males.

The facial defects are often associated with forebrain hypoplasia. Dermatoglyphics reveal distally placed axial triradii. The infants generally fail to thrive, and most succumb during the first few months. As with the other autosomal trisomies, there is an association with advanced maternal age (15).

Trisomy 22

A number of cases have been reported in which there is an extra small acrocentric chromosome that appears to belong to the G group (17, 18). These patients present with a wide variety of congenital defects, but all seem to have ear defects, cleft palate, congenital heart disease and limb defects. Many researchers feel that these patients are trisomic for chromosome 22 (17, 18). The incidence of this disorder is unknown.

Cat-Eye Syndrome

The chromosomal defect of this syndrome is the presence of a small satellited acrocentric chromosome, about half the size of the G group chromosomes. The name "cat-eye" was derived from the presence of vertical colobomata of the iris that resemble the pupils of cats. Patients also have anal atresia and rectovesical fistulas. Mental retardation is not a constant feature of the syndrome (19). Familial occurrence in a mother and a daughter has been reported.

AUTOSOMAL DELETION SYNDROMES

The cri-du-chat syndrome was originally described in 1963 by Lejeune et al (28). The features of the syndrome include a weak cry in infancy (resembling the mewing of a cat), failure to thrive, microcephaly, hypertelorism, antimongoloid slant of the eyes, micrognathia, simian creases and mental retardation (11, 28). Chromosomally, patients have a deletion of the short arm of chromosome 5 (24). Although most cases seem to occur sporadically, there have been reports of multiply affected siblings born to a balanced translocation carrier parent (23).

Karyotypes should therefore be done on the parents of patients with this syndrome to determine the risk of recurrence.

A number of patients with a short arm deletion of chromosome 4 have also been reported. These infants usually show midline fusion defects that include scalp defects, cleft lip, cleft palate and hypospadias. Other clinical features include preauricular dimples, colobomata and seizures (20, 21, 27).

Partial deletion of the long arm of chromosome 18 is responsible for a syndrome that includes the following features: mental retardation, short stature, microcephaly, hypotonia, prominent antihelix or antitragus, nystagmus and a high incidence of congenital heart disease (26, 30).

Several patients have been described with a long arm deletion of chromosome 21. These patients have a high incidence of mental retardation, hypertonia, antimongoloid slant of the eyes, prominent nasal bridge, micrognathia and pyloric stenosis (22).

Patients have also been described with short arm deletions of chromosome 18, short arm deletion of a D group chromosome and short arm deletions of a G group chromosome. The clinical features of the few cases reported with these autosomal deletion syndromes are not consistent enough to define definite clinical syndromes (25, 29).

SEX CHROMOSOME ABERRATIONS

Although some syndromes associated with sex (X and Y) chromosome abnormalities are apparent in the neonate, many do not become apparent until later in life. Some manifestations of these conditions are ambiguous genitalia (such as in true hermaphroditism or mixed gonadal dysgenesis) or somatic abnormalities, such as lymphedema, webbed neck and cubitus valgus (Turner's syndrome). On the other hand, many neonates with ambiguous genitalia have a normal karyotype, e.g, congenital adrenal hyperplasia and the syndrome of testicular feminization.

Examination of the buccal mucosal smear is an important adjunct in determining the sex chromosome pattern of an infant whenever a question arises in the clinical diagnosis. In over 25% of normal female cells, a condensed mass of nuclear chromatin (Barr bodies) (Fig. 14–13) may be detected adjacent to the nuclear membrane. A single Barr body within a cell indicates the presence of two X chromosomes. If more than two X chromosomes are present in a cell, the total number of Barr bodies is one less than the total number of X chromosomes. (Thus, a cell with three X chromosomes contains two Barr bodies.) Since there may be an apparent decrease in the number of chromatin-positive nuclei in normal female infants for the first two days of life because of poor cell selection, this test should be delayed until after this time (36).

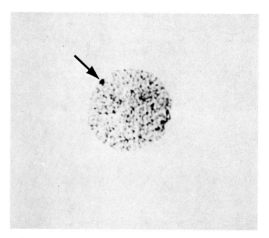

FIG. 14–13. Single Barr body in nucleus of buccal mucosal cell (arrow).

Klinefelter's Syndrome

Klinefelter's syndrome is the most common sex chromosome aberration, with an incidence somewhat over 2:1000 live births. The usual karyotype is 47, but many cases with more than two X chromosomes as well as mosaics have also been found (34).

Although clinically inapparent during the neonatal period, the diagnosis may be suspected if a phenotypic male has chromatin-positive cells in the buccal mucosa. The diagnosis is confirmed by examination of the patient's karyotype.

The complete clinical syndrome is characterized by gynecomastia, small testes with seminiferous tubule degeneration, aspermatogenesis or oligospermia, eunichoid body proportions and mild to moderate mental retardation (37). Dermatoglyphics reveal a low ridge count.

It is believed that the extra X chromosome is due to meiotic nondisjunction of either the sperm or ova. There is an increased incidence of this syndrome with advanced maternal age (35). Mosaicism has been reported, and these patients tend to be less severely involved. Patients with more than two X chromosomes have also been reported, and these tend to have more severe

mental retardation (35). Somewhat more than 20% of patients with features typical of Klinefelter's syndrome have been found to be sex chromatin–negative with a normal 46 XY karyotype (34). The etiology of this "pseudo-Klinefelter's" syndrome is unknown.

Turner's Syndrome

Turner's syndrome is characterized by short stature, sexual infantilism, streak gonads and XO sex chromosome pattern in phenotypic females. It may or may not be apparent in the newborn infant (33, 34, 44). The most striking feature observed at birth is peripheral lymphedema (Fig. 14–14). Other signs include shield-like chest, webbed neck, cubitus valgus, coarctation of the aorta, short fourth metacarpal, multiple pigmented nevi and a low hairline (33). The condition is not usually associated with mental retardation, but it may be associated with specific cognitive deficit (40, 42). There is no correlation with maternal age at conception (33). Many patients have been found with various forms of mosaicism, e.g., 45 XO/46 XX. These patients may show the full-blown syndrome with all the stigmata or may be phenotypically normal or may present with intermediate features. Some of the XO/XX mosaics are fertile (33).

A number of patients have been found to

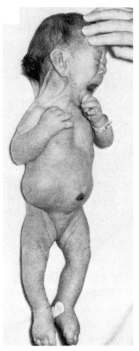

FIG. 14–14. Turner's syndrome in a newborn infant. (Uchida IA, Soltan HC: Evaluation of dermatoglyphics in medical genetics. Pediatr Clin North Am 10:409, 1963)

have deletions of portions of the short arm or long arm of the X chromosomes (33). The clinical stigmata demonstrated in these patients have been variable, in part because many of them have various forms of mosaicism. It is generally felt that a long arm deletion of the X chromosome is associated with streak gonads and a short arm deletion with short stature (33).

A clinical syndrome noted in males who have many of the features of females with Turner's syndrome is usually accompanied by a normal XY male karyotype (43).

Poly X Syndrome

There have been many reports of women with either 47 XXX chromosome constitution or 47 XXX/46XX chromosome constitution. These women are generally normal phenotypically (32). Buccal smears show two Barr bodies. There have also been reports of women with 48 XXXX and 49

XXXXX chromosome constitutions. Among these latter females, there is a higher incidence of mental retardation (32).

XYY Syndrome

The XYY karyotype occurs with a frequency of about 1.8:1000 in newborn surveys. It is difficult to delineate a characteristic phenotype for XYY individuals except for tall stature, which has been a consistent finding (40a).

IDENTIFICATION OF INDIVIDUALS WITH ABNORMAL CHROMOSOMES

The criteria of selection of patients for chromosomal analysis is quite variable. The indications are clear for those patients with recognizable syndromes and their families. Sex chromatin analysis, Y body fluoresence or dermatoglyphic analysis may suffice for patients with specific problems related to sexual ambiguity. Patients with multiple organ system defects, however, should have chromosome studies. It is not within the scope of this chapter to discuss the technical details of the various cytogenetic techniques currently available for studying selected individuals. A listing of the techniques with a brief discussion of the advantages and limitations of some of the techniques follows, and the reader is referred to the references for the technical details.

Sex chromatin studies for the determination of the number of X chromosomes have previously been discussed. In addition, it has been shown that the distal portion of the long arms of the Y chromosome fluoresce with quinacrine mustard or dihydrochloride (47, 52). A combination of sex chromatin staining and Y body fluorescence may be useful in detecting aberrations of the sex chromosomes.

Dermatoglyphic analysis has proven useful as a screening device for most types of chromosomal abnormalities (3, 41).

Two new staining techniques have made possible the identification of specific chromosomes by demonstrating characteristic banding patterns for each individual chromosome. These methods are: 1) the fluorescent staining technique of Caspersson et al (47) and 2) the differential staining (DNA reannealing) technique of Arrighi and T. C. Hsu and various modifications of these methods (45, 48). Further modifications have been used and adapted by others to detect specific chromosomal defects, particularly reciprocal equal translocations, which could not be detected in conventional karyotypes (46, 49, 50, 51, 53).

ANTENATAL DIAGNOSIS

Several disorders may now be detected antenatally by a combination of preconceptional genetic screening and transabdominal amniocentesis. A mass screening program, involving the general population or a specific at risk population, e.g., relatives of affected children, carried out prior to the onset of pregnancy is one means of detecting nonaffected individuals who may transmit a genetic disorder to their offspring. Exemplifying this type of approach is the screening program for Tay-Sach's disease that has been carried out on a wide-scale basis among a high-risk population consisting of those of Ashkenazic Jewish ancestry (57). Normal carriers of the gene for Tay-Sach's disease have decreased serum levels of the enzyme hexosaminidase A, and decreased levels are found in about 1 in 30 individuals of Ashkenazic Jewish ancestry. When two individuals from this group marry each other, approximately 1 in 900 couples is at risk for having an affected fetus (the risk for these couples being 1:4 with each pregnancy).

Knowledge of the risk of having an affected offspring is desirable for any couple planning a pregnancy, and this is especially true in those instances when an affected fetus can be diagnosed antenatally. The following metabolic disorders can be diagnosed antenatally by demonstrating precise enzyme defects:

Acatalasemia
Argininosuccinic aciduria

Chédiak-Higashi syndrome
Citrullinemia
Congenital erythropoietic porphyria
Cystinosis
Fabry's disease
Fucosidosis
Galactosemia
Gaucher's disease
Glucose-6-PD deficiency
Glycogen storage diseases (Types 2–4)
G_{M1} gangliosidoses (Types 1 & 2)
G_{M2} gangliosidoses (Types 1–3)
Homocystinuria
Hyperlysinemia
Hypervalinemia
I-cell disease
Ketotic hyperglycinemia
Krabbe's disease
Lesch-Nyhan syndrome
Lysosomal acid phosphatase deficiency
Mannosidosis
Maple syrup urine disease
Metachromatic leukodystrophy
Methylmalonic aciduria
Mucopolysaccharidoses (Types 1–6)
Niemann-Pick disease
Ornithine-A-keto acid transaminase deficiency
Orotic aciduria
Pyruvate decarboxylase deficiency
Refsum's syndrome
Xeroderma pigmentosum

TRANSABDOMINAL AMNIOCENTESIS

Since the mid 1960s the use of transabdominal amniocentesis for the prenatal detection of genetic disorders has gained widespread importance in genetic counseling. The procedure is performed early in the second trimester of pregnancy and appears to be a safe and accurate method of diagnosing genetic disorders in utero (55). Fibroblast cultures are readily established from amniotic fluid cells within 10 to 20 days (56, 61, 63). These cultures can be used either in delineation of fetal karyotype or in enzymatic studies leading to the diagnosis of an ever-increasing number of biochemical disorders. In addition, uncultured amniotic fluid cells as well as the supernatant fluid can be used to detect certain heritable disorders ante-natally (61, 63).

The types of pregnancies associated with a high risk for genetic disorders in which diagnostic amniocentesis is indicated are as follows:

1. Advanced maternal age
2. Translocation carriers
3. Previous child with chromosomal dis-order
4. Carrier of X-linked disorder
5. Carrier of a biochemical disorder that can be diagnosed by tissue culture techniques or amniotic fluid analyses
6. Previous spontaneous abortion (variable indication)

Advanced maternal age has long been associated with trisomy 21 (Down's syn-drome). Among women aged 21 to 30, the risk of delivering an infant with this dis-order is 1:1500, whereas among women 45 and over, the risk is 1:46 (64). In addition, an increased incidence of other autosomal trisomies and sex chromosomal aneuploidies occurs with advanced maternal age (54, 63, 66).

Translocation carriers with balanced re-ciprocal translocations and centric fusion type translocations have a high risk of pro-ducing offspring with an unbalanced chro-mosomal complement regardless of mater-nal age. Parents with normal chromosomal complements who produce offspring with chromosomal aberrations may not fall into the category of high-risk pregnancy on a statistical basis, but the fear of producing another abnormal child may be so great and difficult to alleviate that diagnostic amnio-centesis may be indicated.

A carrier of an X-linked disorder (e.g., classic hemophilia or G-6-PD deficiency) has a 50% chance of producing an affected infant if the fetus is a male. Metabolic dis-orders that have been diagnosed in utero usually have an autosomal recessive mode of transmission (Lesch-Nyhan syndrome, Hunter's syndrome and Fabry's disease—which have X-linked recessive modes of transmission—are exceptions). Thus, where the possibility of this type of disorder is suspected, there is a one in four chance that the fetus will be affected.

Families with a high incidence of sponta-neous abortion have a 2% to 3% incidence of chromosomal abnormalities (mostly translocations). Karyotype studies prior to conception are indicated; if abnormalities are detected, amniocentesis is indicated (67).

Maternal drug ingestion, x-ray exposure or thyroid disease have not been definitely established as indications for amniocentesis (66).

Chromosomal Analysis of Amniotic Fluid Cell Cultures

Karyotypes of cultured amniotic fluid cells are readily obtained by standard tissue cul-ture techniques (59). However, the use of cells found in amniotic fluid for prenatal sex determination antedates the current cell cul-tivation and chromosome analysis tech-niques. Although a quick sex determination is possible by examining these cells for Barr bodies or fluorescent Y bodies, the accuracy of such determinations has been variable (65). Several explanations for this phenome-non exist: the cells examined may be mater-nal rather than fetal or the cells may be nonviable or bacterial particles may fluo-resce. The consequences of a mistaken sex determination in prenatal diagnosis are obvious. Therefore, it behooves the geneti-cist to examine the karyotypes of cultivated cells in order to accurately predict the fetal sex. Even here, caution should be exercised since Nadler has found that chromosome analyses done ten days after the cultures have been established may reflect the karyo-type of maternal macrophages rather than that of fetal amniotic fluid cells (62). Later determinations are, therefore, advised after the maternal line has died out.

Even after waiting for maternal cells to die and carefully karyotyping the cultures with meticulous technique, errors may oc-cur. In the case of twins, it is possible that only one amniotic sac will be aspirated. With fetal mosaicism, it is possible that only one cell line will be apparent. Con-versely, the presence of a rare heteroploid cell among otherwise diploid cells may lead to confusion in diagnosis. Another phenomenon that has occurred in most laboratories has been the appearance of a variable percentage of tetraploid cells (58, 60). It is not clear whether this is an artefact of tissue culture or whether tetraploid cells actually exist in human amnion.

In the case of maternal carriers of X-linked disorders, fetal sex should be determined by karyotyping cultured fibroblasts. Since in most X-linked disorders it is not possible to determine prenatally whether a male fetus is affected or not, the high risk of abnormality (50%) may be sufficient for many couples to request the termination of pregnancy. In three disorders of this group (Fabry's disease, Lesch-Nyhan and Hunter syndromes) biochemical studies of the fibroblast cultures can be used to ascertain the presence or absence of the disorder in the male fetus (60).

Prior to the availability of diagnostic amniocentesis, a couple at risk for producing offspring with autosomal recessive metabolic disorders could only be advised (once it had been established that the couple were carriers) that the risk of producing such a child was 1:4 with each pregnancy. With the use of fibroblast cultures derived from amniotic fluid cells, it has become possible to determine prenatally whether or not the fetus is affected in an ever-increasing number of heritable disorders. These may be detected by a variety of techniques of enzyme assay.

When an enzymatic determination is indicated, it usually takes four to six weeks to obtain an adequate number of fibroblasts for reliable results. Direct analysis of amniotic fluid or uncultivated cells is not usually advisable for determining enzyme levels (66).

Amniocentesis and Genetic Counseling

The question of termination of pregnancy arises in all cases where prenatal diagnosis indicates an affected fetus. Generally, the decision has been made prior to the performance of the procedure to terminate the pregnancy if an affected fetus is found. It is senseless to subject both mother and fetus to the risks of amniocentesis if the parents do not wish to terminate the pregnancy in the event of a positive diagnosis. A couple contemplating amniocentesis should be advised beforehand of the risks of the procedure (see Ch. 2, High Risk Pregnancy and Fetal Monitoring), the risk of producing an affected offspring, the chances of successful diagnosis and other alternatives, e.g., adoption, artificial insemination, available to them. After the aforementioned has been carefully explained to the patients, amniocentesis should be advised for those couples who desire termination of a pregnancy if an affected fetus is diagnosed. It should be emphasized that the decision to terminate a pregnancy is made by the patients and not by the genetic counselor. It is the counselor's role to provide the patients with as much information as he can to enable them to reach their decisions. Supportive services from such personnel as social workers and psychologists are often invaluable in assisting the patient with the decisions.

Technique of Amniocentesis

Transabdominal paracentesis for the diagnosis of genetic disorders is best performed during the 15th or 16th week of pregnancy. Although the procedure can be performed at a later date, it must be borne in mind that chromosomal analysis usually takes two to three weeks and diagnosis of metabolic disorders four to six weeks.

Prior to removal of amniotic fluid, the patient voids, and the size and location of the uterus is ascertained by palpation. Sonography is helpful in about 50% of cases at this point in the pregnancy. Under sterile conditions, a 22 gauge spinal needle with a stylet is introduced transabdominally into the uterus, and 10 to 20 ml of amniotic fluid is removed and placed in a sterile container.

The fluid is centrifuged, and the cell button is resuspended in nutrient media in Falcon flasks. Cell attachment occurs within one to two days, and cells are grown by standard tissue culture techniques. In this way, sufficient fibroblasts are obtained for chromosome analysis in two to three weeks and for biochemical studies in four to six weeks.

For chromosome studies, the cells are synchronized by trypsinization 24 to 48 hours before harvesting. They are then suspended in nutrient medium, replanted in Falcon flasks and treated with Velban. The cells are then trypsinized and harvested by standard techniques.

For enzyme assays, the cells should be transported to a center that has the proper facilities for performing the particular test (62, 67).

REFERENCES

GENETIC DISORDERS

1. Srb, AM, Owen RD, Edgar RS: General Genetics, 2nd ed. San Francisco, Freeman, 1965
2. Stern C: Principles of Human Genetics, 3rd ed. San Francisco, Freeman, 1973

DOWN'S SYNDROME

3. Alter M: Dermatoglyphic analysis as a diagnostic tool. Medicine (Baltimore) 46:35, 1967
4. Breg WR, Miller OJ, Schnickel RD: Chromosomal translocations in patients with mongolism and in their normal relatives. N Engl J Med 266:845, 1962
5. Carter CO, Evans KA: Risk of parents who have had one child with Down's syndrome (mongolism) having another child similarly affected. Lancet 2:785, 1961
6. Collmann RD, Stoller A: A survey of mongoloid births in Victoria, Australia, 1942–1957. Am J Public Health 52:813, 1962
7. Fitzgerald PH, Lycette RR: Mosaicism in man, involving the autosome associated with mongolism. Heredity (Lond) 16:509, 1961
8. Hall B: Mongolism in newborn infants, an examination of the criteria for recognition and some speculations on the pathogenic activity of the chromosomal abnormality. Clin Pediatr (Phila) 5:4, 1966
9. Oster J: Mongolism. Copenhagen, Danish Science Press Ltd, 1953
10. Polani PE, Hamerton JL, Giannelli F, Carter CO: Cytogenetics of Down's syndrome (mongolism). III. Frequency of chromosome interchanges 4:193, 1965
11. Smith DW: Major Problems in Clinical Pediatrics, Vol VII, Recognizable Patterns of Human Malformations: Genetic, Embryologic,

and Clinical Aspects. Philadelphia, Saunders, 1970
12. Smith GS, Therman EM, Pateau KA, Inhorn SL: Mosaicism in mother of two mongoloids. Am J Dis Child 104:534, 1962
13. Stewart A, Webb J, Hewitt D: A survey of childhood malignancies. Br Med J 1:1495, 1958

AUTOSOMAL TRISOMY SYNDROMES

14. Hsu LYF, Sharpiro LR, Gertner M, Lieber E, Hirschhorn K: Trisomy 22: a clinical entity. J Pediatr 79:12, 1971
15. Nusbacher J, Hirschhorn K: Autosomal anomalies in man. Adv. Teratology 3:1, 1968
16. Pateau K, Smith DW, Therman E, Inhorn SL, Wagner HP: Multiple congenital anomaly caused by an extra chromosome. Lancet 1:790, 1960
17. Smith DW: Autosomal abnormalities. Am J Obstet Gynecol 90:1055, 1964
18. Uchida IA, Ray M, McRae KN, Besant DF: Familial occurrence of trisomy 22. Am J Hum Genet 20: 107, 1968

CAT EYE SYNDROME

19. Schachenmann G, Schnied W, Fraccaro J, Mannine A, Tieplo L, Perona GP, Sartou E: Chromosomes in coloboma and anal atresia. Lancet 2: 290, 1965

AUTOSOMAL DELETION SYNDROMES

20. Arias D, Passarge E, Engel MA, German J: Human chromosomal deletion: two patients with the 4p– syndrome. J Pediatr 76, 1970
21. Carneiro Leao J, Bargman GJ, Leu RL, Kajii T, Gardner LI: New syndrome associated with partial deletion of short arms of chromosome No 4. JAMA 202:434, 1967
22. Challacombe DN, Taylor A: Monosomy for a G autosome. Arch Dis Child 44:113, 1969
23. De Capoa A, Warburton D, Berg WR, Miller DA, Miller OJ: Transolcation heterozygosis: a cause of five cases of the cri du chat syndrome and two cases with a duplication of chromosome number five in three families. Am J Hum Genet 19:586, 1967
24. German J, Lejeune J, MacIntyre MN, De Grouchy J: Chromosomal autoradiography in the cri du chat syndrome. Cytogenetics 3:347, 1964
25. De Grouchy J, Lamy M, Theiffry S, Arthierio M, Salmon C: Dysmorphic complexe avec des oligophrenie: deletion des bras courts d'un chromosome 17-18. Compt Renal. Acad Sci [D] (Paris) 256L:1028, 1963
26. De Grouchy J, Royer P, Salmon C, Lamy M: Deletion partielle des bras longs du chromosome 18. Pathol Biol (Paris) 12:579 1964
27. Hirschhorn K, Cooper HL, Cooper IL, Firschein IL: Deletion of short arms of chromosome 4-5

in a child with defects of midline fusion. Humangenetik 1:479, 1965

28. Lejeune J, LaFourcade T, Berges R, Vialatte J, Boeswillwold M, Seringe P, Turpin, R: Trois cas de deletion partielle des bras courts d'un chromosome 5. Compt Rend Acad Sci [D](Paris) 257:3098, 1963

29. Migeon BR: Familial variant autosomes: new human cytogenetic markers. Bull Johns Hopkins Hosp 116:396, 1965

30. Polani PE: Autosomal imbalance and its syndromes, excluding Down's. Br Med Bull 25:81, 1969

SEX CHROMOSOME ABERRATIONS

31. Barr ML, Sergovich FR, Carr DJ, Shaver EL: The triplo-X female: an appraisal based on a study of 12 cases and a review of the literature. Can Med Assoc J 101:247, 1969

32. Di Cagno L, Franceschini P: Feeblemindedness and XXXX karyotype. J Ment Defic Res 12:226, 1968

33. Ferguson-Smith MA: Review article: Karyotype correlations in gonadal dysgenesis and their bearing on the pathogenesis of malformation. J Med Genet 2:93, 1965

34. Ferguson-Smith MA: Sex chromatin: Klinefelter's syndrome and mental defiiency. In: The Sex Chromatin. Edited by KL Moore. Philadelphia, Saunders, 1966

35. Ferguson-Smith MA, Mace WS, Ellis PM, Dickson M, Sanger R, Race RR: Parental age and the source of the X chromosomes in XXY Klinefelter's syndrome. Lancet 1:46, 1964

36. Hsu LYF, Klinger HP, Weiss J: Influence of nuclear selection criteria on sex-chromatin frequency in oral mucosal cells of newborn females. Cytogenetics 6:371, 1967

37. Klinefelter HF, Reifenstein EC Jr, Albright F: Syndrome characterized by gynecomastica aspermatogenesis A-leydigism and increased excretion of follicle stimulating hormone. J Clin Endocrinol Metab 2:615, 1942

38. Lubs HA, Ruddle FH: Chromosomal abnormalities in the human population: estimation of rates based on New Haven newborn study. Science 169:495, 1970

39. Moore KL, Barr ML: Nuclear morphology, according to sex in human tissues. Acta Anat (Basel) 21:197, 1954

40. Morrey J: Two cytogenetic syndromes. psychologic comparisons. I. Intelligence and specific factor quotients. J Psychiatr Res 2:223, 1964

40a. Nora JJ, Fraser C: Medical Genetics, Principles and Practice. Philadelphia, Lea and Febiger, 1974, p. 67

41. Penrose LS: Finger-print pattern and the sex chromosomes. Lancet 1:298, 1967

42. Shaffer JW: A specific cognitive deficit observed in gonadal dysplasia (Turner's syndrome). J Clin Psychol 18:403, 1962

43. Steiker DD, Mellman WJ, Bongiovanni AM, Eberlein WR, Leboef G: Turner's syndrome in the male. J Pediatr 58:321, 1961

44. Turner HH: A syndrome of infantilism, congenital webbed neck and cubitus valgus. Endocrinology 23:566, 1938

IDENTIFICATION OF INDIVIDUALS WITH ABNORMAL CHROMOSOMES

45. Arrighi FE, Hsu TC: Localization of heterochromatin in human chromosomes. Cytogenetics 10:81, 1971

46. Breg WR, Miller DA, Alldedice PW, Miller OJ: Identification of human translocation chromosomes by quinacrine fluoresence, abstract. Pediatr Res 5:423, 1971

47. Caspersson T, Fech L, Johansson C: Differential binding of alkylating fluorochromes in human chromosomes. Exp Cell Res 67:315, 1970

48. Caspersson T, Lomakta G, Zech L: The 24 fluoresence patterns of the human metaphase chromosomes—distinguishing characters and variability. Hereditas 67:89, 1971

49. Chernay PR, Hsu LYF, Hirschhorn K: Human chromosome identification by differential staining: G. group (21-22-Y). Cytogenetics 10:219, 1971

50. Drets ME, Shaw MW: Specific banding patterns of human chromosomes. Proc Nat Acad Sci USA 68:2073, 1971

51. Patil SR, Merrick S, Lubs HA: Identification of each human chromosome with a modified Giemsa stain. Science 173:821, 1971

52. Pearson PL, Bobrow M, Vosa CG: Technique for identifying Y chromosome in human interphase nuclei. Nature 226:7, 1970

53. Sumner AT, Evans HJ, Buckland RA: New technique for distinguishing between human chromosomes. Nature [New Biol] 232:31, 1971

ANTENATAL DIAGNOSIS

54. Court Brown WM, Law P, Smith PG: Sex chromosome aneuploidy and parental age. Ann Hum Genet 33:1, 1969

55. Gerbie AB, Nadler HL, Gerbie MV: Amniocentesis in genetic counseling. Am J Obstet Gynecol 109:765, 1971

56. Gertner M, Hsu LYF, Martin J, Hirshhorn K: The use of amniocentesis for prenatal genetic counseling. Bull NY Acad Med 46:916, 1970

57. Kaback MM, Zeiger RS: Heterozygote detection in Tay-Sachs disease: a prototype community screening program for the prevention of recessive genetic disorders, In: Sphingolipids, Sphingolipidoses, and Allied Disorders. Edited by BW Volk, SM Aronson. New York, Plenum Press, 1972

58. Kohn G, Robinson A: Tetraploidy in cells cultured from amniotic fluid. Lancet 2:778, 1970

59. Lisgar F, Gertner M, Cherry S, Hsu LY, Hirsch-

horn K: Prenatal chromosome analysis. Nature 225:280, 1970

60. Milunsky A: The Prenatal Diagnosis of Hereditary Disorders. Springfield, Ill, Thomas, 1973

61. Milunsky A, Atkins L, Littlefield JW: Amniocentesis for prenatal genetic studies. Obstet Gynecol 40:104, 1972

62. Nadler HL: Prenatal detection of hereditary disorders. Adv Hum Genet 3:1, 1972

63. Nadler HL, Gerbie A: Present status of amniocentesis in intrauterine diagnosis of genetic defects. Obstet Gynecol 38:789, 1971

64. Penrose LS, Smith GF: Down's Anomaly. London, J&A Churchill, 1966

65. Rook A, Hsu L, Gertner M, Hirschhorn K: Identification of X and Y chromosomes in amniotic fluid cells. Nature 230:53, 1971

66. Taylor AI: Autosomal trisomy syndromes: a detailed study of 27 cases of Edwards' syndrome and 27 of Patan's syndrome. J Med Genet 5:227, 1968

67. Turpin R, Lejeune J: Human Afflictions and Chromosomal Aberrations. London, Pergamon, 1969

withdrawal consists of specific therapy aimed at alleviating major neurologic signs and supportive therapy, e.g., treatment of suspected infection with antibiotics; provision of adequate fluid, electrolytes and calories; and correction of metabolic defects, particularly hypoglycemia and hypocalcemia. The course of heroin withdrawal is usually benign and self-limiting. Those drugs used to control signs must have the minimum amount of toxic side effects and should be used in lowest dosage necessary for the shortest possible period of time.

Paregoric (camphorated tincture of opium) was successfully used in treatment for many years. A dosage of 1 to 3 drops/kg prior to each feeding, gradually tapered, was required for many weeks before therapy could be discontinued. One pitfall with this treatment is that the administration of paregoric to an infant in whom the diagnosis of narcotic withdrawal has been made mistakenly will create an addiction problem where none had existed previously.

Chlorpromazine and phenobarbital have been used more recently with approximately the same degree of success. We have found that phenobarbital, 8 mg/kg/day, divided into three oral doses is effective in controlling manifestations. If vomiting is present, phenobarbital may be administered by the IM route. The full dosage is usually required for three to five days, followed by tapering over another three to five days. The duration of therapy varies with the severity of signs and the infant's response. Chlorpromazine, in a dosage of 2.8 mg/day divided into four oral doses, has been found similar to phenobarbital in efficacy in controlling signs of heroin withdrawal.

Diazepam has also been used successfully in controlling withdrawal (21). A drawback to its use is that the IM preparation has sodium benzoate as a preservative. This chemical interferes with albumin binding of unconjugated bilirubin and may enhance the development of bilirubin encephalopahy in jaundiced infants (26).

Treatment of infants undergoing methadone withdrawal is more difficult. It is hard to control withdrawal manifestations with

TABLE 15–1. Treatment of Neonatal Narcotic Withdrawal

I. Prenatal care of mother in high-risk obstetric clinic
II. Specific Therapy
  A. Narcotic antagonist (for narcotic-induced respiratory depression)
    1. Nalorphine hydrochloride (Nalline), 0.1 to 0.2 mg/kg IV; may be repeated in 10 to 15 minutes
    2. Naloxone (Narcan), 0.005 mg/kg IM.
  B. Alleviation of signs of narcotic withdrawal
    1. Phenobarbital 8 to 10 mg/kg/day in 3 divided oral doses
    2. Chlorpromazine 2.8 mg/kg/day in 4 divided oral doses
    3. Paregoric, 1 to 3 drops/kg orally before each feeding (up to 5 drops/kg for severe methadone withdrawal)
    4. Diazepam, 0.5 mg IM once or twice daily
III. Supportive Therapy
  A. Prophylaxis against gonococcal ophthalmia
  B. Treatment of suspected infection
  C. Adequate fluid and caloric intake (IV if vomiting or diarrhea is present)
  D. Treatment of concurrent metabolic aberrations, such as hypoglycemia or hypocalcemia
  E. Meticulous nursing care

either phenobarbital or chlorpromazine, and paregoric often has to be used. Very large doses (up to 5 drops/kg before each feeding) may be required, and the duration of treatment may last several weeks. We have encountered cases in which even paregoric could not alleviate major signs. In this instance, 0.5 mg of diazepam given intramuscularly is usually effective for 12 to 24 hours.

Excellent nursing care is of special importance. In general, these infants should be handled as little and as gently as possible while they are undergoing withdrawal.

Because of the high incidence of venereal disease in pregnant addicts, eye prophylaxis (with silver nitrate or topical broad spectrum antibiotics such as neomycin) against gonococcal ophthalmia is imperative. Infants of narcotic addicts are also prime candidates for congenital syphilis, and early diagnosis and treatment are necessary.

While the diarrhea that accompanies narcotic withdrawal is usually noninfectious, the etiologic role of an enteric pathogen must be excluded. Prompt diagnosis, specific therapy (in the case of salmonella or entero-pathogenic *E. coli*) and isolation of the infant are necessary to treat the affected infant and prevent a nursery-wide diarrhea epidemic. Evidence indicates that these infants may have an unusually high incidence of intra-uterine pneumonia (20). In suspected or proven respiratory infection, appropriate antibiotics should be administered.

Increased water losses secondary to hyperventilation, sweating and loose stools may lead to dehydration. When possible, ample fluids should be given by mouth. When this is not feasible, fluids should be given intravenously. Weighing the baby daily, especially if he is of low birth weight or ill, is the best means of gauging fluid requirements.

Caloric requirements may be increased especially if the infant is hyperactive or small for gestational age. The IV use of 10% glucose solution may be required as either a partial or total source of the infant's caloric requirements.

PROGNOSIS

Although the medical treatment of acute withdrawal in newborn infants is relatively simple, the long-term outlook is more complicated. Discharging an infant to a home where one or both parents are untreated addicts is not in the infant's best interest. Under New York State law, these infants are legally considered victims of child abuse, and cases must be reported to a central registry. Usually, these infants are discharged either to a foster home or to some other relative, such as the grandmother, until such time that the mother has entered a therapeutic program and is considered capable of properly caring for the infant. Infants born to mothers already enrolled in methadone maintenance or drug free programs are usually discharged to their parents. A very carefully planned medical and sociologic follow-up of these families is mandatory.

Irritability and restlessness may be noted for several months after birth in the methadone infants, and the mothers, whose personal life situations are already tenuous, often find the relationship with their infants strained. With intensive medical, psychologic and sociologic support, follow-up care will be successful in the vast majority of cases.

The long-term biologic effects of fetal exposure to heroin and methadone are not fully known. Because of the high incidence of intrauterine growth retardation, the incidence of abnormal psychomotor development would be expected to be higher in the exposed group than in the population at large. Wilson et al (29) found an increased incidence of behavioral disturbances among children of heroin-addicted mothers.

NONNARCOTIC AGENTS

BARBITURATES

Infants of mothers addicted to barbiturates may develop signs similar to those seen in the narcotic withdrawal syndrome. With a short-acting drug, such as secobarbital, signs may develop shortly after delivery (3). If a long-acting barbiturate, such as phenobarbital, has been used, withdrawal may not be evident until a week after birth, by which time the infant may have been discharged (6).

Treatment consists of the administration of phenobarbital in a dosage similar to that required in narcotic withdrawal. The course of treatment is about 10 to 15 days, with a gradual reduction of dosage after 3 to 5 days.

There are no known neurologic sequelae following neonatal barbiturate withdrawal. However, long-term follow-up is necessary.

ALCOHOL

The chronic use of alcohol during pregnancy is associated with a perinatal mortality rate of 17% (16). Among the survivors, approximately one-third have prenatal and postnatal growth failure associated with microcephaly, craniofacial abnormalities,

15

Drug
Abuse

During the 1960s and early 1970s the use of addictive drugs during pregnancy has become an increasingly serious urban problem in the United States, with an estimated 1500 to 2000 illicit drug users delivering infants each year in New York City alone. Among the drugs more commonly abused during pregnancy are heroin, methadone, barbiturates, cocaine, alcohol, tranquilizers, LSD, marijuana and amphetamines.

Until the early 1970s heroin was the addictive drug most frequently used (with the exception of alcohol) by pregnant addicts. At about this time, methadone, a synthetic narcotic agent that blocks the euphoric effects of heroin and decreases the desire of addicts for this drug gained acceptance in many urban areas as a therapeutic agent for the treatment of heroin addiction (7). In New York City about 35,000 patients were enrolled in methadone treatment programs in 1973. About 8500 of these were women of child-bearing age, many of whom were already pregnant. By late 1973 it was estimated that about 80% of pregnant narcotic abusers in New York City were using either methadone alone (obtained either legally or illegally) or in combination with heroin. In addition, many pregnant women were using such mood affecting nonnarcotic drugs as barbiturates, tranquilizers, alcohol, marijuana, amphetamines and cocaine, and a substantial number of these women were assumed also to be narcotic users.

NARCOTIC AGENTS

OBSTETRIC FACTORS

Both heroin and methadone have profound effects on the pregnancy and on the newborn infant following delivery. With the use of heroin, there is interference with ovulation, irregular menses and a decreased sexual drive, but in spite of this, a substantial number of women addicted to heroin become pregnant. In women who are on methadone maintenance therapy, ovulation and menstrual cycles are usually normal, as is the sexual drive, and many of the pregnancies are planned.

Both drugs cross the placenta, and the fetus like the mother is in danger of becoming addicted following exposure to the drug. Maternal heroin addiction is associated with an unusually high incidence of both intrauterine growth retardation and prematurity. Approximately 50% of the infants born to these mothers have birth weights of less than 2500 g (23, 24, 30, 31). Although faulty maternal diet may be partially responsible for this intrauterine growth failure, experimental evidence implies that heroin per se impedes fetal growth (9, 28). Naeye et al (20) have correlated the excessively high rate of prematurity with intrauterine infection, which is seen with increased frequency in these infants. Infants of mothers on methadone maintenance also tend to have reduced birth weights, but are usually heavier than infants of heroin users (30).

Fetal anoxia with aspiration of meconium is encountered with increased frequency in both groups of infants, especially when maternal drug intake has been abruptly reduced. This is probably due to intrauterine narcotic withdrawal.

The high incidence of veneral disease and hepatitis encountered in pregnant addicts not enrolled in therapeutic programs may have an adverse effect on the fetus and newborn infant.

Although heroin addicts have, over the years, tended to avoid obstetric care, the increasing availability of both methadone and nonmethadone therapeutic programs has increased the number of those seeking prenatal treatment.

NEONATAL PERIOD

Most infants born to narcotic users are vigorous at birth and have Apgar Scores of 7 to 10 (23, 24). Respiratory depression secondary to narcotic overdose is rare, and if it is present, a narcotic antagonist may be administered. Nalorphine hydrochloride (0.1 to 0.2 mg/kg IV) has the disadvantage of worsening the respiratory depression if it is actually secondary to asphyxia rather than to narcotic overdose. Naloxone, which has been administered to a limited number of infants in an IM dosage of 0.005 mg/kg, has the advantage of not worsening respiratory depression caused by asphyxia.

It is much more likely that infants of mothers addicted to both heroin and methadone will develop signs of acute narcotic withdrawal. If withdrawal has begun in utero, signs will occur immediately after delivery. About 50% of infants of mothers using heroin will undergo moderate or severe withdrawal; the remainder have either very mild or no signs. The latter group may reflect a relatively low dosage of drug taken by their mothers. Heroin withdrawal usually appears within the first 24 hours of life and will rarely begin after the third day. The appearance of signs of

methadone withdrawal may be delayed for several days or even weeks. In contrast to infants of heroin users, about 80% exhibit signs that are moderate or severe (23). This greater severity may reflect the high doses the mother receives (usually over 60 mg/day) and the pharmacologic characteristics of the drug.

If the mother is known to be enrolled in a methadone maintenance program, neonatal withdrawal can be anticipated, and there is usually little doubt about the diagnosis. If the mother's narcotic habit is not known to the physician caring for the infant, establishing the correct diagnosis may pose a problem. Many signs of acute withdrawal are nonspecific and may be seen in other conditions such as hypoglycemia, hypocalcemia, intracranial bleeding and meningitis. Withdrawal from nonnarcotic drugs such as barbiturates may also produce a similar clinical picture.

Withdrawal

The two major signs of neonatal narcotic withdrawal are a unique type of coarse, flapping tremor and irritability. Muscular rigidity is a common finding. One-third to one-half of these infants have vomiting, diarrhea, or both.

A shrill, high pitched cry, sneezing and yawning are often present. Excessive sweating, presumably due to a central neurogenic stimulation of sweat glands, is common, even among premature infants (2).

Convulsions are uncommon in infants of heroin-addicted mothers, but are more likely to be encountered in methadone withdrawal and occasionally may be the presenting sign. Myoclonic jerks of the extremities are occasionally seen. Tachypnea, not associated with the respiratory distress syndrome (RDS), is a frequent and early finding. The basis for this sign is unknown. In adult addicts, it is believed to be related to increased sensitivity of the respiratory center to carbon dioxide (19). The phenomenon is associated with a primary respiratory alkalosis.

Infants undergoing withdrawal will suck

on any available object, most often their fists, with unusual vigor. In spite of this they are usually inefficient feeders. Because of their extreme restlessness, skin abrasions secondary to sheet burns are often seen.

Although mortality rates of as high as 94% have been recorded in neonatal heroin withdrawal (14), we have never encountered a death directly attributable to the withdrawal process. Deaths in these infants are usually due either to prematurity, infection or intrauterine asphyxia. Among infants of mothers using methadone, sudden death in the late neonatal period or early infancy have been described (22), the reason for which has not been determined.

Diagnosis

We have used the criteria of Kahn et al (17) to classify the major signs of narcotic withdrawal, which are tremulousness and irritability. In grade I, the signs are recognizable but mild; in grade II, the signs are marked only when the infant is disturbed; and in grade III the signs are marked and occur at frequent intervals even when the infant is undisturbed. In general, signs tend to be more severe and prolonged in infants withdrawing from methadone than in those undergoing heroin withdrawal (23).

Findings. Several interesting phenomena have been observed to be associated with maternal use of heroin during pregnancy. We have found a marked decrease in the incidence of RDS in premature infants of heroin-addicted mothers (10). The reason for this remains unclear, but it has been suggested that opiates may function as enzyme inducers, resulting in an increased production of pulmonary surfactant, whose absence or decreased presence in the lungs of premature infants has been causally linked to RDS.

The incidence of neonatal jaundice also seems to be decreased in this group of infants. There is some experimental evidence that heroin enhances hepatic glucuronyl transferase activity, thus accelerating the conjugation of bilirubin (4).

Quinine, which is often mixed with heroin sold in the street, may also have an effect on bilirubin metabolism. We have seen one G-6-PD deficient infant with quinine present in his urine, who developed hemolytic anemia and jaundice, presumably due to the effect of the quinine on his sensitive RBCs (12).

Because opiates are known to suppress the hypothalamic anterior pituitary axis, we measured serum cortisol concentrations in addicted and nonaddicted women at the time of delivery and in the umbilical venous sera of their offspring. While there was a significant decrease in the cortisol concentration among the addicted women, this effect was not apparent in their offspring (13).

Teratogenic effects of heroin and methadone have not been observed. Abrams (1), however, notes chromosomal breakage in infants of mothers addicted to heroin.

Procedures. In addition to the physical examination, the history is of great importance in establishing the diagnosis of neonatal narcotic withdrawal. In our experience the mother has usually been willing to discuss her drug habit with the physician. While interviewing the mother, a glance at her arms may reveal evidence of needle tracts or scarring, which will be of value should she deny using narcotics.

On some occasions the diagnosis of narcotic withdrawal may be doubtful, or coexisting medical conditions may cause similar signs, and at these times laboratory and radiologic studies may be useful. Metabolites of opium and other addictive drugs may be detected in the urine of the mother or infant by chromatography (5) or radioimmunoassay.

Since tremulousness and irritability may be presenting signs of the hypoglycemia which is common in infants who are small for gestational age, blood glucose determinations in all infants with signs of withdrawal are mandatory (see section Carbohydrate Metabolism, Ch. 12).

Neuromuscular irritability is also a sign of neonatal hypocalcemia (serum calcium

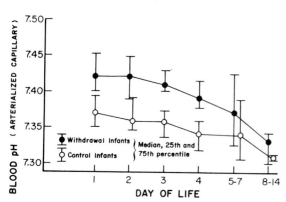

FIG. 15–1. Arterialized capillary-blood pH values in neonates with heroin withdrawal and in normal controls. (Glass et al: N Engl J Med 286:746, 1972)

concentration below 8.0 mg/100 ml). In the interpretation of serum calcium levels, the infant's blood pH should be considered since an alkalotic pH may decrease the concentration of ionized calcium. Whether low levels of ionized calcium are related to neuromuscular signs in this syndrome remains to be determined. Likewise, the total serum protein concentration should be measured when considering the possibility of hypocalcemia.

If there is suspicion of systemic bacterial infection, appropriate cultures (blood, CSF, urine, stool, nose and throat) should be obtained, and the appropriate antimicrobial therapy started.

FIG. 15–2. Capillary blood Pco_2 values in infants with heroin withdrawal and normal controls. (Glass et al: N Engl J Med 286:746, 1972)

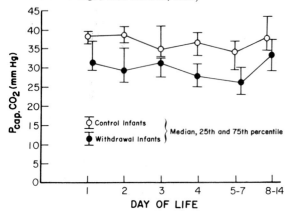

Acid-base studies of the infant's blood aid both in diagnosis and management of drug withdrawal. In the respiratory alkalosis associated with withdrawal-induced tachypnea, the average blood pH value during the first days of life is 7.42 (Fig. 15–1) compared to normal average values of about 7.37. The Pco_2 (Fig. 15–2) is decreased, averaging about 30 mm Hg, compared to a normal neonatal value of about 35 mm Hg (11).

A serologic test for syphilis should be performed on cord bloods of all infants of addicted mothers because of the high maternal incidence of venereal disease.

A normal chest x ray accompanies the tachypnea of narcotic withdrawal. If pneumonia or aspiration of meconium is possible, a chest x ray should be taken.

Treatment

Therapy of neonatal narcotic withdrawal begins with treatment of the pregnant addict (Table 15–1). Antenatal obstetric care at a facility capable of following a high-risk pregnancy—with the proper facilities and staffing for handling an infant underoing withdrawal—is mandatory.

Every effort must be made to have pregnant addicts seek obstetric care as early in pregnancy as possible. Both drug free and methadone maintenance programs are available, and these programs should attempt to identify pregnancy in patients already enrolled at the earliest possible date in order to insure the necessary obstetric care. Whether in a methadone or drug free program, intensive psychiatric and social service counseling are required.

Women already enrolled in methadone programs who become pregnant and are on a high maintenance dosage should have their dosage gradually lowered to 40 to 60 mg/day during the first trimester. Obstetricians treating women who are in methadone maintenance or drug free programs must communicate prior to delivery with the pediatricians who will be caring for the newborn infants.

The actual treatment of neonatal narcotic

withdrawal consists of specific therapy aimed at alleviating major neurologic signs and supportive therapy, e.g., treatment of suspected infection with antibiotics; provision of adequate fluid, electrolytes and calories; and correction of metabolic defects, particularly hypoglycemia and hypocalcemia. The course of heroin withdrawal is usually benign and self-limiting. Those drugs used to control signs must have the minimum amount of toxic side effects and should be used in lowest dosage necessary for the shortest possible period of time.

Paregoric (camphorated tincture of opium) was successfully used in treatment for many years. A dosage of 1 to 3 drops/kg prior to each feeding, gradually tapered, was required for many weeks before therapy could be discontinued. One pitfall with this treatment is that the administration of paregoric to an infant in whom the diagnosis of narcotic withdrawal has been made mistakenly will create an addiction problem where none had existed previously.

Chlorpromazine and phenobarbital have been used more recently with approximately the same degree of success. We have found that phenobarbital, 8 mg/kg/day, divided into three oral doses is effective in controlling manifestations. If vomiting is present, phenobarbital may be administered by the IM route. The full dosage is usually required for three to five days, followed by tapering over another three to five days. The duration of therapy varies with the severity of signs and the infant's response. Chlorpromazine, in a dosage of 2.8 mg/day divided into four oral doses, has been found similar to phenobarbital in efficacy in controlling signs of heroin withdrawal.

Diazepam has also been used successfully in controlling withdrawal (21). A drawback to its use is that the IM preparation has sodium benzoate as a preservative. This chemical interferes with albumin binding of unconjugated bilirubin and may enhance the development of bilirubin encephalopahy in jaundiced infants (26).

Treatment of infants undergoing methadone withdrawal is more difficult. It is hard to control withdrawal manifestations with

TABLE 15-1. Treatment of Neonatal Narcotic Withdrawal

I. Prenatal care of mother in high-risk obstetric clinic

II. Specific Therapy
  A. Narcotic antagonist (for narcotic-induced respiratory depression)
    1. Nalorphine hydrochloride (Nalline), 0.1 to 0.2 mg/kg IV; may be repeated in 10 to 15 minutes
    2. Naloxone (Narcan), 0.005 mg/kg IM.
  B. Alleviation of signs of narcotic withdrawal
    1. Phenobarbital 8 to 10 mg/kg/day in 3 divided oral doses
    2. Chlorpromazine 2.8 mg/kg/day in 4 divided oral doses
    3. Paregoric, 1 to 3 drops/kg orally before each feeding (up to 5 drops/kg for severe methadone withdrawal)
    4. Diazepam, 0.5 mg IM once or twice daily

III. Supportive Therapy
  A. Prophylaxis against gonococcal ophthalmia
  B. Treatment of suspected infection
  C. Adequate fluid and caloric intake (IV if vomiting or diarrhea is present)
  D. Treatment of concurrent metabolic aberrations, such as hypoglycemia or hypocalcemia
  E. Meticulous nursing care

either phenobarbital or chlorpromazine, and paregoric often has to be used. Very large doses (up to 5 drops/kg before each feeding) may be required, and the duration of treatment may last several weeks. We have encountered cases in which even paregoric could not alleviate major signs. In this instance, 0.5 mg of diazepam given intramuscularly is usually effective for 12 to 24 hours.

Excellent nursing care is of special importance. In general, these infants should be handled as little and as gently as possible while they are undergoing withdrawal.

Because of the high incidence of venereal disease in pregnant addicts, eye prophylaxis (with silver nitrate or topical broad spectrum antibiotics such as neomycin) against gonococcal ophthalmia is imperative. Infants of narcotic addicts are also prime candidates for congenital syphilis, and early diagnosis and treatment are necessary.

While the diarrhea that accompanies narcotic withdrawal is usually noninfectious, the etiologic role of an enteric pathogen must be excluded. Prompt diagnosis, specific therapy (in the case of salmonella or entero-pathogenic *E. coli*) and isolation of the infant are necessary to treat the affected infant and prevent a nursery-wide diarrhea epidemic. Evidence indicates that these infants may have an unusually high incidence of intra-uterine pneumonia (20). In suspected or proven respiratory infection, appropriate antibiotics should be administered.

Increased water losses secondary to hyperventilation, sweating and loose stools may lead to dehydration. When possible, ample fluids should be given by mouth. When this is not feasible, fluids should be given intravenously. Weighing the baby daily, especially if he is of low birth weight or ill, is the best means of gauging fluid requirements.

Caloric requirements may be increased especially if the infant is hyperactive or small for gestational age. The IV use of 10% glucose solution may be required as either a partial or total source of the infant's caloric requirements.

PROGNOSIS

Although the medical treatment of acute withdrawal in newborn infants is relatively simple, the long-term outlook is more com-plicated. Discharging an infant to a home where one or both parents are untreated addicts is not in the infant's best interest. Under New York State law, these infants are legally considered victims of child abuse, and cases must be reported to a central reg-istry. Usually, these infants are discharged either to a foster home or to some other relative, such as the grandmother, until such time that the mother has entered a thera-peutic program and is considered capable of properly caring for the infant. Infants born to mothers already enrolled in methadone maintenance or drug free programs are usu-ally discharged to their parents. A very carefully planned medical and sociologic fol-low-up of these families is mandatory.

Irritability and restlessness may be noted for several months after birth in the metha-done infants, and the mothers, whose per-sonal life situations are already tenuous, often find the relationship with their infants strained. With intensive medical, psycho-logic and sociologic support, follow-up care will be successful in the vast majority of cases.

The long-term biologic effects of fetal ex-posure to heroin and methadone are not fully known. Because of the high incidence of intrauterine growth retardation, the inci-dence of abnormal psychomotor develop-ment would be expected to be higher in the exposed group than in the population at large. Wilson et al (29) found an increased incidence of behavioral disturbances among children of heroin-addicted mothers.

NONNARCOTIC AGENTS

BARBITURATES

Infants of mothers addicted to barbiturates may develop signs similar to those seen in the narcotic withdrawal syndrome. With a short-acting drug, such as secobarbital, signs may develop shortly after delivery (3). If a long-acting barbiturate, such as pheno-barbital, has been used, withdrawal may not be evident until a week after birth, by which time the infant may have been discharged (6).

Treatment consists of the administration of phenobarbital in a dosage similar to that required in narcotic withdrawal. The course of treatment is about 10 to 15 days, with a gradual reduction of dosage after 3 to 5 days.

There are no known neurologic sequelae following neonatal barbiturate withdrawal. However, long-term follow-up is necessary.

ALCOHOL

The chronic use of alcohol during preg-nancy is associated with a perinatal mortal-ity rate of 17% (16). Among the survivors, approximately one-third have prenatal and postnatal growth failure associated with microcephaly, craniofacial abnormalities,

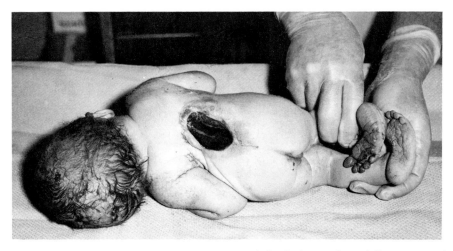

FIG. 15–3. Skeletal abnormalities following use of LSD during pregnancy. (Eller et al: N Engl J Med 283:395, 1970)

cardiac and joint anomalies and altered palmar crease patterns. Direct toxicity of alcohol on the fetus is incriminated (16).

Motor and intellectual developmental delays have been described in this syndrome (28a).

COCAINE

Although we have observed severe signs of withdrawal among infants whose mothers used cocaine during pregnancy, it is not certain whether these manifestations were secondary to the cocaine or to another drug that the mother was concomitantly using.

LSD

There have been several reports (8, 18) of deformed infants born to mothers who were users of lysergic acid dieythylamide (LSD), mostly involving the spine and bony thorax (Fig. 15–3). There is also evidence that the use of LSD during pregnancy may lead to chromosomal breakage (27), but this is not definitely established.

MISCELLANEOUS DRUGS

There is no evidence that the use of either amphetamines or marijuana during pregnancy adversely affects the fetus. Addiction to diazepam may lead to a heroin-like with-

drawal syndrome on the second or third day of life (25).

REFERENCES

1. Abrams C, Liao PY: Chromosomal aberrations in newborns exposed to heroin in utero (abstr). J Clin Invest 51:1a, 1972
2. Behrendt H, Green M: The nature of the sweating deficit of prematurely born neonates. Observations on babies with the heroin withdrawal syndrome. N Engl J Med 286:1376, 1972
3. Bleyer WA, Marshall RE: Barbiturate withdrawal syndrome in a passively addicted infant. JAMA 221:185, 1972
4. Cohen MI, Nathenson G, McNamara H, Litt IF: The mitigating effect of addiction to heroin on neonatal jaundice. J Pediatr 81:899, 1972
5. Cole VP, Kim WK, Eglitis I: Detection of narcotic drugs, tranquilizers, amphetamines, and barbiturates in urine. JAMA 198:349, 1966
6. Desmond MM, Schwanecke RP, Wilson GI: Maternal barbiturate utilization and neonatal withdrawal symptomatology. J Pediatr 80:190, 1972
7. Dole VP, Nyswander ME: A medical treatment for diacetylmorphine (heroin) addiction. JAMA 193:646, 1965
8. Eller JL, Morton JM: Bizarre deformities in offspring of user of lysergic acid diethylamide. N Engl J Med 283:395, 1970
9. Friedler G, Cochin J: Growth retardation in offspring of female rats treated with morphine prior to conception. Science 175:654, 1972

10. Glass L, Rajegowda BK, Evans HE: Absence of respiratory distress syndrome in premature infants of heroin addicted mothers. Lancet 2:685, 1971

11. Glass L, Rajegowda BK, Kahn EJ, Floyd MV: Effect of heroin withdrawal on respiratory rate and acid base status of the newborn. N Engl J Med 286:746, 1972

12. Glass L, Rajegowda BK, Bowen E, Evans HE: Quinine induced jaundice in a G6PD deficient newborn infant. J Pediatr 82:741, 1973

13. Glass L, Rajegowda BK, Mukherjee TK, Roth MM, Evans HE: Effect of heroin on corticosteroid production in pregnant addicts and their fetuses. Am J Obstet Gynecol 117:416, 1973

14. Goodfriend MJ, Shey IA, Klein MD: The effects of maternal narcotic addiction on the newborn. Am J Obstet Gynecol 71:29, 1956

15. Jones KL, Smith DW, Streissguth AP: Further knowledge concerning the fetal alcohol syndrome. Clin Res 22:219A, 1974

16. Jones KL, Smith DW, Ulleland CN, Streissguth AP: Pattern of malformation in offspring of chronic alcoholic mothers. Lancet 1:1267, 1973

17. Kahn EJ, Newmann LL, Polk G: The course of heroin withdrawal syndrome in newborn infants treated with phenobarbital or chlorpromazine. J Pediatr 75:495, 1969

18. Lavy NW, Palmer CG, Merritt AD: A syndrome of bizarre vertebral anomalies. J. Pediatr 69:1121, 1966

19. Martin WR: A homeostatic and redundancy theory of tolerance to and dependence on narcotic analyzing. In: The Addictive States: Proceedings of the Association for Research in Nervous and Mental Disease, December 2, 3, 1966, New York, NY. Edited by A Wikler. Baltimore. Williams & Wilkins, 1968, p 206

20. Naeye RL, Blanc W, Leblanc W, Khatamee MA: Fetal complications of maternal heroin addiction. Abnormal growth infections, and episodes of stress. J Pediatr 83:1055, 1973

21. Nathenson G, Golden GS, Litt IF: Diazepam in the management of the neonatal narcotic withdrawal syndrome. Pediatrics 48:523, 1971

22. Pierson PS, Howard P, Kleber HD: Sudden deaths in infants born to methadone-maintained addicts. JAMA 220:1733, 1972

23. Rajegowda BK, Glass L, Evans HE, Maso G, Swartz DP, Leblanc W: Methadone withdrawal in newborn infants. J Pediatr 81:532, 1972

24. Reddy AM, Harper RG, Stern G: Observation on heroin and methadone withdrawal in the newborn. Pediatrics 48:353, 1971

25. Rementeria J: Personal communication, 1974

26. Schiff D, Chan G, Stern L: Fixed drug combinations and the displacement of bilirubin from albumin. Pediatrics 48:139, 1971

27. Smart RG, Bateman K: The chromosomal and teratogenic effects of lysergic acid diethylamide: a review of the current literature. Can Med Assoc J 99:805, 1968

28. Taeusch HW Jr, Carson W, Wang NS, Avery ME: The effects of heroin on lung maturation and growth in fetal rabbits. J Appl Physiol 34:660, 1973

28a. Tenbrinck MS, Buchin SY: Fetal alcohol syndrome: report of a case. JAMA 232:1144, 1975

29. Wilson GS, Desmond MM, Verniand WM: Early development of infants of heroin-addicted mothers. Am J Dis Child 126:457, 1973

30. Zelson C, Lee SJ, Casalino M: Neonatal narcotic addiction. N Engl J Med 289:1216, 1973

31. Zelson C, Rubio E, Wasserman E: Neonatal narcotic addiction: 10 year observation. Pediatrics 48:178, 1971

16

Care
of the Normal
Newborn Infant
and Psychosocial
Problems

THE NORMAL FULL-TERM INFANT

While the physical design and medical and nursing policies of neonatal nurseries vary from one hospital to another, proper medical care requires that several basic principles be followed. These are usually enumerated in state and municipal health codes.

PHYSICAL DESIGN OF THE NORMAL FULL-TERM NURSERY

The normal full-term nursery should be located on the obstetric floor, close to the mothers' rooms. In many hospitals, rooming-in facilities are available. At least 20 sq ft should be allocated for each bassinet with at least 1½ to 2 ft between bassinets.

A special transitional care area (4) should be set aside for close observation of newborn infants during the critical first 8 to 24 hours of adjustment to postnatal life. This transitional nursery should be either adjacent to the delivery suite or in a prominent location in the normal-neonate nursery area. The unit must be staffed at all times by highly trained nurses capable of recognizing subtle signs of illness. Following stabilization of vital signs, the infant may be transferred to the normal full-term nursery.

At least one room should be set aside as a suspect nursery for clinically well infants who have been exposed to infection. In many institutions, infants who are medically ready for discharge are kept in the nursery for prolonged periods because of maternal social problems, such as drug abuse. An adequate number of bassinets (dependent on the magnitude of the problem in the hospital) should be allocated for these boarder babies.

POLICIES AND STAFFING

The nursery should be under the supervision of a qualified pediatrician. Each infant admitted to the unit must be under the direct care of a physician (either a house officer or a physician in private practice), and each should have an initial complete physical examination within the first 12 hours of life.

The ratio of nursing staff to infants should be at least one to six, and at least one registered nurse must be on duty at all times. This staff must be able to recognize abnormal signs in the infants and should be capable of administering emergency care, e.g., artificial ventilation by bag and mask, until the arrival of a physician.

Each unit should be assigned a medical social worker, who will play an active role in planning for discharge and home care, solving placement problems and enhancing family–staff rapport.

All nurseries must maintain a set of up-to-date written policies governing such procedures as admission, standard care and discharge. In addition, the medical (both house and attending staffs) and nursing staff should hold daily rounds to review the progress of the infants and discuss any problems that may have developed.

Admissions

Infants admitted to the normal nursery should be those at lowest risk for morbidity and mortality. These are infants without obvious signs of illness who weigh 2250 to 4000 g at birth and whose gestational ages are between 37 and 41 weeks (5).

Medical and Nursing Care

Immediately after delivery, 1 mg of vitamin K is injected intramuscularly to prevent hemorrhagic disease, and prophylaxis against gonococcal ophthalmia is administered. Umbilical cord blood is taken in order to perform a serologic test for syphilis and, if necessary, a blood grouping and Coombs' test. The infant should be examined briefly in the delivery room and more thoroughly following admission to the nursery.

Initial cleansing of the infant's skin depends on the prevalence of staphylococcal disease in the nursery. Where this problem is rarely encountered, the infant may be washed with tap water and, if necessary, with a simple cleansing agent such as castile soap. If the infant is bathed with a HCP-containing soap, a thorough rinsing is necessary to prevent the absorption of this potentially neurotoxic agent through the skin.

There is no evidence that applying an antimicrobial agent to the umbilical cord stump helps prevent infection. Exposed to room air and allowed to dry, the stump usually falls off in about ten days.

Circumcision should not be performed before the infant is at least two or three days old. Most complicating medical or surgical problems (in which circumstance elective surgery is contraindicated) appear within the first 48 postpartum hours.

Routine neonatal nursing care includes the measurement of axillary temperature, pulse and respiration every four hours. Weights should be recorded at least two or three times a week. The passage of meconium or stool and urine should be carefully observed and recorded and any deviation from normal reported to the physician. Poor feeding, pallor, jaundice, respiratory distress or any other abnormal sign should also be promptly reported to the physician.

Prevention of Infection

Strict criteria must be met to prevent the spread of infectious disease in the normal nursery. All personnel who handle the infants must wash their hands and arms up the elbow for at least three minutes on entering the nursery and should rewash between infants. While caps and masks are unnecessary, gowns should be worn when entering a room in which infants are in open bassinets.

Nursery personnel should emphasize personal hygiene and skin care. They should be free of respiratory and GI infection. When illness does occur, the employee should be excused from duty in the nursery without penalty. Control of infection is discussed more fully in Chapter 19, Bacterial Infections.

Discharge

The timing of discharge is dependent on both nursing policy and clinical considerations. Even if the infant appears healthy and no medical problem has been noted, it is unwise to discharge the infant before age three days, since problems such as jaundice may not be apparent until this time. If there is any reason for delayed discharge of the mother (such as cesarean section), discharge of the infant is also delayed.

If there are major familial socioeconomic

problems that have not been resolved prior to delivery, the infant should be kept in the nursery until adequate arrangements have been made for home care.

Immediately prior to discharge, the mother should meet with both physician and nurse to discuss future well-baby care, feeding, bathing, skin care and the general management of a newborn infant.

FEEDING

Many basic principles of feeding the newborn infant are discussed in the section Feeding the Low-Birth-Weight Infant, Chapter 12.

Breast Feeding

Little controversy exists over the fact that for normally grown full-term infants, human milk is the ideal complete nutrient (1, 3). While artificial formulas that closely simulate human milk are now available, there are at least two good reasons why breast feeding is superior to artificial feeding. No matter how closely a formula is prepared to resemble human milk, the infant is still exposed to cow's milk protein, whose principal component—casein—is a potential sensitizing agent and which has a low concentration of cystine and high concentrations of phenylalanine and tyrosine. Furthermore, breast feeding eliminates the possibility of contamination, which may occur with artificial feeding, especially under poor sanitary conditions, such as those in "underdeveloped" nations or during periods of war. To this, one may add the possible psychologic advantages to both mother and infant that accompany breast feeding.

The relative unpopularity of breast feeding in today's Western culture is apparent. This reflects several factors, e.g., accessibility to safe artificial formulas and lack of encouragement from family, friends and physicians. The apparent renaissance of breast feeding among the more educated women in the United States is a cause for guarded optimism. However, at the present time, breast feeding is probably practiced by less than 5% of new mothers in the United States.

The mother who elects to breast feed her infant must be well motivated. She should have the support of her family and physician and should not attempt to nurse because of guilt feelings or outside pressures.

During pregnancy, colostrum, which has a higher protein but lower caloric content than human milk, begins to form, and the breast volume increases considerably. Following delivery colostrum continues to be secreted for two to four days before true milk appears. It is advisable to begin nursing as soon as possible after delivery since early nursing tends to clear inspissated colostrum and enhance lactation. Early nursing may also stimulate the production of oxytocic substances, which cause contraction of the uterus after delivery.

Nursing should be attempted at approximately 2½ to 3-hour intervals during the early neonatal period. Adjustment to the infant's needs will come later. A hospital schedule that allows infants to nurse only every 4 hours even if he shows signs of hunger (hunger cry) may result in an exhausted infant incapable of nursing. On the other hand, allowing the infant to nurse whenever there is minimal crying is also contraindicated since he will fail to empty at least one breast.

Even on the first day of life, both breasts should be offered at each feeding for about 5 minutes. By the third day, the infant should be allowed about 15 minutes at one breast (completely emptying it and thus facilitating continuation of the process of lactation). Following this, he should be allowed to nurse at the second breast until satisfied. At the next feeding, the order in which the breasts are offered may be reversed.

Good nursing techniques are vital if breast feeding is to be successful, and the hospital nursing staff who will teach these techniques must be sympathetic and knowledgeable. The infant's lips should be on the areola; the gums should not be allowed to clamp down on the nipple. This is accomplished by the mother grasping the areolar margin between her second and third finger in order to increase nipple protractility. The rooting reflex should be generated prior to nursing in order to insure proper engagement of the nipple and infant's mouth. Gently stroking the mouth with the nipple causes the mouth to turn toward it and initiates insertion. Trying to force the nipple into the mouth without using the rooting reflex may end in failure. Once sucking has begun, the mother may apply some pressure to the areola to enhance the flow of milk into the infant's mouth. The breast should be pressed away from the infant's nose during nursing to facilitate breathing.

The mother should ordinarily be able to produce more than enough milk to supply the infant's nutritional demands. On rare occasions, however, when inadequate milk output results in poor weight gain and irritability, artificial formula feedings should be started. Whether on breast feeding or formula, the infant should receive multivitamin and iron supplementation. If the infant is receiving a formula fortified with iron, the additional administration of iron is not necessary.

While the addition of solid food to the diet is nutritionally unnecessary until at least three or four months of age, it has become customary in the United States to introduce solid food at an extremely early age. This should be discouraged, but from a practical point of view it is virtually impossible to withhold solid food for longer than six to eight weeks.

PSYCHOSOCIAL ASPECTS

Most pregnancies fortunately end in the delivery of a healthy full-term infant. However, the birth of a baby who is compromised because of prematurity or other medical illness is a relatively common occurrence on a busy obstetric service. Even under normal circumstances, the addition of a healthy infant to the family requires many emotional adjustments on the part of the parents. The birth of an abnormal infant has a serious emotional and financial impact that may disrupt familial relationships.

PHYSICIAN–PARENT RELATIONSHIP

Antenatal

It is advisable that the pediatrician who will care for the infant confer with the expectant parents sometime during the pregnancy to discuss and allay some of the anxieties associated with impending parenthood, especially during a first pregnancy. If there is any complication of the pregnancy, such as diabetes mellitus or preeclampsia, or if there is a family history of a genetic disorder, or if a previous pregnancy has been associated with a complicated neonatal course, this interview becomes a necessity. The parents should be reassured that all steps are being taken to achieve a successful outcome and that a qualified pediatrician will be caring for the infant following delivery. Potential benefits should the infant be placed in a special care nursery (as in the case of maternal diabetes mellitus) and special procedures that may be required can be discussed at this time.

Postnatal

Shortly after delivery, the infant's mother should be visited by the physician (either the private pediatrician or house officer) responsible for the infant's medical care. Assuring the mother that her infant is normal and healthy is a pleasant task that helps build affectionate ties between mother and infant. On the other hand, one of the most difficult tasks the pediatrician faces is informing parents that their infant is ill, has a severe congenital defect or has died. If the parents are not already acquainted with the pediatrician, the initial contact may be made by the obstetrician alone or by the obstetrician and pediatrician together. Every attempt should be made to see both parents together as soon after delivery as possible. If the mother is an unmarried minor, or if she is separated from the father, the infant's grandmother or some other responsible member of the family should be present.

Perinatal Death

In the case of fetal or early neonatal death, strong emotional support by the physician is necessary during the initial period of mourning for the dead infant. An attempt must be made to allay parental guilt feelings universally present at this time. A careful explanation of the cause of death is necessary. This usually involves obtaining consent for postmortem examination. Rapid performance of the autopsy and sharing the information thus obtained with the parents is of the utmost importance. In most instances, the parents can be reassured that the next pregnancy will not be accompanied by an increased risk of fetal or neonatal death. If there is any question whether a genetically transmitted disorder caused the infant's death, genetic counseling is mandatory.

Neonatal Illness

The wide spectrum of illness among newborn infants ranges from relatively minor disorders to severely disabling or life-threatening ones. Whenever possible, the physician must emphasize positive possibilities during his initial contact with the parents. In the presence of minor problems, such as hemangiomata or extra digits, the physician must present the findings to the parents, reassure them of their lack of clinical significance and indicate what procedures may be appropriate (such as tying off the extra digits or leaving the hemangiomata alone).

If the infant is born prematurely, the parents should be given a realistic assessment concerning the chances for survival. If RDS occurs, the parents should be told about treatment and prognosis. This situation is usually resolved within a few days, with either recovery or death.

Jaundice (except in severe hemolytic disease) usually does not appear prior to the first postnatal meeting between the parents and physician. If there has been a previous history of hemolytic disease and jaundice, the parents have probably anticipated the problem. In a first child, the abnormal skin color may cause parental anxiety, and the parents should be advised that neonatal jaundice is common, transient and usually not harmful. Warning of possible brain damage in the presence of a relatively low or moderately elevated serum concentration of unconjugated bilirubin may cause unnecessary alarm. If either phototherapy or exchange transfusion is required, more detailed information can be given.

Congenital Anomalies

Informing parents that their newborn infant has a major congenital malformation is an unpleasant duty that has to be faced at some time by all pediatricians. In the case of certain anomalies that mar the appearance of the infant but are potentially curable, the pediatrician must present an optimistic picture. Some of these, such as cleft lip and palate, may cause parental antipathy towards the infant, and considerable effort and understanding are sometimes needed to gain parental acceptance of the infant's condition.

A difficult, sometimes unresolvable situation, arises with the birth of an infant with one or more congenital anomalies that, while not immediately life threatening, will severely handicap the patient and indirectly, his family (6, 10). Examples of this are a mongoloid infant, or one with a myelomeningocele and evidence of neurologic deficit that will likely be permanent. In the case of a mongoloid infant, parental acceptance will vary greatly; certain parents with preconceived ideas may refuse to even look at the infant. On the other hand, some parents may completely accept the infant. Many are willing to take the baby home from the nursery with the intent of institutionalizing it later. The place of the pediatrician is not to make a value judgment, but to try to help the parents make the decision that is best for them. It should be pointed out to the parents, however, that mongoloids have varying levels of intelligence and many are trainable.

A special problem that has aroused great controversy involves the question of obtaining informed consent for procedures that are immediately lifesaving, but which will result in an individual who will be handicapped throughout life (such as an infant with a myelomeningocele or a mongoloid with duodenal atresia). Some hospitals have been able to ease this dilemma for both parents and physicians by the establishment of "Ethics Committees" and weekly "Ethics Rounds" (7). In this way, a consensus of opinion may be used to cope with what is really an unsolvable problem.

After the initial meeting between the pediatrician and parents of the infant requiring special care, an ongoing relationship must be maintained to keep the parents up to date concerning clinical problems and to prepare them for taking the infant home.

ROLE OF THE SOCIAL WORKER

One of the most important staff members of the Neonatal (or Perinatal) Center is the medical social worker, whose major responsibilities include enhancing the parent–physician relationship and supporting the parents during periods of major sociologic and emotional adjustment. The social worker should be assigned to the prenatal clinic to work primarily with medically and sociologically high-risk pregnancies.

There is particular concern for the parent with a disordered family situation, such as an unmarried teenager or a drug abuser, and steps should be taken at the earliest time to resolve psychosocial problems, e.g., enrollment of the drug abuser in a therapeutic program. If adoption or placement in a foster home are anticipated, arrangements should be made well in advance of the date of delivery. Following delivery, the social worker should remain actively involved in management of the mother and infant.

Two basic situations in which the social worker will become initially active in a case only after delivery involve: 1) mothers with

severe psychosocial pathology who have not received prenatal care and 2) newborn infants with unexpected appearance of severe illness. The mother with a high-risk pregnancy receiving prenatal care from a private obstetrician will rarely be seen by a social worker prior to delivery. However, the social worker may be of great supportive value in cases of severe neonatal illness.

The social worker must coordinate communication between medical and nursing staffs, and with various social welfare agencies whose resources are available to the families. There should be at least one regularly scheduled conference per week, attended by medical, nursing and social service staff, in which psychosocial problems of the families of patients are discussed. In addition, the social worker should be encouraged to attend and participate in medical rounds whenever possible.

MOTHER–INFANT SEPARATION

Affectionate ties between mother and newborn infant are formed both during pregnancy and in the early neonatal period. Immediately after delivery of a healthy infant the mother establishes tactile and visual contact, which are important factors in the development of a normal mother–infant relationship, but the birth of a premature or sick infant invariably leads to the physical separation of mother and infant. In the case of a very low birth weight infant, this separation may last for several months.

In the late 1960s, it was observed that separation of the newly born infant from its mother, even for a relatively short time, may lead to a disturbed mother–child relationship (8, 9). At its worst, this is manifested by child neglect and abuse. However, when mothers were allowed relatively free access to their infants in premature nurseries (including handling them within the confines of incubators), there appeared to be a significant improvement in the establishment of affectionate ties between mother and infant. In spite of the increased handling of infants, there was no concurrent increase in the incidence of infection in the nursery. By the mid-1970s, increased participation of parents in caring for their premature and sick newborn infants had become an accepted routine in most nurseries in the United States and Canada.

REFERENCES

CARE OF NORMAL FULL-TERM INFANT

1. Aldrich CA: The advisability of breast feeding: a survey of the subcommittee of the Committee on Maternal and Child Health, National Research Council. JAMA, 135:915, 1947
2. American Academy of Pediatrics: Standards and Recommendations for Hospital Care of Newborn Infants, 5th ed. Evanston, American Academy of Pediatrics, 1971
3. Applebaum RM: The modern management of successful breast feeding. Pediatr Clin North Am 17:203, 1970

4. Desmond MM, Rudolph AJ, Phitaksphraiwan P: The transitional care nursery: a mechanism for prevention medicine in the newborn. Pediatr Clin North Am 13:651, 1966
5. Lubchenco LO, Searles DT, Brazie JV: Neonatal mortality rate: relationship to birth weight and gestational age. J Pediatr 81:814, 1972

PSYCHOSOCIAL ASPECTS

6. Duff RD, Campbell AGM: Moral and ethical dilemmas in the special care nursery. N Engl J Med 289:890, 1973
7. Ethical questions Hippocrates did not have to face. Medical World News, July 14, 1972, p 35
8. Klaus M, Kennell J: Mothers separated from their newborn infants. Pediatr Clin North Am 17:1015, 1970
9. Robson KS, Moss HA: Patterns and determinants of maternal attachment. J Pediatr 77:976, 1970
10. Shaw A: Dilemmas of "informed consent" in children. N Engl J Med 289:885, 1973

17

History, Physical and Neurologic Examinations

HISTORY TAKING IN NEONATOLOGY

There are few areas of clinical medicine in which a detailed history is as significant as in neonatology. For convenience, three separate phases may be considered (Table 17–1).

MATERNAL HISTORY

Maternal history taking should cover all events up to the time of conception, including age, race and previous medical history. It encompasses both maternal and paternal familial histories. At the extremes of age and among primiparous women, neonatal mortality and morbidity are increased. The risk of Down's syndrome increases beyond age 35, especially after age 40. The mother's *height* and *weight* are important; if she is short and thin, the incidence of low birth weight may be significantly increased, perhaps because of relatively decreased cardiac output. Nutritional status is relevent since morbidity and mortality increase with extreme obesity and poorly nourished women tend to have small infants.

Both maternal and neonatal mortality vary widely with *race*. The outlook is far more favorable for Americans of Japanese or Chinese ancestry than for the population in general, but it is worse for Blacks and American Indians. Knowledge of socioeco-

nomics is helpful since a high incidence of perinatal morbidity, mortality and low birth weight has been established among the poor. A specific example is the greater incidence of amnionitis and neonatal pneumonia reported in this group, especially among Blacks and Puerto Ricans.

If the mother has had previous abortions, either spontaneous or induced, she may be at high risk of incurring another loss. A past history of delivery of infants with congenital anomalies, especially if genetically determined (Tay-Sachs disease, translocation mongolism or cystic fibrosis), may indicate a poor prognosis. If there have been stillbirths or perinatal problems, the risk of the present pregnancy is increased. Therefore, the number and outcome of all *previous pregnancies* are significant, as is any occurrence of genetically determined disease.

Information concerning birth weights of infants of previous pregnancies is important. Large infants may reflect maternal diabetes mellitus, and infants who are small for gestational age may indicate an underlying maternal disorder, conceivably genetic.

The maternal history should reveal pertinent illness, such as diabetes mellitus, tuberculosis, rheumatic heart disease, renal, collagen, vascular, metabolic or hematologic disorders. These all influence intrauterine development. Chronic illness, including malnutrition, may lead to increased fetal wastage, intrauterine growth retardation or premature delivery. Some "silent" medical conditions may modify the outcome of the pregnancy. Both pyelonephritis associated with asymptomatic bacteruria and sickle cell trait may be associated with infants of low birth weight.

Maternal and paternal blood type and Rh group should be determined, especially if there was jaundice in previously delivered newborn infants. Similarly, a history of a previous infant developing the respiratory distress syndrome (RDS) is significant because of the predilection for recurrence of this illness in subsequent infants.

OBSTETRIC HISTORY

Two major areas of concern in the history of the present pregnancy include the clinical course of the mother and knowledge of fetal condition gained through limited physical examination and fetal monitoring.

Maternal diet, weight gain, drug ingestion, hematologic or GU status, infectious diseases, metabolic disorders, trauma or acute illness of any type may relate to the outcome of the pregnancy.

Inadequate maternal diet and a poor weight gain during pregnancy may be associated with fetal malnutrition and growth failure. Any drug taken for medicinal purposes will enter the fetal circulation; some such as diphenylhydantoin or corticosteroids, when taken early in gestation, are potential teratogens. Others, when taken during the intrapartum period may have a bearing on the infant's clinical course during the early neonatal period. Addictive drugs, including barbiturates, taken by the mother will often cause fetal addiction, followed by withdrawal symptoms after delivery. Cigarette smoking may decrease the rate of fetal growth. Alcohol ingestion during pregnancy has been associated with congenital anomalies. Preeclampsia and hypertension may be associated with intrauterine growth failure and neonatal hypoglycemia. History of a hemoglobinopathy or anemia in the mother

TABLE 17–1. History Taking in Neonatology

I. Maternal
Age, race, parity and medical history (including familial history of hereditary disorders)

II. Obstetric
Diet, weight gain, drug ingestion (including alcohol and tobacco), infection, preeclampsia, metabolic disorders and fetal monitoring (e.g., L–S ratio, sonography, estriols and fetal ECG)

III. Neonatal
Apgar score, breathing and crying time, initial pallor or cyanosis, resuscitative measures, description of placenta, weight gain, feeding difficulty, specific abnormal signs and time of onset and environmental factors (use of oxygen, incubator care and exposure to infected infants or staff members)

may be associated with a high-risk pregnancy. Urinary tract infection during pregnancy may be associated with fetal infection or poor fetal weight gain. Several infectious diseases in the mother, e.g., syphilis, rubella, cytomegalovirus or toxoplasmosis may have a profound effect on the fetus. Others like h. simplex or varicella may either be teratogenic or lead to postnatal infection. Metabolic and endocrine disorders, such as diabetes mellitus, may be reflected in the fetus and newborn infant. Uncontrolled maternal phenylketonuria may be associated with fetal brain damage. Hypothyroidism or hyperthyroidism in the mother may be related to thyroid malfunction in the fetus. Parathyroid disturbances occurring during pregnancy may lead to abnormal calcium metabolism in the neonate. Maternal trauma may result in amniotic tears and the intrauterine band syndrome.

A careful history of the immediate antenatal period will reveal the duration of labor, type of presentation, whether or not fetal membranes were intact, if there were signs of amnionitis, which drugs and anesthesia were used during the delivery and whether there was passage of meconium-stained amniotic fluid. Opportunities to examine the fetus are limited; a record of changes in fetal heart rate, especially a pattern of "late" fetal bradycardia, may be associated with fetal distress. Results of physical and biochemical tests of fetal function, such as sonography, urinary and serum estriol concentrations, amniotic fluid lecithin–sphingomyelin (L–S) ratios, and estimations of the state of fetal oxygenation during labor should be known to the physician caring for the infant.

Finally, it is important to know the extent of medical care received during pregnancy. Complete lack of prenatal care implies increased risk of illness during the fetal and neonatal periods and early infancy.

NEONATAL HISTORY

Careful observation of the newborn infant beginning at the time of delivery is the most crucial element in following the neonate's clinical course. The postnatal history is also of great importance; especially during the first 48 hours, a history may lead to early, conclusive diagnosis. Valuable information derived in the delivery room includes Apgar score, breathing and crying time, pallor or cyanosis, resuscitative measures taken, passage of urine or meconium, foul-smelling amniotic fluid and a description of the placenta.

Subsequent signs of serious import in the newborn infant include feeding difficulties with failure to gain weight, hypothermia or hyperthermia, pallor, cyanosis, jaundice, diarrhea and vomiting, tremulousness and convulsions, apathy, irritability, cardiac murmur and episodes of apnea. Associated problems vary from mild physiologic changes to severe, often fatal, illness. It is imperative to determine the duration and time of onset. The slightest change in behavior or the mildest of symptoms, as interpreted by the infant's nurse or mother, should be taken seriously and not casually dismissed. Early manifestations of sepsis and meningitis are often subtle and similar to those of such other disorders as hypocalcemia, hypoglycemia, drug withdrawal or intracranial bleeding. These early clues may be all that is necessary to initiate diagnostic procedures and early treatment, even in the absence of more specific signs such as a bulging anterior fontanelle.

Knowledge of sex and racial background may be important. Males have an increased vulnerability to bacterial infections; white infants have a greater incidence of GI anomalies than Blacks, while black infants have an increased incidence of skeletal aberrations.

The age at which a particular sign becomes apparent is important. In general, the earlier the onset of a particular sign, the more severe the disorder. For example, jaundice developing within the first 24 hours of life usually implies a specific etiology (iso-immunization or sepsis) and a more severe outcome than jaundice developing subsequently. The latter usually signifies either a mild hemolytic process or physiologic jaundice. Respiratory distress beginning after the first day of life is by definition *not* RDS; the afflicted infant usually has a better prognosis. The *duration* of a specific finding may be significant; occasional, brief cessations of respiration may be a manifestation of periodic breathing. However, apneic spells that are frequent and prolonged, such as those seen in severe RDS and CNS bleeding, usually indicate an ominous prognosis.

Environmental factors may explain certain problems. Exposure to an inordinately high temperature may be responsible for fever, while exposure to cool air temperatures may be the cause of hypothermia. If the infant is being reared in a humidified environment, the possibility of droplet-borne bacterial infection, e.g., pseudomonas, must be considered. If the concentration of oxygen within an incubator is over 21%, and the infant is premature, the development of retinal vessel and lung toxicity becomes a possibility. Also important in the environmental history is the presence of infection among other infants, mothers and hospital staff.

PHYSICAL EXAMINATION OF THE NEWBORN INFANT

Signs of illness may be subtle in the neonate. Though this is more often the case in premature rather than full-term infants, the necessity of performing a thorough physical examination on all newborn infants, even those apparently well and of normal gestation, cannot be overemphasized.

If the examining physician is not a pediatrician, he must have special training in the care of the newborn infant. Whenever there is any uncertainty as to the findings (especially in the case of a house officer), an experienced physician should be consulted.

EXAMINATION IN THE DELIVERY ROOM

The initial examination must be performed in the delivery room. In the vast majority of cases, this will be done by the physician who delivers the infant. If there is any antenatal indication that the infant may be at high risk, e.g., prematurity, fetal distress, maternal bleeding, malposition or cesarean section, the pediatrician must be notified as much in advance of delivery as possible and should be in attendance to perform the examination.

Of immediate concern to the examiner is the general condition of the infant. Cardiac, respiratory and neuromuscular status must be immediately evaluated, and a prompt decision made about the need for resuscitation. All necessary equipment for this must be available and in good working order. Size of the infant, color, state of consciousness, respiratory patterns and the presence of obvious major congenital anomalies must be determined.

As part of the initial examination, a catheter should be passed through the nasopharynx to rule out the possibility of choanal atresia. If excessive mucus is noted, atresia of the esophagus may be suspected. Passage of a soft rubber catheter into the stomach will confirm its patency. Introduction of a catheter into the stomach is also indicated if obvious abdominal distension is present. Aspiration of more than 30 ml of gastric fluid arouses suspicion of small bowel obstruction. Genitalia must be examined; extremities, spine and anal orifice must be inspected; and respiratory abnormalities should be carefully noted. Labored respirations and chest retractions may point to a diagnosis of RDS in a premature infant

(this would be an unlikely diagnosis in a full-term infant). Meconium staining of the infant's skin or its presence in the mouth may point to the presence of meconium aspiration, pneumonia, pneumothorax or pneumomediastinum. If respiratory distress is accompanied by a scaphoid abdomen, especially with a right apical cardiac impulse, the diagnosis of diaphragmatic hernia should be entertained, and an x ray of the chest taken immediately. If this diagnosis is confirmed, immediate surgical consultation is indicated. The presence of two umbilical arteries in the severed cord must be determined, since the absence of one artery has been associated with a high incidence of congenital anomalies, especially of the GU system. Inspection of the placenta is always indicated and in certain cases may be of extreme importance. An abnormally small or infarcted placenta may bear a relationship to placental dysfunction and intrauterine growth retardation, while an unusually large placenta may occur with hydrops fetalis, diabetes mellitus and certain infections (e.g., congenital syphilis). The presence of amnion nodosum (firm rounded yellowish nodules on the amniotic surface) may indicate renal hypoplasia. Examination of the placenta is especially important in multiple pregnancies, where the number of chorions present will be helpful in determining zygosity. This point should be constantly stressed, since placental examinations are usually superficial and frequently omitted completely.

Examination of the infant in the delivery room should be performed as rapidly as possible in order to limit heat loss and detect potentially lethal abnormalities without delay. Compromised and very small infants should be examined in a warm environment, preferably under a radiant heater.

Once resuscitation (if necessary) has been performed, low-birth-weight infants and distressed full-term infants should be transported immediately to a special care nursery and reexamined following their arrival. The initial investigation of the healthy full-term infant should take place as soon as is practical, certainly within the first

TABLE 17–2. Physical Examination of the Newborn Infant

I. **Observation**
Congenital anomalies, spontaneous movements, state of consciousness, posture, respiratory pattern (regularity, depth and grunt), skin color, irritability or tremulousness, abdominal distension, ascites, passage of urine and stool, excessive salivation and vomiting

II. **Body Measurements and Vital Signs**
Weight, length, head and chest circumference, apical pulse (rate and rhythm), respiratory rate, temperature (axillary) and blood pressure (when indicated)

III. **Skin**
Cyanosis, pallor, jaundice, edema, erythema, telangiectasia, purpura and petechiae, hemangiomas, pustules, sclerema, erythema toxicum, lanugo, milia, mottling, harlequin color change, mongolian spots, dermatoglyphics, sole creases and pigmentation (especially of areola, scrotum and labia)

IV. **Head**
Microcephaly, hydrocephaly, caput succedaneum, cephalhematoma, craniotabes and anterior and posterior fontanelles (size, shape and fullness)

V. **Eyes**
Periorbital edema, mongoloid or antimongoloid slant, conjunctival hemorrhage, cataracts or glaucoma, retinal hemorrhage and hypertelorism

VI. **Ears**
Shape, cartilage, tags, dimples, sinuses, tympanic membrane and bleeding

VII. **Nose**
Patency, midline defects and flaring of alae nasi

VIII. **Mouth and Pharynx**
Cleft lip and palate, micrognathia, macroglossia, epithelial pearls and teeth

IX. **Neck**
Webbing, cysts and fistulous openings, torticollis, thyroid and clavicles

X. **Chest**
Deformities of chest wall, retractions, anteroposterior diameter and size of breast nodules

XI. **Lungs**
Percussion (usually resonant), rales, quality of breath sounds and bowel sounds (diaphragmatic hernia)

XII. **Heart**
Rate, rhythm, quality of heart sounds, thrill and location of apical impulse

XIII. **Blood Vessels**
Quality of peripheral pulses

XIV. **Abdomen and GI Tract**
Shape of abdomen, gross defects (omphalocele, gastroschisis), visible peristaltic waves, venous distension, bowel sounds, palpation of liver, kidney and spleen, abnormal masses and anal orifice (patency, fistulas)

XV. **Genitalia**
Size of penis, location of meatus, descent and size of testes, inguinal hernias, hydroceles, size of labia majora, minora and clitoris and vaginal bleeding and discharge

XVI. **Extremities and Spine**
Absence of portion of limb, syndactyly, extra digits, joint mobility, muscular weakness, hip mobility, bony deformities of lower extremities, constriction rings, spinal defects and fistulous tracts

12 postpartum hours. Prior to performing the examination, the physician should be fully acquainted with the obstetric and past medical history.

INITIAL EXAMINATION IN THE NURSERY

Observation

Observation of the undisturbed infant is the critical feature of the examination (Table 17–2). Although many findings may become apparent on detailed analysis, the appearance of the neonate is the single most useful guide to diagnosis; specifically, it provides a strong indication as to whether the infant is healthy or "sick" (and if so to what degree). It will very often permit the examiner to decide if immediate diagnostic and therapeutic steps must be taken or whether further observation of the infant is in order.

Interpretation of Data

Physical findings, especially vital signs, that are normal for older infants may not be so for a newborn infant, and signs that are normal in a full-term infant may be abnormal for a premature infant. For example, the normal respiratory rate of the neonate (30 to 50 per minute) is higher than that of older infants. Edematous extremities, which may be normal for a premature infant, are pathologic for a full-term infant. The misinterpretation of normal findings may lead to unnecessary, expensive or possibly dangerous diagnostic studies.

Activity

General activity of the infant, his state of consciousness, posture, respiratory patterns, skin color (jaundice, pallor, cyanosis, plethora) and the presence of tremors should be noted. The patient should be observed for evaluation of abdominal distension, passage of urine and stool, excessive salivation and bilious vomiting. A judgment should be made promptly as to which diagnostic and therapeutic procedures are essential.

Body Temperature

Axillary, rather than rectal temperatures should be taken. Axillary temperatures are extremely close to core (deep colonic) temperatures, and the insertion of a thermometer into the rectum is a hazardous procedure that has been known to cause bowel perforation. Constant measurement of the abdominal skin temperature of a small or sick infant with a thermistor probe may yield valuable information about his thermal state and is a convenient and safe approach widely used in special care nurseries.

Skin

The skin is in many cases the most revealing part of the body examined and can promptly alert the clinician to the existence of serious disease. At birth, all infants are covered by a vernix caseosa, which rapidly disappears from all sites except the intertriginous areas. The true premature infant has thin, shiny skin with little or no subcutaneous fat. Some degree of edema may be present over the extremities. Lanugo, which is fine and downy, usually covers the forehead and side of the face. Milia (slightly distended sebaceous glands) are a normal finding often seen on the nose. Like the true premature infant, the low-birth-weight infant, who is of fairly advanced gestational age but whose intrauterine growth has been impaired by fetal malnutrition, shows an absence of subcutaneous fat. His skin texture, however, is less fine and shiny. The normally grown full-term infant has a well-developed layer of subcutaneous fat. Dysmature and many postmature infants show loss of subcutaneous tissue, often with

meconium staining and desquamation of the skin.

Observation of skin color is vital to recognize and treat cyanosis. Acrocyanosis, which is limited to the hands and feet and is of transient duration, is not a pathologic finding, but represents peripheral vasoconstriction occurring as a response to cold stress. Pallor usually indicates acute or chronic blood loss or asphyxia, and it should be promptly investigated. Jaundice that is noted initially during the first 24 hours of life usually indicates a hemolytic process due to a blood group incompatibility. Excessive ruddiness may be a sign of polycythemia, often secondary to an intertwin transfusion. Infants of diabetic mothers exhibit a peculiar ruddiness of the face ("tomato face") together with an unusually large body size.

A few petechiae over the body and conjunctivae may be considered normal, but their presence in large numbers requires a hematologic investigation for thrombocytopenia and other disorders of the coagulation mechanisms. Sepsis and blood group incompatibilities must be considered. Echymoses over the bodies of premature infants, which are associated with difficult deliveries, are not uncommon and do not necessarily indicate a disease state.

Mottling of the skin is not unusual, especially in infants of low gestational age. The harlequin color change is probably associated with a relatively immature autonomic nervous system. A clear line of demarcation between upper and lower portions of the infant is noted when he is turned on one side. When he is turned on the other side, the coloring reverses. This phenomenon disappears when crying is induced. Telangiectasia and "port wine stains" over the eyelids and nape of the neck are of no clinical significance and usually disappear within two years. However, a large port wine stain on the forehead should arouse suspicion of intracranial vascular anomalies, e.g., Sturge-Weber syndrome.

Sclerema, a "woody" hardening of subcutaneous tissues rarely seen on initial examination, is usually associated with sepsis and subnormal body temperature and indicates a dire prognosis. Lymphedema of the hands and feet is a manifestation of Turner's syndrome. Mongolian spots, areas of bluish discoloration over the back, are most often seen in black infants and are of no clinical significance.

Erythema toxicum, or fleabite dermatitis, is a benign condition that may represent a local allergy to amniotic fluid. A macular rash, resembling a flea bite, is present. It is often associated with very small and discrete pustules containing an eosinophilic exudate. This condition must be differentiated from bacterial skin infections (usually staphylococcal), where the pustules are larger and contain bacteria and polymorphonuclear leukocytes (PMNS). Cellulitis, when present, has an angry red appearance. The rash of cutaneous moniliasis is not usually seen until after the first week of life, most often over the diaper area. The cutaneous manifestations of such intrauterine infections as rubella, congenital syphilis, cytomegalovirus and toxoplasmosis may be seen on inspection of the skin. Varicella and h. simplex also have major skin manifestations.

Examination of the soles of the feet and scrotum may aid in estimating gestational age. At term deep transverse skin creases cover the entire sole (which may be less well developed in black than in white infants), and the scrotum is deeply pigmented and well rugated.

The rhagades of congenital syphilis may occasionally be seen in the first few days of life.

Head

The size of the head in relation to the remainder of the body should be noted, and the head circumference (in the greatest frontooccipital diameter) measured and recorded. In some infants who are small for gestational age, the head may appear relatively large in proportion to the body. This may reflect the fact that with intrauterine growth retardation, brain growth is less severely impaired than weight gain or linear growth. Serious congenital anomalies, such as premature closure of sutures (accompanied by an elevated osseous ridge over the site of the synostosis) and scalp defects associated with D-trisomy, must be noted.

Molding of the head is normally present following a vaginal delivery, but not after a cesarean section (unless there has been some progression of labor). With molding, the anterior fontanelle may seem small with overlapping of sutures. Although wide variations in the size of the fontanelle may normally occur, an especially wide open anterior fontanelle (over 2.5 by 2.5 cm) raises a suspicion of hypothyroidism. Caput succedaneum is an edematous area of the scalp (that portion which has been encircled by a dilated cervical ring during labor) with a vague undefined margin. The edema subsides within a few days.

An open posterior fontanelle is normal, and a temporal fontanelle (Catlin's anomaly) is occasionally palpated.

Craniotabes, a thin area of bone that feels like a pingpong ball on palpation, may normally be present. A cephalhematoma results from bleeding between periosteum and bone and is always limited by a suture line. While the blood may become calcified, it is usually reabsorbed within a few weeks. Subaponeurotic bleeding, on the other hand, is not limited by a suture line. This type of bleeding is often related to the use of the vacuum extractor and may be so serious as to present a life-threatening situation. The entire scalp in this case is usually boggy and edematous, and discoloration may be present.

An unusually large head with separated sutures and bulging anterior fontanelle may indicate subdural bleeding (especially in full-term infants with birth trauma) or hydrocephalus.

Transillumination of the skull in a darkened room aids in making the diagnosis and selecting further diagnostic procedures.

Face

Inspection of the face may reveal a great deal of information. Mongolism, cretinism, trisomies D and E, infants of diabetic mothers and infants with renal agenesis may manifest a peculiar type of facies. Other unusual conditions, such as Cornelia de Lange syndrome, have facial manifestations in the newborn infant. The physician must also be alert to such features as hypertelorism, ptosis, midline facial defects and micrognathia.

Eyes

The eyelids must be opened and both eyes inspected (absence of an eye has gone unnoticed on initial physical examination). Eyelid edema, which is a frequent finding, should not preclude an adequate examination. Spontaneous opening and closing of the eyes should be observed. Size of the cornea, lens and eyeballs should be noted, and the eyeballs palpated to detect increased intraocular pressure. Signs of proptosis must not be overlooked. Subconjunctival hemorrhage may normally be present. Mongoloid and antimongoloid folds may have some diagnostic importance. The pupils in all but the most immature group of infants (gestational age of 22 weeks or less) normally react to light. Constricted pupils may reflect maternal narcotic addiction; dilated pupils that do not react to light may indicate midbrain pressure. Coloboma is a commonly found anomaly in which there is a "keyhole" defect of the iris.

The ophthalmoscope should be used to observe the normal red reflex. In examining the retina, it must be remembered that full-term infants and large prematures have a myopia of 6 diopters and that small prematures may have a myopia of 10 to 20 diopters. It may be extremely difficult to visualize the retina in infants of very low gestational age because of the persistence of a normal embryonic membrane, or velum. Petechial hemorrhages of the fundus are commonly seen, reflecting the trauma of delivery. If extensive, they may reflect central nervous pathology, such as asphyxial brain damage and subdural hematoma.

Ears

Abnormally low-set or misshapen ear lobes may be associated with renal anomalies. The amount of cartilage present in the lobe may aid in the determination of gestational age. At 36 weeks the ear lobe is relatively shapeless and pliable, with little cartilage present; at 40 weeks it is rigid, and the cartilage is well formed. The ears often participate in first branchial arch malformations, and a search should be made for abnormal skin tags, dimples and sinuses. Though the tympanic membranes, which are placed horizontally, are difficult to visualize, they should be carefully inspected since erythema and distortion of normal structures may be a reflection of acute otitis media. Fresh bleeding from the middle ear may indicate a basilar skull fracture.

Nose

The newborn infant is an obligate nose breather. Not recognizing choanal atresia, especially if it is bilateral, may have fatal consequences. The diagnosis is made by attempting to pass a catheter through the nares into the nasopharynx. In those cases where the obstruction is membranous, perforation of the membrane by the catheter may be curative. Radiologic examination using a contrast medium will confirm the diagnosis. The nose, together with a cleft palate, may be involved in midline defects of the face. Rhinitis (snuffles) may be a sign of congenital syphilis and may be present during the first week of life, although it is usually encountered at a later date.

Mouth and Pharynx

Cleft lip and palate are usually obvious. However, careful inspection of the oral cavity may reveal a cleft of the soft palate that might otherwise be overlooked. In the Pierre Robin syndrome (macroglosia, micrognathia and cleft palate) care must be taken to maintain an adequate airway. Surgery may be required to stabilize the tongue early in life. The presence of excessive mucus or bilious vomiting may indicate upper GI tract obstruction. An enlarged tongue may be present in cretinism or mongolism or may be the result of a hemangioma.

Moniliasis is rarely seen in the oral cavity

before the end of the first week of life. Epithelial protrusions (Epstein's pearls), which are mucous retention cysts, may normally be seen on the alveolar ridge and palate. Teeth may occasionally be seen, but these are usually poorly formed and should be removed to prevent aspiration. The size of the frenulum may vary markedly and is rarely, if ever, associated with speech or swallowing difficulties. A high-arched palate may be normal. A sucking pad can usually be seen on the inner surface of each cheek.

Neck

A short, poorly mobile neck may indicate the presence of Klippel-Feil syndrome. Webbing of the neck is usually associated with Turner's syndrome. Inspection for branchial cleft cysts and fistulas and pharyngoglossal duct openings should be performed. Neck masses may be caused by a congenitally enlarged thyroid gland or cystic hygroma. Bleeding into the sternomastoid muscle may cause congenital torticollis. Both clavicles should be palpated to exclude the possibility of fracture; crepitation, usually palpated over the fracture site, is most common in very large infants, especially if there has been shoulder dystocia.

Chest

The chest wall should be examined for such abnormalities as pigeon breast or funnel chest. The shape of the chest may reflect the lung volume. With meconium aspiration and air trapping, the anteroposterior diameter of the chest may be increased; in RDS with atelectasis, the anterior-posterior diameter may be decreased, and the chest may appear sunken. Respiratory patterns, including frequency, regularity and depth of respiration should be noted together with the presence of retractions.

Supernumerary nipples are of no clinical significance. Breast nodules become palpable at about 33 weeks and rarely exceed 3 mm at 36 weeks' gestation. By 37 or 38 weeks, they reach 4 mm in diameter and at term measure about 7 mm. Infants who are small for gestational age may have retarded development of their breast nodules.

An extremely prominent chest may suggest diaphragmatic hernia, especially if accompanied by a scaphoid abdomen. A bell-shaped chest is associated with asphyxiating thoracic dystrophy.

Lungs

The newborn infant's normal respiratory rate is 30 to 50 per minute, but wide variations may occur in the absence of pathology. An increase in respiratory rate associated with retractions, expiratory grunt and cyanosis in room air is a sign of RDS. Irregular or shallow respirations may be a sign of hypoxia or CNS damage or bleeding. Periodic breathing may be observed in the premature infant. This consists of two or more periods of breathing per minute, each separated by cessation of respiratory effort for three seconds or more (this may be a manifestation of inadequate oxygenation). Rapid respiration in the absence of respiratory distress may be a manifestation of the syndrome of transient tachypnea of the newborn infant, or it may occur in infants of heroin-addicted mothers who show signs of acute withdrawal.

Percussion of the thin-walled chest of the newborn infant is of limited value and usually elicits a very resonant note. Hyperresonance may indicate pneumothorax-pneumomediastinum or diaphragmatic hernia. Percussion is of no value in determining decreased aeration of the lungs. On auscultation, both phases of respiration may be heard if the infant is quiet. Breath sounds may be transmitted even by a relatively small amount of aerated lung. The presence of rales may be of some value to the physician in distinguishing congenital pneumonia from RDS. Bowel sounds heard in the chest may indicate diaphragmatic hernia.

When chest pathology is suspected, an immediate x ray (both posteroanterior and lateral) is indicated. A delay may be particularly hazardous when a surgical condition, such as a diaphragmatic hernia or pneumothorax is suspected.

Heart

The cardiac rate and rhythm must be determined, and the apical impulse located. The average cardiac rate is 130 to 140 per minute in a newborn infant at rest; however, wide variations are normal, and only those rates under 100 or over 160 may be considered abnormal. An unusually rapid rate may indicate congestive heart failure, paroxysmal supraventricular tachycardia or (very rarely) congenital hyperthyroidism. A very slow rate may indicate hypoxia, CNS injury, or (rarely) congenital heart block. A right apical impulse usually means either dextrocardia or the presence of bowel in the chest displacing the mediastinum.

The "lub-dub" heart sounds heard in the older infant, child and adult are not heard during the neonatal period. The newborn infant has embryocardia, or a "tic-tac" rhythm, in which systole and diastole are of about equal duration.

It is almost impossible to diagnose an enlarged heart by percussion. This should be done radiologically in conjunction with the ECG. Thrills, like very loud murmurs, are usually indicative of a small ventricular septal defect. Soft systolic murmurs are frequently heard during the neonatal period; these are usually related to a ductus arteriosus that has not yet closed. Most of these physiologic murmurs will have diminished or disappeared by the end of the neonatal period.

The quality of heart sounds should be evaluated (e.g., muffled sounds may accompany myocarditis), and splitting of the second sound, if present, should be noted.

A murmur may not be heard in neonatal cardiac disease, which may be suspected solely on the basis of such extracardiac findings as tachypnea and hepatomegaly.

Blood Vessels

Femoral and brachial arteries should be palpated routinely. Generalized poor peripheral pulses indicate insufficient left ventricular output. Diminished femoral pulses may accompany coarctation of the aorta with a patent ductus arteriosus. In hyperthyroidism or a large arteriovenous fistula, the peripheral pulses may be bounding.

When there is a question of cardiovascular disease, blood pressure should be measured in all four extremities. The flush method has its limitations and can only approximate mean arterial pressure. Another method, now commercially available (Arteriosonde*), which is based on the reflection of ultrasonic waves, provides accurate measurement of both systolic and diastolic blood pressures in the neonate. In very ill infants with indwelling umbilical arterial catheters, aortic blood pressure is easily measured directly and may yield valuable information. The range of normal blood pressure values from the second to 12th hour of life is shown in Fig. 17–1.

Abdomen and Gastrointestinal Tract

The shape of the abdomen must be noted. A scaphoid abdomen suggests a diaphragmatic hernia. Abdominal distension may be the presenting sign of intestinal obstruction, perforation of a hollow viscus or ascites. Further inspection may reveal the presence

* Hoffmann-LaRoche Inc., Cranbury, NJ 08512

FIG. 17–1. Mean aortic blood pressure and 95% confidence limits in normal newborn infants during hours 2 to 12 of life. (Kitterman JA, Phibbs RH, Tooley WH: Pediatrics 44:959, 1969)

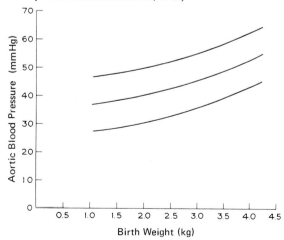

of peristaltic waves that accompany intestinal obstruction. Dilated superficial veins can be a sign of venous obstruction. Diastasis recti, or separation of the lateral rectus muscles, is a nonpathologic condition. Umbilical hernias are generally of no clinical significance and usually heal spontaneously within two years.

Omphalocele and gastroschisis are defects of the abdominal wall through which viscera have herniated. They must be treated as surgical emergencies. Polyps of the umbilical cord should be noted, and the number of umbilical arteries counted.

Palpation of the abdominal wall must be gentle, since absence of abdominal musculature (Eagle-Barrett syndrome) may accompany severe renal and lung anomalies. The edge of the right lobe of the liver may normally be palpated 2 cm below the right costal margin, and the splenic tip may normally be felt below the left costal margin.

The lower poles of both kidneys may be felt on deep palpation. Ascites may accompany hydronephrosis. Intraabdominal tumors (e.g., neuroblastoma, teratoma and ovarian cyst) are rare but must be kept in mind. The position of the anal orifice must be determined. Imperforate anus may be accompanied by a rectovaginal or rectoperineal fistula. The passage of meconium must be noted. If there is any suspicion of intraabdominal pathology, an abdominal x ray is necessary as an adjunct to the physical exam.

Exstrophy of the bladder is a very rare anomaly seen in the suprapubic area.

Genitalia

In the male there is a normal variation in size of the penis, scrotum and testes. An unusually large penis may raise the suspicion of virilizing adrenal hyperplasia. The neonatal prepuce cannot be retracted, but it can be pushed back so that the meatal opening is visible. In hypospadias, the prepuce may be poorly developed; the meatus is usually at the junction of glans and shaft. A first degree hypospadias with the ectopic meatus located in the corona is not uncommon and requires no therapy, since it does not interfere with function.

The testes usually reach the level of the external inguinal ring at 35 to 36 weeks of gestation (the right usually before the left) and therefore may not be palpable in the premature infant. The presence of hydrocele is of little or no clinical significance. Inguinal hernias are rarely seen in the first days of life. Premature infants, however, have a greater chance than full-term infants of eventually developing inguinal hernias, and these are often first noted in the late neonatal period. Inguinal hernias must not be overlooked in female infants, incarceration of the round ligament and ovary being a possible complication. Complete absence of the penis is an extremely rare congenital anomaly.

In the premature female infant, the labia minora and clitoris are quite prominent. In infants of advanced gestational age, the labia majora are more fully developed and pigmented, and hymenal tags are often present. For the first week of life, a mucous vaginal discharge and vaginal bleeding are not uncommon; the latter represents an estrogen withdrawal phenomenon. Masculinization of external genitalia (hypertrophy of the clitoris) occurs in virilizing adrenal hyperplasia and after the therapeutic administration of certain androgenic hormones to gravidas.

Extremities and Spine

Examination of the extremities and spine should reveal such gross abnormalities as absence of a portion of a limb, syndactyly or extra digits. All joints should be flexed and extended in order to detect contractures. The forearms should be pronated and supinated to rule out synostosis of bones of the forearm. Weakness of an upper extremity may be due to fracture of the clavicle or a long bone or to Erb's palsy.

The lower extremities should be examined for tibial bowing, club foot, posterior subluxation of the knee and tibial torsion. Examination of the hips is essential. Inability to completely abduct the hips may arouse suspicion of congenital subluxation or dislocation and a positive Ortoloni's sign (a click felt upon abduction of the hips) aids in confirming the diagnosis.

Phocomelia has been noted after ingestion of thalidomide by the gravida. Constricting rings and congenital amputation of extremities may be the result of amniotic bands.

The spine should be inspected for meningocele and myelomeningocele. Visible or palpable spinal defects, e.g., tufts of hair, palpable absence of laminae, swelling, scoliosis and localized kyphosis, must be noted. The presence of sacrococcygeal teratoma should be obvious.

Fistulous tracts may occur anywhere from the glabella to the sacrum. If overlooked, these may become a portal of entry for bacteria and may lead to recurrent meningitis in later life.

NEUROLOGIC EVALUATION OF THE NEWBORN INFANT

Neurologic examination of the newborn infant, based essentially on muscle tone and various reflexes, is of great importance in evaluating the clinical condition of the infant and estimating gestational age (1, 4, 6). Under normal circumstances, the fetal CNS matures at a fairly constant rate. Myelinization progresses from caudad to cephalad, so that muscle tone and reflexes develop at an earlier time during gestation in the lower than in the upper extremities. Various reflexes begin to appear at a relatively set time during gestation with some individual variation. However, many pathologic factors interfere with normal neurologic maturation and function. These may occur during intrauterine life, during delivery or postnatally. The most common are hypoxia, infection, metabolic disturbances (primarily hypoglycemia), trauma and exposure to various drugs.

Since neurologic maturation of the fetus progresses at a generally fixed rate, the neurologic examination and assessment of land marks is useful in estimating the gestational age of an infant with inappropriate intra-uterine growth when the maternal history is in doubt. The neurologic examination combined with certain external physical characteristics, as described by Dubowitz et al (3), gives an even more accurate estimation of gestational age than the neurologic examination alone (Figs. 17–2 and 17–3 and Table 17–3).

Reasonably accurate knowledge of gestational age may be valuable in management of the infant. Those with intrauterine growth failure are at an increased risk for developing hypoglycemia and at a decreased risk for developing RDS compared to normally grown infants of the same birth weight but lower gestational age. Infants of diabetic mothers may appear to be full term by weight, yet may have the physical and neurologic characteristics of premature infants.

Problems arise, however, when the neurologic examination is used to determine gestational age in infants with intrauterine growth retardation. By modifying the infant's reflex activity, birth shock may make it difficult to perform a completely valid neurologic examination during the first hours of life. Intrauterine hypoxia (and possibly hypoglycemia) may also affect the neurologic exam. Schulte et al (8) have shown that undergrown infants, especially those of severely toxemic mothers, have abnormal neurologic findings with a high incidence of lethargy and hypotonia.

PHYSICAL MEANS OF ASSESSING GESTATIONAL AGE

Since the myelinization of peripheral nerves (both motor and sensory) progresses at a fixed rate during gestation, nerve conduction velocities increase with advancing postconceptional age (2). These nerve conduction velocities are apparently not affected by intrauterine hypoxia and have been shown to correspond fairly well with gestational age. In nurseries where such measurements can be made, they are a useful aid in assessing gestational age when this information is required.

Even in the presence of certain neurologic

Neurologic sign	Score*					
	0	1	2	3	4	5
A Posture†						
B Square window	90°	60°	45°	30°	0°	
C Ankle dorsiflexion	90°	75°	45°	20°	0°	
D Arm recoil†	180°	90–180°	<90°			
E Leg recoil†	180°	90–180°	<90°			
F Popliteal angle†	180°	160°	130°	110°	90°	<90°
G Heel-to-ear†						
H Scarf sign†						
I Head lag†						
J Ventral suspension‡						

*If score differs on two sides, take the mean.
†Infant in supine position
‡Infant suspended in prone position, examiner's hand (two hands for large infant) supporting the chest

FIG. 17–2. Techniques of assessment of neurologic criteria. **A.** With infant quiet: 0, limbs extended; 1, slight flexion hips and knees, arms extended; 2, stronger flexion legs, arms extended; 3, arms slightly flexed, legs flexed and abducted; 4, full flexion of limbs. **B.** Hand flexed on forearm between examiner's thumb and index finger; enough pressure applied to get as full flexion as possible (infant's wrist must not be rotated); angle between hypothenar eminence and ventral aspect of forearm measured and graded. **C.** Foot dorsiflexed onto anterior aspect of leg (examiner's thumb on sole of foot, other fingers behind leg); enough pressure applied to get as full flexion as possible; angle between dorsum of foot and anterior aspect of leg measured and graded. **D.** Forearms flexed for 5 seconds, then fully extended by pulling on hands, then released; arms return briskly to full flexion (2), return to incomplete flexion or response is sluggish (1) or remain extended or move randomly (0). **E.** Hips and knees flexed for 5 seconds, then extended by traction on feet, then released; hips and knees return to full flexion (2), return to incomplete flexion (1) or exhibit minimal or no movement (0). **F.** With pelvis flat on examining couch, thigh held in knee-chest position (examiner's left index finger and thumb supporting the knee), leg is extended by gentle pressure from examiner's right index finger behind ankle, and popliteal angle measured and graded. **G.** Baby's foot drawn as near as it will go without forcing it to head; distance between foot and head and degree of extension at knee measured and graded according to diagram (note that knee is left free and may draw down alongside abdomen). **H.** Infant's hand put around neck and as far posteriorly as possible around opposite shoulder; maneuver assisted by lifting elbow across body: 0, elbow reaches opposite axillary line; 1, elbow between midline and opposite axillary line; 2, elbow reaches midline; 3, elbow will not reach midline. **I.** Infant pulled slowly by his hands (or arms, if very small) toward sitting position (with small infant, examiner's hand may initially support head); position of head in relation to trunk noted: 0, complete lag; 1, partial head control; 2, head maintained in line with body; 3, head brought anterior to body. **J.** Degree of extension of back, amount of flexion of arms and legs and relation of head to trunk noted and graded according to diagram. (Dubowitz LMS et al: J Pediatr 77:1, 1970)

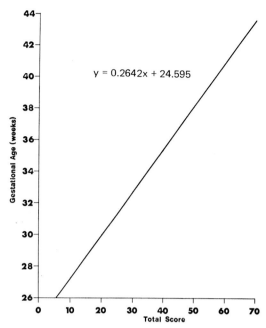

$$y = 0.2642x + 24.595$$

FIG. 17–3. Scoring system for neurologic criteria. For scoring, see Fig. 17–2. (Dubowitz LMS et al: J Pediatr 77:1, 1970)

NEUROLOGIC EXAMINATION

The neurologic examination should be undertaken when the infant is awake and quiet, preferably following a feeding. The examination may require several repetitions, especially if the infant becomes "uncooperative."

INSPECTION

The general state of activity and level of alertness are good indicators of neurologic status. Lethargy and hypotonia may be signs of cerebral hypoxia, hypoglycemia, hypermagnesemia, hypocalcemia, intracranial bleeding or infection; an unusually agitated state occurring with increased muscle tone may be an indication of narcotic withdrawal.

The infant should be inspected for gross neurologic abnormalities, such as microcephaly or hydrocephaly, meningocele, encephalocele or myelomeningocele.

abnormalities, the EEG may be useful (within a 2-week range) in estimating gestational age (2, 5), but this interpretation should be made only by a physician expert in reading neonatal EEGs.

TABLE 17–3. Scoring System for External Criteria

External Sign	Score*				
	0	1	2	3	4
Edema	Obvious edema of hands and feet; pitting over tibia	No obvious edema of hands and feet; pitting over tibia	No edema		
Skin texture	Very thin, gelatinous	Thin and smooth	Smooth; medium thickness; rash or superficial peeling	Slight thickening; superficial cracking and peeling, especially of hands and feet	Thick and parchment-like; superficial or deep cracking
Skin color	Dark red	Uniformly pink	Pale pink; variable over body	Pale; only pink over ears, lips, palms or soles	
Skin opacity (trunk)	Numerous veins and venules clearly seen, especially over abdomen	Veins and tributaries seen	A few large vessels clearly seen over abdomen	A few large vessels seen indistinctly over abdomen	No blood vessels seen
Lanugo (over back)	No lanugo	Abundant; long and thick over whole back	Hair thinning especially over lower back	Small amount of lanugo and bald areas	At least ½ of back devoid of lanugo
Plantar creases	No skin creases	Faint red marks over anterior half of sole	Definite red marks over > anterior ½; indentations over < anterior ⅓	Indentations over > anterior ⅓	Definite deep indentations over > anterior ⅓

Nipple formation	Nipple barely visible; no areola	Nipple well defined; areola smooth and flat, diameter < 0.75 cm	Areola stippled, edge not raised, diameter < 0.75 cm	Areola stippled, edge raised, diameter > 0.75 cm
Breast size	No breast tissue palpable	Breast tissue on one or both sides, < 0.5 cm diameter	Breast tissue both sides; one or both 0.5–1.0 cm	Breast tissue both sides; one or both > 1 cm
Ear form	Pinna flat and shapeless, little or no incurving of edge	Incurving of part of edge of pinna	Partial incurving whole of upper pinna	Well-defined incurving whole of upper pinna
Ear firmness	Pinna soft, easily folded; no recoil	Pinna soft, easily folded; slow recoil	Cartilage to edge of pinna, but soft in places; ready recoil	Pinna firm, cartilage to edge; instant recoil
Genitals Male	Neither testis in scrotum	At least one testis high in scrotum	At least one testis right down	
Female (with hips ½ abducted)	Labia majora widely separated, labia minora protruding	Labia majora almost cover labia minora	Labia majora completely cover labia minora	

* If score differs on two sides, take the mean. (Dubowitz et al: J Pediatr 77:1, 1970)

Posture

The posture that the infant assumes may be useful in the assessment of gestational age. At 24 weeks' gestation, an infant placed in a supine position rolls over on his side (lateral decubitus position). By 28 weeks he usually remains on his back with total extension of all extremities. By 32 weeks, with some increase in tone of the lower extremities, there is some flexion at the hips and knees. By 34 weeks the infant assumes a froglike position, and there is good flexion of the lower and extension of the upper extremities. By 36 or 37 weeks, the infant begins to maintain his forearms flexed at the elbows, and by term there is total flexion of all extremities when the infant is in a supine position.

Spontaneous Movements

Spontaneous movements can be of some help in assessing maturity. Generalized athetoid type of movement is noted in relatively immature infants. As the infant becomes more mature, movements tend to be more localized.

The inability to move an upper extremity may indicate Erb's palsy or fracture of the humerus. Facial nerve palsy is most usually related to forceps trauma, but it may be secondary to a central lesion.

Muscular Activity

Abnormal muscular activity should be noted. Tremulousness may be a manifestation of hypoglycemia, hypocalcemia, systemic infection or narcotic withdrawal. On the other hand, it may be also seen with relative frequency in infants who are small for gestational age and in whom no disease is apparent. Seizure activity is more difficult to detect in the neonatal period than at any other time. Such abnormal movements as jerking of an extremity, blinking or eye rolling, sudden assumption of a tonic posture or unusual chewing activity may be signs of seizures (see section Neonatal Seizures, Ch. 9).

EVALUATION OF MUSCLE TONE

Recoil

Following careful inspection, an evaluation of the infant's muscle tone should be undertaken. Under normal circumstances, recoil (the ability of the extremity to return to its flexed position after passive stretching and release) is first noted in the lower extremities at about 32 weeks and is strong at 34 weeks. Recoil begins to appear in the upper extremities at 36 to 37 weeks and is quite strong at term.

Heel-to-Ear and Scarf Maneuvers

The heel-to-ear maneuver is based on increasing resistance that is met with progressing gestational age as the heel of the leg extended at the knee is brought into approximation with the ipsilateral ear. This becomes difficult at 34 weeks and almost impossible at 37 weeks.

In the scarf maneuver, the infant's hand is grasped by the examiner and drawn across his chin to the opposite shoulder. This becomes fairly difficult to perform by 36 weeks because of increasing muscle tone in the arms.

Suck

The sucking reflex normally begins to appear at about 24 weeks and is usually coordinated with swallowing at about 34 weeks. A poor sucking reflex in a relatively mature infant may be associated with intrauterine hypoxia, infection or hypoglycemia.

Moro

The Moro reflex is usually complete but easily exhaustible by about 28 weeks. Its absence after this gestational age is usually indicative of neurologic impairment.

Grasp

The grasp reflex appears at about 24 to 28 weeks; by 37 weeks it is strong enough to lift the infant off the examining surface.

Rooting

The rooting reflex (head turning in the direction of stimulation about the mouth) also appears at 24 to 28 weeks and becomes strong by about 33 weeks.

Automatic Walking

The automatic walking reflex is elicited by holding the infant upright and tilted slightly forward, keeping the soles of his feet in contact with a solid surface. A "walking" motion of the legs (placing one leg in front of the other) begins to appear at 33 weeks. By 37 weeks the infant walks on tiptoes, and by 40 weeks he walks on his soles.

The neurologic examination can provide a wealth of information concerning the clinical condition of the neonate. It is therefore extremely important that the physician caring for newborn infants be familiar with its performance.

REFERENCES

1. Amiel-Tison C: Neurological evaluation of the maturity of newborn infants. Arch Dis Child 43:89, 1968
2. Dreyfus-Brisac C: The EEG of the premature infant and fullterm newborn: In: Neurological and EEG Correlative Studies in Infancy. Edited by P Kellaway, J Peterson. New York, Grune & Stratton, 1964, p 186
3. Dubowitz LMB, Dubowitz V, Goldberg C: Clinical assessment of gestational age. J Pediatr 77:1, 1970
4. Koenigsberger MR: Judgment of fetal age. I. Neurologic evaluation, Pediatr Clin North Am 13:823, 1966
5. Parmelee AH, Schulte FJ, Akiyama Y, Wenner WH, Schulz MA, Stern E: Maturation of EEG activity during sleep in premature infants. Electroencephalogr Clin Neurophysiol 24:319, 1968
6. Robinson RJ: Assessment of gestational age by neurologic examination. Arch Dis Child 41:437, 1966
7. Schulte FJ, Michaelis R, Linke I, Nolte R: Motor nerve conduction velocity in term, preterm, and small-for-dates newborn infants. Pediatrics 42:17, 1968
8. Schulte FJ, Schrempf G, Hinze G: Maternal toxemia, fetal malnutrition, and motor behavior of the newborn. Pediatrics 48:871, 1971

18

Mechanisms
of
Infection

PERINATAL INFECTION

Infections caused by both bacterial and non-bacterial microorganisms may occur during fetal life, in the intrapartum period and following delivery (5, 7, 8, 10). Although advances have been made in both diagnosis and treatment of perinatal infections, they still account for significant morbidity and mortality.

FETAL

Nonbacterial

The mechanism of transplacental passage of nonbacterial infectious agents is unknown. For the large majority of cases, maternal viremia is not associated with fetal infection. However, a few maternal viral infections, such as rubella, cytomegalovirus, h. simplex, varicella and group B coxsackie virus are known to affect the fetus and are frequently teratogenic; others, such as infectious hepatitis, influenza and mumps, have been incriminated, but no precise relationship has been established. Many fetuses of mothers infected with rubella, cytomegalovirus and h. simplex remain unaffected, whereas others develop virologic and serologic evidence of the infection without its clinical findings. The principal manifestations of fetomaternal infection are summarized in Table 18–1, and the intervals during intrauterine or postnatal development when specific organisms can affect progeny are shown in Figure 18–1.

Certain protozoal infections, such as toxoplasmosis and malaria, may also affect the fetus. As in viral infections, the mechanism of transplacental passage of the infectious agent is poorly understood.

Bacterial

Amniotic infection with bacterial agents is relatively common. It may occur with membranes either ruptured or intact and is associated with increased fetal wastage, premature labor and increased incidence of neonatal morbidity and mortality. Its incidence is highest among gravidas of the lowest socioeconomic classes (16).

Gram-negative bacteria such as E. coli, which are normally found in the vagina, may ascend in the presence of either intact or ruptured membranes into the amniotic fluid. Clinical evidence of amnionitis in the mother (fever, leukocytosis or fetid vaginal discharge) may or may not be present. The maternal response to infection is migration of leukocytes across the decidua capsularis, chorion laeve and amnion into the amniotic fluid. In the placenta the maternal leukocytes migrate to the chorion from the intervillous space toward the amniotic cavity. The fetal response starts after the maternal reaction and includes leukocytic aggregation and migration to those aspects of umbilical vessels close to the amniotic cavity.

Signs of Infection

Clinical signs of infection begin in the fetus when contaminated fluid is swallowed. The

TABLE 18–1. Fetomaternal Infection

Disease	Time of Transmission	Teratogenic Effects	Other Manifestations	Laboratory Diagnosis
Rubella	1st trimester; early second trimester (problematical)	Cataracts, glaucoma, retinopathy, microphthalmia, microcephaly, congenital heart disease	Thrombocytopenia, hepatosplenomegaly, hepatitis, pneumonia, bone destruction, encephalitis, growth retardation	HI antibody, viral isolation from body fluids
Toxoplasmosis	1st trimester	Microcephaly, hydrocephaly, cerebral calcifications, chorioretinitis	Encephalitis, myocarditis, hepatosplenomegaly, jaundice, diarrhea, vomiting, convulsions	CF, HI antibody, IgM-FTA specific antibody
Cytomegalovirus	Throughout pregnancy	Microcephaly, cerebral calcifications	Same as toxoplasmosis	Neutralizing or CF antibody, isolation of virus from urine, inclusion-bearing cells in urine
Herpes simplex	1st trimester (transplacental); intrapartum (transplacental); ascending and direct contact	Chorioretinitis, microcephaly, microphthalmia	Cutaneous lesions (vesicles), visceral involvement (granulomas)	Neutralizing or CF antibody, isolation of virus from chorioallantoic membrane tissue culture, growth of virus on rabbit cornea
Varicella	1st trimester and intrapartum	Chorioretinitis, microcephaly, limb deformities	Skin lesions, encephalomyocarditis, visceral involvement	Growth of virus on tissue culture, CF antibody
Group B coxsackie virus	1st trimester and late in pregnancy	Provisional assn.: GU anomalies, hare lip, cleft palate, congenital heart disease, CNS anomalies, pyloric stenosis	Encephalomyocarditis, pneumonia	Neutralization and CF antibody, growth of virus on tissue culture
Syphilis	Second half of pregnancy	Delayed effects on eyes, ears, teeth, joints, CNS	Osteochondritis, jaundice, hepatosplenomegaly, lymphadenopathy, rhagades, anemia	Darkfield exam. for spirochetes, FTA–ABS, TPI immobilization
Listeria	Intrapartum	Not known	Sepsis, meningitis, hepatitis, diffuse granulomatosis	Isolation of bacteria from blood, urine or pus
Gonococcus	Last trimester and at delivery	Not known	Sepsis, conjunctivitis, panophthalmitis	Gram stain and culture (Thayer-Martin medium)
Tuberculosis	Rarely transplacental; usually following delivery	Not known	Fever, anemia, pulmonary and systemic dissemination	Isolation of organism from gastric washing or maternal lesions, PPD unreliable during neonatal period

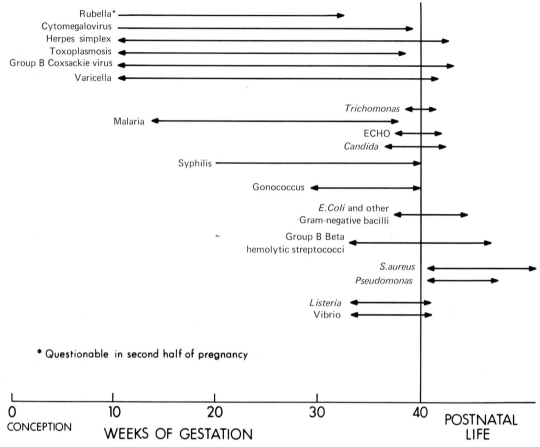

FIG. 18–1. Time of acquisition of perinatal infections.

fluid may be aspirated into the lungs and spread to the bloodstream, meninges and middle ear (otitis media).

Fetal infection may occur in the absence of ruptured membranes, especially in listeriosis and candidiasis. Loss of viability of the membranes, especially at the lower poles, may be at least a partial explanation of the phenomenon. Rupture may be imperceptible, or the membranes may have degenerated or necrosed, as demonstrated by biopsy of intact membranes. The combination of impaired membranous viability at the lower uterine pole and fetal descent prior to onset of labor permit organisms to enter the amniotic fluid before apparent rupture. However, the role of prolonged rupture of membranes as a predisposing factor cannot be minimized.

Inflammatory processes in fetal lung and membranes have been observed after brief intervals of rupture of membranes, ranging from a few minutes to six hours, but the frequency increases with longer intervals. It is often difficult to evaluate the inflammation present in fetal membranes, since it may also represent a response to hypoxia or to meconium in amniotic fluid.

Inflammatory response, including placental vasculitis, is also associated with a high incidence of prematurity. Therefore a triad of prematurity, infection and chorioamnionitis may be envisioned.

AMNIOTIC INFECTION SYNDROME

The presence of polymorphonuclear neutrophil leukocytes (PMNs) in the alveoli of the lung represents spread of infection from the amnion and is an integral part of the amniotic infection syndrome. In most fetal and neonatal deaths secondary to congenital pneumonia, inflammation of the placental membranes is seen. To the pathologist, fluid —or any inert material—in the lungs favors the diagnosis of infection; in contrast vernix caseosa may be aspirated in the absence of infection. Meconium may be aspirated into the lungs following an episode of fetal asphyxia. Although it enhances bacterial infection, it may be found in regions of the lung where pneumonic reaction is absent.

Inflammatory response in the chorion, amnion and umbilical cord is a diagnostic criterion in intrauterine infection. The specificity of these changes, however, is uncertain; hence the pathogenetic significance originally attributed to such findings is now moot. From a practical point of view such findings are rarely available in sufficient time to aid clinical management.

Various diagnostic tests based on these findings are described. Amnion mounts, microscopic examination of the umbilical cord (6), chorionic imprints (17) and studies of aspirated gastric contents for bacteria (4) and inflammatory cells (18) have all been used in an attempt to diagnose fetal infection. Most of the tests have not gained acceptance because of practical problems or because of the frequency of false results.

NEONATAL

Formidable rates of morbidity and mortality continue to be associated with systemic bacterial infection (sepsis and meningitis) in newborn infants, despite the availability of an ever-expanding list of potent antimicrobial agents. Case fatality rates vary from 25% to 60%. This generally unfavorable outlook reflects several problems: signs of systemic infection are nonspecific in the neonate and may easily be mistaken for a variety of metabolic and hematologic disorders. The clinical features of meningitis and sepsis in older children and adults are absent among newborn infants. Fever, for example, is a rare manifestation of infection, and when it occurs, it is more prevalent in full-term than in premature infants.

Hypothermia is a much more frequently encountered finding. Signs of meningeal irritation that are typical among older age groups, such as nuchal rigidity or tenderness of hamstring muscles, are rare among newborn infants except as terminal manifestations. The wide range of total white blood cell counts (4,000 to 30,000/mm^3) usually precludes the diagnostic value of this test, except for extreme values. The history may be helpful but is often misleading.

Such predisposing maternal factors as prolonged rupture of membranes (over 18 hours), prolonged labor even with membranes intact, fever (which may be associated with a purulent vaginal discharge) and pyelonephritis are often associated with chorioamnionitis, congenital pneumonia and sepsis. Instrumentation and operative extraction may also predispose to infection. Males are more commonly infected than females, and premature infants more than full-term infants. Rates of infection are highest among those individuals from the poorest socioeconomic background (16).

The pediatrician's awareness of predisposing prenatal factors is critical since the history may provide distinction between infection and other illnesses with similar clinical manifestations, e.g., hypoglycemia. It should be stressed, however, that the majority of newborn infants in the high-risk category do not have demonstrable infection.

There are, however, other factors leading to a poor prognosis. Newborn infants exhibit multiple impairments of their immunologic mechanisms that may lead to an increase both in incidence and in severity of infections. This is especially true among premature infants and includes complications with opsonization, complement levels and serum immunoglobulin concentrations (see section Perinatal Immunology). Many of the organisms (especially nonbacterial ones) typically found among infected newborn infants are not sensitive to any known therapeutic agent except on an experimental basis. For example, h. simplex, toxoplasma, cytomegalovirus and coxsackievirus are rarely amenable to therapy, whereas such bacterial agents as pseudomonas, enterococci and various members of the enterobacteriaciae family may be only partially sensitive to the antibiotic agents presently available. For these reasons even an early diagnosis of systemic infection will lead to death in a certain proportion of these infants, primarily because of the etiologic agent.

Apart from the problem of host defects, a variety of postnatal challenges predisposes the neonate to infection. Umbilical cord contamination; exposure to carriers of pathogens among the medical and nursing staff (especially handborne infection); cross infection from other infants in the nursery; contamination of IV infusions, incubators (2), ventilators (13) and humidifying devices (3, 19); circumcisions; umbilical blood vessel catheters; and even exposure to an infected mother who is a source of pathogens are all hazards facing the newborn infant (Table 18–2).

Although exposure to pathogenic organisms in utero is responsible for a substantial number of neonatal infections, they may also be acquired during parturition or postnatally (Fig. 18–2). Contact with such organisms of the birth canal as varicella, h. simplex and vibrio may result in neonatal infection. The infant may become infected postnatally from a variety of environmental sources. Certain organisms such as h.

simplex or *L. monocytogenes* may be responsible for either prenatal or postnatal infection.

Physical Examination

Several physical findings are frequent in systemic infection of the newborn infant, but few if any of them are unique to this condition. Hepatomegaly, splenomegaly, cyanosis, abdominal distension, jaundice, lethargy, irritability, omphalitis, rapid respirations and coagulation disorders should draw the attention of the examiner to a possible diagnosis of sepsis. Inflammation of the tympanic membranes, pustules, cellulitis and conjunctivitis may be findings of localized infection but may also be associated with generalized infection. Increased intracranial pressure, as manifested by a bulging anterior fontanelle, is usually a late sign of meningitis. Sclerema or doughy hardening of the skin is generally a terminal finding (Fig. 18–3).

It must be assumed that any infant with some or all of the signs described is likely to have a generalized infection. A detailed examination and diagnostic investigation may clearly lead to another diagnosis as the sole basis for the observed signs. Even if another abnormality is identified, sepsis may still be present. A "sepsis work-up" (see section Laboratory Studies) is indicated if suspicion of systemic infection exists.

After the diagnostic tests have been completed, therapy directed against the most likely causative organisms with parenteral administration of antibiotics should be promptly initiated. It may appear after the results of laboratory tests have become available and after the infant's clinical course has been evaluated for several days that infectious disease is not present. If this is the case, antibiotic therapy can be stopped. The risk to the infant of this approach is minimal compared with the hazard of aggravating an ongoing, progressive infection caused by an agent that may have responded to commonly used antibiotics. If the cultures suggest that the infection is due to an organism not sensitive to the origi-

TABLE 18–2. Factors Predisposing to Systemic Infection In the Newborn Infant

Antenatal
  Prolonged rupture of membranes over 24 hours
  Frank maternal infection, e.g., amnionitis
  Unexplained maternal fever
  Poor maternal socioeconomic status
  Prematurity
  Untreated maternal venereal disease
  Maternal diabetes mellitus (?)

Postnatal
  Generalized debilitation
  Congenital anomalies, e.g., myelomeningocele,
    pilonidal fistula
  Central venous catheters
  Breaks in skin
  Contaminated water reservoirs and soap
    dispensers
  Inadequate handwashing by nursery staff
  Transmission of illness from infected infant or
    staff nursery member or parent
  Overcrowding of nursery

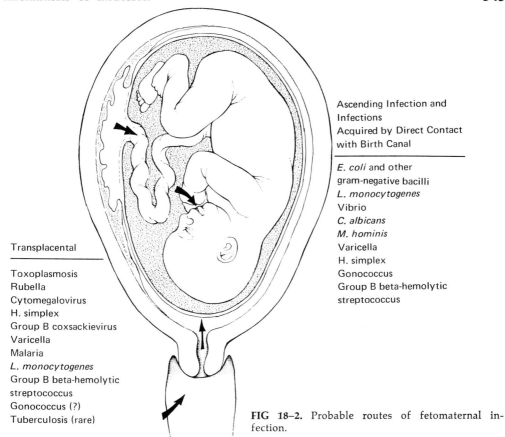

Ascending Infection and
Infections
Acquired by Direct Contact
with Birth Canal

E. coli and other
gram-negative bacilli
L. monocytogenes
Vibrio
C. albicans
M. hominis
Varicella
H. simplex
Gonococcus
Group B beta-hemolytic
streptococcus

Transplacental

Toxoplasmosis
Rubella
Cytomegalovirus
H. simplex
Group B coxsackievirus
Varicella
Malaria
L. monocytogenes
Group B beta-hemolytic
streptococcus
Gonococcus (?)
Tuberculosis (rare)

FIG 18–2. Probable routes of fetomaternal infection.

nally chosen antibiotic preparation, the proper substitution can then be made.

Laboratory Studies

A wide range of studies is useful in establishing a diagnosis of systemic infection in the newborn infant, including:

Blood cultures drawn from a peripheral vein (if possible)

Lumbar puncture (plate specimen immediately on culture medium)

Cultures of nose, throat, umbilicus, stool, external auditory canal, gastric fluid (if maternal amnionitis or prolonged rupture of membranes is present) and skin lesions

Clean-catch (or suprapubic) urine specimen for culture and microscopic examination

Hemoglobin or hematocrit
Total and differential WBC
Platelet count

ESR

C-reactive protein (valid only in first 48 hours of life)

Chest x rays (skull films if toxoplasmosis or cytomegalovirus is suspected)

Serologic test for syphilis

Serum immunoglobulin levels (IgM and IgA)

Specific fluorescent antibody tests, when indicated, e.g., FTA–IgM for syphilis

Acid-base studies
Bilirubin
Electrolytes
Blood glucose

The complete blood count is of limited diagnostic value. A falling hemoglobin or hematocrit level may be a reflection of hemolysis or bleeding secondary to disseminated intravascular coagulation (DIC), which may accompany infection. A diagnostic evaluation for DIC is warranted under these circumstances. The white blood cell

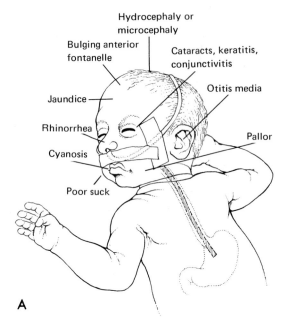

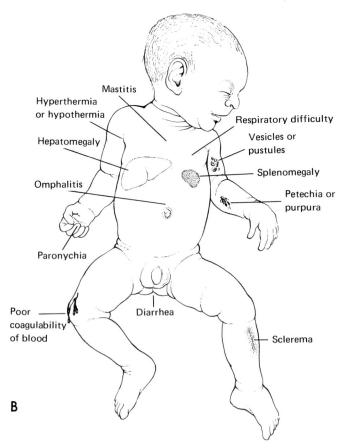

FIG. 18–3. Signs of neonatal infection. **A.** Craniofacial signs. **B.** Bodily signs.

count (WBC) and differential count are also of limited value in establishing a diagnosis. Extremely low levels, 4,000/mm³ or less, may suggest endotoxemia or other massive infection; a marked leukocytosis of 30,000 mm³ or greater may also indicate infection. Any value between these extremes may be normal for newborn infants. The normal differential count during the first few days of postnatal life is similar to that seen in school age children and adults, with a predominance of PMNs. A relative absence of PMNs may reflect severe infection, as may a "shift to the left" (a predominance of immature forms of PMNs) or a marked neutrophilia. Toxic granulations in PMNs and an increased number of band forms may also suggest sepsis. However, these tests may not be helpful in far-advanced stages of infection.

The microanalytic technique for determining erythrocyte sedimentation rate (ESR) is a simple although nonspecific test that aids in the diagnosis of bacterial infection in the neonatal patient. In our hands ESR values of over 6 mm/hour during the first days of life and over 12 mm/hour by the end of the first month of life are usually associated with systemic bacterial infection (11).

The C-reactive protein is another nonspecific test for infection that can be utilized only during the first two days of life since all newborn infants normally develop elevated levels by the third or fourth day. This test is positive in approximately two-thirds of infected infants prior to the third day of life (12).

Elevated umbilical cord serum IgM levels were considered to be a major sign of fetomaternal (nonbacterial) infection in early studies (20, 24). However, several surveys show that high levels (over 15 to 20 mg/100 ml) occur among those babies who are not infected, whereas other newborn infants with congenital infection, such as rubella, may have low levels (15). Our own experience with this test is disappointing, and we observe with considerable frequency levels over 15 to 20 mg/100 ml among normal neonates. The test may be more valuable if repeated on sera drawn during the first few days of life. Infected infants usually demonstrate increasing concentrations, whereas values decline or remain constant in noninfected infants.

Cultural evidence is necessary in order to

FIG. 18–4. Factors predisposing to neonatal infection.

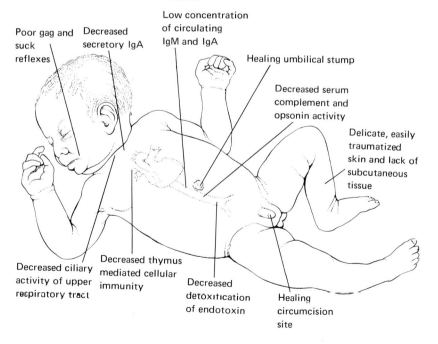

Poor gag and suck reflexes

Decreased secretory IgA

Low concentration of circulating IgM and IgA

Healing umbilical stump

Decreased serum complement and opsonin activity

Delicate, easily traumatized skin and lack of subcutaneous tissue

Decreased ciliary activity of upper respiratory tract

Decreased thymus mediated cellular immunity

Decreased detoxification of endotoxin

Healing circumcision site

make a definitive diagnosis of bacterial infection. Blood cultures must be routinely obtained when sepsis is suspected. A negative culture does not rule out the diagnosis; neither does a single positive culture offer absolute proof. Ideally, two or three cultures should be obtained; however, the fulminating course of sepsis in the newborn child, together with technical difficulties in obtaining blood specimens, often makes this goal difficult or impossible. However, if multiple cultures are taken and all are positive for the same organism, the diagnosis is a certainty. Urine cultures should be obtained to rule out the diagnosis of pyelonephritis, which may be an isolated infection or a concomitant finding with sepsis. Microscopic examination of the urine alone is inadequate, since WBCs may be present in the absence of infection and vice versa. (Methods used for collection of urine in the newborn infant are discussed in the section Urinary Tract Infection, Ch. 19.)

Cultures of the nares, throat and umbilicus are of less value, especially after the second day of life, since colonization with S. aureus and E. coli is common. Cultures of the external auditory canal or gastric fluid (following prolonged rupture of the membranes) may be of greater diagnostic value. Pathogenic organisms and PMNs in the aspirates from either of these two sites may be valuable in identifying sepsis of antenatal origin. Stool cultures are appropriate especially when enteropathogenic E. coli or salmonella are suspected. Isolation of these organisms should be followed by serologic typing and determination of antibiotic sensitivity.

The importance of lumbar punctures cannot be overstated. They must be performed whenever sepsis is suspected since about one-third of septic infants also suffer from meningitis. It must be emphasized that cultures of cerebrospinal fluid (CSF) must be processed immediately after the lumbar puncture since delays may lead either to false negative results or to the growth of contaminants that may be mistaken for pathogenic organisms.

A technique used in many medical centers

is the fluorescent antibody test. In the newborn period it is especially useful for identification of enteropathogenic E. coli and gonococci. Special microscopic equipment is required for this test, and questions about the specificity of results have been raised. It is a rapid procedure, and a negative result is especially helpful. As with the gram stain method, it is a screening procedure and should not be regarded as a substitute for culture and definitive isolation techniques.

Radiologic studies are of some value in the diagnosis of infectious disease. When pneumonia is suspected chest x rays are helpful in determining the extent of involvement but do not aid in establishing etiology. Skull films are helpful in identifying the intracranial calcifications often seen with toxoplasmosis or cytomegalovirus. X rays of the long bones aid in the identification of rubella or congenital syphilis.

It is evident that a rational approach to the diagnosis and treatment of neonatal infection depends on a high index of suspicion backed by history, physical findings and laboratory data. Presumably the condition is diagnosed and treated far more often than it is proved, and until more specific tests become available, this state of affairs is likely to continue. Since generalized infection is usually treatable, it is axiomatic that virtually any newborn infant—especially a premature one—who is regressing, e.g., lethargic and feeding poorly, be evaluated for diagnosis of sepsis.

PERINATAL IMMUNOLOGY

During the late 1960s and early 1970s great advances were made in understanding host defense mechanisms against infection. To evaluate the immunologic capabilities of the fetus and newborn infant, it is necessary to review the major events in the immunologic pathway:

Afferent Limb:
Slowing of blood flow, margination (adherence of WBCs to vascular endothelium), diapedesis (tissue migration of WBCs),

chemotaxis (migration of WBCs toward incitant), opsonization (damage to incitant), phagocytosis by WBCs and lysis of organisms within WBCs.

Processing:

Stimulation of lymphocytes and activation of humoral and cellular antibody.

AFFERENT LIMB

Slowing of blood flow is the initial event following antigenic invasion of such areas as the skin and lungs, followed by margination or adherence of WBCs to the vascular endothelium and diapedesis (migration of WBCs through tissues). Chemotaxis, or specific migration of WBCs toward the incitant, is followed by opsonization, or damage to the incitant. The latter event is mediated through opsonins, which are either nonspecific or specific antibodies of the IgM or IgG class. Complement must be present for all of the events described to occur. The final phases of the afferent limb are phagocytosis (ingestion by WBCs) and lysis or dissolution of the antigens within the WBCs. Inherited deficiency of certain intraleukocytic enzymes involved in lysis of antigens leads to conditions such as chronic granulomatous disease.

PROCESSING

The next series of events includes stimulation of lymphocytes and activation of both humoral (antibody) and cellular (delayed hypersensitivity) capability. The former is mediated by B cells (bursal or bone marrow in origin), which have the potential for antibody synthesis and secretion; they may eventually be transformed into plasma cells. Delayed hypersensitivity is mediated by T (thymic) lymphocytes, which are limited in their capacity to synthesize and secrete antibody. They do, however, play a major role in the elimination of intracellular organisms such as tubercle bacilli, salmonellae, viruses and fungi; skin sensitivity to antigens such as purified protein derivative (PPD); and homograft rejection. Both B and T cells frequently cooperate in effecting host defense mechanisms.

CLASSES OF IMMUNOGLOBULINS

Five classes of immunoglobulins are known (Table 18–3). Most of the antibody in serum and confined extravascular fluid (e.g., CSF, synovial fluid, aqueous humor) is of the IgG variety; in contrast, surface fluids such as mucus, tears and succus entericus contain predominantly IgA and IgE antibody. The role of IgD is unknown. The IgM class includes isohemagglutinins, endotoxin and Forssman antibody. The IgE class consists mainly of reagins, or atopic antibodies, which combine with circulating basophils or tissue mast cells to effect the release of such chemical mediators as histamine, slow-reacting substance A (SRS-A), bradykinin and

TABLE 18–3. Immunoglobulins

Antibody	Primary Location(s)	Function
IgG	Serum, CSF, synovial fluid anterior chamber of eye	Humoral immunity to many infectious agents
IgM	Serum	Absent or present in low concentrations in normal neonates; elevation may be a response to fetomaternal infection
IgA	Serum, saliva, colostrum	Absent or present in low concentrations in normal neonates; salivary IgA protects against respiratory tract infections; colostral IgA may decrease enteropathogenic *E. coli* infection
IgE	Serum, bronchial washings	Mediates hypersensitivity reactions; probably rare in neonates
IgD	Serum	Function unknown at any age; elevated in pregnancy

TABLE 18–4. Serum IgG Levels in Relation to Gestational Age in Normally Grown, Single Birth Neonates*

Gestational Age (weeks)	Number of Neonates	Median Level (Range)	10th Percentile	90th Percentile
40	24	1088 (348–2000)	489	1740
30–39	30	935 (135–2975)	406	1453
32–35	55	850 (270–2150)	380	1462
28–31	21	595 (200–2505)	277	1400
27 or less	14	430 (128–980)	150	872

* All determinations on umbilical cord sera. All results expressed in mg/100 ml.

serotonin. They are also skin-fixing antibodies.

Organs capable of synthesizing antibody include the liver, spleen, lymph nodes and other lymphid tissue and bone marrow. The thymus may play a coordinate role with these other tissues, particularly the bone marrow.

FETAL LIFE

Immunologic maturation is an ongoing process that begins early in fetal life (26, 53) and continues through the perinatal period, infancy and early childhood (25, 38).

At 7 to 8 weeks of gestation round lymphocytes can be demonstrated in the peripheral circulation. By 12 weeks the total lymphocyte count is approximately 1,000/mm³, and by 20 to 25 weeks, 10,000/mm³. Interferon production parallels the increase in peripheral lymphocytes.

The fetal thymus is derived from the second and third branchial pouches. By the eighth week of gestation it differentiates into a cortex and medulla, and small lymphocytes (T cells) are found.

The spleen appears at the 5th week of gestation; lymphocytes appear in this organ at 12 weeks, and IgM and IgG synthesis are demonstrable by immunofluorescence by the 21st week. A few primary follicles and red pulp with collections of lymphocytes can be seen at birth, whereas germinal centers develop postnatally.

Lymph nodes appear at the end of the first trimester but are poorly differentiated;

germinal centers are absent at birth. Plasma cells are virtually absent (about 1% of adult levels) in the bone marrow, spleen and lamina propria of the intestine in normal newborn infants. Their presence in more than minimal numbers indicates fetal infection (28).

Functional competence of splenic lymphocytes is demonstrable after the 16th week of gestation, and that of the thymus between 12 and 16 weeks when tested by phytochemagglutinin (PHA) transformation. tion. This test, however, is nonspecific and does not measure complete functional maturation of the lymphocyte.

Complement synthesis starts at 10 to 14 weeks of gestation and reaches about one-half of adult levels at term (22, 36).

The concentration of circulating IgG increases with advancing gestational age after the 20th week (Tables 18–4 and 18–5); this is primarily a reflection of antibody that has been passively acquired from the maternal circulation. About 5% to 10% of the IgG is probably synthesized by the fetus. Although some investigators have observed that a substantial proportion of infants with intrauterine growth failure have significantly decreased umbilical cord serum concentrations of IgG (45, 56), we have not found this to be true (35).

Neither IgA nor IgM cross the placenta into the fetal circulation. They are present in only a small proportion of newborn infants and usually in low concentrations. These levels reflect synthesis by the fetus in response to some type of antigenic stimulus

(24, 25, 27, 43, 52). Studies of α2-haptoglobin and isohemagglutinin may determine whether IgM is of maternal or fetal origin.

We have been able to detect IgD in only 8% of neonates who were tested (35). The biologic role of this class of immunoglobulins is not known. Secretory IgA is usually absent in the saliva in the neonatal period (41).

The fetus has an excellent capacity for forming antibody; this function, however, is limited by its protected environment, which limits its exposure to antigenic stimuli, and by passive acquisition of antibody from the mother (36, 51). Second and third trimester antibody response to *T. pallidum* (23) and toxoplasma (33, 44) has been recognized for many years, and formation of antibody against rubella may occur as early as 112 days' gestation (31). The capacity of premature infants (birth weights 1320 to 1900 g) to form antibody against both experimental ϕ X 174 phage and naturally occurring coxsackievirus is marked and is consistent with the ability of the fetus to synthesize antibody (44, 55).

Most of the fetal antibody at the time of delivery has been passively transferred across the placenta from the maternal circulation.

The types of antibody that cross the placenta in high titer, i.e., those in which the fetomaternal titers are about equal, include tetanus, diphtheria and scarlet fever antitoxin; antistaphylococcal antibody (Rantz); Rh-blocking antibody; and antibody to poliomyelitis, h. simplex, toxoplasma, anthropod-borne encephalitis, hepa-titis, measles, mumps, rubella, rickettsia, *Histoplasma capsulatum* and influenza virus. Cytotoxic (HL-A) and salmonella flagellar antibodies also cross the placenta. Low cord titers of antibody include those to *H. influenza*, *T. pallidum*, and *H. pertussis*. There is no demonstrable transmission of salmonella and *E. coli* somatic (O) antibodies, skin-sensitizing antibody (reagin), heterophil and complete Rh antibody.

Antibodies that cross the placenta are primarily of the IgG variety, whereas those that do not usually belong to the IgM family. For example H antibodies to *S. typhosa* and other gram-negative organisms pass the placental barrier, whereas those of the O type do so poorly (51). The former are of the IgG class, the latter of the IgM class. In general, viral antibodies are efficiently transmitted. For unexplained reasons types 1 and 2 polioantibodies are passed in a higher titer than are type 3 (42).

NEONATAL PERIOD

The process of birth has no direct effect on immunologic maturation. However, removal from the protected uterine environment exposes the infant to bacteria, viruses and a host of other antigenic stimuli.

Serum Antibodies

The presence of antibodies in their serum along with limited exposure is responsible for the rarity of such diseases as poliomyelitis, measles, mumps, rubella and diphtheria in newborn infants. Newborn infants are

TABLE 18–5. Serum IgA and IgM Levels in Relation to Gestational Age in Normally Developed, Single Birth Neonates*

Gestational Age (weeks)	Number of Neonates	IgA Level			IgM Level		
		Mean	Range	Percent Undetectable	Mean	Range	Percent Undetectable
40	24	6.6	0–46	71	17	0–41	25
36–39	30	3.3	0–23	81	9.5	0–69	37
32–35	55	6.5	0–51	78	7.8	0–43	47
28–31	21	2.2	0–17.5	86	4.4	0–34	71
27 or less	14	10	0–58	75	3.0	0–17	75

* All determinations on umbilical cord sera. All results expressed in mg/100 ml. (Evans et al: Am J Clin Pathol 56:514, 1971)

particularly susceptible to staphylococcal disease. Neonatal streptococcal illness, especially to group B organisms, has also been well described. The presence of pertussis antibody in neonatal serum is variable.

Even in the presence of demonstrable antibody titer, pertussis may occur in the neonatal period.

Antibodies that traverse the placenta decline at a variable rate; however, since most of them are of the IgG class, the average half-life is 25 to 28 days.

The response of the newborn infant to immunizations is variable and affected by such factors as route of administration, dosage, timing, gestational or postnatal age and birth weight. The degree of pre-existing antibody (of maternal origin) may both influence these results and explain the generally poor neonatal response to pertussis (50) and poliomyelitis vaccine (21, 48). That other factors are operative is suggested in one study (47) by the immunoparalysis noted during the first 24 hours of life in response to pertussis antigen, even though passively transmitted antibodies were absent or present in low titer.

Poor antibody response to certain infections (ECHO 9, 18 and adenoviruses 1, 2 and 8) have been reported (32). This is in contrast to the marked response noted with other viral infections.

IgA (hemagglutinating) antibodies to ECHO virus and neutralizing antibody against poliovirus are found in newborn infants who are breast fed (21). These antibodies have greater resistance to gastric acidity than do serum antibodies and persist for two to three months after birth. In contrast, only traces of coproantibody (poliovirus neutralizing antibody) are found in the stools of bottle-fed newborn infants. Although there is ten times as much IgA in cow's as in human milk, there is little antiviral or bactericidal antibody. The protective effect of these two milks may be approximately the same.

The antibody content of colostrum is of significant value only during the first few days postpartum. This interval, however, may be sufficient for protection of the infant by preventing penetration of the gut wall by gram-negative bacteria until the lamina propria begins to synthesize IgA. Human colostrum is protective against O-111, O-55 and other serotypes of E. coli.

Blocking Antibodies

"Blocking antibodies" of maternal origin, perhaps representing desensitization, are found in the newborn infant. Since they are of the IgG class, they are passively transferred across the placenta. In contrast reaginic or atopic antibody (IgA and IgE) are not transferred even when present in high titer in the mother.

Since IgE is rarely present in newborn infants, they do not give a positive skin reaction with anti-IgE antigen. In spite of this, newborn infants, including those born prematurely, react with passively transferred adult reaginic antibody in a Prausnitz-Küstner test. A competent immediate hypersensitivity mechanism exists at birth, but there is insufficient skin-fixed IgE to react with anti-IgE antigen.

The postnatal development of immunoglobulins varies according to the class. For IgG there is a decline over a two to three-month period, leading to a transient state of "physiologic hypogammaglobulinemia." Among premature infants who begin extrauterine life with low IgG concentrations, extremely low levels may be observed at age two to six months; whether this is of clinical significance in predisposing to infection is unknown. Concentrations of IgA rise gradually following birth and may not reach adult levels until the tenth birthday. Adult levels of IgM on the other hand may be attained by age two (25).

Delayed Hypersensitivity

The synthesis of secretory IgA begins about the ninth or tenth day and reaches adult levels by the ninth week. Levels of secretory and serum IgA are not correlated.

At birth there is evidence of partially developed delayed hypersensitivity (26). Although data are limited, it appears that skin grafts are rejected more slowly in the neonatal period than in later life. Skin testing for Rhus, milk and egg protein hypersensitivity during the first week of life is positive. At a high dosage the response to 2,4-dinitrofluorobenzene (2,4-DNFB) is excellent in experimental animals (54). Hypersensitivity to drugs as well as to streptococcal nucleoprotein and salmonella antigens are rare. By age two to three weeks, fullterm infants respond to immunization with Bacille de Calmette-Guérin (BCG) vaccine, developing a positive tuberculin test within two to ten weeks (39). A slightly depressed reaction is noted among premature infants.

Inflammatory Response

The inflammatory response of the neonate is beset by two problems. The first of these is the delayed transition from the initial outpouring of PMNs to a predominance of mononuclear cells; the other is the relative excess of eosinophilic neutrophils in the initial response (29).

Circulating PMNs are more numerous in newborn infants than in older infants, children, or adults. The mean concentration at birth is about $18,000/mm^3$, with a normal range of about 9,000 to 30,000. By one week the mean is about $12,000 \ mm^3$, with a range of about 5,000 to 21,000. There is increased enzymatic activity within these cells, as shown by degradation of nitroblue tetrazolium to formazan (46).

A deficiency of phagocytosis in the newborn infant has been demonstrated by in vitro studies of engulfment of carbon particles and *E. coli* in premature infants (40); this phagocytic deficiency also extends to *S. aureus* and *S. marcescens*. The opsonic capacity of neonatal serum is deficient, related in part to low levels of complement (31, 37). The deficiency may be corrected by addition of complement and IgM maternal serum fractions for *E. coli* (31). Suspension of the newborn infant's leukocytes in adult serum produces a similar result, followed by normal opsonization and phagocytosis.

Newborn infants also have an impaired ability to detoxify large quantities of endotoxin.

Nonspecific Mechanisms

Nonspecific protective mechanisms against infection have been less frequently studied. However, there is evidence that the cough, gag and other reflexes and ciliary movements that are of major importance in the prevention of respiratory tract infections in older children and adults are poorly developed in newborn infants (Fig. 18–4). Asphyxia further impairs these protective mechanisms.

The very thin and easily penetrated skin of premature infants may also be a predisposing factor in neonatal infection. Disruption of the skin, as in the healing umbilical wound or soft tissue injury after an instrument delivery or following circumcision, provides another potential route of infection.

The placenta itself with several layers intervening between mother and fetus may be considered to be a nonspecific but important part of the fetal defense mechanism. As term approaches, the placenta "thins out," facilitating placental penetration by pathogenic microorganisms.

REFERENCES

PERINATAL INFECTION

1. Alford CA, Schaefer J, Blankenship WJ, Straumfjord JV, Cassady G: A correlative immunologic, microbiologic and clinical approach to the diagnosis of acute and chronic infections in newborn infants. N Engl J Med 277:437, 1967

2. American Journal of Diseases of Children: Water bugs in the bassinet. Editorial 101:273, 1961

3. Bassett DCJ, Thompson SAS, Page B: Neonatal infections with Pseudomonas aeruginosa associated with contaminated resuscitation equipment. Lancet 1:78, 1965

4. Beargie R, Armstrong S, Weddle R: Pus cells containing bacteria in stomachs of newborns, abstract. Clin Res 20:108, 1972

5. Bernischke K: Routes and types of infection in the fetus and newborn. Am J Dis Child 99:714, 1960

6. Bernischke K, Clifford SH: Intrauterine bacterial infection in the newborn infant. Frozen sections of the cord as an aid in every detection. J Pediatr 54:11, 1959

7. Blanc WA: Amniotic infection syndrome. Pathogenesis, morphology, and significance in circumnatal mortality. Clin Obstet Gynecol 2:705, 1959

8. Blanc WA: Pathways of fetal and early neonatal infection. Viral placentitis, bacterial and fungal chorioamnionitis. J Pediatr 59:473, 1961

9. Blankenship WJ, Cassady G, Schaefer J, Straumfjord J, Alford CA Jr: Serum gamma-M globulin responses in acute neonatal infections and their diagnostic significance. J Pediatr 75:1271, 1969

10. Eichenwald HF, Shinefield HR: Viral infections of the fetus and of the premature and newborn infant. Adv Pediatr 8:249, 1962

11. Evans HE, Glass L, Mercado C: The microerythrocyte sedimentation rate in newborn infants. J Pediatr 76:448, 1970

12. Felix NS, Nakajima H, Kagan BM: Serum C-reactive protein in infections during the first six months of life. Pediatrics 37:270, 1966

13. Fierer J, Taylor PM, Gezon HM: Pseudomonas aeruginosa epidemic traced to delivery room resuscitators. N Engl J Med 276:991, 1967

14. Florman AL, Teubner D: Enhancement of bacterial growth in amniotic fluid by meconium. J Pediatr 74:111, 1969

15. McCracken GH, Hardy JB, Chen TC, Hoffman LS, Gilkeson MR, Sever JL: Serum immunoglobulin levels in newborn infants. Survey of cord and follow-up sera from 123 infants with congenital rubella. J Pediatr 24:383, 1969

16. Naeye RL, Blanc WA: Relation of poverty and race to antenatal infection. New Engl J Med 283:555, 1970

17. Overbach AM, Daniel SJ, Cassady G: The role of umbilical cord histology in the management of potential perinatal infection. J Pediatr 76:22, 1970

18. Ramos A, Stern L: Relationship of premature rupture of the membrane to gastric fluid aspirate in the newborn. Am J Obstet Gynecol 105:1247, 1969

19. Sever JL: Possible role of humidifying equipment in spread of infections from the newborn nursery. Pediatrics 24:50, 1959

20. Stiehm ER, Ammann AJ, Cherry JD: Elevated cord macroglobulins in the diagnosis of intrauterine infections. N Engl J Med 275:971, 1966

PERINATAL IMMUNOLOGY

21. Adcock E, Green H: Poliovirus antibodies in breast-fed infants. Lancet 2:662, 1971

22. Adinolfi M: Levels of two components of complement (C'4 and C'3) in human fetal and newborn sera. Dev Med Child Neural 12:306, 1970

23. Alford CA, Polt SS, Cassady GE, Straumfjord SV, Remington JS: Gamma M fluorescent treponemal antibody in the diagnosis of congenital syphilis. N Engl J Med 280:1086, 1969

24. Alford CA, Schaefer J, Blankenship WJ, Straumfjord JV, Cassady G: A correlative immunologic, microbiologic and clinical approach to the diagnosis of acute and chronic infections in newborn infants. N Engl J Med 277:437, 1967

25. Allansmith M, McClellan BH, Butterworth G, Maloney JR: The development of immunoglobulin levels in man. J Pediatr 72:276, 1968

26. August CS, Berkel AI, Driscoll S, Merler E: Onset of lymphocyte function in the developing human fetus. Pediatr Res 5:539, 1971

27. Brasher AW, Hartley TF: Quantitation of IgA and IgM in umbilical cord serum of normal newborn infants. J Pediatr 74:784, 1969

28. Bridges RA, Condie RM, Zak SJ, Good RA: The morphological basis of antibody formation, development during the neonatal period. J Lab Clin Med 53:331, 1959

29. Bullock JD, Robertson AF, Bodenbender JG, Kontras SB, Miller CE: Inflammatory response in the neonate re-examined. Pediatrics 44:58, 1969

30. Cohen SM, Ducharme CP, Carpenter CA, Deibel R: Rubella antibody in IgG and IgM immunoglobulins detected by immunofluorescence. J Lab Clin Med 72:760, 1968

31. Davis AT, Blum PM, Quie PG: Studies on opsonic activity for E coli in premature infants after blood transfusion. Program and Abstracts, Atlantic City, Soc Ped Res, 1971, p 233

32. Eichenwald HF, Kossevalov O: Immunologic responses of premature and full term infants to infection with certain viruses. Pediatrics 25:829, 1960

33. Eichenwald HF, Shinefield HR: Antibody production by human fetus. J Pediatr 63:870, 1963

34. Evans HE, Millian SJ, Glass L: Antibody titers to measles, rubella, and poliomyelitis in umbilical cord serum. Obstet Gynecol 42:596, 1973

35. Evans HE, Akpaka SO, Glass L: Serum immunoglobulin levels in premature and full-term infants. Am J Clin Pathol 56:416, 1971

36. Fireman P, Zuchowski DA, Taylor PM: Development of human complement system. J Immunol 103:25, 1969

37. Forman ML, Stiehm ER: Impaired opsonic activity but normal phagocytosis in low-birth-weight infants. N Engl J Med 281:926, 1969

38. Fulginiti VA, Sieber OF, Claman HN, Merrill DA: Serum immunoglobulin measurement during the first year of life and in immunoglobulin deficiency states. J Pediatr 68:723, 1966

39. Gainsford W, Griffiths MS: BCG vaccination in the newborn: Preliminary report. Br Med J 2:702, 1951

40. Cluck L, Silverman WA: Phagocytosis in premature infants. Pediatrics 20:951, 1957

41. Haworth JC, Dilling L: Concentration of IgA

globulin in serum, saliva and nasopharyngeal secretions of infants and children. J Lab Clin Med 67:922, 1966

42. Keller R, Dwyer JE, Oh W, D'Amodio M: Intestinal IgA neutralizing antibodies in new-born infants following poliovirus immunization. Pediatrics 43:330, 1969

43. McCracken GH Jr, Chen TC, Hardy JB, Tzan N: Serum immunoglobulin levels in newborn infants. I. Evaluation of a radial diffusion plate method. J Pediatr 74:378, 1969

44. Makela O, Lapinleimu K, Kostianen E: Timing of different virus neutralising 19S and 7S antibody in natural Coxsackie infections of newborn babies and adluts. Clin Exp Immunol 3:269, 1968

45. Papadatos C, Papavengelou GL, Alexio D, Mendris J: Serum immunoglobulin G levels in small-for-dates newborn babies. Arch Dis Child 45:570, 1970

46. Park BH, Holmes B, Good RA: Metabolic activities in leukocytes of newborn infants. J Pediatr 76:237, 1970

47. Provenzano RW, Wetterlow LH, Sullivan CL: Immunization and antibody response in the newborn infant. I. Pertussis inoculation within 24 hours of birth. N Engl J Med 273:959, 1965

48. Rannon L, Goldblum N, Skalska P, Gotlieb A: Antibody response of newborns to formalinised poliomyelitis vaccine (Salk type). Am J Hygiene 72:244, 1960

49. Sabin AB, Feldman HA: Persistence of placentally transmitted antibodies in normal children in relation to diagnosis of congenital toxoplasmosis. Pediatrics 4:660, 1949

50. Sako W: Studies on pertussis immunization. J Pediatr 30:29, 1947

51. Smith RT, Eitzman DV, Catlin ME, Wirtz EO, Miller BE: The development of the immune response, characterization of the response of human infant and adult to immunization with salmonella vaccines. Pediatrics 33:163, 1964

52. Stiehm ER, Fuldenberg HH: Serum levels of immune globulins in health and disease. Pediatrics 37:715, 1966

53. Toivanen P, Rossi T, Hirvonen T: Immunoglobulins in human fetal sera at different stages of gestation. Experientia 24:527, 1969

54. Uhr JW: Development of delayed-type hypersensitivity in guinea pig embryos. Nature 187:957, 1960

55. Uhr JW, Dancis J, Franklin EC, Finkelstein MS, Lewis EW: The antibody response to bacteriophase ΦX174 in newborn premature infants. J Clin Invest 41:1509, 1962

56. Yeung CY, Hobbes JR: Serum γG-globulin levels in normal, premature, postmature and 'small-for-dates' newborn babies. Lancet 1:1167, 1968

19

Bacterial Infection

BACTERIAL MENINGITIS AND SEPSIS

Bacterial meningitis usually occurs secondary to sepsis in the newborn infant; consequently both entities will be considered together. Pathogenesis is discussed in Chapter 18, Mechanisms of Infection, and the highlights of the history, physical examination and laboratory investigation in the first section of that chapter, Perinatal Infection. Meningitis occurs in roughly 1.5:1000 live births among premature infants and about one-third as frequently among full-term births. The frequency of sepsis varies from 1:1000 to 5:1000 live births (9).

The initial exposure to the infectious agent may occur either prepartum or postpartum. Prolonged rupture of membranes, amnionitis and unexplained fever in the mother may predispose the infant to sepsis and meningitis (7, 9). Postnatally, a wide variety of factors may lead to these conditions, especially among debilitated and premature infants. Breaks in the skin secondary to venipuncture, IM injections or even tape; contaminated incubator water reservoirs, soap dispensers and pieces of resuscitative equipment (8); inadequately scrubbed hands of physicians, nurses and technicians; illness among nursery personnel; and spread of disease from other infants are some of the factors that predispose newborn infants to serious bacterial infection.

In infants with congenital anomalies of the· CNS, such as myelomeningocele, risk of meningitis is especially high. Even such seemingly minor anomalies as a pilonidal fistula communicating with the spinal canal may predispose to meningitis.

Host defense mechanisms may be defective, especially among premature infants, but other special problems exist in regard to the pathogenesis of meningitis. The relative ease of penetration of the blood-brain barrier by bacteria has been presumed to be one factor predisposing the newborn infant to meningitis. However, direct proof of this is lacking. In the same manner, the GI tract mucosal barrier may also be penetrated with relative ease, leading to sepsis and meningitis caused by both normal and abnormal bacterial flora. The latter may result from antibiotic therapy leading to suppression of *E. coli* or other organisms with resultant overgrowth of fungi or pseudomonas.

The most common bacteria responsible for meningitis in the neonate are *E. coli* and other coliform bacilli, which comprise about two-thirds of all cases of neonatal sepsis and meningitis.* Pseudomonas, *S. aureus*, enterococci, Listeria, Achromobacter and virtually any gram-negative bacillus must be regarded as a potential causative agent. In a previous era when puerperal sepsis was common, β-hemolytic streptococcal infection was common in the newborn infant. A recrudescence of neonatal sepsis and meningitis due to group B streptococci has been widely encountered in the late 1960s and 1970s.

Salmonella may either cause local GI disease in the infant or be responsible for sepsis and meningitis. Among this group the most important serotypes are *S. paratyphi* B, *S. enteritidis*, *S. typhimurium*, *S. panama*

* See Appendix A, Addendum 5.

and *S. habana*, which account for 80% of the cases of meningitis. Others that may be important are *S. newport*, *S. thompson*, *S. heidelberg*, *S. infantis*, *S. saintpaul* and *S. blockley*.

Vibrios are thin gram-negative flagellated rods that are very mobile and appear to vibrate. They grow best under anaerobic conditions, ferment lactose slowly and may be morphologically confused with coliform organisms. Antigens of the O type determine two major types, and antisera may be used for agglutination and identification.

CLINICAL COURSE

The illness may fulminate, with death following the apparent onset of signs by only a few hours, or the course may be prolonged for two weeks or longer. Typically the newborn infant exhibits subtle signs, especially "poor feeding" as reported by an experienced nurse or a multiparous mother. Such complaints are relatively common in the nursery, but the clinician is well advised to heed them. A detailed review of the perinatal history plus a careful examination of the infant is indicated.

Virtually any sign of illness in newborn infants may be associated with sepsis and meningitis, including jaundice, apnea, hypoglycemia, neuromuscular irritability, lethargy, diarrhea and vomiting, poor cry and suck, loss of the Moro reflex, petechiae, purpura and bleeding, sclerema, convulsions, poor feeding and hepatosplenomegaly—all arouse the suspicion of generalized infection but yet may be associated with numerous other conditions (9, 10). The clinician is then on the horns of a dilemma. If he seriously considers sepsis and meningitis, he is obliged to subject the infant to a lengthy, expensive and often technically difficult evaluation. At the conclusion he may still be unable to localize the site of infection, much less identify a causative organism, even provisionally. If he overlooks the possibility of sepsis, the patient's life is imperiled and even if he survives, sequelae such as mental retardation may ensue. Most clinicians prefer to err on the side of "overdiagnosis" and

will evaluate a newborn infant for sepsis and meningitis even when evidence is relatively sparse. This seems to be justified in view of the nonspecificity of findings. To complicate matters, sepsis and meningitis may exist in a newborn infant in the absence of even the vaguest signs.

LABORATORY DIAGNOSIS

The diagnostic evaluation for neonatal infection is discussed in Chapter 18, in the section Perinatal Infection. In establishing a bacteriologic diagnosis, care must be taken not only in obtaining specimens of blood and CSF, but also in processing them properly and in interpreting results.

Ideally, blood cultures should be drawn from a peripheral vein following careful preparation of the skin with an iodine compound. Use of the femoral vessels for obtaining a specimen for blood culture is to be condemned because of the potential danger of septic arthritis of the hip joint associated with the procedure. No more than 1 ml of blood should be withdrawn, with a ratio of blood to culture medium, e.g., trypticase soy broth, of 1:10. A single positive blood culture may represent only bacteremia without sepsis (1) or skin contamination. However, even this single observation cannot be disregarded, and the clinician may be justified in making a diagnosis of sepsis if the patient's condition warrants (4). If an organism such as *S. epidermidis* is recovered, the probability of contamination is likely. Other bacteria, e.g., *E. coli* and enterococci, are more likely to be true pathogens. Two or more blood cultures from which the same organism is isolated are almost always confirmatory of a diagnosis of sepsis.

Because of the plethora of information that can be extracted from a complete examination of CSF, every attempt must be made to perform an atraumatic lumbar puncture. Success in this procedure depends mainly on correctly positioning the infant and using a proper needle. The procedure is best done under a radiant heater, especially for a low-birth-weight infant. Although we have had optimum results with the infant in the lateral decubitus position, other clinicians prefer the sitting position. Since the distance between skin and dura is very short, a 1-in. No. 23 spinal needle should be used.

Macroscopic examination of the CSF may yield valuable information. A xanthochromic color is present in about 50% of cases, representing hemolyzed erythrocytes (the presence of which is secondary to the normal trauma of delivery). A turbid or cloudy fluid may represent the pleocytosis of meningitis; frankly bloody fluid may represent either subarachnoid bleeding or a traumatic tap. If the latter, the fluid tends to clear as it is collected in three test tubes.

The fluid may be permitted to drop directly on the surface of culture medium plates, thus avoiding the risk of contamination and expediting the processing. In addition a second blood agar plate may be streaked and antibiotic sensitivity discs added immediately. Should growth occur, a preliminary assessment of antibiotic sensitivity is available in 16 to 24 hours. If the fluid has not been immediately plated in this manner, no more than 15 minutes should elapse before it is streaked on culture medium. A useful combination is blood, chocolate agar and eosin-methylene blue (EMB) plates.

A microscopic examination should also be performed immediately. The presence of 30 or more white blood cells per cubic millimeter (in a blood-free specimen) usually indicates meningitis. These cells, predominantly PMNs, may be as high as 10,000/mm³. The fluid should be centrifuged, and a Gram stain performed on a smear of the sediment. If bacteria are present in the fluid, the procedure provides an accurate clue as to what antibiotic preparation to try first.

The glucose concentration of the fluid should be measured concurrently with a blood glucose determination. Under normal conditions the CSF glucose concentration is about two-thirds that of the blood; a significant decrease in this ratio is usually associated with bacterial meningitis.

The protein concentration of the CSF of a newborn infant may normally be as high as 200 mg/ml. Therefore a value that would be regarded as markedly elevated for an older infant or child may be normal for a newborn infant.

THERAPY

Following the diagnostic tests but prior to availability of results, both general and specific therapy should be initiated. The infant should not be fed orally; instead, an IV infusion should be started. A thermoneutral environment should be maintained with careful monitoring of the infant's temperature. The state of hydration must be carefully followed, and frequent measurements must be made of acid-base and electrolyte status. Oxygen should be used as indicated. If there is evidence of seizure activity, phenobarbital therapy should be started. In recalcitrant cases, agents such as diazepam (Valium) may be required to overcome seizures. Jaundice should be carefully evaluated and treated.

Antibiotic therapy should be started pending the identification of specific microorganisms. A combination of kanamycin, 15 mg/kg/day in two divided IM doses, and ampicillin, 150 to 200 mg/kg/day given intravenously, provides the widest antimicrobial spectrum against bacteria that are commonly responsible for neonatal sepsis and meningitis. There is some indication, however, that a dose of 20 mg/kg/day of kanamycin may be necessary to provide adequate therapeutic blood levels (5a). Therapy is continued for at least one week and usually longer, depending on the infant's clinical and bacteriologic response. If the isolated organism is identified as *E. coli* or a related member of the enterobacteriaceae family (which is true in 70% to 80% of cases of neonatal sepsis and meningitis), this antibiotic regimen can usually be continued. If a pseudomonas is isolated, gentamicin or carbenicillin is the primary drug of choice. For *S. aureus*, one of the semisynthetic penicillins such as oxacillin (150 mg/kg/day) is the primary antibiotic used. The final choice of antibiotic preparations, however, should be based on both in vitro sensitivities of the offending organism and the clinical response of the patient.

OTITIS MEDIA

Although otitis media has long been known to affect both premature and full-term infants, its clinical diagnosis is relatively uncommon. It has been encountered rather frequently at postmortem examination, often associated with sepsis, meningitis and gastroenteritis (15, 17). In the preantibiotic era, most of these infections were caused by gram-positive organisms, but in recent years such gram-negative organisms as *E. coli, P. aeruginosa* and klebsiella have been implicated (12, 13, 16). This distribution of etiologic agents reflects the general trend observed in neonatal sepsis.

Ordinarily otitis media is not diagnosed in the neonatal period for several reasons. First, careful examination of tympanic membranes often is not performed by house officers or other physicians assigned to the nursery. Visualization of the tympanic membrane may be difficult because of plugging of the external auditory canal with debris consisting of vernix and meconium. The canal is small and the tympanic membrane is in a relatively horizontal position when compared to their size and orientation in an older child or adult. When visualized, landmarks may be difficult to interpret because of dullness, erythema and thickening. A pneumatic otoscope may demonstrate poor mobility of the membrane, providing an additional diagnostic clue (14).

CHARACTERISTICS

The incidence of otitis media is higher in premature than in full-term infants, with about one-third of all cases occurring in the former group (12). As with other types of neonatal infection, there is a preponderance among male progeny. Bottle-fed infants are more prone to this illness than those who are breast fed, possibly because of the protection conferred by secretory IgA in breast milk (11). Hypothermia rather than fever may be a presenting sign, especially in premature infants. Onset occurs most frequently during the winter months.

Nonspecific findings such as diarrhea, vomiting and anorexia may be the only signs of illness. Rhinorrhea, the most frequent finding, occurs in as many as 71% of cases and irritability in 48% (12). The WBC is rarely of diagnostic value.

Tympanocentesis yields bacteria in up to 86% of cases. Organisms recovered with relative frequency are *E. coli, S. aureus, K. pneumoniae, H. influenzae, P. aeruginosa* and *Proteus* species; *D. pneumoniae* and *S. viridans* also have been recovered. The Gram stain of ear aspirates may be of value in the initial selection of antibiotic agents (12).

MANAGEMENT

As in other bacterial infections, antibiotic selection should be based on the in vitro antimicrobial sensitivity of the offending organism. Ampicillin alone is effective in approximately 60% of all cases, but *P. aeruginosa, Klebsiella, S. aureus* and *Proteus* organisms often show resistance to this agent. About 83% of bacterial isolates are reported to be sensitive to a combination of kanamycin and ampicillin (12).

Poor response to treatment is more common in neonatal otitis media than in the disease seen in older age groups. Some of these failures represent superinfection with a resistant organism.

Treatment should be initiated by IM administration of kanamycin, 15 to 20 mg/kg/day in two divided doses, and ampicillin, 150 to 200 mg/kg/day, preferably administered by the IV route. Oral administration of ampicillin in the newborn infant usually is unreliable. Continuation of therapy should be based on cultural evidence, especially if an organism is isolated from middle ear exudate, blood or CSF. If no definitive organism is isolated, ampicillin and kanamycin should be continued for ten days. Even with this regimen, there is a failure rate of over 20%. When such potentially nephrotoxic drugs as kanamycin and gentamycin are used, the urine should be examined frequently for casts, red blood cells and protein. In some patients who have organisms resistant to systemic antibiotic therapy, corticosteroid-containing eardrops have been helpful, provided the tympano-centesis site remained open (12).

INFECTIOUS DIARRHEA

Viral, fungal and bacterial infections of the GI tract may cause diarrhea in the newborn infant. Diarrhea also may be a nonspecific manifestation of any infection ranging from sepsis to otitis media; it frequently has a noninfectious etiology.

Bacterial agents capable of causing neonatal diarrhea include *E. coli*, salmonella, *Pseudomonas sp.*, *Klebsiella sp.*, enterobacteriaceae, *P. morganii*, *S. aureus*, Group B β-hemolytic streptococci and paracolon bacilli.

A fungal agent that causes diarrhea is *C. albicans*, and agents of viral etiology include ECHO, coxsackievirus and adenovirus.

ETIOLOGY

There are no characteristics of the stool specimen that permit an exact etiologic diagnosis. Two or more stool specimens should be obtained for bacteriologic, and when feasible virologic, study. Fluorescent antibody (FA) study for enteropathogenic *E. coli* provides a rapid screening test (29), but culture is needed for definitive diagnosis and for antibiotic sensitivity testing. Because of antigenic overlap, the precise interpretation of the results of FA testing is often difficult. When suspicion of generalized infection arises, two or more blood cultures should be taken, and the same evaluation utilized as in the approach to sepsis (lumbar puncture, complete blood count, ESR, urinanalysis and cultures) may be required.

When several infants develop diarrhea simultaneously, isolation of the causative organism and identification of a carrier or contaminant are mandatory. The hands of

nursing and medical staff, soap dispensers, water reservoirs of incubators and milk formulas should all be tested for the presence of pathogenic bacteria.

COMPLICATIONS

In severe infectious diarrhea, complications may include shock, major electrolyte and acid-base disturbances, bacteremia, pneumonia, peritonitis and encephalopathy. Renal vein thrombosis with enlargement of one or both kidneys, shock and hematuria may also occur. Cortical vein thrombosis with resulting seizures, coma and paresis may occur secondary to severe dehydration. Perianal excoriation, anal prolapse, intussusception, abdominal distention and sclerema are possible complications.

The postpartum incidence and severity of infectious diarrhea has been reduced markedly in recent years in the United States. This may reflect improvements in infant formula preparation and nursing techniques. Unknown factors may also have been contributory.

Enteropathogenic E. coli

The most common bacterial agents responsible for neonatal diarrhea are the enteropathogenic *E. coli* (19, 21, 22). The incubation period for the illness is usually 2 to 12 days but may be less than 1 day. Only about 10 of the 145 or more serogroups of this organism are of etiologic significance in the production of diarrhea among neonates.

Two pathogenic mechanisms are postulated, based on studies in animals and adult volunteers. The organism may penetrate the intestinal wall, especially the colon, giving rise to a dysentery-like profile of blood, mucus and inflammatory cells in the stool (22, 30). In some cases an enterotoxin is elaborated, with diarrhea occurring after an average incubation of 26 hours, compared with only 11 hours in the invasive form.

Multiplication of the organism occurs in the jejunum and ileum as well as in the stool. There are usually no systemic manifestations of the disease. A far greater number of organisms is required to cause illness in older children and adults than in small infants.

The bacteria contains two types of antigens (1): 1) the O type is attached to the body of the cell and known as the somatic antigen and 2) the H type attached to the flagella and known as the flagellar antigen.

Diarrhea due to *E. coli* is more common in industrialized than in rural or primitive countries because of the decrease in breast feeding and the increase in hospital-delivered infants in the former countries (26, 27). Colostrum and breast milk contain antibodies to *E. coli* (24) and may play a protective role against the development of this illness. It is encountered more frequently in tropical than nontropical countries, but climate per se is not a major causative factor.

Type A and B organisms both are capable of causing disease, with type B serotypes usually encountered with greater frequency. While about ten serotypes have been associated with clinical disease, the one most often encountered is 0111:B4 (25).

Clinical features include lethargy, anorexia and weight loss, which may be significant and precede the diarrhea. Before the passage of watery stools, clinical symptoms may closely resemble those of sepsis and meningitis. Among premature and other debilitated infants, the mortality rate may be significant (23, 30).

With the occurrence of diarrhea in a neonatal nursery, the possibility of this organism being the etiologic agent must be rapidly proved or excluded. Screening tests using the FA technique in both symptomatic and asymptomatic infants may be valuable (29). The presence of large numbers of organisms in the stool will suggest the diagnosis, so that specific measures may be taken both to treat the affected infant and prevent a widespread epidemic.

Affected infants should be isolated, with nursing staff assigned to no other duties. Disposable gloves should be used when handling the infants.

Specific antimicrobial therapy should be started immediately. The drugs of choice are

neomycin, 50 to 100 mg/kg/day, or colistin 3.5 to 5.0 mg/kg/day in four divided doses administered orally. The latter agent is preferred if drug sensitivities are not available when treatment is begun since neomycin-resistant strains are more frequently encountered than those resistant to colistin. Another effective antibiotic is gentamicin, administered orally in the dose of 5 to 20 mg/kg/day. The duration of antibiotic therapy is about one week and is discontinued after three stool cultures on consecutive days are negative. Correction of fluid, electrolyte and acid-base disturbances are also required.

Shigella

Shigella enteritis is relatively uncommon among newborn infants. In part, this may be due to difficulty in isolation of the organism because of inefficient media. However, the introduction of Hoentgen-Enteric agar and other special media may increase the frequency of isolation. Nursery outbreaks with fatalities have been described (28). The fecal–oral route is the principal mode of transmission, with relatively few organisms required. The clinical picture is nonspecific with diarrhea beginning on the second or third day after exposure.

Together with nonspecific treatment, the antibiotic of choice is ampicillin, 150 to 200 mg/kg/day given intravenously. Antibiotic therapy must, however, be based both on in vitro sensitivity of the organism and clinical response of the infant. Once the diarrhea has subsided, the antibiotic may be administered orally.

Salmonella

Salmonellosis is a more frequently observed cause of neonatal diarrhea than is shigellosis (20). This may partly be due to the ready growth of salmonella organisms on culture medium. It is also more likely to invade the bloodstream (rare in shigella). Specific treatment is kanamycin, 15 to 20 mg/kg/day in two divided doses, or ampicillin, 150 to 200 mg/day by the IV route. This should be used even if the infection is localized to the GI tract. Antimicrobial therapy should be continued for 10 to 14 days. As in diarrhea caused by enteropathogenic *E. coli*, strict isolation techniques must be observed for diarrhea caused by shigella or salmonella.

Salmonella have numerous reservoirs and may be a contaminant of food products.

Pseudomonas

Pseudomonal diarrhea may be seen in conjunction with sepsis, meningitis, ulcerative dermatitis, granulocytopenia and thrombocytopenia. Intestinal infection may be complicated by perforation resulting in peritonitis, sepsis and death. Gentamicin (3 mg/kg/day) administered in two divided IM doses is the antibiotic agent of choice. Carbenicillin, in an IV dose range of 300 to 400 mg/kg/day has also been effective.

As with all potential pathogens, this organism may be carried asymptomatically. Incubator reservoirs and aerosols are usually the source of this pseudomonas, but the feces of carriers are also an important reservoir of infection.

Other Organisms

S. aureus, Klebsiella pneumonia, paracolon bacilli, vibrios and *Proteus* are other bacteria that can cause diarrhea in the newborn infant (21). Candidiasis of the GI tract, associated with oral candidiasis may also be a cause. Various enteric viruses (e.g., ECHO, coxsackievirus, adenoviruses) are also responsible for diarrhea in the newborn infant (31).

OSTEOMYELITIS

Although osteomyelitis is diagnosed with relative infrequency among newborn infants, it is nevertheless of clinical importance. The prompt diagnosis and treatment of this disorder may prevent death or serious disability. A possible reason for the infrequency of the diagnosis of this disease is that signs are often atypical in the newborn

infant, and many cases may not be identified.

ETIOLOGY

Osteomyelitis may occur as a complication of sepsis (34, 35). It may also follow such localized infections as paronychia, pyoderma or breast abscess. Femoral puncture, with introduction of bacteria into the hip joint, may lead to this condition (32). Trauma to the skin and subcutaneous tissues, as in the case of an IV infusion that has infiltrated, may result in osteomyelitis.

The most frequently encountered organism is *S. aureus*, but gram-negative organisms, such as proteus (36, 38), klebsiella (33) and pseudomonas may be etiologic agents. Streptococci, which were much more frequently encountered in the preantibiotic era than they are today, may also cause neonatal osteomyelitis. The increased prevalence of this organism noted in the late 1960s and early 1970s, has not been specifically associated with osteomyelitis.

As in later life, the principal areas involved are the ends of long bones, most often the proximal end of the femurs. Hip, knee and shoulder joints may all be involved. Bones of the skull may also be affected, especially after localized infection (37). In any single patient, multiple bone lesions may appear, often associated with soft tissue or visceral involvement.

CLINICAL MANIFESTATIONS

Swelling over the involved bony site is the most important sign of infection. Tenderness is usually difficult to evaluate in the newborn infant, and erythema may be absent. Occasionally obvious abscess formation is present. Beyond this, there is a wide variation in the clinical picture. Systemic signs may be minimal; the infant may eat well, gain weight and remain afebrile even in the presence of a positive blood culture. At the other extreme, a typical picture of neonatal sepsis may rapidly emerge, with either hypothermia or fever, anorexia, vomiting, diarrhea and lethargy as prominent findings. Untreated, the disease may be relatively mild, and bone healing may occur with involucrum formation; however, permanent and severe deformities, especially of the hip joint, may be noted if the infant survives without therapy. In contrast, a virulent course of generalized sepsis, dehydration, acidosis and death may ensue if the condition remains undiagnosed and untreated.

DIAGNOSTIC STUDIES

X-ray examination of the involved area may help to distinguish soft tissue involvement from osteomyelitis. However, early in the course of the disorder bony involvement may not be noted on x ray. Even in the presence of a positive x ray, it is virtually impossible to differentiate between relatively benign lesions and those with a virulent course.

Two or more blood cultures should be obtained from veins not immediately adjacent to the soft tissue lesion. However, if the infant appears ill enough to warrant immediate antimicrobial therapy, one culture must suffice. Superficial cultures of the nares, throat, umbilicus, breasts and any cutaneous lesions should be obtained since they may reveal the causative organism.

A total and differential WBC count should be performed, although this may be normal in the presence of osteomyelitis. However, an elevated micro-ESR may give a clue as to the seriousness of the illness.

TREATMENT

Antibiotic therapy should be based both on sensitivity studies of the offending organism and on clinical response of the patient. In the presence of *S. aureus*, a semisynthetic penicillin such as methicillin is the drug of choice. Therapy should be continued for at least four weeks, with at least two weeks of this being by the IV route.

In addition to antibiotics, drainage of purulent material is essential. Immobilization of the affected extremity must also be attempted.

As with any other serious infectious disease in the newborn infant, supportive therapy must include the maintenance of fluid, acid-base and electrolyte balance and the provision of temperature control and optimal oxygenation.

URINARY TRACT INFECTION

Urinary tract infection in the newborn infant is associated to a variable extent with either bacteremia or congenital anomalies. It may also occur as an isolated problem. It is more frequently observed in premature than in full-term infants and may or may not be accompanied by signs of illness.

The frequency of bacteriuria in surveys of asymptomatic newborn infants has been reported to range from 0.1% to 25% (39, 41, 42, 46, 48), depending on the methods of collection. Edelmann et al (40) have found bacteriuria to be present in 0.7% of full-term and 2.9% of premature infants, with the majority being asymptomatic. With suprapubic puncture, the prevalence rates are very low, usually well under 1%. In contrast, collections of voided urine yield high rates of significant bacterial colonization. This latter finding is apparently due to contamination of the specimen.

There is no sex-related difference in the prevalence of urinary tract infection in newborn infants despite the marked predilection for females at all other ages. This difference may be attributed to the relative importance of hematogenous dissemination among neonates compared with the ascending route of infection that is more common beyond the neonatal period.

The most common offending organism by far is *E. coli*. However, other gram-negative bacilli frequently responsible for neonatal sepsis and meningitis also cause urinary tract infection, e.g., klebsiella, enterobacter and paracolon bacillus. In cases where congenital urinary tract anomalies are present, more than one pathogen, including *S. aureus* may be recovered. In a similar manner, the presence of less commonly encountered gram-negative bacilli, such as pseudomonas or *P. mirabilis*, suggests the presence of a congenital anomaly.

CLINICAL MANIFESTATIONS

While signs are frequently absent in infants with urinary tract infection, almost any abnormality may be associated with this diagnosis. Jaundice, anorexia, vomiting, diarrhea and weight loss are well-known findings. Occasionally, a diaper rash may be the only associated sign. A grayish skin color, convulsions and paralytic ileus have also been observed. Endotoxemia-like characteristics with circulatory collapse may occur, as well as hepatic necrosis and hemolytic anemia. Whenever systemic infection is suspected in a newborn infant, a urinalysis including bacterial culture is mandatory. Reciprocally all neonates with a documented urinary tract infection should be evaluated for systemic infection. In addition, an investigation for congenital GU anomalies should be undertaken after the acute episode is under control.

DIAGNOSIS

The diagnosis of urinary tract infection in newborn infants is predicated upon bacteriologic examination of the urine, with the major problem being the collection of specimens under aseptic conditions. Even with meticulous technique in collecting urine in sterile plastic bags, bacterial contamination is not uncommon. A colony count of 10^4/ml or greater will raise the suspicion of urinary tract infection. Counts of 10^3/ml also require a repeat study. Since the clean catch collection of urine in newborn infants is essentially a screening procedure, such findings warrant further study of the urine, and cannot in themselves be considered diagnostic of urinary tract infection. Diagnosis is best accomplished by suprapubic bladder puncture (43–45, 47) rather than by bladder catheterization. If properly performed, there is practically no morbidity associated with this procedure, and the presence of bacteria of any type and number (with the possible exception of such skin contaminants as *S.*

epidermidis) is indicative of urinary tract infection.

An increased number of leukocytes in the urine (five or more white blood cells in a high-power field) may be associated with urinary tract infection in newborn infants. However, a diagnosis cannot be made on this finding alone; it must be made on a bacteriologic basis. This general principle applies not only to the neonate, but to all age groups.

There is no generally accepted definition of pyuria, and no clear correlation exists between the number of WBCs and the bacterial colony count of the urine.

URINE COLLECTION

Clean Catch

Edelmann et al (40) describe the following method for collecting urine in sterile plastic bags. After cleaning the perineum with green soap, it is rinsed with sterile saline and patted dry with a sterile gauze pad. A sterile plastic urine collector is affixed, and examinations at five to ten-minute intervals are made to see if voiding has occurred. If a stool is passed, or if the infant has not voided within 60 to 90 minutes, the entire procedure is repeated and a new bag applied.

Suprapubic Bladder Puncture

Suprapubic bladder puncture should be performed with the infant supine in a frog position. If at all possible, the puncture should be performed at least two hours after the last voiding. Percussion of the bladder may help confirm that the infant has not recently voided. The suprapubic area is cleansed with iodine and alcohol, and the index finger of one hand (gloves do not have to be worn) is placed over the symphysis pubis. A 1.5-in. No. 21 or 23 needle, attached to a 20-ml syringe is inserted into the bladder to a depth of about 2 cm. As soon as a decrease in resistance is encountered, the barrel of the syringe is gently drawn back, and urine is aspirated (Fig. 19–1). In order to prevent voiding when the needle pierces the skin, an

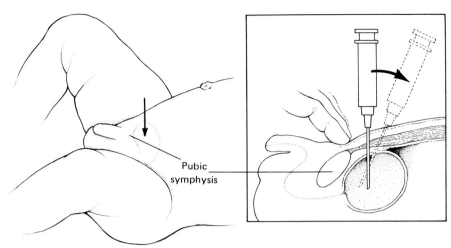

FIG. 19–1. Suprapubic bladder puncture.

assistant may occlude the urethra in the male by compressing the penis and in the female by inserting a finger into the rectum and pressing anteriorly. A portion of the aspirated urine should be centrifuged and a Gram stain performed on the sediment (39). The presence of any bacteria must arouse suspicion of urinary tract infection.

Whether the urine is collected by a clean catch method or by suprapubic bladder puncture, it must be plated immediately after collection on a culture medium, since bacteria will reproduce rapidly in nonrefrigerated urine. If necessary, the urine specimen may be refrigerated for up to one hour.

THERAPY

Specific antimicrobial therapy for urinary tract infection must be based on bacterial sensitivity studies. However, if clinical circumstances warrant, therapy may be initiated immediately, pending laboratory results. Since the offending organism is usually an *E. coli* or other gram-negative bacillus, ampicillin, kanamycin, or both, are the most frequently used antibiotics. Treatment should be continued for ten days to two weeks or longer, depending on clinical and bacteriologic progress. In cases that are due to *E. coli*, in vitro resistance to these antibiotic agents may require the use of another drug, such as gentamicin or colistin. However, urinary concentrations of antibi-

otics may be so high that therapy may be successful even if there is in vitro resistance to the organism.

Negative urine cultures following the cessation of antibiotic therapy and a clinically well patient are the obvious goals of therapy. As is true in later life, prolonged therapy of six weeks to several months may be required, especially with mixed infection and underlying congenital anomalies. The latter may require surgical intervention in order to eliminate the infection.

An intravenous pyelogram (IVP) should be performed on all infants with urinary tract infection after symptoms have subsided, as well as in those with persistent infection. If the IVP is abnormal or questionable, further diagnostic studies such as voiding cystourethrogram and on occasion, cystoscopy, should be undertaken in order to investigate the possibility of any underlying congenital anomalies of the GU tract.

PNEUMONIA

Pneumonia that occurs within the first 24 hours of life or is noted on postmortem examination following fetal death is defined as the congenital variety. The disorder often occurs as a sequel to prolonged rupture of membranes (50, 51) and chorioamnionitis. Its incidence is highest in patients of lowest socioeconomic status, and a disproportion-ately high number of affected infants are premature. Pneumonia secondary to aspira-tion of meconium containing amniotic fluid by hypoxic fetuses is discussed in the sec-tion Meconium Aspiration, Ch. 6.

Following colonization of the amniotic cavity, microorganisms may enter tracheal and lung fluid, setting up a focus of infec-tion in the lungs (see section Perinatal Infec-tion, Ch. 18). Concomitant involvement of the middle ears and paranasal sinuses may occur. If the fetus survives, the onset of respirations will spread the infection to alveolar spaces. Systemic spread of the in-fection with or without meningitis may also occur.

In the presence of a suggestive history, tachypnea, retractions and crepitant râles strongly suggest congenital pneumonia. Occasionally it is difficult to differentiate congenital pneumonia from RDS on clinical grounds.

DIAGNOSIS

Clinical diagnosis may be made on the basis of physical examination, i.e., chest x ray and isolation of pathogenic bacteria from gastric fluid following delivery, or from a deep throat culture. While a WBC count is usu-ally of little value in the diagnosis of con-genital pneumonia, the ESR may be ele-vated.

At postmortem examination, the lungs appear firm and relatively airless, but there are no distinctive findings on gross pathology. A polymorphonuclear leukocytic (PMN) infiltration is usually seen; occasion-ally, the infiltration is hemorrhagic (49). Pathogenic bacteria can usually be re-covered from the lungs, and the inability to isolate bacteria may suggest a mycoplasmal or viral etiology.

If clinical signs of pneumonia appear after the first day of life, it is probable that the illness has been acquired postnatally. Etiology may be either infectious (bacterial or viral) or secondary to aspiration of feed-ings, especially in a debilitated or premature infant. The reflux of gastric fluid into the

lungs through a tracheoesophageal fistula may also result in a chemical pneumonia.

Specific therapy of both congenital and postnatally acquired pneumonia consists of using antibiotics aimed at eradicating the causative bacteria. Until positive cultures can be isolated, ampicillin and kanamycin may be administered parenterally in the same dosage employed for the treatment of neonatal sepsis.

Antimicrobial drugs should be adminis-tered in the presence of aspiration pneu-monia, since both the formula and meco-nium are potential culture media.

Nonspecific supportive therapy such as oxygen, IV administration of fluids and warmth, is also required.

BACTERIAL COLONIZATION

Since newborn infants are especially suscep-tible to bacterial infection, knowledge of the prevalence of various microorganisms nor-mally comprising the flora of the skin and respiratory tract is of clinical importance. Since Bloomfield's report in 1922 (52), sev-eral investigations in this area have yielded widely varying results (60–63). This may reflect differences in sampling methods, bac-teriologic techniques and incomplete evalua-tion of multiple host and environmental fac-tors that may influence the flora. For several years we have investigated in detail bacte-rial colonization of newborn infants under a variety of environmental conditions (53–58). Our findings may be of value in both early diagnosis and treatment of bacterial infection in the neonate.

During intrauterine life, the fetus nor-mally lives in a bacteria-free environment; it is not until after birth that the colonization of deep and superficial sites with a variety of microorganisms begins.

The throat and nasopharynx usually re-main bacteria free for 12 to 18 hours follow-ing delivery. If the amniotic membrane has been ruptured for a prolonged period of time (especially 18 hours or more) bacterial colonization is apparent earlier, often shortly after birth. This latter circumstance may be associated with an increased incidence of congenital pneumonia (50).

Colonization of the umbilicus occurs somewhat more rapidly than that of the respiratory tract. During the first three days of life, colonization of this site by *S. epidermidis, E. coli*, enterobacter and other bacilli is more extensive than nasal colonization by the same organisms. The administration of systemic antibiotics decreases the frequency of colonization at both sites, especially among premature infants. The application of topical antimicrobial agents to the umbilicus reduces colonization of this site by *S. aureus* and *S. epidermidis;* however, this is associated with a "rebound" or increase in nasal colonization with *E. coli* and enterobacter.

The external auditory canal has a lower colonization rate than other superficial sites. The finding of potentially pathogenic bacteria and PMNs at this location may be of diagnostic significance (64).

Bacterial colonization appears to be affected by the season of the year. During the summer months, the prevalence of *E. coli* reaches a peak, while colonization with *S. aureus* decreases and colonization with nonhemolytic streptococci increases in the autumn. The pattern of colonization is, in general, not influenced by the birth weight or sex of the newborn infant. The major exception to this is *S. aureus*.

S. AUREUS COLONIZATION

Of special importance in the neonatal nursery is a knowledge of the patterns of colonization with *S. aureus,* since this organism has been associated with serious skin and systemic infections (see section Staphylococcal Disease). Over the years, the frequency of staphylococcal colonization of the newborn infant has been reported to range from 0% to 100%, with clinical infection often observed where the colonization rate was high. Several factors appear to modify the prevalence of staphylococcal colonization. Daily bathing with hexachlorophene (HCP) markedly diminishes both the prevalence of staphylococcal colonization and

overt disease. (Toxicity of HCP for the newborn infant is discussed in the section Staphylococcal Disease.) However, there may be increased colonization or overgrowth of gram-negative bacilli on the skin and in the respiratory tract (59). Other factors, such as prematurity and high ambient humidity are associated with an increased prevalence. Careful handwashing by the nursery staff and exclusion from the nursery of personnel with staphylococcal lesions are two measures that may be beneficial in decreasing the frequency of staphylococcal colonization of infants.

ENVIRONMENTAL CONTROL PROCEDURES

The role of specific environmental control measures in the modification of neonatal bacterial colonization is difficult to evaluate. The use of masks and hairnets, once absolutely mandatory in premature nurseries, has largely been abandoned. Gowning procedures have been relaxed in nursery areas containing incubators since several studies have failed to show any advantage, at least under experimental conditions (55, 65), and many experienced clinicians feel that fewer restrictions lead to more frequent and thorough examination of infants.

Many measures have been advocated for controlling bacterial colonization and subsequent clinical illness in newborn infants. Some, such as the use of prophylactic antibiotics, the application of topical antimicrobial agents to the umbilicus, washing of the nursery walls and the sterilization of linen, are of dubious value. Other measures, such as thorough handwashing between examinations and bathing the infants with HCP to prevent staphylococcal colonization, are of proven value.

The elimination of overcrowding in the nursery may reduce the possibility of cross infection.

Often, the source of bacteria is a contaminated piece of equipment or water reservoir (Table 19–1). Frequent bacterial cultures are necessary to prevent spread of potentially pathogenic bacteria to infants from these sources.

TABLE 19–1. S. Aureus, Characteristics and Disease Range

Toxins and Enzymes	Antigens	Bacteriophage Groups	Disease Range
α hemolysin (dermonecrosis)	Polysaccharide A	Group I: 29, 52, 52A, 79, 80, 81	Skin:
			Impetigo
β hemolysin	Antigen A	Group II: 3A, 3B, 3C,	Carbuncles
γ hemolysin	Capsular antigen	55, 71	Scalded skin syndrome
Coagulase—free bound	Polyglycerophosphate	Group III: 6, 7, 42E,	Ritter's Disease
Fibrinolysin		47, 53, 54, 75, 77, 83A	Sepsis
Hyaluronidase		Group IV: 42D	Meningitis
Penicillinase		Miscellaneous 187	Pneumonia
(β-lactamase)			Otitis media
Enterotoxin			Osteomyelitis
Lipase			Pyarthrosis
DNAase			Endocarditis
Protease			Pericarditis
			Sinusitis
			Mastoiditis
			Mastitis

Finally, the clinician must be aware that an ecologic disturbance occurs and a "microbiologic price" must be paid when a specific organism is suppressed. For example, when the growth of S. aureus is suppressed with HCP, an overgrowth of gram-negative organisms that are themselves potentially pathogenic may occur, and these may even be more resistant than S. aureus to commonly used antibiotics. The need to maintain normal flora, which is itself a host defense mechanism, is therefore as apparent in newborn infants as it is in other age groups (66).

STAPHYLOCOCCAL DISEASE

Staphylococcal infection is of great clinical importance during the neonatal period and early infancy. The bacteriology, epidemiology, clinical manifestations and treatment have been the subject of major investigative interest (68, 70, 75, 79, 84–86, 89–91). The organisms are ubiquitous and difficult to control, and there is a wide spectrum of observed disease, not only among the affected infants, but also among hospital personnel and older family members.

Pathogenic staphylococci are gram-positive, catalase-producing microorganims that grow readily on most routinely available agar media. Their colonies are often pigmented white (albus), yellow (aureus) or

orange (citreus). Microscopic examination following a Gram stain reveals grapelike clusters of gram-positive cocci.

The ability of staphylococci to survive and grow in a variety of environments, including such hostile ones as within PMNs and monocytes, is related to various capsular antigens and to several toxins and enzymes produced and extracted by these bacteria. Nursery equipment and supplies that are a potential source of pathogenic bacteria include respirators and resuscitators, suction apparatus, humidifying equipment, faucet aerators, squeeze bottles of benzalkonium chloride and sterile water, HCP soap dispensers, sink traps, laryngoscope blades, endotracheal tubes, umbilical vessel catheters and surgical gowns. It is, however, difficult to ascribe a particular degree of virulence or predilection for organ involvement to any one specific bacterial product. Usually it is the capsule that probably retards phagocytosis. The presence of hemolysins and catalase may add to the virulence of the illness. Another factor that often impedes treatment of staphylococcal disease is the high frequency of abscess formation.

Host defense mechanisms against pathogenic staphylococci are not clearly delineated, but both humoral mechanisms and delayed hypersensitivity appear to be involved. The inoculum size and physical defects in the host, such as poor ciliary action of the respiratory tree and thermal injury to the skin are also of prime importance. Newborn infants localize staphylococci poorly, but the basis for this is unknown.

Most staphylococcal disease observed in newborn infants is caused by *S. aureus*. Of these, surface infections, such as Ritter's disease, impetigo and mastitis, are of the greatest clinical importance. They may proceed to systemic involvement of the infant and may be transmitted to other infants, to hospital personnel and to the infant's family. Often they are a reflection of asymptomatic carriage or clinical illness among these latter groups.

The classification of *S. aureus* is based primarily on bacteriophage groups and antibiotic sensitivity patterns. The relative clinical importance of these groups has varied over the years. Group I, especially phage types 80 and 81, was the most important group prior to 1961. In the early 1970s, group III appears to be most closely associated with nosocomial infections.

IMPETIGO NEONATORUM

Impetigo neonatorum appears as a vesicular eruption as early as the second or third day of life; its appearance, however, may be delayed for up to two to four weeks after birth. The vesicles may appear anywhere on the skin. They vary considerably in their number and size, with the diaper and intertrigenous areas most frequently involved.

The vesicles contain a turbid fluid and are usually surrounded by an area of erythema that must be differentiated from the rash of erythema toxicum, which is self-limiting and requires no specific therapy. In addition to the vesicles, breast abscesses, furuncles and omphalitis may also be seen. Upon healing, scarring is rarely encountered.

OTHER FORMS OF STAPHYLOCOCCAL SKIN DISEASE

Group II staphylococci are associated with several types of severe skin disease. Ritter's disease is a form of neonatal exfoliative dermatitis. Lyell's disease (toxic epidermal necrolysis) occurs after the neonatal period

(two months to five years). Two other forms of staphylococcal skin disease are encountered in the neonatal period: 1) a scarletiniform rash and 2) bullous impetigo. Along with Ritter's disease, these two entities are usually caused by a phage type 71 bacteria (84), which can usually be isolated from the skin, upper respiratory tract and eyes.

Exfoliative disease (Fig. 19–2) starts abruptly with erythema; facial edema is often present. During the first two days of the illness, the superficial epidermal layers begin to wrinkle and peel, and the Nikolsky sign is positive. Large flaccid bullae containing clear fluid appear. Desquamation continues for three to five days, and by seven to ten days there is complete recovery, provided antimicrobial therapy is adequate.

The scarletiniform rash markedly resembles the streptococcal rash of scarlet fever

FIG. 19–2. Newborn infant with scalded-skin syndrome in the exfoliative stage. (Melish ME and Glasgow LA: N Engl J Med 282:1114, 1970)

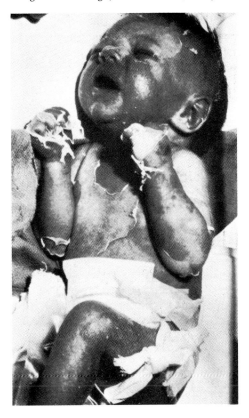

found in older children. Desquamation occurs about four to five days after the appearance of the rash, and Nikolsky's skin sign is rarely if ever present.

In bullous impetigo the lesions are clearly demarcated, and erythema is absent. The trunk and diaper areas are most typically involved, and the lesions have been known to affect circumcision sites. As in scarletiniform disease, Nikolsky's sign is absent.

The antibiotic therapy for this group of diseases is essentially the same as that for impetigo neonatorum.

OTHER ORGAN SYSTEMS

Besides involvement of the skin and its appendages, *S. aureus* may be responsible for a wide range of disease in the newborn infant, including sepsis and meningitis. Staphylococcal pneumonia may be complicated by the formation of pneumatocele and pneumothorax, requiring the insertion of a chest tube. The most common cause of osteomyelitis in the newborn infant is *S. aureus*, but it ranks relatively low as a cause of otitis media. Other diseases caused by this organism and occasionally encountered in the neonatal nursery are enterocolitis, parotitis, sinusitis, endocarditis and pericarditis.

EPIDEMIOLOGY OF STAPHYLOCOCCAL DISEASE

The appearance of staphylococcal skin disease in the neonatal nursery may be associated with a high rate of nosocomial staphylococcal infection throughout the entire hospital (71, 73, 75, 87, 89). In this case, one or more members of the nursery staff are often asymptomatic (or occasionally symptomatic) carriers of this bacteria. Impetigo neonatorum may occur following a break in good nursery technique, such as improper handwashing and overcrowding of infants.

Therapy

Treatment of staphylococcal disease requires systemic antibiotics, preferably semi-synthetic penicillin preparations such as oxacillin, since most offending organisms found in the neonatal period are penicillinase producing and therfore resistant to penicillin G. Oxacillin in an average daily dosage of 150 mg/kg/day given in four to six divided doses parenterally, is an example of initial therapy. Further treatment should be based on sensitivity testing.

HCP and Neuropathologic Disease

The bathing of newborn infants with HCP gained wide popularity during the mid-1960s and coincided with a decrease in the incidence of staphylococcal disease (77, 78). At a symposium conducted in 1972 (74, 76, 81), evidence was presented that indicated a cause and effect relationship between HCP washing and decreased staphylococcal colonization and disease. One report, however, showed that the decrease in colonization of newborn infants was unrelated to the use of HCP (82). Our own long-term studies of factors influencing bacteriologic colonization of newborn infants have shown considerable variation in the prevalence of *S. aureus* over the years in a nursery utilizing only minimal applications of dilute HCP and not employing routine bathing.

In 1971 evidence was presented that associated the topical use of HCP with neuropathologic lesions in newborn experimental animals (72, 82). Because of this finding most clinicians took a cautious approach to the use of HCP.

In 1974 important data were presented showing a marked association between HCP bathing and neuropathologic lesions in human newborn infants (88). Postmortem examinations were performed on brains of infants who were bathed with HCP and subsequently expired. Lesions that were vacuolar in nature and located in the reticular formation and other brainstem areas were found in 63% (19 of 30) of infants bathed three or more times with HCP. Less than 1% (2 of 220) of infants bathed less than three times with 3% HCP, or exposed to 100-fold dilutions of 3% HCP, showed these lesions. The frequency of lesions was related, at least in part, to the birth weight of the infants. All of the neonates weighing less than 1400 g who were bathed in 3% HCP three or more times showed these lesions. There were no specific clinical signs associated with them.

With the presentation of evidence of animal experience in the early 1970s that HCP is capable of causing brain damage, the U.S. Food and Drug Administration placed restrictions on its use (75). In the light of conclusive reports of neuropathologic lesions in newborn humans secondary to the use of 3% HCP, even more rigid limitations are likely to be enforced.

At present HCP should be restricted to personnel handwashing and to two daily applications of 3% HCP on normal skin of neonates, followed by thorough washing. In centers not experiencing problems with staphylococcal skin or systemic disease, surveillance, avoidance of overcrowding, use of the cohort system, thorough handwashing with HCP or an iodophor and prompt isolation and therapy in the event of disease appear warranted.

Control in the Nursery

Other measures such as washing infants with iodine or quaternary amine–containing soaps may also be valuable in decreasing the frequency of both staphylococcal illness and skin disease.

The control of epidemics of staphylococcal skin disease in the nursery depends largely on the severity of the illness encountered, the physical arrangement of the nursery and the nursery census (usually a reflection of the birth rate). If the birth rate is relatively low and there is an underutilization of bassinets, the affected room or rooms can be closed to new admissions. After all of the affected infants have been discharged, these areas may be reopened. When the disease is virulent and separation of newly born infants from those already infected is impossible, temporarily closing the obstetric service may be advisable. If adequate separation of new admissions from infants already infected is for some

reason impossible, the use of daily prophylactic baths with a soap containing an antistaphylococcal agent may be a second-best alternative. The use of prophylactic antistaphylococcal antibiotics in these infants may also be of some value. An experimental approach used during the severe staphylococcal epidemics of the early 1960s is the colonization of the nares with strains of minimally pathogenic staphylococci, such as 502A (67), which interfere with colonization by more virulent strains of *S. aureus*. Since clinically significant lesions have been ascribed to 502A (69, 80), this approach is no longer in clinical use.

GONOCOCCAL INFECTION

Although gonococcal ophthalmia neonatorum has long been recognized as a major public health problem, recent evidence implies that maternal gonorrheal infection may produce systemic gonorrheal infection in the fetus (95). Since eye prophylaxis with either silver nitrate or a topically applied antibiotic agent has all but eliminated conjunctivitis, the gonococcal amniotic infection syndrome may be of greater clinical significance than the former condition. With an increase in the incidence of gonococcal infection throughout the United States, a rise in the number of newborn infants at risk can be anticipated.

GONOCOCCAL OPHTHALMIA

The causative organism of gonorrheal conjunctivitis is *Neisseria gonorrhoeae*, a gram-negative intracellular diplococcus that is found in the vaginal canal and cervical floor of infected mothers. The organism ferments glucose, but not maltose or sucrose, and is oxidase positive. The bacteriologic diagnosis is not always straightforward, and the organism may be confused with *Mima polymorpha* or other nonpathogenic neisseriae.

The disorder is acquired during passage through the birth canal, when the offending organism comes in contact with the infant. There is recent evidence, however, that in-

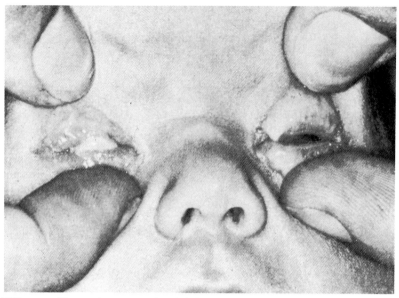

FIG. 19–3. Neonatal gonococcal ophthalmia. (Medical World News, Feb. 25, 1972)

fection may be acquired in utero from contact with infected amniotic fluid (4).

The major manifestation of gonococcal conjunctivitis is a purulent eye discharge that is usually first noted on the second or third day of life (Fig. 19–3). Edema of the eyelids and conjunctival erythema are also seen. It is virtually impossible to differentiate this condition from chemical or viral conjunctivitis on clinical grounds alone. While chemical conjunctivitis (usually secondary to silver nitrate installation) generally is noted during the first 48 hours of life and viral conjunctivitis between the 4th and 14th day, the incubation period of *N. gonorrhoeae* is so variable that the time of onset cannot be reliably used as a differentiating point.

With proper treatment, complete regression of signs occurs. If left untreated, the infection attacks the deep layers of the cornea, leading to ulceration and corneal opacification. A panophthalmitis may ensue, with resultant loss of vision.

The diagnosis is established on a bacteriologic basis. Because of the virulence of gonococcal conjunctivitis, a Gram stain and culture should be carried out on each case of conjunctivitis seen in the newborn infant.

The use of Thayer-Martin medium is recommended since it is selective for the recovery of the organism.

Fluorescent antibody examination may be of some value, but should be used with caution, since there is some antigenic overlap with other organisms.

Prevention

Prior to the institution of chemoprophylaxis, the incidence of gonococcal ophthalmia was as high as 10%. Since no therapy existed at that time, this condition was a major cause of blindness and hospitalization of small infants.

There are three available methods of prophylaxis. The Crede method (94) consists of the installation of one drop of 1% silver nitrate in each eye. This was the first method used, and it is still extremely effective today (92, 93). One possible drawback is the fact that the silver nitrate itself may lead to a chemical conjunctivitis that requires differentiation from gonococcal conjunctivitis. Disastrous accidents have also been associated with the use of more highly concentrated solutions, which are toxic to the eyes.

The application of topical antibiotics following delivery is another commonly used method of eye prophylaxis. Chemical conjunctivitis is rare, and the method is generally effective. Neomycin is the most commonly used agent. Penicillin ointment is rarely used today. Although there is no direct evidence that it is a sensitizing agent, the possibility exists, and its use has been discouraged.

Penicillin when administered parenterally immediately after birth has long been known to protect against gonococcal conjunctivitis. Several problems, however, are associated with its use. It is a less convenient form of prophylaxis than the topical medications, and furthermore, the organism has become progressively less sensitive to penicillin over the past 20 years.

When the discontinuation of eye prophylaxis was attempted in a low-risk population on an experimental basis in the 1950s (96), several cases appeared, and the trial was halted. The use of eye prophylaxis is now universally mandated by state laws. Because of the increasing prevalence of gonorrhea, any attempt to discontinue eye prophylaxis would undoubtedly lead to widespread resurgence of the disease.

Therapy should consist of the administration of aqueous penicillin, 50,000 U/kg/day in two divided IM doses for 7 to 10 days, plus frequent topical applications of neomycin solution (at least every 1 to 2 hours) for the 24 hours after the onset of clinical signs. Consultation with an experienced ophthalmologist is advisable in this situation, as it is in any other condition in which there is potential loss of vision.

GONOCOCCAL AMNIOTIC INFECTION

Handsfield et al (95) have studied 14 infants with signs of clinical sepsis in whom *N. gonorrhoeae* were isolated from orogastric aspirates. Twelve of these infants were premature, and delivery usually followed prolonged rupture of membranes and chorioamnionitis in the mother.

Because of the inherent dangers associated with generalized gonococcal infection acquired in utero, it is essential that all pregnant women be routinely cultured for

gonorrhea several times during pregnancy and treated adequately if infection is discovered.

Since this condition was recognized for the first time in the early 1970s, the complete clinical spectrum and methods of therapy have not been completely elucidated.

CONGENITAL SYPHILIS

Prior to the antibiotic era, the incidence of congenital syphilis was extremely high, affecting 1% to 2% of all infants born in the United States. With the introduction of penicillin, a marked decline occurred. In 1964 the incidence of congenital syphilis in New Orleans was reported to be less than 0.1%. While rarely seen during the mid-1960s, an increasing incidence has now become apparent, consistent with the overall increase in the number of cases of venereal disease occurring in the adult population of the United States at this time (99, 100, 102).

Virtually an entire generation of physicians trained in the United States has only minimal experience in the diagnosis and treatment of this disease; these doctors may well be faced with a recrudescence of congenital syphilis in the near future.

The infection is usually transmitted from mother to fetus during the second half of pregnancy. The etiologic agent, the spirochete *Treponema pallidum*, is transmitted by hematogenous spread across the placenta into the fetal circulation. If the agent crosses at an earlier time no inflammatory response is elicited. Severity of fetal infection is roughly equivalent to that in the mother. With successive pregnancies, fetal infection becomes progressively milder.

DIAGNOSIS

On the basis of a positive serologic test for syphilis (STS) on maternal and cord blood specimens the diagnosis is suspected. The mother may have a biologic false positive test, but these are usually of low titer and occur later in pregnancy. This possibility should be considered especially among drug addicts in whom a biologic false positive test may reflect hepatitis. A negative test on maternal blood, however, does not necessarily exclude the possibility of congenital syphilis, whereas a positive test on the infant's cord blood does not necessarily confirm the diagnosis. If the maternal infection has been acquired late in pregnancy with little time for seroconversion (as in a case we have observed at Harlem Hospital Center), the fetus may still become infected in the presence of a negative maternal STS. A repeat STS on maternal blood taken three to six weeks after delivery and serial testing of a suspect neonate may clarify this point.

Conversely the vast majority of cord blood STS determinations, e.g., fluorescent treponemal antibody-absorption test (FTA-ABS) or venereal disease research laboratory test (VDRL), represent passive transmission from treated maternal cases that have not undergone conversion to seronegativity. Serial follow-up of these infants will reveal a gradual decline in titer of one-half every month (approximately the half-life of IgG, which is the immunoglobulin class of these passively acquired antibodies). Elevation of serum IgM (20 mg/100 ml or more) is nonspecific and not reliable in diagnosis (see section Perinatal Immunology, Ch. 18). In contrast, the IgM–FTA-ABS test is specific and efficient (97, 100), particularly in asymptomatic cases prior to appearance of clinical signs, but again, with late infection even this test may be negative.

Since the earliest clinical signs of congenital syphilis may be delayed for one week to three months, the importance of a serologic diagnosis and serial antibody titer determinations becomes apparent. With the recent recrudescence of venereal disease, the clinician's index of suspicion must always be high. It is probably the best policy to obtain a routine STS on all umbilical cord sera.

CLINICAL SIGNS

Coryza, often with a blood-tinged discharge (snuffles), is usually the first clinically recognized sign of neonatal syphilis. A maculopapular eruption then appears, most prominent on the palms, soles and face.

Occasionally this rash is noted at birth. In rare instances vesicular or bullous eruptions may appear on the soles or palms. Later, perioral scars or rhagades may occur. Hepatosplenomegaly is almost always observed. Bleeding, jaundice, anemia and lymphadenopathy are all nonspecific findings. In general, both cutaneous and systemic findings become apparent from the 2nd through the 12th week of life (101). Pseudoparalysis, secondary to epiphyseal separation of a long bone may be present. Asymptomatic involvement of the CNS occurs transiently, reflected by pleocytosis and protein elevation.

Radiologic findings may be noted even in the fetus prior to delivery. These include osteochondritis and periostitis, particularly of long bones, such as the femur, and epiphyseal separation. The presence of these early findings is a helpful diagnostic tool that precedes the appearance of clinical signs.

Numerous manifestations occur in later months and years (97a); defects in vision and hearing, dental anomalies, orthopedic deformities and eventual general paresis are all late signs of congenital syphilis.

In the differential diagnosis of congenital syphilis, one must include erythroblastosis fetalis, sepsis, cytomegalovirus and toxoplasmosis.

Pathologic lesions include a large placenta with an increase in connective tissue; mononuclear cells in the chorionic villi may be seen with phase microscopy. Spirochetes may be demonstrated with a silver impregnation technique in the placenta and in numerous organs, e.g., liver, lung, adrenals. Gummas may also be seen. Extramedullary hematopoiesis and thickened alveolar walls with lymphocytes and plasma cells sometimes occur, as may an infiltrate similar to that found in the submucosal tissue of the nose associated with snuffles. Numerous osseous lesions occur especially at the ends of long bones.

THERAPY

The primary reason for the decreased incidence of congenital syphilis over the past 30 years (despite an upswing in the late 1960s and early 1970s) is the widespread availability of penicillin therapy for the gravida. Penicillin crosses the placenta, with consequent treatment of the infected fetus. However, therapy directed to the mother is not sufficient. Treatment of the newborn infant for congenital syphilis is mandatory. The organism may persist in the tissues and body fluids of the fetus in spite of maternal therapy. Similarly, suspected infection is often treated when the sole evidence is a positive cord blood STS, even though most of these signify only passive transfer of antibody across the placenta. This is usually done in cases where it is likely that the mother may not bring the infant back for routine well baby care. The need for follow-up evaluation of all infants with positive cord blood serologies, whether treated or not, cannot be overemphasized.

Treatment of the infant is based on maintaining continuous blood levels of penicillin for seven days. This may be done by giving a single injection of benzathine penicillin (50,000 U/kg), or by giving daily injection of aqueous penicillin (total dosage of at least 100,000 U/kg) over a seven to ten day period. Erythromycin could be used as an alternate therapeutic agent; this is rarely if ever necessary since penicillin hypersensitivity in the neonatal period is virtually unknown.

Treatment failure with the recommended dosage of penicillin has only been reported once in the literature (98).

Initial penicillin therapy may lead to a Herxheimer reaction in the newborn infant, including fever and a rash; despite this, therapy should be continued.

TETANUS NEONATORUM

Neonatal tetanus is a rare entity in the United States today. However, it remains a major cause of neonatal mortality in many of the underdeveloped areas of the world (105-107).

The causative microorganism is a gram-positive anaerobic spore-bearing bacillus present in the intestinal tract of such herbivores as horses or cattle; it may also be found in the intestines of adult man, especially among farm workers.

Two toxins are produced by all of the subgroups, but only one of these, tetanospasmin, is significant in disease production. Clinical signs of the illness reflect the affinity of this toxin for the CNS. There is no natural immunity to the disease, and patients recovering from it are susceptible to reinfection. Umbilical venous serum antibody concentrations are proportional to maternal levels.

The site of entry among neonates is the umbilicus that has become contaminated, with infants of nonimmunized mothers being at risk. The incubation period of the illness is one to two weeks.

Fever, irritability, poor feeding, muscle stiffness and convulsions herald the onset of the illness. These signs are followed by trismus, risus sardonicus, tenseness of muscles and abdominal rigidity. Nuchal rigidity, opisthotonus, clonic jerking and tightened fists are also typical. Death may ensue because of bronchopneumonia, respiratory arrest, exhaustion, hypoxic brain damage or a combination of these factors.

Among survivors improvement is slow, with a decrease in signs over a three to seven-day period and recovery over one to two months.

Definitive diagnosis depends on anaerobic isolation of the causative organism, *Clostridium tetanus*, from the site of entrance.

TREATMENT

Therapy involves the administration of human tetanus immune globulin, 1000 to 3000 U, intramuscularly, or equine tetanus antitoxin; its purpose is to bind circulating toxin that has not yet affected the CNS (104). Aqueous penicillin, 100,000 U/kg given intramuscularly every 12 hours, may help to eradicate the bacillus but is not helpful in combating the toxin.

Sedation and muscle relaxants of various types, including barbiturates, chlorpromazine, tribromoethanol, diazepam and magnesium sulfate have been used. Endotracheal intubation and the use of assisted ventilation may be required. Intravenous alimentation is usually necessary.

The infant should be disturbed as little as possible. Meticulous nursing care plays a large role in survival. Mortality rates are now about 45% to 50%, compared to 75% to 90% in previous eras. Survival rates of 100% have been noted with the use of diazepam (103). An infant who has survived this disease does not acquire immunity and should receive tetanus toxoid.

On rare occasions, especially in a heroin-addicted mother, tetanus may occur during the last trimester of pregnancy. Based on anecdotal evidence and one case that we have seen, maternal toxin does not appear to affect the newborn infant.

LISTERIOSIS

Listeria monocytogenes is a small, motile, pleomorphic, non-spore-forming gram-positive bacillus that is ubiquitously distributed among birds and mammals. There is, however, no known dissemination from animals to humans. While listeria infection may lead to abortion in pregnant animals, there is no evidence that this occurs in humans. In general, infection most commonly occurs in debilitated patients and has a special predilection for the pregnant individual.

There are three recognized routes of transmission of Listeria infection from mother to fetus. In cases of maternal illness (manifestations of which are fever, chills, sore throat, myalgia and diarrhea) transplacental transmission may occur. This form of illness may end in fetal death. Aspiration of infected amniotic fluid and direct contact with a cervical or vaginal lesion during delivery are other modes of transmission. In addition, Listeria infection is sometimes (but rarely) acquired postnatally from contact with nasal, GI and mucous membrane discharge of already infected infants (108).

The clinical picture in the newborn infant is indistinguishable from that of other systemic bacterial infections. Meningitis is most characteristic (109), but petechiae, hepatosplenomegaly, severe respiratory distress secondary to pneumonia, seizures,

diarrhea and vomiting have all been reported. Manifestations of illness may be apparent at birth or may be delayed for one to two weeks. Among the latter group a gradual, progressively more severe illness may be seen with bronchopneumonia as the major finding.

The definitive diagnosis is established by identification of the organism in the urine and blood of the infant and mother. In addition, a Gram stain of meconium may reveal the organism.

L. monocytogenes may be confused bacteriologically with β-hemolytic streptococci and diphtheroids. Listeria, however, gives a positive catalase test, whereas the other two do not.

On rare occasions dark red or livid papules may be seen in the oropharynx or skin. These represent miliary granulomas, which can be found in the liver, spleen, adrenal glands, lung, GI tract and CNS on postmortem examination.

L. monocytogenes is sensitive to a wide variety of antibiotics. Lavetter et al (109) and Nelson et al (110) have had excellent results with ampicillin. Definitive therapy, however, should be based on antibiotic sensitivity tests. In general, the route and duration of therapy are the same as for sepsis and meningitis.

GROUP B STREPTOCOCCAL INFECTIONS

During the late 1960s and 1970s the potential significance of group B β-hemolytic streptococci in the pathogenesis of neonatal sepsis and meningitis has been recognized (111–115, 117). Just as gram-negative bacilli replaced staphylococci during the early 1960s as the major bacterial pathogens in the nursery, group B streptococci may in future years occupy this position (116).

ETIOLOGY AND PATHOGENESIS

Group B streptococci can be isolated from vaginal and cervical cultures of 10% to 20% of asymptomatic pregnant women; the organism may also be isolated from urethral cultures of their asymptomatic male partners (115).

Whereas most other perinatal bacterial infections are associated with premature rupture of membranes, maternal fever, low socioeconomic status and obstetric trauma, this is not the case with group B streptococci. Indeed, white middle-class families seem to be the predominant group involved. Moreover there may be a decided preponderance of female neonates involved, again the reverse of the usual trend with other organisms.

The basis for the increased appearance of this pathogen is unknown. Asymptomatic carriage has not increased, nor has the use of antibiotics enhanced their emergence. These organisms are all susceptible to penicillin as they have been in the past. Speculations have been offered that decreased bathing with HCP may have allowed their emergence. Likewise it may be that placental transfer of type specific group B streptococcal M-type antibodies is impaired. Data are insufficient to draw conclusions.

The neonatal cases that have been described have been due to ascending colonization and infection during parturition.

Infections with group B streptococci may lead to abortion, sepsis or meningitis in the offspring. In these respects it is similar to *L. monocytogenes*.

Two distinct clinical patterns in the newborn infant have thus far emerged (115, 116). In some infants there is early onset of respiratory distress with tachypnea, grunt, cyanosis and apnea, suggestive of RDS. Chest x rays usually reveal pneumonia. Hypotension and coma are common. Mortality rates are 70% or higher. The organism can be recovered from blood, skin, nasopharynx, CSF and meconium. In the second type there is a delay of 1 to 12 weeks. The onset is more gradual; apnea is rare, but lethargy and fever are common. A bulging anterior fontanelle is seen in the majority of cases, and about one-fifth have nuchal rigidity. Mortality is 14% to 18%. The organism is recovered from the blood and CSF but not usually from other sites.

The organism in each form may be somewhat different. In the acute, early illness group B I is the primary offender but in the delayed variety group B III is most common. The latter type of illness may be acquired from adult carriers other than the mother, or the infant may become colonized at birth, remain asymptomatic for a few weeks and then develop meningitis. The acute form is acquired during parturition.

The definitive diagnosis is made from isolation of the organism from cultures of blood, CSF, gastric fluid and various superficial sites. It can be grown easily on blood agar and other culture media. An early presumptive diagnosis based on Gram stain of specimens from the rectum and nasopharynx in symptomatic infants during the early hours of life may lead to rapid institution of therapy and an increased survival rate.

Identification of gravidas and their spouses carrying these organisms can be followed by penicillin therapy leading to apparent eradication of the etiologic agent. In communities with an especially marked frequency of this pathogen among newborn infants, systematic examination of gravidas and subsequent treatment may be justified, especially in view of the severity of the neonatal infection. Experience is still too limited to permit recommendations in this regard.

The organisms thus far isolated have been susceptible to penicillin, ampicillin and methicillin. The unfavorable outcome in the acute cases reflects the rapidity of dissemination of the organism perhaps associated with an undefined host defect. In the delayed type the illness, although it includes meningitis, appears more indolent and less severe. The clinician is presented with a more suggestive array of signs, and the response to therapy is usually satisfactory.

PERINATAL TUBERCULOSIS

Fetal tuberculosis may be acquired by transplacental passage of the tubercle bacillus from a mother with miliary disease. Postnatally, it may be transmitted by contact with an infected nurse, mother or other family member; even a circumcision site has been reported as the portal of entry (125).

CONGENITAL

Congenital tuberculosis is rarely seen today. Even with placental involvement the fetus is usually spared. About 100 cases of congenital tuberculosis have been recorded in the literature, and approximately one-third of these infants died soon after birth (122). Infection may be widespread, with involvement of multiple organ systems. Since the offending organisms enter the fetus through the umbilical vein, the liver is often the first organ to be affected. There is subsequent involvement of the lungs, brain, spleen and other organs secondary to bloodstream or lymphatic dissemination.

At birth the tuberculin reaction is usually negative (120, 124). Tuberculin sensitivity is not transmitted from mother to fetus since it reflects cellular rather than humoral immunity. In rare cases the mother's tuberculin reaction may be negative. Onset of symptoms in the newborn infant may be abrupt, accompanied by pneumonia, melena or overwhelming toxemia. However, there may be a delay of six to eight weeks or even to three months before clinical manifestations appear. Fetal or very early neonatal deaths rarely occur.

The criteria for diagnosis of this rare form of tuberculosis are proof of infection in both mother and infant, with no postpartum contact between the two. We are aware of two cases that occurred in New York City between 1969 and 1972 (119, 123).

POSTNATAL

Management of the newborn infant whose mother either has active or inactive tuberculosis is a much more commonly encountered problem. If the mother has open cavitary disease, separation from the infant is mandatory until her sputum cultures become negative. If the mother is under treatment but has a negative sputum culture, two alternatives are available concerning treatment of her infant. The first is administration of Bacille de Calmette-Guérin (BCG) vaccine (121), and the other is prophylactic administration of isoniazid (INH) syrup (average dose 10 mg/kg/day; range, 5 to 20 mg/kg/day) to the infant for one year. Both methods have advantages and disadvantages (118). With administration of BCG the diagnostic value of the tuberculin test is lost, at least for a few years. However, when there are indications that the infant may be lost to follow-up examination or doubt exists that daily medication will be administered, this approach is probably the only alternative.

The advantages of daily administration of INH are that the tuberculin test may still be utilized as a diagnostic tool and that the drug is usually safe and effective. The major disadvantage is that the mother may forget to give the medication to a seemingly well child. If the organism is INH-resistant, the efficacy of the therapy is problematic. However, in many such cases among adults recovery occurs despite in vitro resistance.

If the mother's disease is arrested, no prophylactic therapy for the infant is indicated. If the infant has not received BCG vaccine, tuberculin testing should be performed every three months, and the mother should have chest x rays taken three and six months postpartum.

Routine administration of BCG vaccine to newborn infants is indicated only under special circumstances, such as in developing countries where the incidence of tuberculosis is especially high or among certain ethnic groups susceptible to tuberculosis.

Our own experience at Harlem Hospital, using INH therapy in infants with tuberculous mothers, has been favorable. Families have been cooperative and overt disease has not developed among the infants.

REFERENCES

BACTERIAL MENINGITIS AND SEPSIS

1. Albers WH, Tyler CW, Boxerbaum B: Asymptomatic bacteremia in the newborn infant. J Pediatr 69:193, 1966
2. Berman PH, Banker BQ: Neonatal meningitis: a clinical and pathological study of 29 cases. Pediatrics 38:6, 1966

3. Eickhoff TC, Klein JO, Daly K, Ingall D, Finland M: Neonatal sepsis and other infections due to group B hemolytic streptococci. N Engl J Med 271:1221, 1964

4. Franciosi RA, Favara BE: Single blood culture for confirmation of diagnosis of neonatal septicemia. Am J Clin Pathol 57:215, 1972

5. Gluck L, Wood HF, Fousek MD: Septicemia of the newborn. Pediatr Clin North Am 13:1131, 1966

5a. Howard JB, McCracken GH Jr: Reappraisal of kanamycin usage in neonates. J Pediatr 86:949, 1975

6. McCracken GH Jr: Group B streptococci. The new challenge in neonatal infections. J Pediatr 82:703, 1973

7. McCracken GH Jr, Shinefield HR: Changes in the pattern of neonatal septicemia and meningitis. Am J Dis Child 112:33, 1966

8. Moffet HL, Williams T: Bacteria recovered from distilled water and inhalation therapy equipment. Am J Dis Child 114:7, 1967

9. Overall JC Jr: Neonatal bacterial meningitis. J Pediatr 76:499, 1970

10. Young CY: Hypoglycemia in neonatal sepsis. J Pediatr 77:812, 1970

OTITIS MEDIA

11. Ammann AJ, Stiehm ER: Immune globulin levels in colostrum and breast milk, and serum from formula and breast-fed newborns. Proc Soc Exp Biol Med 122:1098, 1966

12. Bland RD: Otitis media in the first six days of life: diagnosis, bacteriology, and management. Pediatrics 49:187, 1972

13. Feigin RD, Klein JO: Otitis media in the premature infant: a report of two cases. Pediatrics 34:122, 1964

14. Jaffe BF, Hurtado F, Hurtado E: Tympanic membrane mobility in the newborn (with seven months follow-up). Laryngoscope 80:36, 1970

15. Johnson WW: A survey of middle ears: 101 autopsies of infants. Ann Otol Rhinol Laryngol 70:377, 1961

16. McLellan MS, Strong JP, Abdo CJ, Tomerlin CG: Otitis media in a permature infant. Am J Dis Child 116:439, 1968

17. McLellan MS, Strong JP, Johnson QR, Dent JH: Otitis media in premature infants. A histopathologic study. J Pediatr 61:53, 1962

INFECTIOUS DIARRHEA

18. Bettelheim KA, Taylor J: Soluble antigens of enteropathogenic Escherichia coli. Ann NY Acad Sci 176:301, 1971

19. Cramblett HG, Azimi P, Haynes RE: The etiology of infectious diarrhea in infancy, with special reference to enteropathogenic E coli. Ann NY Acad Sci 176:80, 1971

20. Epstein HC, Hochwald A, Ashe R: Salmonella infections in the newborn infant. J Pediatr 38:723, 1951

21. Grady GF, Keusch GI: Pathogenesis of bacterial diarrheas (Part I). N Engl J Med 285:831, 1971

22. Grady GF, Keusch GI: Pathogenesis of bacterial diarrheas (Part II). N Engl J Med 285:891, 1971

23. Jacobs SE, Holzel A, Wolman B, Keen JH, Miller V, Taylor J, Gross RJ: Outbreak of infantile gastroenteritis caused by Escherichia coli 0114. Arch Dis Child 45:656, 1970

24. Kenny JF, Boesman MI, Michaels RH: Bacterial and viral coproantibodies in breast-fed infants. Pediatrics 39:202, 1967

25. Kessner DM, Shaughnessy HJ, Googins J, Rasmussen CM, Rose NJ, Marshall AL Jr, Andelman SL, Hall JB, Rosenbloom PJ: An extensive community outbreak of diarrhea due to enteropathogenic Escherichia coli 0111:B4. I. Epidemiologic studies. Am J Hygiene 76:27, 1962

26. Mata LJ, Urrutia JJ: Intestinal colonization of breast-fed children in a rural area of low socioeconomic level. Am NY Acad Sci 176:93, 1971

27. Neter E: Enteropathogenic Escherichia coli enteritis. Pediatr Clin North Am 7:1015, 1960

28. Salzman TC, Scher CD, Moss R: Shigellae with transferable drug resistance: outbreak in a nursery for premature infants. J Pediatr 71:21, 1967

29. Shaughnessy HJ, Lesko M, Dorigan F, Forster GF, Morrissey RA, Kessner DM: An extensive community outbreak of diarrhea due to enteropathogenic Escherichia coli 0111:B4. II. A comparative study of fluorescent antibody identification and standard bacteriologic methods. Am J Hygiene 76:44, 1962

30. South MA: Enteropathogenic Eschericia coli disease: new developments and perspectives. J Pediatr 79:1, 1971

31. Yow MD, Melnick JL, Blattner RJ, Stephenson WB, Robinson NM, Burkhart MA: The association of viruses and bacteria with infantile diarrhea. Am J Epidemiol 92:33, 1970

OSTEOMYELITIS

32. Asnes R, Arendar GM: Septic arthritis of the hip: a complication of femoral venipuncture. Pediatrics 38:837, 1966

33. Berant M, Kahana D: Klebsiella osteomyelitis in a newborn. Am J Dis Child 118:634, 1969

34. Dennison WH: Hematogenous osteitis in the newborn. Lancet 2:477, 1965

35. Howard PJ: Sepsis in normal and premature infants with localization in the hip joint. Pediatrics 20:279, 1957

36. Levy HL, O'Connor JF, Ingall D: Neonatal osteomylitis due to Proteus mirabilis. JAMA 202:582, 1967

37. Levy HL, O'Connor JF, Ingall D: Bacteremia, infected cephalhematoma, and osteomyelitis of the skull in a newborn. Am J Dis Child 114:649, 1967

38. Nelson DL, Hable KA, Matsen JM: Proteus mirabilis osteomyelitis in two neonates. Am J Dis Child 125:109, 1973

URINARY TRACT INFECTION

39. Braude H, Forfar JO, Gould JC, McLeod JW: Cell and bacterial counts in the urine of normal infants and children. Br Med J 4:697, 1967

40. Edelmann CM, Ogwo JE, Fine BP, Martinez AB: The prevalence of bacteriuria in full-term and premature newborn infants. J Pediatr 82:125, 1973

41. Hodgman JE, Schwartz A, Thrupp LD: Bacteriuria in the premature infant. Pediatr Res 1:303, 1967

42. Littlewood JM: White cells and bacteria in voided urine of healthy newborns. Arch Dis Child 46:167, 1971

43. Monzon OT, Ory EM, Dobsen HD, Carter E, Yow EM: A comparison of bacterial counts of the urine obtained by needle aspiration of the bladder, catheterization and mid-stream voided methods. N Engl J Med 259:764, 1958

44. Nelson JD, Peters PC: Suprapubic aspiration of urine in premature and term infants. Pediatrics 36:132, 1965

45. Newman CGH, O'Neill P, Parker A: Pyuria in infancy, and the role of suprapubic aspiration of urine in diagnosis of infection of the urinary tract. Br Med J 2:277, 1967

46. O'Brien NG, Carroll R, Donovan DE, Dundon SP: Bacteriuria and leucocyte excretion in the newborn. J Ir Med Assoc 61:267, 1968

47. Pryles CV, Atkin MD, Morse TS, Welch KJ: Comparative bacteriologic study of urine obtained from children by percutaneous suprapubic aspiration of the bladder and by catheter. Pediatrics 24:983, 1959

48. Randolph MF: Screening for bacteriuria in the newborn nursery: collection of the suitable urine specimen. J Pediatr 79:463, 1971

PNEUMONIA

49. Bernstein J, Wang J: The pathology of neonatal pneumonia. Am J Dis Child 101:350, 1961

50. Calkins LA: Premature spontaneous rupture of the membranes. Am J Obstet Gynecol 64:871, 1952

51. Naeye RL, Blanc WA: Relation of poverty and race to antenatal infection. N Engl J Med 283:555, 1970

BACTERIAL COLONIZATION

52. Bloomfield AL: Adaption of bacteria to growth on human mucous membranes with special reference to the throat flora in infants. Bull Hopkins Hosp 33:61, 1922

53. Evans HE, Akpata SO, Baki A: Factors influencing the establishment of the neonatal bacterial flora. I. The role of host factors. Arch Environ Health 21:514, 1970

54. Evans HE, Akpata SO, Baki A: Factors influencing the establishment of the neonatal bacterial flora. II. The role of environmental factors. Arch Environ Health 21:643, 1970

55. Evans HE, Akpata SO, Baki A: A bacteriologic and clinical evaluation of gowning in a premature nursery. J Pediatr 78:883, 1971

56. Evans HE, Akpata SO, Baki A: Relationship of the birth canal to the bacterial flora of the neonatal respiratory tract and skin. Obstet Gynecol 37:94, 1971

57. Evans HE, Akpata SO, Baki A, Glass L: Annual variation in prevalence of S. aureus in the flora in newborn infants. Arch Environ Health 26:275, 1973

58. Evans HE, Akpata SO, Baki A, Glass L: Bacterial flora of newborn infants in the external auditory canal and other sites. NY State J Med 73:1071, 1973

59. Forfar JC, Gould J, Maccabe A: Effect of hexachlorophene on incidence of staphylococcal and gram-negative infection in the newborn. Lancet 2:177, 1968

60. Hardyment, AF, Wilson RA, Cockcraft W Johnson B: Observations on the bacteriology and epidemiology of nursery infections. Pediatrics 25:906, 1960

61. Light IJ, Sutherland JM, Cochran ML, Sutorius J: Ecologic relation between S. aureus and Pseudomonas in a nursery population. N Engl J Med 278:1243, 1968

62. Sarkany I, Gaylarde C: Skin flora in the newborn. Lancet 1:589, 1967

63. Sarkany I, Gaylarde C: Bacterial colonization of the skin of the newborn. J Pathol 95:115, 1968

64. Scanlon J: The early detection of neonatal sepsis by examination of liquid obtained from the external ear canal. J Pediatr 79:247, 1971

65. Sinclair J, Silverman W: Evaluation of precautions before entering a neonatal unit. Pediatrics 40:900, 1967

66. Sprunt K, Redman W: Evidence suggesting importance of role of interbacterial inhibition in maintaining balance of normal flora. Ann Intern Med 68:579, 1968

STAPHYLOCOCCAL DISEASE

67. Boris M, Shinefield HR, Romano P, McCarthy DP, Florman AL: Bacterial interference and protection against recurrent intrafamilial staphylococcal disease. Am J Dis Child 115:521, 1968

68. Baldwin JN, Rheins MS, Sylvester RF Jr, Shaffer TE: Staphylococcal infections in newborn infants. III. Colonization of newborn infants by Staphylococcus pyogenes. J Dis Child 94:107, 1957

69. Blair EB, Tull AH: Multiple infections among newborns resulting from colonization with

staphylococcus aureus 502A. Am J Clin Pathol 52:42, 1969

70. Dixon RE, Kaslow RA, Mallison GF, Bennett JV: Staphylococcal disease outbreaks in hospital nurseries in the United States—December 1971 through March 1972. Pediatrics 51:413, 1973

71. Ehrenkranz NJ: Bacterial colonization of newborn infants and subsequent acquisition of hospital bacteria. J Pediatr 76:839, 1970

72. Gaines TB, Kimbrough RD: The oral and dermal toxicity of hexachlorophene in rats. Toxicol Appl Pharmacol 19:375, 1971

73. Gezon HM, Rogers KD, Thompson DJ, Hatch TF: Some controversial aspects in the epidemiology of hospital nursery staphylococcal infections. Am J Public Health 50:573, 1960

74. Gezon HM, Thompson DJ, Rogers KD, Hatch TF, Rycheck RR, Yee RB: Control of staphylococcal infections and disease through the use of hexachlorophene bathing. Pediatrics (Suppl) 51:331, 1973

75. Gillespie WA, Simpson K, Tozer RC: Staphylococcal infection in a maternity hospital: epidemiology and control. Lancet 2:1075, 1958

76. Gluck L: A perspective on hexachlorophene. Pediatrics 51:400, 1973

77. Gluck L, Wood HF: Effect of an antiseptic skin care regimen on reducing staphylococcal colonization in newborn infants. N Engl J Med 265:1177, 1961

78. Gluck L, Wood HF: Staphylococcal colonization in newborn infants with and without antiseptic skin care. N Engl J Med 268:1265, 1963

79. Hardyment AF: The baby and his staphylococci. Lancet 2:700, 1966

80. Houck PW, Nelson JD, Kay JL: Fatal septicemia due to staphylococcus aureus 502 A. Am J Dis Child 123:45, 1972

81. Kaslow RA, Dixon RE, Martin SM, Mallison GF, Goldmann DA, Lindsey JD II, Rhame FS, Bennett JV: Staphylococcal disease related to hospital nursery bathing practices—a nationwide epidemiologic investigation. Pediatrics 51:418, 1973

82. Kimbrough RD, Gaines TB: Hexachlorophene effects on the rat brain: studies of high doses by light and electron microscopy. Arch Environ Health 23:114, 1971

82. Light IJ, Sutherland JM: What is the evidence that hexachlorophene is not effective? Pediatrics 51:345, 1973

83. Lockhart J, Simmons HE: Hexachlorophene decisions at the FDA. Pediatrics 51:430, 1973

84. Melish ME, Glasgow LA: The staphylococcal scalded skin syndrome. N Engl J Med 282:1114, 1970

85. Mortimer E, Lipsitz R, Wolinsky E, Gonzaga A, Rammelkamp G: Transmission of staphylococci between newborns. Am J Dis Child 104:289, 1962

86. Shaffer TE, Baldwin JN, Rheins MS, Sylvester RF Jr: Staphylococcal infections in newborn infants. I. Study of an epidemic among infants and nursing mothers. Pediatrics 18:750, 1956

87. Shaffer TE, Baldwin JN, Wheeler EE: Staphylococcal infections in nurseries. In Advances in Pediatrics, Vol 10. Chicago, Year Book Med Pub, 1958, p 243

88. Shuman RM, Leech RW, Alvord EC: Neurotoxicity of hexachlorophene in the human: I. A clinicopathologic study of 248 children. Pediatrics 54:689, 1974

89. Simon HJ, Allwood-Paredes J, Trejos A: Studies on neonatal staphylococcal infection. I. Ecology and prevention in a maternity hospital in El Salvador. Pediatrics 35:254, 1965

90. Simon HJ, Yaffe SJ, Gluck L: Effective control of staphylococci in a nursery. N Engl J Med 265:1171, 1961

91. Williams CPS, Oliver TK Jr: Nursery routines and staphylococcal colonization of the newborn. Pediatrics 44:640, 1969

GONOCOCCAL INFECTION

92. Barsam PC: Specific prophylaxis of gonorrheal ophthalmia neonatorum. N Engl J Med 274:731, 1966

93. Committee on Fetus and Newborn: Standards and Recommendations for Hospital Care of Newborn Infants, 5th ed. Evanston, American Academy of Pediatrics, 1971, p 103

94. Crede CSF: Die Verhutung der Augenentzundung der Neugeborenen. Arch Gynaekol 17:50, 1881

95. Handsfield HH, Holmes KK, Hoelson WA: Gonocccal amniotic infection syndrome. Clin Res 20:233, 1972

96. Mellin GW, Kent MP: Ophthalmia neonatorum: is prophylaxis necessary? Pediatrics 22:1006, 1958

CONGENITAL SYPHILIS

97. Alford CA, Polt SS, Cassady GE, Straumfjord JV: IgM-fluorescent treponemal antibody in the diagnosis of congenital syphilis. N Engl J Med 280:1086, 1969

97a. Fiumara NJ, Lessell S: Manifestations of late congenital syphilis. Arch Dermatol 102:78, 1970

98. Hardy JB, Hardy PH, Oppenheimer EH, Ryan SJ, Sheff RN: Failure of penicillin in a newborn with congenital syphilis. JAMA 212:1345, 1970

99. Hoffman OD, Herweg JC: Status of serological testing for congenital syphilis. J Pediatr 71:686, 1967

100. Mamunes P, Budell JW, Steward RE, Cave VG, Andersen JA: Early diagnosis of neonatal syphilis. Am J Dis Child 120:17, 1970

101. Oppenheimer EH, Hardy JB: Congenital syphilis in newborn infant: clinical and pathological observations in recent cases. Johns Hopkins Med J 129:63, 1971

102. Wilkinson RH, Heller RM: Congenital syphilis: resurgence of an old problem. Pediatrics 47:27, 1971

TETANUS NEONATORUM

103. Gedukoglu G, Yalcin I, Aggen A, Cakin I: Diazepam therapy in tetanus. Summaries of the scientific papers IX Mediterranean and Middle Eastern Pediatric Congress, 1973, p 23

104. McCracken GH, Dowell DL, Marshall FN: Double-blind trial of equine antitoxin and human immune globulin in tetanus neonatorum. Lanect 1:1146, 1971

105. Nourmand A, Ghavami A, Ziai M, Tahernia AC: Tetanus neonatorum. Iran Clin Pediatr 9:609, 1970

106. Ogbeide MI: Problems of neonatal tetanus in Lagos. J Trop Pediatr 12:71, 1966

107. Tompkins AB: Neonatal tetanus in Nigeria. Br Med J 1:1382, 1958

LISTERIOSIS

108. Florman AL, Sundararajan VL: Listeriosis among nursery mates. Pediatrics 41:784, 1968

109. Lavetter A, Leedom JM, Mathies AW, Ivler D, Wehrle PF: Meningitis due to Listeria monocytogenes. A review of 25 cases. N Engl J Med 285:598, 1971

110. Nelson JD, Shelton S, Parks D: Antibiotic sensitivity of Listeria monocytogenes and treatment of neonatal listeriosis with ampicillin. Acta Pediatr Scand 56:151, 1967

GROUP B STREPTOCOCCAL INFECTIONS

111. Baker CJ, Barrett FF, Gordon RC, Yow MD: Suppurative meningitis due to streptococci of Lancefield group B: a study of 33 infants. J Pediatr 82:724, 1973

112. Barton LL, Feigin RD, Lins R: Group B beta hemolytic streptococcal meningitis in infants. J Pediatr 82:719, 1973

113. Bergqvist G, Hurvell B, Thal E, Vaclavinkova V: Neonatal infections caused by group B streptococci. Relation between the occurrence in the vaginal flora of term pregnant women and infection in the newborn infant. Scand J Infect Dis 3:209, 1971

114. Eickhoff TC, Klein JO, Daly AD, Ingall D, Finland M: Neonatal sepsis and other infections due to group B beta-hemolytic streptococci. N Engl J Med 271:1221, 1964

115. Franciosi RA, Knostman JD, Zimmerman RA: Group B streptococcal neonatal and infant infections. J Pediatr 82:707, 1973

116. McCracken GH Jr: Group B streptococci: the new challenge in neonatal infections. J Pediatr 82:703, 1973

117. Rogers KB: Neonatal meningitis and pneumonia due to Lancefield group B streptococci. Arch Dis Child 45:147, 1970

PERINATAL TUBERCULOSIS

118. Avery ME, Wolfsdorf J: Diagnosis and treatment: approach to newborn infants of tuberculous mothers. Pediatrics 42:519, 1968

119. Cohen SN: Personal communication, 1972

120. David SF, Finley SC, Hare WK: Congenital tuberculosis. J Pediatr 57:221, 1960

121. Kendig EL Jr: BCG vaccine in management of infants born of tuberculous mothers. N Engl J Med 281:520, 1969

122. Morrison JE: Fetal and Neonatal Pathology, 3rd ed. New York, Appleton-Century-Crofts, 1970, p 609

123. Steiner M: Personal communication, 1972

124. Voyce MA, Hunt AC: Congenital tuberculosis. Arch Dis Child 41:299, 1966

125. Wolff E: Ueber Zircumzisionstuberkulose. Klin Wochenschr (Berl) 58:1531, 1912

20

Nonbacterial Infection

TORCH SYNDROME

The acronym, "ToRCH syndrome" (toxoplasmosis, rubella, cytomegalovirus and h. simplex), is applied to a group of nonbacterial diseases capable of infecting the fetus during the first trimester of pregnancy or later and causing a wide range of teratogenic changes. All have several features in common: they may cause mild or inapparent illness in the mother, and except on an experimental basis, none are amenable to specific therapy. Rubella alone of this group (in 1975) is largely preventable through programs of active immunization.

With the exception of rubella, the frequency and degree of fetal damage following exposure to the causative organism (as well as to other potential teratogenic organisms, such as Group B coxsackieviruses and varicella virus) is unknown and may be so low as to discourage recommendation of therapeutic abortion when maternal illness is diagnosed during the first trimester.

Elimination of these diseases through widespread immunization appears to offer the only future solution for combatting their teratogenic potential.

CONGENITAL RUBELLA

Since Gregg's discovery in 1941 that maternal rubella during the early part of pregnancy is associated with an increased incidence of cataracts (13), deafness and congenital heart disease, a wealth of knowledge has accumulated. Much information

was gathered after the severe rubella epidemic of 1964, in which the incidence and severity of congenital anomalies appeared to exceed those of previously observed epidemics (34, 35). Because the rubella virus had been first isolated and grown in 1961 (25), study of the 1964 epidemic was greatly facilitated. It was not long after this that a successful vaccine against rubella became commercially available (22).

The rubella virus is generally grouped with the myxovirus family. The agent is moderately large (150 to 200 mμ) in diameter and is inactivated by extremes of pH, heat and chemical reagents. It produces interference with other viral agents, such as ECHO 11, on several lines of tissue culture and a cytopathic effect on rabbit kidney and cornea. The basic effects of the virus are inhibition of mitosis, increased number of chromosomal breaks and a subnormal number of cells due to interference with cell division, with resultant hypoplasia of organs (2, 24, 26).

TRANSMISSION TO THE FETUS

The maternal illness is mild and the rash nonspecific. In the absence of an epidemic the diagnosis may be overlooked in the mother.

The transplacental passage of rubella virus occurs predominantly during the first trimester of pregnancy, especially during the first four weeks. In fact fetal infection almost invariably follows first trimester infection in the mother. However, several investigators (14, 38) have observed congenital rubella in infants whose mothers developed the infection during the second trimester of pregnancy. Another mechanism of fetal infection may be transmission from the maternal genital tract with ascent into the amniotic cavity (32).

Unlike the mild form of the disease seen in older children and adults, the fetus is severely affected, with the virus being capable of damaging almost all organ systems. Lesions are found in the endometrium, placenta, embryo and fetus. Progressive sclerosing villous inflammation may account for vascular anomalies and failure of intrauterine growth. Angiopathy is observed in chorionic and embryonic tissue recovered at an early stage in gestation (6).

The virulence of the disease in the fetus and its extremely benign postnatal course may be related to the virus–antibody–host interaction. In postnatal infection the rise in serum antibody concentrations following infection is associated with a rapid disap-pearance of virus from the tissues. This is not true, however, in fetal infection, in which the virus may be recovered from several sites for weeks, months and even years after infection, despite rising antibody titers. The reason for viral persistence has not yet been explained.

CLINICAL MANIFESTATIONS

The infant with congenital rubella exhibits many physical signs that aid in establishing the correct diagnosis shortly postpartum (20). These findings, in the approximate order of frequency, include hepatomegaly and hepatitis (8), splenomegaly (17), extramedullary hematopoiesis (Fig. 20–1), congenital heart disease (patent ductus arteriosus, ventricular septal defect, atrial septal defect and pulmonic stenosis—12, 17, 30, 33, 37, 39), myocardial necrosis, hypoplastic abdominal aorta (31), eye defects (cataracts and glaucoma), thrombocytopenia (27, 42), interstitial pneumonitis, adenopathy, bone lesions (27, 31, 36), CNS lesions (microcephaly, encephalitis and hearing loss—19, 29), anemia, abnormal dermatoglyphics (1), GU abnormalities (polycystic kidney, duplications of collecting systems—21) and GI abnormalities (esophageal and jejunal atresia —9).

The most severely affected infants exhibit microcephaly (secondary to involvement of the CNS early in gestation), thrombocytopenia and severe growth retardation. Findings of thrombocytopenic purpura may carry a particularly poor prognosis. The overall mortality rate of infants with normal platelet counts is about 10%; however, it rises to about 35% among thrombocytopenic infants with purpura.

A very strong correlation exists between intrauterine growth failure and neurologic deficits, perhaps owing to the fact that in the severe form of the disease both somatic growth and brain development (41) are markedly impaired. From a long-term point of view, language and speech development may also be impaired (40).

The development of diabetes mellitus,

FIG. 20–1. Blueberry muffin lesions in an undergrown term infant with congenital rubella who died at one week of age. (Hodgman JE et al: Pediatr Clin North Am 18:713, 1971)

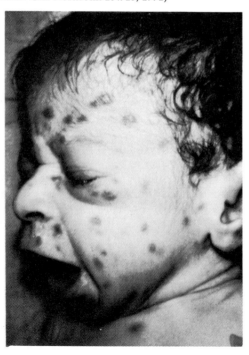

secondary to pancreatic involvement has also been described (3, 10, 11, 18).

DIAGNOSIS AND TREATMENT

Although the diagnosis of congenital rubella is made largely on a clinical basis, especially during epidemic periods, laboratory studies may be of great value. A throat, urine or CSF culture that yields rubella virus confirms the diagnosis.

As with other viral fetomaternal infections, the class and level of antibody are of diagnostic importance, e.g., IgM antibody, which is found in umbilical cord blood or very early in postnatal life, usually reflects fetal infection and active antibody response. Later these antibodies may be replaced with IgG antibodies that have been synthesized by the infant. In infants with congenital rubella a mixture of maternal IgG and fetal IgM antibody is present at birth. The former declines over one to three months, whereas IgM increases to a peak at six months and declines at one year. The infant's IgG level gradually rises, reaching a plateau at one year and remaining at that level thereafter.

Distinction between IgM and IgG class antibodies can be made on the basis of 2-mercaptoethanol incubation, which causes a decline in the value for IgM antibodies but does not affect those of the IgG class. Sucrose gradient columns can also be used to separate the two classes.

Positive titers for hemagglutination-inhibition (HI) or complement-fixing antibody (which are of the IgG class) may be significant on one of several scores (6). If these antibodies decline at a predicted rate (half-life is 24 to 28 days), it is likely that they represent a passive transfer of maternal antibodies in the absence of fetal infection. A slow decline or a stable titer (especially of HI antibody) may signify active response and recovery from infection. Persistently high titers may indicate active, continuing, chronic infection. Frequently, the infant with congenital rubella demonstrates impairment of immunologic mechanisms (5, 23).

Placental permeability to maternal IgG antibodies occurs after the first trimester. Fetal antibody synthesis begins at about the 18th to 20th week of fetal life. It is possible that both of these classes of antibodies play a role in the neutralization of rubella virus in fetal serum.

No specific therapy is available for either fetal or neonatal rubella. Among gravidas with serologic conversion (a fourfold increase in HI antibody titer) during the first trimester of pregnancy, 90% had viral isolation from the fetus (28). Therapeutic abortion is perhaps the most satisfactory approach once a definitive diagnosis has been made in the mother. Gamma globulin administration does not appear to be of much value. It has, however, been recommended when the patient declines abortion.

Once the diagnosis is suspected or confirmed in the newborn patient, isolation should be attempted, since the infant, if indeed infected, continues to shed the virus. It is mandatory that pregnant nursing and medical staff be excluded from caring for the infant.

Treatment is supportive in the neonatal period. Digitalization is indicated when congestive heart failure ensues. Platelet transfusions are of limited value in bleeding secondary to thrombocytopenia.

For those patients who survive the neonatal period, rehabilitation should be initiated as early as possible. Special programs are available for those patients with audiovisual and psychomotor defects secondary to fetal rubella.

PREVENTION

Rubella is now a potentially preventable disease. With widespread use of the effective vaccines developed in the mid-1960s, congenital rubella may become a disease of the past. Immunization of both male and female children should be performed either prior to or on entering school. Immunization should *not* be done in women of childbearing age, since the live virus in the vaccine has the potential of affecting the fetus, and in fact such transmission has been proved with isolation of the vaccine strain from the placenta, decidua and fetus. A susceptible female may be safely vaccinated in the immediate postpartum period, however, as long as conception will not occur for two or more months (16).

At present the efficacy of rubella vaccine is being reassessed in the light of reports (4, 15) of "breakthroughs," or cases occurring among susceptible pregnant females and other adults in communities with nearly complete herd immunity following immunization of children. Instances of congenital rubella have not as yet been reported. No change in current recommendations regarding childhood rubella immunization is warranted at present.

CYTOMEGALOVIRUS INFECTION

Cytomegalovirus is responsible for an ever-broadening spectrum of disease, especially among newborn infants and adults with an immunologic deficiency.

The infectious agent is a medium-sized

FIG. 20–2. Intranuclear inclusion body characteristic of cytomegalovirus infection in desquamated epithelial cell. (Diosi P et al: Lancet 2:1064, 1967)

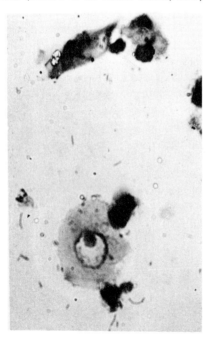

virus, 60 to 120 mμ in diameter, that is DNA containing and heat sensitive; it readily grows on human fibroblast tissue culture. The pathognomonic finding is that of an eosinophilic or basophilic inclusion body (Fig. 20–2) in either the nucleus or cytoplasm. Such cells may be found in nearly all organs of the body and can be recovered from urine and saliva of affected newborn patients.

Maternal infection may occur at any time in gestation from the fourth week to the last trimester (54). The virus invades the fetus during this period by hematogenous spread across the placenta. The severity of illness is proportional to the duration of fetal infection as reflected by the increase in fetal IgM concentrations that generally follow first and second (but not third) trimester infections. Fetuses infected prior to the third trimester usually exhibit severe neurologic and somatic involvement (54, 55).

In general, mothers with cytomegalovirus tend to be younger than the noninfected childbearing population and are often primiparous. Maternal illness may not be clinically apparent, or it may mimic infectious mononucleosis, with fever, lymphadenopathy, malaise and skin rash as presenting signs. A greater than normal incidence of abortion may be associated with fetal infection (43, 46).

The role of the father has been emphasized because of the isolation of high concentrations of cytomegalovirus from the semen of asymptomatic males. This may signify that venereal transmission plays a role in fetal acquisition of this disorder (52).

CLINICAL MANIFESTATIONS AND TREATMENT

Principal signs of cytomegalovirus in the newborn infant are similar to those found in other fetomaternal infections. Jaundice and hepatomegaly are very common findings. Involvement of the CNS usually results in microcephaly with subsequent mental retardation (44). If the CNS is not involved at parturition, it will remain free of infection during the postnatal period. Thrombocytopenia and petechiae are hematologic manifestations. In mild cases, facial petechiae may be the only manifestations of this disease. Although cytomegalovirus usually does not affect subsequent pregnancies, its occurrence (congenitally acquired) in siblings is documented (48).

The teratogenic range of this disease is wide and includes the first branchial arch syndrome (about 25% of cases), occasional cleft palate, high-arched palate, micrognathia, congenital heart disease (tetralogy of Fallot, pulmonary valvular stenosis, ventricular and atrial septal defects), club foot, inguinal hernia, omphalocele and diastasis recti abdominis; CNS malformations other than microcephaly such as hydrocephalus, microgyria, cerebellar aplasia, encephalomalacia, optic atrophy, cystic lesions and periventricular calcifications may be attendant manifestations (44, 53). These calcifications, which are apparent on the skull x ray cannot be distinguished from those observed in congenital toxoplasmosis. It is estimated that each year 5000 infants born in the United States develop mental retardation because of cytomegalovirus (49).

The basic diagnostic modalities are serologic testing (CF and neutralizing antibody that are of the IgG class and may be passively transmitted to the fetus), measurements of cord serum IgM concentrations and most specifically immunofluorescent testing for cytomegalovirus IgM antibody (FA–IgM) in cord serum (50). The latter test measures active response by the fetus to infection and may be positive even in the absence of other serologic signs, or viruria, or both. Virologic testing (histologic studies of cells in urinary sediment for typical inclusion bodies) and viral isolation from urine, saliva and throat cultures are also imperative diagnostic procedures. However, these cells may be absent in both the congenital and acquired forms of the disease. Some major pitfalls in diagnosis are that viruria may be found in 1% to 2% of noninfected newborn patients (58). Conversely, viruria may be absent among infected infants. When present, neonatal viruria may

continue up to the eighth month of age (57, 58).

Treatment of cytomegalovirus infection in the neonate is essentially symptomatic. Antiviral agents such as cystosine arabinoside, 5-fluorouracil and deoxyuridine (45, 49, 53, 56) have been employed, but there is insufficient information to evaluate these preparations. They are highly toxic agents, potency is uncertain, and therefore case selection, as with h. simplex, is difficult. The live vaccine currently (1975) undergoing field trials is a promising new approach to the prevention of this infection (48).

CONGENITAL TOXOPLASMOSIS

Congenital toxoplasmosis is a disease caused by an organism (*Toxoplasma gondii*) of uncertain classification which is usually considered to be a protozoa. It is grown readily in tissue culture, such as HeLa cells and chick embryos, but not in artificial media. The organism, an obligate intracellular parasite about 3 to 6 mμ long, was discovered in 1908 in rabbits and in rodents known as gondii. In 1938 Wolf et al (67) demonstrated the presence of meningoencephalitis among infected newborn infants and were able to transmit the disease from their brain tissue to mice. In 1941 Pinkerton and Weinman (62) and Sabin (65) demonstrated that the organism is a cause of disease in adults. In addition to hydrocephalus, retinitis and encephalitis were demonstrated in the infants. In 1952 Sabin and Feldman developed a dye titer antibody test for toxoplasmosis (66).

Maternal illness may occur at any time during pregnancy and is nonspecific. The earlier in gestation the infection occurs, the greater the severity of illness and likelihood of involvement of the fetal brain and eyes. Involvement during the latter part of pregnancy predisposes the fetus to a more generalized infection with relative sparing of the CNS. No matter in what stage of pregnancy infection occurs, placental involvement is a prerequisite for fetal infection. If the maternal infections occur very early, prior to placental development, the fetus presumably will be completely spared.

Congenital infection is more severe than the acquired form for several reasons: transmission is intravenous, the number of parasites to which the fetus is exposed is greater, and organisms are transmitted in a proliferative phase of growth.

Maternal infection, as demonstrated by a rise in antibody titer, does not necessarily lead to infection or clinical illness in the fetus. A survey of 47 infected pregnant women in France showed that 28 (60%) of their offspring had neither infection nor clinical illness, 12 (25%) had infection without illness, and only 7 (15%) had both infection and clinical evidence of illness (59).

The infection having occurred during a given pregnancy, it will not recur during future pregnancies. Exceptions to this have been reported, however (61). Maternal infection may be acquired from contact with infected cats or by the ingestion of raw or poorly cooked meat.

The incidence of congenital toxoplasmosis ranges from 1:500 to 1:1300 in the United States (60a). Black and Puerto Rican gravidas are more likely than Caucasians to reach childbearing age with positive dye test antibody titers. This finding probably reflects socioeconomic status.

It has been estimated that congenital toxoplasmosis may be responsible for 2% of the severe mental retardation that occurs in the United States.

NEONATAL ILLNESS

The signs of toxoplasmosis in the newborn infant are variable, but they often include pneumonia, hepatosplenomegaly, petechiae, jaundice, hydrocephalus, anemia, chorioretinitis and a maculopapular eruption. Although clinical signs may be apparent at birth, onset may be delayed for as long as several months. The combination of unexplained jaundice and hepatosplenomegaly in a neonate may raise suspicion of toxoplasmosis, as well as other fetomaternal infections.

The classic triad of chorioretinitis, cerebral calcification and hydrocephaly (or occasionally microcephaly) occurs in only 60% or less of infants with clinical evidence of the disease. Bilateral chorioretinitis developing within a few weeks after birth is the single most common finding (86% in one series—60) with CSF abnormalities (pleocytosis and increased protein content the next most common [63%]). Some distinction is made between the septic (or generalized) and neurologic forms of the disease; each, however, has a mortality rate of about 12% in the neonatal period. With CNS involvement, severe neurologic sequelae are common. Mental retardation, convulsions and hydrocephaly or microcephaly are found in 60% to 80% of the cases.

LABORATORY DIAGNOSES AND THERAPY

The dye titer, CF, HI and neutralization tests are all measurements of the IgG class of antibodies and may therefore reflect passive transmission of maternal antibodies. If the Sabin–Feldman test titer is 1:128 or less in both maternal and umbilical cord sera, the probability of infection is unlikely. If the titer is 1:256 or greater, toxoplasmosis becomes a strong diagnostic possibility. The diagnosis is confirmed if the titer rises during the first three months of postnatal life.

The indirect FA–IgM test described by Remington (63) suggests active infection and is therefore a more specific test (especially on a single determination) than any of the IgG-related antibody tests.

The temporal course of the various IgG-related antibody titers differs. The dye titer develops promptly but lasts for several years, whereas the CF titer does not begin to rise until a few months after infection and then declines fairly rapidly. A newborn infant is therefore likely to have a positive dye titer but a negative or very low CF titer. The level of the latter varies with the distribution of the lesion; it tends to be low (1:4 or less) with generalized infection but is likely to be much higher if CNS disease is predominant. The basis of this phenomenon is unknown.

Avoidance of undercooked meat and contact with pet cats may be helpful in preventing this potentially lethal illness.

Two chemotherapeutic agents are available for the treatment of toxoplasmosis: 1) pyrimethamine, 1 mg/kg/day in two divided oral doses (after two to four days this dose may be halved and continued for about one month), and 2) sulfisoxazole, in an oral dose of 100 mg/kg/day. The latter drug must not be given in the presence of hyperbilirubinemia. This drug combination shows considerable synergy in vitro, but there is unfortunately no proof of its efficacy among newborn infants. However, the very high risk of disability and death warrants the use of this combination.

The major side effect of pyrimethamine is platelet depression and anemia that can be prevented by the administration of folinic acid.

HERPES SIMPLEX (HERPESVIRUS HOMINIS)

The DNA-containing *Herpesvirus hominis*, about 75 mμ in diameter, is readily grown on tissue culture and chorioallantoic membranes. It is transmissible to rabbits and guinea pigs, causing keratoconjunctivitis and encephalitis. The two antigenic types are oral (type 1) and genital (type 2). The latter type is responsible for the vast majority of neonatal lesions (73, 74). The frequency of neonatal infection varies from 1:3,200 to 1:30,000 live births in the United States (72, 73, 76).

There are three possible routes of transmission. Transplacental passage may lead to abortion, fetal death or congenital anomaly, such as microcephaly or microphthalmia, especially if the infection has occurred early in gestation (70, 76). Disseminated disease with secondary skin involvement may also be observed. Another route of transmission occurs during parturition, particularly after prolonged rupture of the membranes; secondary systemic spread may follow cutaneous and mucous membrane involvement. A third possibility is droplet transmission

from the respiratory tract of the mother or member of the nursery staff to the neonatal skin or mucous membranes.

The quantity of infectious material in maternal genital lesions may influence the eventual severity of the disease in the infant. Immaturity (based on animal experiments) may be another factor that determines the severity of the infection.

Although cesarean section has been utilized as a means of avoiding transmission of the infection in the presence of maternal genital lesions, it has not always been successful. This emphasizes the role of transplacental transmission.

IMMUNE MECHANISMS

Antibodies against *Herpesvirus hominis* (of the IgG type) are almost universally present in umbilical cord sera in about the same titer as in maternal sera, but they apparently provide the infant with incomplete protection. This lack of protection may be due to the fact that the virus is disseminated by infected WBCs and may also account for the fact that the mortality rate cannot be correlated with antibody titer. Among infected infants, IgM antibody synthesis may not begin for two weeks to two months and may have a poor neutralizing capacity. However, the presence of this type of antibody may be of diagnostic value. Antibodies to each of the two types (oral and genital) cross react but may not be mutually protective.

In addition to serologic differences, the two types differ in cytopathogenic effect in tissue culture, plaque production, mouse neurovirulence and other laboratory properties. Cellular immunity impairment may also be important in neonatal infection, as demonstrated by the high prevalence of *Herpesvirus hominis* infection in Wiskott–Aldrich syndrome.

CLINICAL MANIFESTATIONS

Diagnosis is made on clinical grounds by the appearance of vesicular lesions (Fig. 20–3). Up to 25% of cases, however, may remain

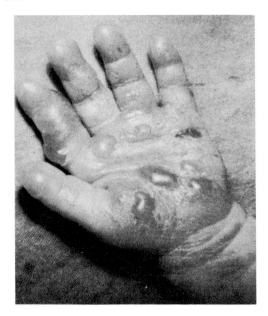

FIG. 20–3. Vesicular lesions involving the palm and fingers of a premature infant with h. simplex infection. (Hodgman JE et al, Pediatr Clin North Am 18:713, 1971)

undetected until postmortem examination.

Signs of disseminated infection may occur from birth to six days. Nonspecific findings of vomiting, anorexia, diarrhea, poor weight gain, hypoactivity, respiratory distress, bleeding and fever may be present. Conjunctivitis and jaundice are sometimes noted. Central nervous system findings include bulging anterior fontanelle, opisthotonus, convulsions and coma. Microcephaly, microphthalmia, hydrocephaly, porencephalic cysts, intracranial calcifications and chorioretinitis may be noted. Examination of the CSF may reveal pleocytosis and an elevated protein level. In about one-third of disseminated cases, vesicular skin lesions are found over various parts of the body. Ulceration and crusting may occur after rupture, with occasional bacterial superinfection. Conjunctival and corneal lesions are encountered less frequently than cutaneous lesions.

Localized infection may involve only the skin and mucous membranes. In addition to the vesicles an erythema multiforme type of picture may be seen, as well as lesions resembling incontinentia pigmenti. The appearance of these localized lesions may be delayed for 10 to 14 days, in contrast to a more rapid appearance in generalized disease.

In the disseminated form of the disease (about one-third of which cases occur in premature infants), mortality may be over 80% (72). Death may be secondary to disseminated intravascular coagulation (DIC) (which may occur in 40% of cases), hypoglycemia, hypoadrenalism and encephalitis.

Infection with *Herpesvirus hominis* should be considered in the differential diagnosis of pneumonia, incontinentia pigmenti and hypoadrenalism when there is no other known etiologic agent.

Cytologic findings of multinucleated giant cells and intranuclear inclusions in cell scrapings from vesicles and ulcers, fluorescent antibody detection (71) or organisms on smear or biopsy are useful laboratory aids in confirming the diagnosis. Elevated levels of serum IgM in the infants point nonspecifically to a viral infection.

At postmortem examination, the liver and adrenal glands are most frequently involved, with the brain, trachea, lung, esophagus, stomach, kidneys, spleen, pancreas, heart and bone marrow also involved. Typical lesions include areas of focal necrosis surrounded by an inflammatory response. Epithelial cells show both nuclear and cytoplasmic changes. The latter include eosinophilic intranuclear inclusions, multinucleated giant cells and degeneration. Eosinophilic inclusion bodies surrounded by "halos" (Fig. 20–4) are observed in the nucleus (72).

THERAPY

The general supportive therapy for infants with *Herpesvirus hominis* infection consists of warmth, proper oxygenation, IV administration of fluids, heparinization in the presence of DIC, and antibiotic administration to treat secondary infections. Use of gamma globulin is ineffective (72).

Herpesvirus hominis infection, however,

is the one life-threatening neonatal viral disease in which chemotherapeutic agents are of some potential value. Agents that have been used include 5-iodo-2'-deoxyuridine (IDU), in a dosage of 50 to 100 mg/kg/day for 4 to 5 days (68), and cytosine arabinoside, 2 mg/kg/day given intravenously over 6 to 12-hour periods for 5 to 7 days (69). Another experimental approach utilizes an agent capable of inducing interferon production, such as Poly I:C. Both IDU and cytosine arabinoside are extremely toxic, and their efficacy in combating neonatal *Herpesvirus hominis* infection has never been clearly demonstrated. The number of cases suitable for such treatment is small, and the course of the untreated disease is variable. Use of these agents must still be considered experimental.

GROUP B COXSACKIEVIRUSES

Group B coxsackieviruses are small (25 to 30 mμ) RNA-containing viruses that are grown readily in tissue culture and which cause typical neuropathologic signs in mice.

FETAL INFECTION

Transplacental and infant to infant transmission of Group B coxsackieviruses usually occur during local epidemics of this group of disorders and have been reported from various parts of the world (80, 81).

When maternal infection occurs during the first trimester, the virus may have a teratogenic effect on the fetus (77, 78). Genitourinary anomalies, such as hypospadias, epispadias, cryptorchidism and hydrocele, are associated with maternal infection with coxsackieviruses B2 and B4; infection with coxsackievirus A9 has been associated with pyloric stenosis, hare lip and cleft palate, while a variety of congenital cardiac disorders have been described following maternal infection with coxsackieviruses B3 and B4. Musculoskeletal and CNS anomalies have also been implicated as sequelae of coxsackievirus infection. Infants

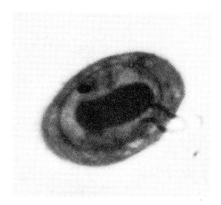

FIG. 20–4. Cell from urine sediment of a neonate with h. simplex infection showing intranuclear inclusion body surrounded by a halo. (Florman et al: JAMA 222:130, 1973. Copyright, American Medical Association.)

with congenital anomalies secondary to first trimester coxsackievirus infection usually show evidence of intrauterine growth retardation.

A variety of clinical signs appears in the infected infant within the first eight or nine days of life. Anorexia, weight loss, diarrhea, vomiting, pallor, jaundice, irritability, respiratory distress and hepatomegaly may all be encountered. Myocarditis associated with cardiac enlargement, tachycardia and ST segment and T-wave changes are often seen on the ECG (79). Aseptic meningitis with pleocytosis (usually 100–1000 mononuclear cells /mm³) and elevated CSF protein is a frequent finding. The clinical course varies from gradual recovery over a one to two-week period to rapid deterioration leading to death.

A presumptive diagnosis is based on the combined findings of aseptic meningitis and myocarditis in a newborn infant. The virus may be isolated from the feces in almost all cases and from the throat in about one-half of all cases. At postmortem examination it can be isolated from the brain and myocardium. Elevated or rising antibody titers are frequently found (82).

There is no specific therapy for the treatment of coxsackievirus infection. Digitalization may be helpful if congestive heart failure is present.

RESPIRATORY VIRUS INFECTIONS

Occasionally infants with cough, rhinorrhea and mild respiratory distress are seen in the nursery. Even after exhaustive evaluations the specific etiology of the infection may not be ascertained. If no bacterial agent is isolated, and no other noninfectious cause for the signs (such as RDS) is found, the diagnosis may be made by exclusion of a viral respiratory tract infection. Although no specific therapy is yet available for this group of illnesses, many attempts have been made recently to isolate the underlying viral agents. Some of the viruses that have been isolated are the respiratory syncitial virus (84), ECHO (85, 86), parainfluenza (88), influenza (83), adenoviruses (87) and coxsackievirus (see section Group B Coxsackieviruses).

INFLUENZA

Of special interest are the influenza viruses, since epidemics occur with regular frequency in the North American continent. During an epidemic of Hong Kong influenza in Montreal in the winter of 1971–72, Bauer et al (83) encountered three cases among newborn infants whose disease was acquired from infected nursery personnel. Although the initial respiratory signs were dramatic, the clinical courses were benign and all of the infants recovered. (This suggests that the neonate has the immunologic capacity required for spontaneous recovery.)

While transplacental passage of influenza virus has been reported (89), it has no proven teratogenic effect. Most cases in the neonatal period are acquired through direct contact with infected adults or other infants.

Tissue culture and serologic studies are required to isolate viral respiratory pathogens.

The best way to prevent these illnesses from occurring in newborn infants is to exclude all adults with respiratory virus infections from the nursery.

ECHO VIRUS

At least five serotypes of ECHO virus are associated with illness in the newborn infant (85, 86). Although no teratogenic effects are associated with this group of virus, transplacental infection apparently can occur. Affected infants, however, usually acquire the infection postnatally.

A wide range of signs and severity of illness is associated with ECHO virus infection. Type 9 causes meningoencephalitis, which can terminate in death of the infant. Types 14 and 19 can cause hepatic necrosis and death. A milder type of infection with occasional fever and respiratory symptoms has been described with type 22 infection. Type 17 causes lethargy, anorexia, fever and rash.

In its most severe form, neonatal ECHO virus infection may resemble coxsackievirus and Herpesvirus infection, all of which are characterized by anorexia, hypotonia, hypothermia, respiratory distress with cyanosis and apnea, jaundice, disseminated intravascular coagulation and abnormal liver function tests. Hepatic and adrenal necrosis and encephalitis may occur in all of these illnesses. However, a vesicular rash distinguishes Herpesvirus infection from the other two.

There is no effective treatment, and a definitive diagnosis is usually not available until the infant has either recovered or died.

VARICELLA

Maternal varicella may affect the fetus in two ways. More commonly, a maternal infection in the weeks just prior to delivery may result in neonatal infection. Transmission of the virus to the fetus either transplacentally or by direct contact during delivery may result in neonatal disease, ranging in severity from extremely mild to fatal (90, 92).

A less commonly encountered form of fetal varicella occurs when the mother is infected during early pregnancy (91, 93), a period of organogenesis. The teratogenic effects of first trimester varicella infection are growth retardation, microphthalmia, cataracts, limb deformities and atrophic skin with scarring. Meningoencephalitis, chorioretinitis and Horner's syndrome are other recognized manifestations of this form of varicella.

NEONATAL HEPATITIS

Neonatal hepatitis refers to a group of inflammatory diseases of the liver caused by either infectious or noninfectious agents. It is usually first encountered between the third and sixth week of life. However, it may occasionally be seen within the first 48 hours postpartum, in which case it is commonly associated with such intrauterine infections as rubella, toxoplasmosis and cytomegalovirus. Hepatitis may also be observed in such bacterial diseases as sepsis and listeriosis. Often the infectious agent cannot be isolated, even after extensive diagnostic studies. However, the hepatitis B antigen, which is a probable cause of hepatitis in older children and adults has been implicated in neonatal hepatitis (94, 97, 102). In a group of 25 neonates and older infants with hepatitis in Athens, Greece (98), 9 of the patients had disease associated with this antigen, the course of which was not only more severe than that of the disease not associated with this agent, but which also paralleled in severity the course in patients over 50 years of age.

Two of the affected infants died, and two more developed cirrhosis. In three cases exchange transfusion was the probable route of transmission, and in the others it was felt that transmission was either by the oral-fecal route or through breast milk. The relative importance of placental transmission of hepatitis B antigen is unknown. Since there is a marked delay (100 to 120 days) in the appearance of hepatitis B antigen in newborn infants, a point can be made against transplacental passage as the primary mode of transmission of the disease. The isolation of hepatitis B antigen from umbilical cord serum, however, strengthens the possibility of intrauterine transmission. A possible mode of transmission might be secondary to maternal bleeding into the fetal circulation, present in about 6% of pregnancies.

Hepatitis due to other causes tends to be less severe. Congenital syphilis as a cause of hepatitis is rarely encountered today. Hepatitis B-related antigens, such as Milan antigen (100), may be causally related to hepatitis. Such noninfectious etiologies as galactosemia, hereditary tyrosinemia (95), genetically determined α-1-antitrypsin deficiencies (100) and possibly certain anesthetic agents may be responsible for the production of hepatitis (103). In addition, there is an apparent increased incidence of hepatitis among infants with Down's syndrome and the trisomy E syndrome.

DIAGNOSIS AND TREATMENT

The diagnostic evaluation of infants in whom hepatitis is suspected is difficult, and there is often a problem in distinguishing it from biliary atresia. The radioactive rose bengal test is described as a means of differentiating the two conditions, but the necessary collections of urine and stool are difficult to obtain and the test is successful only in the hands of a few competent investigators (96, 101). Tests of liver function may show evidence of combined obstruction and hepatocellular damage in both conditions. Measurements of serum glutamic pyruvic transaminase (SGPT) may be of some value. The normal level of this enzyme in neonatal serum is 10 to 90 units/100 ml. Slight elevations (100 to 300 units/100 ml) suggest an obstructive process, while levels over 300 units/100 ml suggest hepatocellular damage. However, overlap of values is often encountered. Elevations of serum levels of two enzymes, γ-glutamyl transpeptidase and 5-nucleotidase, may indicate biliary obstruction.

Biopsy studies of the liver during the late neonatal period often are not conclusive in distinguishing the two diseases. Multinucleated giant cells, which are often seen, reflect the regenerative capacity of the liver and occur in about 65% of hepatitis cases and in 10% to 15% of cases of biliary atresia. Ductal proliferation is a reliable sign of extrahepatic biliary atresia. An operative cholangiogram often differentiates the two conditions.

The specific etiologic agent of the hepatitis is amenable to therapy only in limited instances. In congenital syphilis, administration of penicillin is a specific treatment, as is a galactose-free diet in galactosemia. In other instances treatment must be geared to sound general medical management.

Isolation procedures should be instituted in the presence of such communicable infectious agents as rubella and hepatitis B antigen-associated hepatitis. The hepatitis B antigen may remain long after the jaundice has disappeared, with a mean duration of about 13 months.

Following recovery from neonatal hepatitis, careful long-term monitoring is indicated, since posthepatic cirrhosis is always a possibility.

UNCOMMON INFECTIONS

MYCOPLASMA

Mycoplasmas are unique microorganisms, in that they resemble both bacteria and viruses. Like bacteria they respond to antibiotic therapy and can be grown on artificial media (but only of a particularly enriched type). However, they are smaller than bacteria (but larger than viruses) and lack cell walls.

These organisms (primarily *M. hominis* type I), including the T or tiny strains, are often isolated from the female GU tract (104). A possible association has been made between their presence and spontaneous abortion, premature rupture of the membranes, prematurity and decreased birth weight (105). Since many of the mothers who are infected with mycoplasma also have gonococcal disease, trichomoniasis and urinary tract infection and are of low socioeconomic status, the exact role of this organism remains uncertain.

Although colonization with *M. hominis* may occur in up to 15% of newborn infants, actual disease is rare (107). Sacker et al (108) reported one case in which *M. hominis* was isolated both from a skin abscess in the infant and the mother's genital tract. The organism has also been associated with neonatal conjunctivitis (106).

The diagnosis is made by observing the very small colonies growing on a specially enriched agar medium. Their growth is very slow, and they often will not be observed for several weeks. A magnifying glass is needed to identify them. Typically they have a "fried egg" appearance with a dark center and grow below the surface of the agar.

CANDIDIASIS

Neonatal infection with *Candida albicans* usually occurs secondary to maternal vulvovaginitis. This yeastlike fungus is usually transmitted during descent through the birth canal, although amniotic infection has also been reported (111, 112). It may also be transmitted postnatally through contaminated nipples and other objects.

The most commonly encountered lesion is oral thrush, in which a whitish exudate develops on the oral mucosa. Passage of the organism in the stool may be associated with a perianal candidal dermatitis. Skin lesions may also appear anywhere on the body. More serious complications, such as invasion of deep tissues and the bloodstream, are rare in newborn infants (109, 110).

Diagnosis is made by microscopic identification of the organism (Fig. 20–5). This is done by suspending a scraping of the exudate in a drop of 10% sodium hydroxide solution. *Candida albicans* can also be grown on Sabouraud's culture medium.

Neonatal candidiasis can best be prevented by treatment of maternal vulvovaginitis. Treatment of oral candidiasis in the newborn infant consists of oral administration of 100,000 units of nystatin solution, three or four times daily for about one week. The skin lesion may be treated by topical application of nystatin ointment. Occasionally amphotericin B is administered topically.

MALARIA

Congenital malaria infection is rare in the United States. Even in cases of advanced illness in the mother, the fetus is usually spared. Fetal transmission is thought to be secondary to fetomaternal transfusion. When cases occur, they are usually of the falciparum variety and responsive to chloraquine therapy.

Diagnosis may be made on the basis of demonstration of the parasite within the RBC and the presence of specific FA-IgM in the infant's serum (114).

There have been two reported cases of malaria due to exchange transfusion in the neonatal period (113, 115). These were associated with anemia and hepatosplenomegaly and responded to treatment.

TRICHOMONAS VAGINALIS

Trichomonas vaginalis, a flagellated protozoa, is a major cause of vaginitis among premenopausal adult females and has also been reported as an etiologic agent in neonatal vaginitis (116, 118).

The organism is transmitted directly to the infant during delivery from an infected birth canal. Because the neonatal vagina shows a maternal estrogen effect during the first days of life, the vaginal epithelium is similar to that of the adult and provides a suitable environment for proliferation of the microorganism.

The infant may be an asymptomatic carrier of the organism or may develop vaginitis either as an isolated finding or together with urinary tract infection.

Diagnosis is made either by demonstration of the organism on direct smear with Giemsa's stain or on wet smear following culture in Diamond's medium (117).

Successful treatment has been reported in full-term infants using metronidazole, 50 mg orally, every eight hours for five days. This drug, however, is carcinogenic in

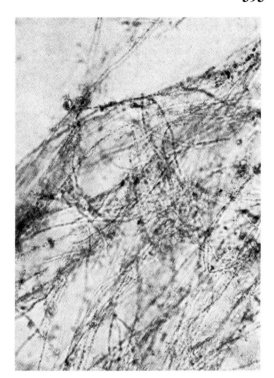

FIG. 20-5. Smear of meconium with mycelia of *C. albicans.* (Sonnenschein et al: Am J Dis Child 107:260, 1964. Copyright, American Medical Association.)

rodents and mutanogenic in bacteria, and must be regarded as potentially dangerous in humans (117a).

REFERENCES

CONGENITAL RUBELLA

1. Achs RMD, Harper RG, Siegel M: Unusual dermatoglyphic findings associated with rubella embryopathy. N Engl J Med 274:148, 1966
2. Boue A, Boue JG: Effects of rubella virus infection on the division of human cells. Am J Dis Child 118:45, 1969
3. Bunnel CE, Monif GRG: Interstitial pancreatitis in the congenital rubella syndrome. J Pediatr 80:465, 1972
4. Chang IW, Des Rosiers S, Weinstein L: Clinical and serologic studies of an outbreak of rubella in a vaccinated population. N Engl J Med 283:246, 1970
5. Claman HN, Suvatte V, Githens JH, Hathaway WE: Histiocytic reaction in dysgammaglobulinemia and congenital rubella. Pediatrics 46:89, 1970

6. Cooper LZ, Matters B, Rosenblum JK, Krugman S: Experience with a modified rubella hemagglutination inhibition antibody test. JAMA 207:89, 1967

7. Driscoll SH: Histopathology of gestational rubella. Am J Dis Child 118:49, 1969

8. Esterly JR, Oppenheimer EH: Pathological lesions due to congenital rubella. Arch Pathol 87:380, 1969

9. Esterly JR, Talbert JL: Jejunal atresia in twins with presumed congenital rubella. Lancet 1:1028, 1969

10. Forrest JM, Menser MA, Burgess JA: High frequency of diabetes mellitus in young adults with congenital rubella. Lancet 2:332, 1971

11. Forrest JM, Menser MA, Harley JD: Diabetes mellitus and congenital rubella. Pediatrics 44:445, 1969

12. Fortuin NJ, Morrow AG, Roberts WC: Late vascular manifestations of the rubella syndrome. Am J Med 51:134, 1971

13. Gregg NM: Congenital cataract following german measles in the mother. Trans Ophthalmol Soc Aust (1941) 3:35, 1942

14. Hardy JB, McCracken GH, Gilkeson MR, Sever JL: Adverse fetal outcome following maternal rubella after the first trimester of pregnancy. JAMA 207:2414, 1969

15. Horstmann DM, Liebhaber H, Le Bouvier GL, Rosenberg DA, Halstead SB: Rubella: reinfection of vaccinated and naturally immune persons exposed in an epidemic. N Engl J Med 283:771, 1970

16. Horstmann DM, Liebhaber H, Kohorn EJ: Postpartum vaccination of rubella-susceptible women. Lancet 2:1003, 1970

17. Jeresaty RM, Russell WR: Hepatosplenomegaly and heart disease in congenital rubella syndrome. Pediatrics 39:36, 1967

18. Johnson GM, Tudor RB: Diabetes mellitus and congenital rubella infection. Am J Dis Child 120:453, 1970

19. Karmody CS: Subclinical maternal rubella and congenital deafness. N Engl J Med 278:809, 1968

20. Menser MA, Dorman DC, Kenrick KG, Purvis-Smith SG, Slinn RF, Dods L, Harley JD: Congenital rubella: long-term follow-up study. Am J Dis Child 118:32, 1969

21. Menser MA, Robertson SEJ, Gillespie AM, Murphy AM: Renal lesions in congenital rubella. Pediatrics 40:904, 1967

22. Meyer HM Jr, Parkman PD, Hobbins TE, Ennis FA: Clinical studies with experimental live rubella virus vaccine (strain HPV-77): evaluation of vaccine-induced immunity. Am J Dis Child 115:648, 1968

23. Michaels RH: Immunologic aspects of congenital rubella. Pediatrics 43:339, 1969

24. Naeye RL, Blanc W: Pathogenesis of congenital rubella. JAMA 194:1277, 1965

25. Parkman PD, Buescher EJ, Artenstein MS: Recovery of rubella virus from army recruits. Proc Soc Exp Biol Med 111:225, 1962

26. Plotkin SA, Vaheri A: Human fibroblasts infected with rubella virus produce a growth inhibitor. Science 156:659, 1967

27. Rausen AR, London RD, Mizrahi A, Cooper LZ: Generalized bone changes and thrombocytopenic purpura in association with intrauterine rubella. Pediatrics 36:264, 1965

28. Rawls WE, Desmyter J, Melnick JL: Serologic diagnosis and fetal involvement in maternal rubella. JAMA 203:627, 1968

29. Rorke LB, Spiro AJ: Cerebral lesions in congenital rubella syndrome. J Pediatr 70:243, 1967

30. Rowe RD: Maternal rubella and pulmonary artery stenosis: report of 11 cases. Pediatrics 32:180, 1963

31. Rudolph AJ, Singleton EB, Rosenberg HS, Singer DB, Phillips CA: Osseous manifestations of the congenital rubella syndrome. Am J Dis Child 110:428, 1965

32. Seppälä M, Vaheri A: Habitual rubella infection of the female genital tract. Lancet 1:46, 1974

33. Siassi B, Emmanouilides GC: Hypoplasia of the abdominal aorta associated with the rubella syndrome. Am J Dis Child 120:476, 1970

34. Siegel M, Fuerst HT, Duggan W: Rubella in mother and congenital cataracts in child. JAMA 203:632, 1968

35. Siegel M, Fuerst HT, Guinee VF: Rubella epidemicity and embryopathy. Am J Dis Child 121:469, 1971

36. Singleton EB, Rudolph AJ, Rosenberg HS, Singer DB: Roentgenographic manifestations of the rubella syndrome in newborn infants. Am J Roentgenol Radium Ther Nucl Med 97:82, 1966

37. Tang JS, Kauffman SL, Lynfield J: Hypoplasia of pulmonary arteries in infants with congenital rubella. Am J Cardiol 27:491, 1971

38. VesiBari J: Rubella antibodies in infants whose mothers had rubella during the 2nd and 3rd trimesters of pregnancy. Scand J Infect Dis 3:1, 1971

39. Vince DJ: The role of rubella in the etiology of supravalvular aortic stenosis. Can Med Assoc J 103:1157, 1970

40. Weinberger MM, Masland MW, Asbed RA, Sever JL: Congenital rubella presenting as retarded language development. Am J Dis Child 120:125, 1970

41. Zausmer E: Congenital rubella: pathogenesis of motor deficits. Pediatrics 47:26, 1971

42. Zinkham WH, Medearis DN, Osborn JE: Blood and bone marrow findings in congenital rubella. J Pediatr 71:512, 1967

CYTOMEGALOVIRUS INFECTION

43. Berenberg W, Nankervis G: Long-term follow-up of cytomegalic inclusion disease of infancy. Pediatrics 46:493, 1970

44. Collaborative study: CMV infection in the northwest of England. Arch Dis Child 45:513, 1970

45. Conchie AF, Barton BW, Tobin J O'H: Congenital cytomegalovirus infection treated with idoxuridine. Br Med J 4:162, 1968

46. Diosi P, Babuscese L, Nevinglooschi O, Kun-Stoicu G: Cytomegalic infection associated with pregnancy. Lancet 2:1063, 1967

47. Elek SD, Stern H: Development of a vaccine against mental retardation caused by cytomegalovirus in utero. Lanset 1:1, 1974

48. Embil JA, Ozere RL, Haldane EV: Congenital cytomegalovirus infection in two siblings from consecutive pregnancies. J Pediatr 77:417, 1970

49. Hanshaw JB: Congenital cytomegalovirus infection: a fifteen year perspective. J Infect Dis 123:555, 1971

50. Hanshaw JB, Steinfeld HJ, White CJ: Fluorescent-antibody test for cytomegalovirus macroglobulin. N Engl J Med 279:566, 1968

51. Kraybill EN, Sever JL, Avery GB, Movassaghi M: Experimental use of cytosine arabinoside in congenital cytomegalovirus infection. J Pediatr 80:485, 1972

52. Lang DJ, Kummer JF: Demonstration of cytomegalovirus in semen. N Engl J Med 287:756, 1972

53. McCracken GH, Shinefield HR, Cobb K, Rausen AR, Dische MR, Eichenwald HF: Congenital cytomegalic inclusion disease. Am J Dis Child 117:522, 1969

54. Monif GRG, Egan EA, Held B, Eitzman DV: The correlation of maternal cytomegalovirus infection during varying stages in gestation with neonatal involvement. J Pediatr 80:17, 1972

55. Nankervis GA, Cox FE, Kumar ML, Gold ME: A prospective study of maternal cytomegalovirus and its effect on the fetus, abstract. Pediatr Res 6:385, 1972

56. Plotkin SA, Steller H: Treatment of congenital cytomegalic inclusion disease with antiviral agents. In: Antimicrobial Agents and Chemotherapy. Edited by GL Hobby. Bethesda, American Society For Microbiology, 1969, p 373

57. Starr JG, Gold E: Screening of newborn infants for cytomegalovirus infection. J Pediatr 73:820, 1968

58. Starr JG, Bart RD Jr, Gold E: Inapparent congenital cytomegalovirus infection: clinical and epidemiologic characteristics in early infancy. N Engl J Med 282:1075, 1970

CONGENITAL TOXOPLASMOSIS

59. Couvreur J: Prospective study of acquired toxoplasmosis in pregnant women with a special reference to the outcome of the foetus. In Hentsch D (ed): Toxoplasmosis. Bern: H Huber Publishers, 1971, p 119

60. Eichenwald HF: Congenital toxoplasmosis. A study of 150 cases. Am J Dis Child 94:411, 1957

60a. Fuchs F, Kimball AC, Kean BH: The management of toxoplasmosis in pregnancy. Clin in Perinatology 1:407, 1974

61. Langer H: Repeated congenital infection with toxoplasma gondii. Obstet Gynecol 21:318, 1963

62. Pinkerton H, Weinman D: Toxoplasma infection in man. Arch Pathol 30:374, 1940

63. Remington JS, Desmonts G: Congenital toxoplasmosis: variability in the IgM-fluorescent antibody response and some pitfalls in diagnosis. J Pediatr 83:27, 1973

64. Robertson JS: Excessive perinatal mortality in a small town associated with evidence of toxoplasmosis. Br Med J 1:91, 1960

65. Sabin AB: Toxoplasmic encephalitis in children. JAMA 116:801, 1941

66. Sabin AB, Feldman HA: Dyes and microchemical indicators of a new immunity phenomenon affecting a protozoan parasite (Toxoplasma). Science 108:660, 1948

67. Wolf A, Cowen D, Paige B: Toxoplasmic encephalomyelitis. Am J Pathol 15:657, 1939

HERPES SIMPLEX

68. Charnock EL: Five IDU in neonatal HSV encephalitis. J Pediatr 76:459, 1970

69. Chow A, Foerster J, Hryniuk W: Cytosine arabinoside therapy for herpes virus infections. Antimicrob Agents Chemother 10:214, 1970

70. Florman AL, Gershon AA, Blacket PR, Nahmias AJ: Intrauterine infection with Herpes simplex virus. Resultant congenital malformations. JAMA 225:129, 1973

71. Gardner PS, McQuillin J, Black MM, Richardson J: Rapid diagnosis of herpes virus hominis infection in superficial lesions by immunofluorescent antibody techniques. Br. Med J 4:89, 1968

72. Hanshaw JB: Herpesvirus hominis infections in the fetus and newborn. Am J Dis Child 126:546, 1973

73. Nahmias AJ, Alford CA, Korones SB: Infection of the newborn with Herpesvirus hominis. Adv Pediatr 17:185, 1970

74. Nahmias AJ, Dowdle WR, Josey WC, Naib FM, Lavonne MP, Luci C: Newborn infection with Herpesvirus hominis types 1 and 2. J Pediatr 75:1194, 1969

75. Miller DR, Hanshaw JB, O'Leary DS, Hnilicka JV: Fatal disseminated herpes simplex virus infection and hemorrhage in the neonate. J Pediatr 76:409, 1970

76. South MA, Tompkins WAF, Morris R, Rawls WE: Congenital malformation of the central nervous system associated with genital type (type 2) herpes virus. J Pediatr 75:13, 1969

GROUP B COXSACKIEVIRUSES

77. Brown GC, Evans TN: Serologic evidence of Coxsackievirus etiology of congenital heart disease. JAMA 199:183, 1967

78. Brown GC, Karunas RS: Relationship of congenital anomalies and maternal infection with selected enteroviruses. Am J Epidemiol 95:207, 1972

79. Burch GE, Sun SC, Chu KC, Sohal RS, Colcolough HL: Interstitial and Coxsackie B. myocarditis in infants and children. JAMA 203:55, 1968

80. Javett SN, Heymann S, Mundel B, Pepler WJ, Lurie HI, Gear J, Measroch V, Kirsch Z: Myocarditis in the newborn infant: a study of an outbreak associated with Coxsackie Group B virus infection in a maternity home in Johannesburg. J Pediatr 48:1, 1956

81. Rantakallio P, Lapinleimu K, Mantyparvi R: Coxsackie B 5 outbreak in newborn nursery with 17 instances of serious meningitis. Scand J Infect Dis 2:17, 1970

82. Sieber OF Jr, Kilgus AH, Fulginiti VA, Pearlman D: Immunological response of the newborn infant to Coxsackie B-4 infection. Pediatrics 40:444, 1967

RESPIRATORY VIRUS INFECTIONS

83. Bauer CR, Elie K, Spence L, Stern L: Hong Kong influenza in a neonatal unit. JAMA 223:1233, 1973

84. Berkovich S, Taranko L: Acute respiratory illness in the premature nursery associated with respiratory syncytial virus infections. Pediatrics 34:753, 1964

85. Berkovich S, Kibrick S: ECHO 11 Outbreak in newborn infants and mothers. Pediatrics 33:534, 1964

86. Berkovich S, Pangon J: Recoveries of virus from premature infants during outbreaks of respiratory disease. The relationship of ECHO virus type 22 to disease of the upper and lower respiratory tract in the premature infant. Bull NY Acad Med 44:377, 1968

87. Chanock RM, Parrott RH: Acute respiratory disease in infancy and childhood: present understanding and prospects for prevention. Pediatrics 36:21, 1965

88. Moscovici C, LaPlaca M, Amer J: Respiratory illness in prematures and children: illness caused by parainfluenza type 3 virus. Am J Dis Child 102:91, 1961

89. Yawn DH, Pyeatte JC, Joseph JM, Eichler SL, Bunuel RG: Transplacental transfer of influenza virus. JAMA 216:1022, 1971

VARICELLA

90. Abler C: Neonatal varicella. Am J Dis Child 107:492, 1964

91. LaForet E, Lynch CL Jr: Multiple congenital defects following maternal varicella. N Engl J Med 236:534, 1947

92. Neustadt A: Congenital varicella. Am J Dis Child 196:96, 1963

93. Savage MO, Mossa A, Gordon RR: Maternal varicella infections as a cause of fetal malformations. Lancet 1:352, 1973

NEONATAL HEPATITIS

94. Cossart YE, Hargreaves FD, March SP: Australia antigen and the human fetus. Am J Dis Child 123:376, 1973

95. Gaull GE, Rassin DK, Solomon GE, Harris RC, Sturman JA: Biochemical observations on so-called hereditary tyrosinemia. Pediatr Res 4:337, 1970

96. Ghadimi H, Sass-Kortsak A: Evaluation of the radioactive rose bengal test for the differential diagnosis of obstructive jaundice in infants. N Engl J Med 265:351, 1961

97. Gillespie A, Dorman D, Walker-Smith JA, Yu JS: Neonatal hepatitis and Australia antigen. Lancet 2:1081, 1970

98. Matsomiotis N: Personal communication, 1973

99. Nezelof C: Histological findings in neonatal hepatitis. Am J Dis Child 123:299, 1972

100. Porter CA, Haynes D, Mowat AP, Williams R: Etiologic factors in neonatal hepatitis. Am J Dis Child 123:300, 1972

101. Sharp HL, Krivit W, Lowman JT: The diagnosis of complete extrahepatic obstruction by rose bengal I^{131}. J Pediatr 70:46, 1967

102. Smithwick EM, Go SC: Hepatitis-associated antigen in cord and maternal sera. Lancet 2:1080, 1970

103. Thaler MM, Gellis SS: Studies in neonatal hepatitis and biliary atresia. II. The effect of diagnostic laparotomy on long-term prognosis of neonatal hepatitis. Am J Dis Child 116:262, 1968

MYCOPLASMA

104. Braun P, Klein JO, Lee YH, Kass EH: Methodologic investigation and prevalence of genital mycoplasmas in pregnancy. J Infect Dis 121:391, 1970

105. Braun P, Lee YH, Klein JO, Marcy SM, Klein TA, Charles D, Levy P, Kass EH: Birth weight and genital mycoplasmas in pregnancy. N Engl J Med 284:167, 1971

106. Jones DM, Tobin BM: Neonatal eye infections due to *Mycoplasma hominis*. Br Med J 3:467, 1968

107. Klein JO, Buckland D, Finland M: Colonization of newborn infants by mycoplasmas. N Engl J Med 280:1025, 1969

108. Sacker I, Walker M, Brunell PA: Abscess in newborn infants caused by mycoplasma. Pediatrics 46:303, 1970

CANDIDIASIS

109. Dvorak A, Gavaller B: Congenital systemic candidiasis. N Engl J Med 274:540, 1966

110. Koenig UD: Fatal bronchopulmonary moniliasis in premature infant. Dtsch Med Wochenschr 96:818, 1971

111. Lopez E, Aterman K: Intra-uterine infection by candida. Am J Dis Child 115:663, 1968

112. Sonnenschein H, Taschdjian OL, Clark DH: Congenital cutaneous candidiasis. Am J Dis Child 107:260, 1964

MALARIA

113. Czapek EE, Barry DW, Gryboski JD: Malaria in an infant transmitted by transfusion. JAMA 204:549, 1968

114. Harvey B, Remington JS, Sulzer AJ: IgM malaria antibodies in a case of congenital malaria in the United States. Lancet 1:333, 1969

115. Mallin WS, Alter AA, Ritz ND, Dempsey L: Posttransfusion malaria in a newborn. Postgrad Med 54:219, 1973

TRICHOMONAS VAGINALIS

116. Al-Salihi FL, Curran JP, Jung-Shung W: Neonatal trichomonas vaginalis: report of three cases and review of the literature. Pediatrics 53:196, 1974

117. Diamond LS: The establishment of various trichomonads of animals and man in axenic cultures. J Parasitol 43:488, 1957

117a. The Medical Letter, 17:53, 1975

118. Trussell RE, Wilson ME, Longwell FH, Laughlin KA: Vaginal trichomoniasis, complement fixation, puerperal morbidity and early infection of the newborn infants. Am J Obstet Gynecol 44:292, 1942

21

Pharmacology

SANFORD N. COHEN
SARASWATHY K. GANAPATHY

Most women take between four and ten drugs during pregnancy. Since virtually any drug taken by a pregnant woman can cross the placenta and enter the fetus, concern over the potential effect of maternal drug exposure upon both the fetus and the newborn infant is reasonable. The effect upon the fetus of drugs administered to the pregnant woman depends on the period of gestation in which they are given. Early in development, teratogenesis and fetal loss are the major hazards; in the more mature fetus and in the newly born infant, the major hazards involve alterations of the function of systems necessary to sustain life during the perinatal period. There is also a hazard that the slow action of some agents administered to pregnant women will cause effects that will not be manifested until later in the infant's life. An example of this is adenocarcinoma of the vagina developing in adolescent daughters of women who were treated with diethylstilbestrol for high risk pregnancy (29a).

THE PLACENTA

There are six major placental types based on the number of tissue layers that separate maternal from fetal blood (17). In the earliest stages of human gestation, the placenta is epitheliochorial (the maternal and fetal circulations are separated by six layers of tissue), but the developed human placenta is hemochorial (the trophoblast is directly exposed to maternal blood).

Soon after implantation, the embryonic trophoblast gives rise to villi, fingerlike structures having a central mesodermal core that contains blood vessels. The villi in the basal area form the placenta by proliferating and invading the endometrium of the uterus. Other early villi have no functional significance and degenerate rapidly. Maternal vessels, eroded by the invading trophoblastic tissues, form pools of blood within the uterine wall, and these pools later coalesce to form a large lake—the intervillous space. Thus, the placenta is a fetal structure consisting of numerous highly vascular villi that are bathed directly by maternal blood in the intervillous space.

Maternal uterine arterial blood enters the intervillous space via the spiral arterioles. In the intervillous space, only the trophoblastic basement membrane and the fetal capillary endothelium separate maternal from fetal blood. Fetal blood enters the villi via the umbilical arteries. Blood that has passed through the villous capillaries is collected into placental veins, which converge to form the umbilical vein that returns it to the fetus. It has been estimated that an area of ten square meters of villous surface is in contact with maternal blood in the placenta, and the exchange of materials between maternal and fetal circulation takes place across this large area (17).

Substances may be transported across the

placenta by one or several of the following mechanisms: 1) simple diffusion, 2) facilitated diffusion, 3) active transport, 4) pinocytosis, and 5) breaks in villi. The primary mechanism by which substances cross the placenta seems to be simple diffusion. The transfer of a substance by this mechanism occurs in the direction of a concentration gradient and is governed by the same physicochemical processes that operate in other biologic membranes (43).

It is possible that some placental transport also occurs by facilitated diffusion, which allows equilibrium to occur across the membrane more rapidly than would be possible by simple diffusion alone. Active transport may play a role in the passage of some nondrug chemicals from maternal to fetal circulation, but it is unlikely that it is involved in drug transport to a major degree. This mechanism involves the expenditure of metabolic energy and results in the transfer of a compound against a concentration gradient. Neither pinocytosis nor breaks in villi are thought to provide significant access for materials from maternal to fetal circulation.

Various physicochemical factors influence diffusion across the placental membrane. These factors include ionization constants, lipid solubility and molecular weight of the drug, concentration gradient, pH and protein binding. Some factors that influence the diffusion of materials across the placental membranes are intrinsic to the placenta itself. These include blood flow, placental area and thickness and pathologic changes that influence the anatomic configuration of the placenta and the intervillous space (1).

PHARMACOLOGIC AGENTS

PLACENTAL TRANSFER OF SPECIFIC GROUPS

Steroid Hormones

A female fetus may become masculinized in utero as a result of maternal exposure to androgens, progestins or stilbestrol early in pregnancy. This effect may be minimal, re-sulting in slight clitoral enlargement, or it may be so complete as to produce a pseudo-hermaphrodite. Furthermore, it is possible that a fetus of either sex could be stimulated to undergo premature skeletal maturation by these hormonal agents, and should this happen, the individual might never achieve his full stature.

The high incidence of cleft palate in certain strains of mice following the use of adrenocortical steroids in the pregnant female is not seen in man. Sporadic cases of cleft palate have been reported in human infants born to mothers receiving these agents during pregnancy. However, a firm association has not yet been confirmed (11).

Antithyroid Drugs

When propylthiouracil or similar agents are administered to pregnant women for the treatment of hyperthyroidism, relative maternal hypothyroidism may occur and the fetus may be stimulated to produce an excessive amount of thyroid-stimulating hormone. When this occurs, the infant may be born with a goiter. The thyroid status of such infants must be established soon after birth since they may be either euthyroid, hypothyroid or hyperthyroid (61). The main hazard of a goiter to a newborn infant is due to its potential to produce respiratory embarrassment. However, when antithyroid drugs lead to fetal hypothyroidism, brain damage may occur if the hypothyroidism is not diagnosed soon after birth.

Radioactive iodine has been implicated in the production of congenital abnormalities when given early in pregnancy and is capable of destroying the fetal thyroid gland and producing permanent hypothyroidism when given later. Furthermore, it is possible that thyroid tumors may occur later in life in those individuals exposed to radioactive iodine during fetal life (77). Thus, this agent is contraindicated throughout pregnancy.

Anticancer Drugs

One would expect that cancer chemotherapeutic agents would be teratogenic since they interfere with the proliferation of developing tissues. However, they have been used extensively during pregnancy in recent years and have produced much less fetal toxicity than was anticipated either from theoretic considerations or from the results of animal experiments (65). The folic acid antagonists seem to be the only members of this group of drugs that are teratogenic to a significant degree. It is possible that abortion occurs in almost all cases after the administration of some other potent antimetabolites used commonly in the treatment of neoplastic conditions, thus obscuring the true incidence of toxicity to the developing organism.

Aminopterin, a potent antifolic acid agent, may produce either intrauterine death or a clearly defined picture of congenital anomalies when given early in pregnancy. The complex of anomalies that occurs includes cranial dysplasia, a broad nasal ridge and low set ears.

Whenever the use of other chemotherapeutic agents has been implicated in the production of anomalies, it has always been after treatment of the mother during the first trimester of pregnancy. Agents that have been associated with teratogenesis in some cases include 6-mercaptopurine, chlorambucil, triethylene melamine, busulfan, nitrogen mustard and cyclophosphamide.

Anticonvulsants and Tranquilizers

The widespread use of thalidomide early in pregnancy led to an epidemic of congenital anomalies in the early 1960s that is now referred to as "the thalidomide tragedy" (71). It is probably familiar to all of those involved in the care of newborn infants. Thalidomide was introduced as an "ideal" hypnotic and sedative drug since it was not associated with direct toxicity to the recipient and did not have the respiratory depressant action of the barbiturates and other hypnotic drugs. The thalidomide tragedy initiated much of the current concern over drug administration in pregnancy. Other hypnotic drugs have not been implicated in the production of fetal anomalies, but the barbiturates and phenothiazines may produce side effects in the infant.

The anticonvulsant, diphenylhydantoin may be responsible for congenital anomalies in human beings. Cleft lip or cleft palate, or both, may occur with higher frequency in infants born to mothers who have received this drug (39). A hemorrhagic diathesis has also been reported in the offspring of mothers taking diphenylhydantoin, but the relationship of the drug to this abnormality has not been defined. The bleeding in such cases is usually controlled by the administration of vitamin K (42). Another anticonvulsant, trimethadione has also been reported to cause an increased incidence of fetal loss and congenital anomalies (26).

Antihypertensive Agents

There are no reports implicating any drugs in this class in the production of congenital anomalies. However, several of the antihypertensives in common use are dangerous to the fetus and may lead to neonatal depression and other side effects.

Anticoagulants

The coumarin anticoagulants, such as dicoumarol and warfarin, cross the placenta and enter the fetus readily. They do not produce teratogenic effects early in pregnancy, but they may produce hypoprothrombinemia, intrauterine death and fetal or neonatal hemorrhage if administered late in pregnancy. Since these complications may occur even in the absence of prolonged maternal prothrombin time, the fetus may have an increased susceptibility to the action of coumarin anticoagulants.

Heparin does not cause either anticoagulant effects or hemorrhage in the fetus or neonate after it is administered to the mother. It is believed that the heparin molecule is too large and complex to cross the placenta into the fetus. Heparin should be used in the place of coumarin anticoagulants when continuous anticoagulant therapy is necessary late in pregnancy.

Vitamin K

Vitamin K₃ (menadione) is one of the drugs that can induce hemolysis in individuals who have a genetically determined deficiency of glucose-6-phosphate dehydrogenase (G-6-PD) activity in their red blood cells. The administration of this agent late in the third trimester of pregnancy can result in the development of serious neonatal hyperbilirubinemia after the infant is born if the infant has G-6-PD deficiency. Furthermore, if large doses of this synthetic vitamin are administered, hemolysis and hepatotoxicity may occur in the newborn infant, even in the absence of a genetic abnormality. Naturally occurring vitamin K (K₁) does not seem to have this effect.

Hypoglycemic Agents

Insulin is the safest hypoglycemic agent for the treatment of a pregnant diabetic. The various oral hypoglycemic agents have either been connected with fetal loss, teratogenesis or poor control of diabetes during pregnancy (61). This is true for the sulfonylureas (tolbutamide, chlorpropamide) and the biguanides (phenformin).

Prolonged depression and symptomatic hypoglycemia have been reported in an infant whose mother had taken chlorpropamide during pregnancy to control her "mild diabetes" (78). The infant's serum chlorpropamide level at 77 hours of age (when he was still depressed) was reported to be "well within the adult therapeutic range." He was treated with exchange transfusion on the fifth day of life and made a dramatic recovery within six hours after the procedure. This infant was both extrasensitive to the adult blood level of the drug with which he was born and unable to inactivate or excrete it during the first five days of life.

Antipyretic Preparations

Two derivatives of salicylic acid are commonly used for antipyresis and analgesia: a salt of acetylsalicylic acid (aspirin) and salicylamide. Taken immediately prior to parturition, aspirin can cause hypoprothrombinemia and neonatal bleeding. There have been a number of reports of congenital salicylate intoxication in the infants of mothers who had ingested unusually large amounts of the drug near term. The aniline derivatives may lead to the development of methemoglobinemia or hemolytic disease in newborn infants. (The latter is produced in those patients with G-6-PD deficiency but not in normal individuals.) Thus, preparations containing acetanilid, acetampinophen or phenacetin should probably be avoided during pregnancy.

Diuretics

Neonatal thrombocytopenia has been associated with the use of thiazide diuretics during pregnancy. However, there is no evidence that chlorothiazide depresses the production of platelets in the bone marrow. Many of the cases of neonatal thrombocytopenia occurring after maternal chlorothiazide exposure are probably due to the presence in the maternal circulation of antiplatelet antibodies that cross the placenta and affect the fetal platelets.

Drugs of Abuse

Heroin and methadone are addictive narcotic agents used by many women during pregnancy. The syndrome of neonatal narcotic withdrawal has become a common one in many areas and is discussed fully in Chapter 15, Drug Abuse.

Excessive cigarette smoking has been implicated in the causation of intrauterine growth retardation. Carboxyhemoglobin, which is formed when hemoglobin is exposed to carbon monoxide, is found in greater amounts in smokers than in nonsmokers. Exposure of pregnant rabbits to carbon monoxide decreases birth weight and increases neonatal mortality, which indicates that carbon monoxide in tobacco smoke may be at least partially responsible for the reduced birth weight found in infants of smokers (2).

There is no conclusive evidence that LSD

or marijuana act as teratogens in spite of an early report that LSD induces chromosome breaks in leukocyte culture.

DRUGS IN BREAST MILK

Many drugs and drug metabolites are excreted in breast milk. The concentration of each of these in milk depends upon many of the same physicochemical factors that control both the passage of drugs through the placenta and the fat content of the milk, and upon other maternal factors, such as intramammary pressure (12).

Some drugs will be destroyed in the infant's gastrointestinal (GI) tract if they are ingested in milk, e.g., polypeptide hormones and epinephrine. Many others are either present in milk in very small quantities or do not have adverse effects upon the infant when ingested early in life. On the other hand, narcotic analgesics, some oral contraceptives, anticoagulants, hypnotics and tranquilizers have been implicated in the production of a toxic effect in nursing infants (12).

It is well known that environmental contaminants, e.g., DDT and methyl mercury, are excreted in milk. The transmission of toxic substances to the infant via this route may be an important factor in the production of serious illness in some patients and requires further investigation.

EFFECTS OF DRUGS ADMINISTERED DURING LABOR

In our search to improve the infant's chance for a full life, it is important to recognize that drugs administered to a woman in labor may have profound effects upon the fetus just prior to birth and upon the newborn infant soon after delivery. These effects may result in "depression" of the infant, either immediately after birth as reflected in the Apgar score or within the next several days as reflected in unusual behavior patterns (15). The choice of drugs and timing of doses during labor should thus be influenced by our knowledge of the potential hazards of the various agents in common use.

INHALATION AGENTS

A number of inhalation agents are used alone or in combination to provide analgesia or anesthesia late in the course of labor. These include nitrous oxide, cyclopropane, diethyl ether, halothane and others. Nitrous oxide and cyclopropane are used most frequently.

The effects of nitrous oxide and cyclopropane on both the fetus and newborn infant are difficult to evaluate because these agents are almost always used in combination with other analgesics or with hypnotic and sedating drugs. Furthermore, these other drugs, such as barbiturates and ataractics, all tend to potentiate the depressant effect of the inhalation agents. Nevertheless, it is possible to state that neither nitrous oxide nor cyclopropane alone leads to significant neonatal depression when administered to the mother in analgesic concentrations (43). However, an infant born following maternal anesthesia with 75% or more nitrous oxide, or with more than 5% cyclopropane for over seven minutes, may be seriously depressed. The immediate (and obvious) depression may last only several minutes, but the true duration of the drug-induced depression (in behavioral terms) is not known.

BARBITURATES

Sedation, amnesia and anesthesia during labor have all been achieved over the years through the use of various barbiturates. The use of barbiturates during labor has, however, been recently curtailed because of the profound "depression" of the sleepy infants delivered following labors managed with them. This effect may be prolonged and may interfere with the infant's feeding while in the newborn infants' nursery (33). Long-term behavioral effects have also been noted in experimental animals and in human infants following the administration of barbiturates to the mother during pregnancy (18). Chronic use of these agents during pregnancy may lead to signs of barbiturate withdrawal in the newborn infant (9, 18), and it has been suggested that neonatal hemorrhagic disease may occur in infants born to mothers who took large doses of phenobarbital during their pregnancy (42).

There are many reports in the literature that detail the possible hazards of the liberal use of barbiturates during labor (15). All barbiturates cross the placenta rapidly (43), and infants born within several hours of the administration of barbiturates to the mother have significant blood barbiturate levels throughout their early neonatal life. Barbital, amobarbital and phenobarbital all appear to accumulate within fetal brain tissue and to remain there in high concentration for more than two days (53). The ultrashort-acting barbiturate, thiopental, commonly used as an intravenous (IV) general anesthetic may produce immediate depression in infants delivered by cesarean section, but it is probably no more of a problem in this regard than are inhalation agents (20). Thiopental passes to the fetus even during normal labor, but possibly as a result of its concentration within the fetal liver rather than the brain, it does not appear to lead to immediate neonatal depression when administered for vaginal deliveries (24). However, the possibility that it may produce altered behavior later during the neonatal period has not been excluded, and it is not used widely for usual obstetric deliveries.

AGENTS THAT PRODUCE REGIONAL ANESTHESIA

Local anesthetics are all chemically similar to cocaine. They can be divided into two major subgroups—esters and amides. The esters, e.g., procaine, are generally characterized by a fairly long latent period between administration and action, a relatively short duration of action and a relatively poor ability to penetrate tissues. The amides, on the other hand, act more rapidly and longer and can penetrate tissues better. This group, which includes lidocaine, prilocaine, bupivocaine and mepivacaine, is widely used to provide obstetric anesthesia. When any of these agents are used to produce spinal anesthesia, maternal hypotension may occur with a consequent reduction in uteroplacental blood flow. It may be possible to prevent this hazardous situation by the rapid IV infusion of a balanced electrolyte solution prior to the administration of the anesthetic agent (37).

Whether administered by the epidural route or as a paracervical block, the amide drugs all pass through the placenta to the fetus and remain in the infant long after birth. Their effects upon the fetus vary from none to profound depression and even to perinatal death. If a paracervical block is to be used for delivery, a dilute solution (0.25% bupivocaine or its equivalent) should be administered. Perinatal complications increase in frequency as the dose is increased (7, 27).

TRANQUILIZER-SEDATIVES

Chlorpromazine has been used to relieve anxiety, to potentiate analgesics and to prevent nausea and vomiting during labor. None of the published data has been gathered in a controlled study, so there is little basis for any conclusions concerning its efficacy or safety in obstetric use, but there have been reports of acute maternal hypotension and of neonatal respiratory depression after its use, and it probably should not be used during labor. If chlorpromazine is used, it may lead to abnormalities in the infant's capability to control its body temperature after birth. Extrapyramidal signs of phenothiazine intoxication have also been observed in infants born to mothers receiving the drug.

Promethazine, another of the phenothiazine tranquilizers, is better noted for its mild sedative effects than for its effects in psychotic or otherwise agitated patients. It is used widely to produce sedation during labor, but it may increase pain sensitivity in some patients (41). Its rate of excretion by the infant after birth is not known, but it does not seem to have an adverse effect.

However, it should be used in minimal sedating doses and as early in labor as possible.

The newer benzodiazepine drug, diazepam, may have a real advantage for use in labor since it seems to decrease the need for potent analgesic agents (25). It should be used sparingly, however, since it is known to localize in neonatal brain tissue (74) and to produce hypotonia (58), poor temperature control (50) and exaggerated perinatal hypercarbia and acidosis (69).

ANTIHYPERTENSIVE AGENTS

The standard drugs used to treat maternal hypertension may lead to adverse effects in the newborn infant. Reserpine, which produces lethargy and nasal congestion in neonates, may be a significant threat due to the infant's inability to breathe through its mouth, and guanethadine may produce α-adrenergic and ganglionic blockade with subsequent hypotension and diarrhea. These agents should be used sparingly in pregnant women. They should not be used at all for the treatment of late third trimester toxemia. Magnesium sulfate is the agent of choice late in pregnancy, but the newborn infant must be carefully watched for lethargy, flaccidity and recurrent apnea following its use. The depressant effects of the magnesium ion upon the infant may be prolonged, especially following IV administration to the mother.

POTENT ANALGESICS

There has been a great deal of confusion and misunderstanding concerning the use of narcotic analgesics during labor. Because of the numerous reports that such use of morphine leads to the birth of severely depressed infants, it has all but disappeared from use on most obstetric services, being replaced by meperidine and other synthetic agents. It is now clear, however, that when equianalgesic doses are administered by the same route and when the time interval between the dose and delivery is optimal, morphine is probably no more hazardous to the

infant than are these newer synthetic potent analgesics (43).

Meperidine produces depression of the newborn infant if the drug is administered to the mother intramuscularly between one and three hours before delivery. However, if it is given intramuscularly within one hour of delivery, no significant depression of the infant occurs (62). If larger than usual doses are administered, if the drug is given intravenously or if the drug is combined with a barbiturate, the "safe period" will be less than one hour and the chances are greater that the infant will be depressed.

In general, it is sufficient to maintain a narcotized infant's respirations while keeping him warm, and pharmacologic treatment is rarely indicated. If any narcotic antagonist therapy seems indicated, naloxone should be administered. Since nalorphine and levallorphan are both respiratory depressants whose effect on neonatal respiratory depression may be erratic, neither should be administered to depressed neonates.

Pentazocine, a newer synthetic analgesic, has not been evaluated thoroughly for safety during labor as yet. It appears in cord blood soon after it is administered to the mother (8), however, and it may lead to immediate neonatal depression (40). There seems to be no role for this agent in the management of routine labor.

MISCELLANEOUS AGENTS

Many interesting case reports and clinical studies concerning the effects of a number of miscellaneous agents upon the newborn infant tend to emphasize the potential hazard to the newborn infant created by the administration of *anything* to the mother during labor. The intravenous administration of the β-adrenergic blocking drug propranolol led to the delivery of seriously depressed infants in four out of five cases in one study (73). This drug should not be used during labor, except in extraordinary situations. When ketamine was administered intravenously for obstetric anesthesia, mild fetal acidosis, maternal apnea and mild hypertension occurred in many cases. Its use also resulted in immediate neonatal depression in more than one-half of the cases (35). This agent does not seem to be a valuable addition for obstetric use.

CLINICAL PHARMACOLOGY DURING THE NEONATAL PERIOD

Drugs have therapeutic effects either by virtue of their ability to alter human physiology and chemistry or because they are selectively toxic to invading organisms or tumor cells. To be an effective systemic therapeutic agent a drug must first gain access to the body and come in contact with its site of action. To be clinically useful a drug must be eliminated from the body rapidly enough so that toxic quantities do not build up during a course of therapy. Drugs can be eliminated either by metabolic alteration of the molecule into inactive derivatives prior to excretion or by excretion of the active drug itself. Thus four basic processes (absorption, distribution, metabolism and excretion) govern the clinical effectiveness and safety of therapeutic agents.

A better understanding exists today than ever before of the parameters that must be considered when administering drugs to the newborn infant, but safe and effective pharmacotherapy in newborn infants remains problematic. The following section contains both some basic pharmacologic principles involved in planning therapeutic regimens and a discussion of drugs that are frequently used in the newborn nursery population.

ABSORPTION

The process by which a drug enters the body from its site of administration is called absorption. The rate of absorption of a drug is dependent to a large degree upon the nature of the drug and the route of administration, but various host factors may also be extremely important in controlling this rate. Orally administered medications are poorly absorbed in the presence of vomiting and diarrhea, while topical preparations that are not absorbed under usual circumstances may be detected in the blood after they are applied to the skin of a newborn infant, absorption then being possible because of the immaturity of the stratum corneum (66).

The absorption of drugs given by other than parenteral routes is especially variable in the newborn infant. Therefore, parenteral administration is preferred for systemic therapy in neonates.

Administration of a drug via the subcutaneous route is not recommended for therapy of newborn infants for several reasons: the volume that can be administered without compromising the blood flow to overlying skin is limited; the possibility exists of causing damage to adjacent tissues due to the concentrated or caustic nature of the injected material; and absorption may vary due to poor circulation to peripheral areas. The latter is especially important in sick neonates and in very immature infants whose poor peripheral circulation is compromised further by hypothermia.

The use of repeated intramuscular injections in newborn infants has similar potential drawbacks. These include poor peripheral circulation in sick infants and a limitation both in the number of injections that can be given safely into the small muscle mass of the infant and in the amount of material that can be given in each dose. Despite these drawbacks, however, the intramuscular route is usually safe and adequate to provide sufficient drug in the circulation for the treatment of disease.

A drug injected intravenously bypasses all of the factors that affect absorption and enters the circulation directly. Certain parenteral preparations can, however, lead to untoward effects when given intravenously due to the physicochemical properties of the active agent as well as the buffers, preservatives, and other additives. Thus, the use of highly concentrated solutions or those with sclerosing properties can lead to thrombophlebitis or to a sloughing of tissues from infiltration around the site of injection; the IV administration of paraldehyde may lead to acute pulmonary difficulty due to the aggregation of droplets of this water-insoluble agent within pulmonary blood vessels; the aminoglycoside antibiotics, e.g., kanamycin and streptomycin, may interfere with breathing when administered in high doses intravenously because they have a curariform action at high blood concentrations (75); and the injection of drugs via umbilical vessel catheters may either cause serious liver damage (umbilical vein) or marked renal or extremity ischemia (umbilical artery) (70). When appropriate precautions are taken, however, the IV route is safe for the treatment of seriously ill infants.

DISTRIBUTION

After absorption, drugs become distributed between the intravascular compartment and the various body organs and tissues (28). The exact distribution of a drug at a given time after a dose depends on both the patient's physiology and the physicochemical properties of the drug itself. Early organ distribution of any drug is found to be almost directly related to the blood flow to individual organs or tissues (56), but the final distribution of a drug (and its concentration in various tissues) is governed by such factors as the pH of the patient's body fluids, the patient's size and weight, the proportion of the total body water that is intracellular, the lipid solubility of the drug, its ionization constant and the extent to which the drug is bound to plasma albumin or to other body proteins (28). Thus, the final distribution of a specific drug and its sites of highest concentration must be determined experimentally.

A factor of major importance in considering drug distribution in infants is the relationship of plasma protein binding to safe drug therapy. Drugs in the intravascular compartment are bound in varying degrees to the plasma proteins, especially to albumin. This bound component of a drug is neither pharmacologically active nor readily diffusable. The molecules that are bound to albumin represent an internal reservoir of the drug, and alterations in the plasma albumin concentration can have a profound effect on the size of this potential reservoir and on the concentration of the drug in various tissues. Thus, the relative hypoalbuminemia associated with low gestational age must be taken into account when suggesting therapeutic regimens for premature infants; otherwise, toxic drug concentrations may build up in their tissues due to the small size of their plasma reservoir compartment.

When several drugs compete for protein-binding sites, the distribution of one or more of them may be altered, as may the distribution of bilirubin that is also bound to protein. This drug–bilirubin interaction represents a unique hazard for neonatal patients and is an example of the effect of distribution on the action of a compound. Premature infants treated with sulfisoxazole have developed kernicterus when their serum bilirubin concentrations were well below the usual dangerous range (63) because the bilirubin displaced from plasma-binding sites by the sulfonamide gained access to the brain where it had a cytotoxic effect (49).

METABOLISM

Most therapeutic agents are highly lipid-soluble chemical compounds that are filtered by the glomerulus. Some drugs are reabsorbed so completely in the renal tubules that they would persist in the body in an active form for weeks or even months if there were not other mechanisms available to assist in their excretion (6). There are enzymes capable of catalyzing the conversion of such compounds into more polar, water-soluble metabolites that can be eliminated from the body in the urine. Occurring mainly in the liver, these enzymes lead to the oxidation, reduction, hydrolysis or conjugation of active drugs to excretable products.

Newborn infants of most mammalian species, including man, carry out drug metabolism reactions at a diminished rate (19). As a consequence of this, a drug that requires metabolism before it can be eliminated from the body may have a longer and more intense action in infants than would be predicted from studies on more mature individuals. Thus it is essential to know whether a drug must be metabolized prior to elimination from the body before an appropriate dosage schedule can be suggested for its use in newborn infants. Chloramphenicol is one of the few antibacterial agents that must be metabolized in the body before it is excreted. Used extensively for several years to treat premature and full-term infants, it was administered according to a dosage regimen adjusted only for the patients' weight and not for their immaturity, and a number of infants succumbed to its toxic effects because they were not capable of metabolizing it into water-soluble derivatives rapidly (76). Our current understanding of the factors that led to this tragedy should allow us to avoid such accidents in the future.

EXCRETION

Most drugs and drug metabolites are eliminated from the body in the urine. The rate of excretion of drugs in the urine may either be limited by the ability of the liver to metabolize them or by the ability of the kidney to filter and excrete them. Since drug metabolism proceeds very slowly, and since the renal blood flow, glomerular filtration rate (GFR) and tubular function are all diminished in newborn infants, the urinary excretion of drugs is generally delayed during the neonatal period. When newborn infants are to be given drugs that are excreted unchanged in the urine, such as the penicillins and the aminoglycoside antibiotics, e.g., streptomycin and kanamycin, adjusting the dose for the tendency of these drugs to accumulate within the body will minimize the possibility that toxic concentrations will be reached in the patient.

Some drugs reach high concentrations in the bile and are eliminated in the feces. Nafcillin, a semisynthetic penicillin, is eliminated in this way, but it still tends to build up in the newborn infant when large doses are administered. This indicates either that

biliary excretion is diminished or that enterohepatic recirculation is increased during the neonatal period (47). It is also possible that a combination of decreased excretion and increased reabsorption is responsible for this observation.

Some of the doses and regimens recommended in Table 21–1 (see end of chapter) were derived from information on the pharmacokinetics of the drugs in newborn infants, while others are recognized to be safe and effective for use in newborns because of empirical observations gathered over many years. These are the only two bases for recommending drug doses for the most-immature patients. It is no longer acceptable to use the commonly available formulas to derive such doses since we know now that the effect of a drug in the body is governed by its distribution, metabolism and excretion rather than by the weight or size of the patient.

SPECIFIC GROUPS OF DRUGS

ANTIBIOTIC AGENTS

The Penicillins

The antibacterial spectrum of penicillin G includes all non-penicillinase-producing gram-positive cocci, most gram-positive bacilli, pathogenic gram-negative cocci and the spirochetes. Penicillin interferes with bacterial cell wall formation by inhibiting the synthesis of mucopeptides. It is frequently used with a drug that is effective against gram-negative bacilli in the treatment of sepsis neonatorum of undetermined etiology.

Penicillin is excreted in the urine without prior metabolism, and hence excretion is the main factor that controls serum levels. The neonate excretes the drug much more slowly than do older children, and relatively small doses of the drug result in therapeutic blood levels. Six hours after an intramuscular dose of 22,000 IU/kg, the mean serum level in full-term infants was 5.45 μg/ml, whereas in children from 3 to 13 years it was 0.005

μg/ml (6). Thus the daily recommended dose in the newborn infant is 50,000 IU/kg administered intramuscularly in divided doses every 12 hours.

Penicillin is vitually nontoxic when administered in usual doses, but seizures may be produced by very high levels in the cerebrospinal fluid (CSF), and these levels are sometimes reached when a large dose is administered rapidly in the presence of meningitis. Thus, IV administration of penicillin should be done at a carefully controlled rate to the infant with meningitis. Penicillin is usually administered by the intramuscular route, but when IV infusions are being given for other reasons, the drug may be administered by the intravenous route.

Semisynthetic Penicillins

Methicillin, oxacillin, cloxacillin, dicloxacillin and nafcillin have all been effective in the treatment of infections caused by penicillinase-producing staphylococci. From 20% to 55% of staphylococci isolated in some European countries are now methicillin resistant, but methicillin-resistant staphylococci have not been isolated commonly in the United States, and methicillin resistance does not seem to be a major problem here in the mid 1970s. This drug should be replaced with one of the others, however, when serious staphylococcal infections occur in institutions where resistant organisms have become common.

Cloxacillin and dicloxacillin should not be administered to jaundiced infants since at therapeutic concentrations they may displace bilirubin from albumin-binding sites (48).

Ampicillin, another semisynthetic penicillin, has a broader antibacterial spectrum than other penicillins, and while not effective against penicillinase-producing organisms, it is effective against many gram-negative bacilli. Some authors suggest that ampicillin be used instead of penicillin G in the therapy of neonatal sepsis of unknown etiology (29). The choice of which drug to use for an infant in a particular nursery should be based upon the antibiotic sensitivity of the bacteria isolated commonly from infants there.

The excretion of most of these drugs and the factors that govern their serum levels are similar to those of penicillin G (10). Nafcillin is excreted mainly in the bile, but its elimination from the newborn infant is slow nonetheless, and reduced doses are indicated (47).

The Cephalosporins

The members of this group of antibiotics bear a strong resemblance to the penicillins in their chemical structure, mechanism of action, low potential for toxic reactions and possible cross sensitivity. The cephalosporins have a broader spectrum than most penicillins and are effective against many gram negative bacilli and penicillinase-producing staphylococci. Penicillin-resistant staphylococci may be sensitive to cephalosporin, but many develop resistance to this drug after brief exposure. This resistance is related to the production of cephalosporinase, an enzyme analagous to penicillinase.

Cephalothin, the most commonly used drug in this group, is useful for the treatment of *E. coli* infections in neonates when the organisms are resistant to both kanamycin, gentamicin, and ampicillin.

Since the cephalosporins are excreted in the same manner as the penicillins, low doses can be used to produce prolonged therapeutic serum levels in newborn infants (59).

The Aminoglycosides

This group includes kanamycin, gentamicin, streptomycin and neomycin. These drugs act directly on bacterial ribosomes with inhibition of protein biosynthesis. Drugs in this group must be given parenterally when used for the treatment of systemic disease because they are not absorbed from the gastrointestinal tract.

Kanamycin is effective against many of the gram-negative organisms that are commonly pathogenic in the newborn infant and is used in conjunction with penicillin as the combination of choice for the treatment of sepsis of unknown etiology in this age group. It may be used to treat infection with enteropathogenic E. coli and must be given orally for this purpose.

Neomycin, once the drug of choice for the elimination of enteropathogenic strains of E. coli, is no longer preferred because of the emergence of many resistant strains.

Gentamicin has an even broader antibacterial spectrum than kanamycin. It is especially useful for the treatment of infections due to pseudomonas organisms that are resistant to other antibiotics. Its use should be limited to the treatment of pseudomonas infections or of diseases caused by other organisms that are resistant to less toxic antibiotics.

This drug should be used with caution in jaundiced infants, since it may increase the risk of bilirubin encephalopathy (16a).

The main indication for the use of streptomycin in the newborn period is congenital tuberculosis, a very rare entity. It is always used in combination with isoniazid for this purpose.

The aminoglycosides have a prolonged half-life in infants since they are excreted by glomerular filtration and GFR is diminished in immature infants. The average serum half-life of kanamycin is 8.9 hours in premature infants and 2 hours in adults (4). Therapeutically effective serum concentrations of kanamycin (15 to 25 μg/ml) may thus be produced and maintained in newborn infants without the production of significant toxicity by the intramuscular administration of 7.5 to 10 mg/kg every 12 hours. Some authors even suggest that a dose as low as 5 mg/kg every 12 hours is effective in neonates (4). Kanamycin has a curarelike action when present in very high concentrations (75) and should not be used intravenously as a routine. However, it seems reasonably safe to administer the usual therapeutic doses by this route when indicated.

The aminoglycosides may be toxic either

to the eighth cranial nerve, leading to vertigo or deafness, or to the kidney, leading to proteinuria and azotemia. Ototoxicity does not appear to occur in immature infants who are treated with the recommended doses of kanamycin for up to 14 days (21). However, proteinuria, cylindruria and mild azotemia may occur in some infants after the first few days of kanamycin therapy, and the administration of the drug should be stopped if they appear. There is no evidence that permanent renal damage results if the nephrotoxic effects are discovered early and the drug is discontinued promptly.

The Polymixins

Colistin (polymyxin E) is the only member of this group of antibiotic agents that is recommended for use in newborn infants. Its use should be limited to the treatment of infections caused by organisms resistant to other antibiotics since it has a narrow margin of safety when administered parenterally. It is not absorbed from the gastrointestinal tract and is the drug of choice for the elimination of enteropathogenic E. coli. It must be given orally for this purpose. Colistin is excreted unchanged in the urine, but in contrast to other antibiotics, its serum half-life in the newborn infant does not differ significantly from its half-life in adults (5). The basis for this apparent paradox has not been explained as yet. A dose as low as 1.5 mg/kg/day, administered in divided doses intramuscularly every 12 hours, has been found to be effective for the treatment of infections in newborn infants. However, the drug is nephrotoxic, and urinalyses and tests for azotemia must be performed every few days during therapy. In all cases, the course of therapy with colistin should not exceed seven to eight days.

Tetracyclines

Tetracyclines, when administered either to pregnant women or newborn infants, are localized in the mineralized portions of long bones and teeth. This leads to impaired growth rates, fluorescence of long bones and yellow staining of teeth. This group of drugs, therefore, should not be administered either during pregnancy or the newborn period.

Isoniazid

Isoniazid (INH) is the most widely used tuberculostatic agent. It has been recommended for the treatment of overt disease, for the treatment of asymptomatic tuberculin reactors and even for prophylaxis in infants who are likely to be exposed repeatedly to persons with active tuberculosis (3). INH is recommended as one drug in the combination of choice for the treatment of overt congenital tuberculosis and should be part of any therapeutic regimen for tuberculosis in the neonatal period. No serious toxic reactions have been reported to occur in newborn infants after INH administration, but since it requires metabolic alteration before it can be excreted efficiently and since blood levels cannot be measured practically on very small volumes of blood it may tend to build up to a dangerous degree in some infants (16). Thus its safety in the newborn infant has not been established firmly enough to recommend that it be administered *prophylactically* during the first month of life.

CARDIAC GLYCOSIDES

Congestive heart failure and paroxysmal supraventricular tachycardia are currently the only two indications for the use of digitalis preparations in newborn infants. Current concepts of the pathophysiology of respiratory distress syndrome and hydrops fetalis indicate that there is no rational basis for the administration of digitalis glycosides in these conditions.

Digoxin is the digitalis glycoside of choice for the treatment of neonates because it is absorbed well, acts rapidly and is excreted in a relatively short time. A therapeutic regimen can be planned rigorously, rapid results can be expected once therapy is begun, and any toxic effects that occur during therapy will diminish rapidly when the dose is readjusted.

Digoxin is eliminated from the body in the urine in the active form. Some data suggest that there may be an inactive metabolite in the urine as well. Excretion of the drug after it is administered to newborn infants may be delayed by the infants' hepatic and renal immaturity (67). Furthermore, there may be increased myocardial sensitivity to the effects of digitalis glycosides in the newborn period (36). The recommended dose of digoxin for newborn infants is, therefore, slightly lower than that recommended for older infants (34).

ANTICONVULSANTS AND SEDATIVES

The effect of these drugs upon the infant when they are administered to the mother late in pregnancy has already been discussed. However, certain drugs in this group are also indicated for treatment of the neonate itself, and this aspect will be discussed here.

Phenobarbital is the most commonly used drug of this group in the newborn infant. The indications for its use include seizures and neonatal narcotic withdrawal. It is very effective in reducing or stopping seizure activity due to causes other than hypoglycemia or other metabolic derangements, which must be treated by correcting the underlying metabolic abnormality rather than with anticonvulsants. It is also effective in reducing the hyperactivity and irritability that are characteristic of infants of narcotic-addicted mothers.

In some centers, phenobarbital is administered to prevent the development of hyperbilirubinemia or to treat those infants who are already jaundiced (38, 39). The action of phenobarbital in this situation depends upon its ability to induce the activity of the enzyme that catalyzes the conjugation of bilirubin with glucuronic acid in the liver (68). However, since this drug acts to increase the activity of many enzymes in the body, it may have widespread effects that have not been defined to date, and it therefore should not be used freely during the neonatal period in the absence of seizures or of a history of maternal addiction with withdrawal.

Chlorpromazine can be administered instead of phenobarbital to alleviate the signs of neonatal narcotic withdrawal (32). It is not an anticonvulsant, however, and should not be prescribed for the treatment of convulsive seizures.

Diazepam (injectable Valium) has been recommended as an anticonvulsant (54) and for the management of neonatal narcotic withdrawal (44). However, it has not been shown to be clearly superior to phenobarbital or paraldehyde for treating seizures during the newborn period and is probably no more effective than phenobarbital or chlorpromazine in controlling withdrawal signs. Furthermore it contains a substantial amount of benzoate, an ion that is known to displace bilirubin from its binding sites on albumin (13). Further investigation is needed to evaluate whether parenteral diazepam is useful during the newborn period and whether it predisposes infants to bilirubin encephalopathy before it is used widely to treat infants during the first week of life.

Paregoric (camphorated tincture of opium) has been used widely in the past to treat drug withdrawal in the newborn period (see section Treatment, Ch. 15). Paregoric should not be used in the treatment of diarrhea in young infants, however, since it does not suppress fluid losses in such an instance, but may only mask the severity of these losses.

DIURETICS

The indications for diuretic therapy during the neonatal period include congestive heart failure and suspected acute renal failure. In the first instance diuretics are used as adjuncts to digoxin therapy, and in the second they are used as part of a therapeutic trial to determine whether fluid intake should be restricted or not.

Meralluride, a mercurial diuretic, acts by interfering with the reabsorption of sodium in both the proximal and distal convoluted tubules of the kidney. The mercurials do not act efficiently in the presence of a diminished GFR, and the onset of diuresis following a dose of meralluride may therefore be delayed in young infants. In recent years, mercurials have been largely supplanted by ethacrynic acid and furosemide.

Ethacrynic acid and furosemide act mainly upon the reabsorption of sodium in the loop of Henle. Their action is not as dependent upon the GRF as is the mercurial's, and they may act very rapidly even during the neonatal period. However, both of these drugs can inhibit the binding of small molecules by albumin and are potentially hazardous if given to infants during the first few weeks of life (14, 57). Furthermore, both can produce deafness if administered intravenously, and this route of administration should always be avoided if possible (52, 64).

The thiazide diuretics should not be used to treat infants during the first week of life since they may displace bilirubin from its albumin-binding sites (14). Furthermore, they are photosensitizing agents and might cause adverse reactions among infants treated with phototherapy. It is also possible that their carbonic anhydrase–inhibiting activity can prolong the period of recovery from birth asphyxia, especially among small and other weak infants.

An osmotic agent, such as mannitol, should be the first choice when a therapeutic trial with a diuretic agent is indicated to define the state of an oliguric infant's renal function during the first week of life. Thereafter, either ethacrynic acid or furosemide should probably be used.

CONCLUSION

The use of drugs to treat the most-immature patients safely is less of a problem to pediatricians today than ever before. However, developmental pharmacology has not yet reached a stage where clinicians can depend routinely on the safety of new therapeutic agents that are introduced into general clinical use. There will have to be a great increase in our knowledge of perinatal

TABLE 21-1. Dosage of Commonly Used Drugs

Drug	Dose	Route	Indication
Antibiotics			
Ampicillin (29)	< 24 hr, 100 mg/kg divided into 2 doses > 24 hr, 150–200 mg/kg divided into 3 doses	IM or IV	Infection with organism sensitive to drug
Cephalothin (60)	50 mg/kg/24 hr divided into 4 doses	IM or IV	Infection with organism sensitive to drug
Cloxacillin (60)	50 mg/kg/24 hr divided into 4 doses	Oral*	Infection with penicillinase-producing staphylococci
Colistin (22)	1.5–5 mg/kg/day divided into 2 doses	IM or IV	Infection with organism sensitive to drug (pseudomonas)
Gentamicin (45)	< 1 wk, 5 mg/kg/day divided into 2 doses > 1 wk, 7 mg/kg/day divided into 3 doses	IM	Infection with organism sensitive to drug (pseudomonas)
Isoniazid (3)	10–20 mg/kg/day single dose	Oral or IM	Congenital tuberculosis
Kanamycin (21)	10–15 mg/kg/day divided into 2 doses	IM	Sepsis of unknown etiology
Methicillin (55)	< 24 hr, 200 mg/kg/day divided into 2 doses > 24 hr, 200–400 mg/kg/day divided into 3 doses	IM or IV	Infection with penicillinase-producing staphylococci
Nafcillin (60)	20–40 mg/kg/day divided into 2 doses	IM or IV	Infection with penicillinase-producing staphylococci
Neomycin (22)	50–100 mg/kg/day divided into 3 to 4 doses	Oral	Gastroenteritis due to or asymptomatic infection with entero-pathogenic E. coli
Oxacillin (55)	50–200 mg/kg/day divided into 6 doses	IM or IV	Infection with penicillinase-producing staphylococci
Penicillin G (31)	20,000–50,000 IU/kg/day divided into 2 doses	IM or IV	Sepsis of unknown etiology, congenital syphilis, gonorrhea
Streptomycin (3)	40 mg/kg/day divided into 2 doses	IM	Congenital tuberculosis
Cardiac			
Digoxin (34, 67)	**Digitalizing dose** 30–40 μgm/kg —premature 40–50 μgm/kg —term 70 μgm/kg —> 2 wks (½ total dose immediately; remainder in 2 divided doses at 4 to 6 hr intervals) **Maintenance dose** ⅓–¼ of total digitalizing dose, in 2 divided doses daily	IM or IV	Congestive heart failure; supraventricular paroxysmal tachycardia
Anticonvulsants			
Phenobarbital (60, 46)	8–12 mg/kg/day divided into 3–4 doses	IM or IV Oral or IM	Convulsions Neonatal narcotic withdrawal
Chlorpromazine (46)	2.5–4.5 mg/kg/day divided into 3–4 doses	Oral or IM	Neonatal narcotic withdrawal
Paregoric (46)	1–3 drops/kg every 4–6 hrs including prn	Oral	Neonatal narcotic withdrawal
Diuretics (30)			
Mercurials	0.125–0.5 ml/dose	IM or IV	Congenital heart failure
Ethacrynic acid	1 mg/kg/dose	IV	Oliguria possibly due to decreased renal blood flow
Furosemide	1 mg/kg/dose	IM or IV	Oliguria possibly due to decreased renal blood flow

* Only oral preparation available.

physiology and of the interaction of drugs with the infant's physiologic systems before new drugs can be introduced with rational recommendations for their use in newborn infants. Hopefully, the drugs mentioned in this section will provide for most clinical situations so that there will be little need to use newer drugs in infants before the appropriate studies have been completed.

REFERENCES

1. Asling J, Way EL: Placental transfer of drugs. In: Fundamentals of Drug Metabolism and Drug Disposition. Edited by BN La Du, HG Mandel, EL Way. Baltimore, Williams & Wilkins, 1971

2. Astrup P, Trolle D, Olsen HM, Kjeldsen K: Effect of moderate carbon-monoxide exposure on fetal development. Lancet 2:1220, 1972

3. Avery ME, Wolfsdorf I: Diagnosis and treatment approaches to newborn infants of tuberculous mothers. Pediatrics 42:519, 1968

4. Axline SG, Simon HJ: Clinical pharmacology of antimicrobials in premature infants: I. Kanamycin, streptomycin and neomycin. Antimicrob Agents Chemother 4:135, 1964

5. Axline SG, Yaffe SJ, Simon HJ: Clinical pharmacology of antimicrobials in premature infants: II. Ampicillin, methicillin, oxacillin, neomycin, and colistin. Pediatrics 39:97, 1967

6. Barnett HL, McNamara H, Shultz, S, Tompsett R: Renal clearances of sodium penicillin G, procaine penicillin G, and inulin in infants and children. Pediatrics 3:418, 1949

7. Beazley JM, Taylor G, Reynolds F: Placental transfer of bupivacaine after paracervical block. Obstet Gynecol 39:2, 1972

8. Beckett AH, Taylor JF: Blood concentrations of pethidine and pentazocine in mother and infant at time of birth. J Pharm Pharmacol 19 [Suppl]:50S, 1967

9. Bleyer WA, Marshall RE: Barbiturate withdrawal syndrome in a possibly addicted infant. JAMA 221:185, 1972

10. Boe RW, Williams CPS, Bennett JV, Oliver TK Jr: Serum levels of methicillin and ampicillin in newborn and premature infants in relation to postnatal age. Pediatrics 39:194, 1967

11. Bongiovanni AM, McPadden AJ: Steroids during pregnancy and possible fetal consequences. Fertil Steril 11:181, 1960

12. Catz CS, Giacoia GP: Drugs and breast milk. Pediatr Clin North Am 19:151, 1972

13. Cohen SN, Fern LM: The displacement of albumin-bound bilirubin by benzoate: a hazard of the use of diazepam in newborn infants, abstract. Pediatr Res 6:404, 1972

14. Cohen SN, Ganapathy SK: Previously unpublished observations

15. Cohen SN, Olson WA: Drugs that depress the newborn infant. Pediatr Clin North Am 17:835, 1970

16. Cohen SN, Weber WW: Newborn infants of tuberculous mothers—further comment. Pediatrics 43:303, 1969

16a. Cohlan SQ, Bevelander G, Tiamsic T: Growth inhibition of prematures receiving tetracyclines: Clinical and laboratory investigation of tetracycline-induced bone fluorescence. Amer J Dis Child 105:453, 1963

16b. Cukier JO, Seungdamrong S, Odell JL, Odell GB: The displacement of albumin-bound bilirubin by gentamicin, abstract. Pediatr Res 8:399, 1974

17. Dancis J: The placenta. J Pediatr 55:85, 1959

18. Desmond MM, Schwanecke RP, Wilson GS, Yasunaga S, Burgdorff I: Maternal barbiturate utilization and neonatal withdrawal symptomatology. J Pediatr 80:190, 1972

19. Done AK: Perinatal pharmacology. Ann Rev Pharmacol 6:189, 1966

20. DuPlessis JME, DuToit HJ, Harrison GC, Craig C: The effect of intra-uterine environment and anaesthetic factors on the condition of the baby after Caesarean section. S Afr Med J 42:757, 1968

21. Eichenwald HF: Some observations on dosage and toxicity of kanamycin in premature and full term infants. Ann NY Acad Sci 132:984, 1966

22. Eichenwald HF, Shinefield HR: Antimicrobial therapy in the neonatal period. Pediatr Clin North Am 8:509, 1961

23. Finland M: Hospital-acquired infections: the problems of methicillin-resistant staphylococcus aureus and infections with Klebsiella pneumonia. Am J Med Sci 264:207, 1972

24. Finster M, Morishima HO, Mark LC, Perel JM, Dayton PG, James LS: Tissue thiopental concentrations in the newborn. Anesthesiology 36:155, 1972

25. Flowers CE, Rudolph AJ, Desmond MM: Diazepam (Valium) as an adjunct in obstetric analgesia. Obstet Gynecol 34:68, 1969

26. German J, Ehlers KH, Kowal A, DeGeorge FV, Engle MA, Passarge E: Possible teratogenicity of trimethadione and paramethadione. Lancet 2:261, 1970

27. Goddard WB: Fetal monitoring in a private hospital. Observation of fetal bradycardia following paracervical block anesthesia. Am J Obstet Gynecol 109:1145, 1971

28. Goldstein A, Aronow L, Kalman SM: Principles of Drug Action. New York, Harper & Row, 1968

29. Gotoff SP, Behrman RE: Neonatal septicemia. J Pediatr 76:142, 1970

29a. Herbst AL, Ulfelder H, Poskanzer DC: Adenocarcinoma of the vagina: Association of maternal stillbestrol therapy with tumor appearance in young women. N Engl J Med 284:878, 1971

30. Herrin JT, Crawford JD: Use of diuretics in children. Mod Treat 7:466, 1970

31. Huang NN, High RH: Comparison of serum levels following the administration of oral and parenteral preparations of penicillin to infants and children of various age groups. J Pediatr 42:657, 1953

32. Kahn EJ, Neumann LL, Polk G-A: The course of the heroin withdrawal syndrome in newborn infants treated with phenobaribtal or chlorpromazine. J Pediatr 75:495, 1969

33. Kron RE, Stein M, Goddard KE: Newborn sucking behavior affected by obstetric sedation. Pediatrics 37:1012, 1966

34. Levine OR, Blumenthal S: Digoxin dosage in premature infant. Pediatrics 29:18, 1962

35. Little B, Chang T, Chucot L, Dill WA, Enrile LL, Glazko AJ, Jassani M, Kretchmer H, Sweet AY: Study of ketamine as an obstetric anesthetic agent. Am J Obstet Gynecol 113:247, 1972

36. Marini A, Sereni F, Bottino D: Digoxin dosage in newborn animals and infants. Pediatrics 30:332, 1960

37. Marx GF, Cosmi EV, Wollman SB: Biochemical status and clinical condition of mother and infant at Cesarean section. Anesth Analg (Cleve) 48:986, 1969

38. Maurer HM, Wolff JA, Finster M, Poppers PJ, Pantuck E, Kuntzman R, Conney AH: Reduction in concentration of total serum-bilirubin in offspring of women treated with phenobarbitone during pregnancy. Lancet 2:122, 1968

39. Meadow SR: Congenital abnormalities and anticonvulsant drugs. Proc R Soc Med 63:48, 1970

40. Miller GW: Intramuscular analgesia with pentazocine during labor. J Am Osteopath Assoc 70:555, 1971

41. Moore J, Dundee JW: Alterations in response to somatic pain associated with anaesthesia. V. The effect of promethazine. Br J Anaesth 33:3, 1961

41a. Morselli PL, Garattini S, Sereni F: Basic and Therapeutic Aspects of Perinatal Pharmacology. New York, Raven Press, 1975

42. Mountain KR, Hirsh J, Gallus AS: Neonatal coagulation defect due to anticonvulsant drug treatment in pregnancy. Lancet 1:265, 1970

43. Moya F, Thorndike V: Passage of drugs across the placenta. Am J Obstet Gynecol 84:1778, 1962

44. Nathenson F, Golden GS, Litt IF: Diazepam in the management of the neonatal narcotic withdrawal syndrome. Pediatrics 48:523, 1971

45. Nelson JD, McCracken GH Jr: The current status of gentamicin for the neonate and young infant. Am J Dis Child 124:13, 1972

46. Neumann LL: Drug abuse in pregnancy. In: Drug Addiction in Youth, 3rd ed. Edited by E Harms. New York, Pergamon, 1973

47. O'Connor WJ, Warren GH, Mandala PS, Edrada LS, Rosenman SB: Serum concentrations of nafcillin in newborn infants and children. Antimicrob Agents Chemother 4:188, 1964

48. Odell GB: Personal communication, 1973

49. Odell GB: The dissociation of bilirubin from albumin and its clinical implications. J Pediatr 55:268, 1959

50. Owen JR, Irani SF, Blair AW: Effect of diazepam administered to mothers during labour on temperature regulation of neonate. Arch Dis Child 47:107, 1972

51. Peckham CH, King RW: A study of intercurrent condition observed during pregnancy. Am J Obstet Gynecol 87:609, 1963

52. Pillay VKG, Schwartz FD, Aimi K, Kark RM: Transient and permanent deafness following treatment with ethacrynic acid in renal failure. Lancet 1:77, 1969

53. Ploman L, Persson BH: On the transfer of barbiturates to the human foetus and their accumulation in some of its vital organs. J Obstet Gynaecol Br Commonw 64:706, 1957

54. Rose AL, Lombroso CT: Neonatal seizure states. A study of clinical, pathological and electro-encephalographic features in 137 full-term babies with a long-term follow-up. Pediatrics 45:404, 1970

55. Schaffer AJ, Avery ME: Diseases of the Newborn, 3rd ed. Philadelphia, Saunders, 1971, p 871

56. Schanker LS: Drug absorption. In: Fundamentals of Drug Metabolism and Drug Disposition. Edited by BN Ladu, HG Mardel, EL Way. Baltimore, Williams & Wilkins, 1971

57. Sellers EM, Koch-Weser J: Kinetics and clinical importance of displacement of warfarin from albumin by acidic drugs. Ann NY Acad Sci 179:213, 1971

58. Shannon RW, Fraser GP, Aitken RG, Harper JR: Diazepam in preeclamptic toxaemia with special reference to its effect on the newborn infant. Br J Clin Pract 26:271, 1972

59. Sheng KT, Huang NN, Promadhattavedi V: Serum concentration of cephalothin in infants and children and the placental transmission of the antibiotic. Antimicrob Agents Chemother 4:200, 1964

60. Shirkey HC: Drug Therapy. In: Textbook of Pediatrics. Edited by WF Nelson, VC Vaughan III, RJ McKay. Philadelphia, Saunders, 1971, p 237

61. Shnider SM: A review. Fetal and neonatal effects of drugs in obstetrics. Anesth Analg (Cleve) 45:372, 1966

62. Shnider SM, Moya F: Effects of meperidine on the newborn infant. Am J Obstet Gynecol 89:1009, 1964

63. Silverman WA, Andersen DH, Blanc WA, Crozier DN: A difference in mortality rate and incidence of kernicterus among premature infants allotted to two prophylactic antibacterial regimens. Pediatrics 18:614, 1956

64. Slone D, Jick A, Lewis GP, Shapiro S, Miettinen OS: Intravenously given ethacrynic acid and gastrointestinal bleeding. JAMA 209:1668, 1969

65. Sokal JE, Lessman EM: Effects of cancer chemotherapeutic agents on the human fetus. JAMA 172:1765, 1960

66. Solomon LM, Esterly NB: Neonatal dermatology. I. The newborn skin. J Pediatr 77:888, 1971

67. Soyka LF: Clinical pharmacology of digoxin. Pediatr Clin North Am 19:241, 1972

68. Stern L, Khanna NN, Levy G, Yaffe SJ: Effect of phenobarbital on hyperbilirubinemia and glucuronide formation in newborns. Am J Dis Child 120:26, 1970

69. Suonio S, Kauppila A, Jouppila P, Linna O: The effect of intravenous diazepam on fetal and maternal acid-base balance during and after delivery. Ann Chir Gynaecol Fenn 60:52, 1972

70. Symansky MR, Fox HA: Umbilical catheterization: indications, management, and evaluation of the technique. J Pediatr 80:820, 1972

70a. Symposium on Drug Therapy in the Neonate. Clinics in Perinatology. Philadelphia, Saunders, March 1975

71. Taussig HB: A study of the German outbreak of phocomelia. The thalidomide syndrome. JAMA 180:1106, 1962

72. Trolle D: Decrease of total serum-bilirubin concentration in newborn infants after phenobarbitone treatment. Lancet 2:705, 1968

73. Tunstall ME: The effect of propranolol on the onset of breathing at birth. Br J Anaesth 41:792, 1969

74. van der Kleijn E, Wijffels CCG: Whole-body and regional brain distribution of diazepam in newborn Rhesus monkeys. Arch Int Pharmacodyn Ther 192:255, 1971

75. Weinstein L: Antibiotics. In: The Pharmacological Basis of Therapeutics, 4th ed. Edited by LS Goodman, A Gilman. New York, Macmillan, 1970, p 1287

76. Weiss CF, Glazko AJ, Weston JK: Chloramphenicol in the newborn infant: a physiologic explanation of its toxicity when given in excessive doses. N Engl J Med 262:787, 1960

77. Yaffe SJ: Some aspects of perinatal pharmacology. Ann Rev Med 7:213, 1966

78. Zucker P, Simon G: Prolonged symptomatic neonatal hypoglycemia associated with maternal chlorpropamide therapy. Pediatrics 42:824, 1968

22

Signs of Neonatal Illness

RESPIRATORY DISTRESS

Unusually rapid or labored respirations in the neonate are often secondary to pulmonary pathology. However, cardiovascular disease, acute blood loss, systemic infections, various metabolic disorders, CNS disease and certain severe congenital anomalies may all be associated with respiratory abnormalities as summarized in the accompanying list.

Differential Diagnosis of Tachypnea and Respiratory Distress

Transient tachypnea
Narcotic withdrawal
Respiratory response to metabolic acidosis
Congenital anomalies of respiratory tract
    Choanal atresia
    Laryngeal and tracheal atresia and stenosis
    Pulmonary hypoplasia
    Pulmonary lymphangiectasis
    Congenital lobar emphysema
    Lung cysts
    Tracheoesophageal fistula
Acquired pulmonary disease
    Respiratory distress syndrome (RDS)
    Meconium aspiration
    Congenital pneumonia
    Aspiration pneumonia
    Pneumothorax and pneumomediastinum

    Bronchopulmonary dysplasia and oxygen toxicity
Nonpulmonary causes
    Acute blood loss
    Cardiac disease
    Surgical conditions of GI tract

The normal newborn infant ordinarily has shallow and irregular respirations, with a rate varying from 30 to 50 per minute, and short bursts of rapid breathing are not uncommon. In premature infants, periodic breathing with short periods of apnea followed by spontaneous resumption of normal respiration may be the dominant pattern.

TRANSIENT TACHYPNEA

The syndrome of transient tachypnea of the newborn infant may occasionally be seen in infants (usually full-term) who are otherwise well. A respiratory rate of up to 120 per minute may be seen for the first few days of life in the absence of any obvious abnormality. Chest x rays often show prominent perihilar streaking, which may represent distended lymphatics. The etiology is unknown, but delayed resorbtion of fetal lung fluid is suggested as a possible mechanism (6).

NARCOTIC WITHDRAWAL

Unusually rapid respirations during the first four or five days of life are noted in infants of heroin-addicted mothers. The infants, who show signs of acute narcotic with-

---

The section Cyanosis (p. 421 ff) was prepared by Drs. Welton M. Gersony and Carl N. Steeg.

drawal, have respiratory rates averaging about 70 and often as high as 120 per minute (5). The respirations are not labored, and the infants are well oxygenated in room air. A primary respiratory alkalosis is often associated with this hyperventilation. The underlying mechanism may be the increased sensitivity of the respiratory center to carbon dioxide that accompanies heroin withdrawal.

METABOLIC ACIDOSIS

Infants exposed to chronic intrauterine hypoxia may be born with severe metabolic acidosis. If pulmonary function is normal (many of the infants are undergrown but relatively mature by gestational age), hyperventilation may be noted during the first day of life. This respiratory mechanism permits infants to eliminate carbon dioxide, thus raising their blood pH. In the same manner, newborn babies with metabolic acidosis secondary to diarrheal disease may increase their respiratory rate in order to eliminate carbon dioxide.

CONGENITAL ANOMALIES OF RESPIRATORY TRACT

Choanal Atresia

Since the newborn infant is an obligate nose breather, bilateral choanal atresia (bony or membranous) may accompany cyanosis and severe respiratory difficulty in the neonatal period. If insertion of an oral airway relieves these signs, this diagnosis must be suspected. Suspicion is further raised by the inability to pass a nasal catheter, and the definitive diagnosis is made by inserting methylene blue into the nostrils and not recovering it in the pharynx or by radiologic examination following insertion of radiopaque dye into the nostrils. Continued use of an oral airway until definitive operative repair can be performed alleviates distress.

Laryngeal and Tracheal Atresia and Stenosis

Congenital malformations of the larynx and trachea are uncommon causes of respiratory distress. Congenital laryngeal and tracheal atresia are rare and associated with gasping respirations and inability to move air into the lungs. Tracheostomy may be lifesaving with the former condition; tracheal atresia is generally fatal.

Laryngeal stenosis is associated with a relatively high-pitched cry and expiratory stridor, signs that present from birth. The deformity is usually several millimeters distal to the vocal cords and requires tracheostomy. Laryngeal webs, which are more common, usually are at the level of the vocal cords. In addition to the inspiratory stridor, the infant often has a hoarse cry. The degree of respiratory embarrassment is proportional to the degree of obstruction. Direct laryngoscopy is necessary to make the diagnosis.

Laryngomalacia is a commonly observed benign cause of inspiratory stridor, which may be present at birth and persist for weeks or months. Inspiratory stridor is caused by collapse of a weak larynx on inspiration (secondary to poorly developed cartilage). On direct laryngoscopy, an omega-shaped epiglottis that is drawn toward the larynx on inspiration may be noted. Treatment is conservative, and the stridor subsides when the larynx becomes firmer, usually by the second year of life. Stenosis of the trachea may be present with a relatively low-pitched stridor. Intrinsic defects of the membranous or cartilagenous portions of the trachea may be present, or the stenosis may be due to an extrinsic lesion, such as a tumor or vascular ring. A markedly enlarged thyroid, as seen following maternal ingestion of iodide, may impinge on the trachea and cause respiratory embarrassment.

Tracheostomy may be insufficient to relieve the respiratory distress, and subtotal thyroidectomy may be lifesaving. Functional tracheal stenosis may occur with tracheomalacia, which is secondary to a delay in maturation of tracheal cartilage. The obstruction is usually inspiratory if the upper portion of the trachea is involved and expiratory if the intrathoracic portion is involved. Although specific therapy may be necessary to correct the causes of intrinsic or extrinsic tracheal stenosis, tracheomalacia is usually self-limiting and requires no specific therapy.

Pulmonary Agenesis and Hypoplasia

Bilateral agenesis of the lungs is rare and universally fatal. Survival with gasping respirations for several minutes after birth is reported (2). Unilateral agenesis of a lung is a less rare anomaly.

Hypoplastic lungs are associated with severe respiratory distress in the early neonatal period, with death usually ensuing shortly after birth. Other congenital anomalies, such as diaphragmatic hernia and renal agenesis or hypoplasia with "Potter's facies," should raise suspicion of lung hypoplasia.

Congenital Pulmonary Malformations

Congenital pulmonary lymphangiectasis has an extremely high mortality rate and is often associated with total anomalous pulmonary venous drainage (3). Congenital cystic adenomatoid malformation of the lung is a rare form of cystic disease of the lung that is usually unilateral and amenable to surgical intervention.

Congenital lobar emphysema may manifest as respiratory distress either in the immediate neonatal period or in early infancy. This diagnosis can be confirmed by chest x ray; lobectomy is curative.

Congenital lung cysts are a rare cause of tachypnea and respiratory distress. Those which communicate with the bronchial tree may be observed within the first week of life and usually require surgical treatment.

Esophageal Atresia and Tracheoesophageal Fistula

Respiratory distress may be an early sign in infants with esophageal atresia and tracheoesophageal fistula. The earliest distress is associated with aspiration of the excessive mucus trapped in the proximal esophageal segment. If the condition goes unrecognized and feedings are attempted, the infant may develop respiratory distress from the aspiration of formula. Reflux of gastric fluid from the stomach into the tracheobronchial tree may result in a chemical pneumonitis.

ACQUIRED PULMONARY DISEASE

Most neonatal respiratory distress however, is not based on congenital malformations. Obstetric history, careful examination of the infant and chest x rays are all of great importance in establishing diagnosis.

Respiratory Distress Syndrome

The respiratory distress syndrome (RDS) is the most important cause of dyspnea in premature infants (see section Respiratory Distress Syndrome, Ch. 6). It is rarely observed (except in infants of diabetic mothers) after a gestation of more than 37 weeks. Third trimester bleeding, diabetes mellitus and intrauterine hypoxia all predispose the premature infant to RDS. Maternal use of narcotics, however, even in combination with a shortened gestational period, seems to protect the infant from developing RDS (4). Determination of the lecithin-sphingomyelin (L–S) ratio in the amniotic fluid aids in the prediction of susceptibility to RDS. Respiratory signs usually appear shortly after delivery. Tachypnea, retractions, cyanosis in room air and expiratory grunt are the cardinal presenting signs. Breath sounds are often diminished, but this cannot be used as a diagnostic criterion. Râles are usually absent.

The chest x ray may reveal lung fields that have taken on a "ground glass" appearance, and an air bronchogram effect may be present. These findings reflect the atelectasis associated with RDS. The signs may exacerbate or subside within several hours. Although the diagnosis of RDS is usually made with relative ease, conditions like adrenal and hepatic bleeding and congenital pneumonia may be attended by respiratory signs similar to those of RDS.

Meconium Aspiration

Aspiration of meconium, amniotic fluid or maternal blood either in utero or during delivery may present with moderate to severe respiratory distress (see section Meconium Aspiration, Ch. 6).

Congenital Pneumonia

Congenital pneumonia may occur in infants of mothers with amnionitis, prolonged labor or rupture of membranes or urinary tract infection. Although signs of congenital pneumonia may occasionally be confused with those of RDS, the infant should be vigorously treated with antimicrobial therapy if it is felt that the pulmonary problem is infectious.

Aspiration Pneumonia

The sudden onset of dyspnea in an infant who has previously been asymptomatic may be the result of several causes. Aspiration of formula, especially in infants of low gestational age with poor sucking reflexes must always be considered. Regurgitation of gastric contents with aspiration, both in infants who are nipple and tube fed, may predispose to respiratory signs.

Pneumothorax

Pneumothorax especially if large and bilateral may be manifested by dyspnea in a previously healthy infant. A chest x ray is required to establish the diagnosis.

Bronchopulmonary Dysplasia and Oxygen Toxicity

Bronchopulmonary dysplasia (Wilson-Mikity Disease) is a cause of respiratory distress that may occur in relatively immature infants who have survived the first days of life. Pulmonary damage secondary to oxygen toxicity may also be observed in infants who have received supplementary oxygen therapy. These two conditions are discussed in Chapter 6.

Postnatal Pneumonia

Acquired infectious pneumonias are usually not seen until several days or weeks after delivery. These may be caused by a variety of infectious agents and usually present with rapid, labored respirations.

NONPULMONARY CAUSES OF RESPIRATORY DISTRESS

Acute, intrapartum bleeding may present with gasping, labored respirations (air hunger), associated with pallor and rapid pulse (see section Pallor).

Dyspnea may also be a primary symptom of congestive heart failure, secondary either to congenital cardiac disease or more rarely to viral myocarditis. In the presence of left-sided cardiac failure, cardiomegaly is present, and signs of pulmonary edema may be present on physical examination. The sudden onset of a shocklike picture together with retractions of the chest wall and gasping respirations may occur in such severe forms of congenital heart disease as hypoplastic left heart syndrome and preductal aortic coarctation when the ductus arteriosus, which has been the major source of blood flow to the lungs, closes.

Gastrointestinal insult, such as sudden perforation of a viscus or volvulus may present with severe dyspnea. Renal vein thrombosis and adrenal hemorrhage may have similar respiratory symptoms. A wide variety of illnesses, both pulmonary and nonpulmonary, can produce dyspnea in the neonate. Prompt recognition and treatment of the underlying condition will reduce morbidity and mortality in a significant number of infants.

CYANOSIS *

The cyanotic neonate presents the physician with a disturbing challenge to his diagnostic acumen. Many lesions can produce cyanosis, and often it is not clear which major organ system is primarily involved (13, 14) (Fig. 22–1). A practical approach to establishment of the etiology of cyanosis is necessary to institute appropriate therapy.

At first appearance, there may be difficulty in deciding whether an infant is actu-

* The section Cyanosis was prepared by Drs. Welton M. Gersony and Carl N. Steeg.

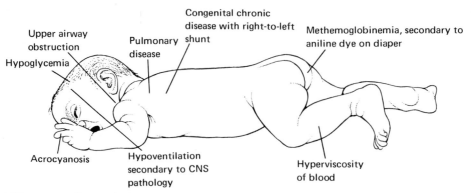

FIG. 22–1. Differential diagnosis of cyanosis.

ally cyanotic. Central cyanosis occurs only when at least 5 g/100 ml of reduced or abnormal hemoglobin are present in the capillary blood. Obviously, the higher the total hemoglobin content in the individual patient, the less the percentage of oxygen desaturation that is necessary to reach the significant level of reduced hemoglobin. The newborn infant with a high hemoglobin concentration may sometimes appear plethoric enough to justify the suspicion that cyanosis is present: contrariwise, an anemic baby may not appear cyanotic even with severe arterial unsaturation. To add to the confusion, babies in the immediate neonatal period may have peripheral cyanosis secondary to either vasomotor instability or exposure to low environmental temperatures without arterial desaturation.

Only two mechanisms account for true central cyanosis: 1) the replacement of normal hemoglobin with significant amounts of reduced hemoglobin that cannot combine with oxygen and 2) the entrance of unsaturated blood from the systemic venous return into the systemic arterial circulation. The latter may result either from intracardiac or intrapulmonary shunting of deoxygenated blood into the systemic arterial circulation. Also to be considered is abnormal pulmonary ventilation—diminished perfusion resulting from primary pulmonary disease.

Pulmonary complications. Upper airway obstruction precipitates cyanosis by the same basic mechanism responsible for CNS cyanosis: overall alveolar hypoventilation due to reduced pulmonary ventilation. Ob-

struction may occur from the nares to the carina. Among congenital abnormalities the important diagnostic possibilities are choanal atresia, vascular ring, laryngeal web or cyst, hypoplasia of the mandible with glossoptosis (Pierre-Robin syndrome) and tracheomalacia. Common acquired causes include vocal cord paresis, obstetric injury to cricothyroid cartilage and foreign body.

In practice, however, structural abnormalities in the lungs due to intrapulmonary disease are more frequently a basis for cyanosis among neonates than is upper airway obstruction. Respiratory distress syndrome, atelectasis or pneumonia cause inflammation, collapse and fluid accumulation in the alveoli, and incompletely oxygenated blood reaches the systemic circulation.

Cardiac complications. Congenital heart disease is responsible for cyanosis when obstruction to right ventricular outflow accounts for intracardiac right-to-left shunts, or when complex anatomic defects that are unassociated with pulmonic stenosis cause admixture of pulmonary and systemic venous return within the heart. The former conditions are associated with decreased pulmonary blood flow, while the latter usually result in pulmonary overvascularity. However, a number of neonates who are cyanotic secondary to true right-to-left shunts do not have organic heart disease.

CNS complications. Irregular, shallow breathing secondary to CNS depression results in a reduced alveolar ventilation and an abnormally low alveolar oxygen tension. In these circumstances, alveolar P_{CO_2} is elevated and Pa_{O_2} is reduced. Intracranial hemorrhage accounts for most of these cases.

Hematologic complications. Methemoglobinemia, either congenital or acquired, is a rare cause of cyanosis in the newborn infant. Recognizable cyanosis occurs in affected babies when 15% of the total hemoglobin is replaced by methemoglobin. Aniline derivatives and nitrites are the poisons that account for most reported cases of the acquired disease, and once suspected the diagnosis is easily established by spectrophotometry. Minute amounts of these toxic substances absorbed even through skin are capable of producing clinically significant methemoglobinemia. Treatment consists of methylene blue administration.

Cyanosis may also attend any overwhelming illness in the neonate, such as sepsis, meningitis, erythroblastosis fetalis or disseminated intravascular coagulation. This is due to involvement of the cardiovascular, respiratory, hematologic systems or CNS with the basic disease.

INITIAL CLINICAL APPRAISAL

The key to successful initial evaluation of the cyanotic neonate is careful observation of the infant's breathing pattern. Weak, irregular respiration, often associated with a weak suck reflex, convulsions and general depression, strongly suggests a CNS etiology. The infant with primary cardiac or pulmonary disease, on the other hand, displays vigorous, labored respiration with tachypnea. Differential diagnosis between pulmonary and cardiac cyanosis may be difficult, especially within the first few days of life. The baby with congenital heart disease will often become more deeply cyanotic with crying, whereas the infant with lung disease will more likely turn pinker as a result of increased pulmonary ventilation. The presence of a significant heart murmur suggests a cardiac basis for cyanosis, but unfortunately, from a diagnostic standpoint, several of the more severe cardiac defects do not manifest a murmur Physical examination of the lungs may be helpful in the detection of pulmonary disease, but a specific diagnosis is usually not established until a chest x ray has been evaluated.

Surprisingly, babies with methemoglobinemia will frequently be asymptomatic despite rather severe cyanosis. Deterioration eventually will occur if the patient remains untreated. The absence of cardiac or pulmonary findings in an alert cyanotic newborn infant should always suggest this condition.

Once the physician has carefully excluded pulmonary, CNS and hematologic disease as the cause of cyanosis and has become reasonably convinced that the origin is cardiac, he reaches still another major diagnostic hurdle. He must decide if the cyanosis is due to cardiac failure and pulmonary congestion associated with acyanotic heart disease or to a defect primarily associated with cyanosis. True cyanotic heart disease is more likely in the neonate with deep cyanosis than in older infants (one to three months of age) with congestive heart failure and only mild unsaturation.

The most convenient classification—the one most likely to result in accurate clinical differentiation of cyanotic heart disease—is based on pulmonary blood flow. Although radiologic interpretation of the routine chest films as to the magnitude of pulmonary blood flow will be accurate in many instances, on all too numerous occasions a borderline "increased" or "decreased" description is the most that can be accepted with confidence. In a questionable situation the presence of a small cardiac silhouette is more likely to be associated with decreased pulmonary flow; cardiomegaly, together with other clinical features of congestive heart failure, is more likely when pulmonary flow is increased. Once the physician has made a roentgenologic evaluation, he is ready to use the ECG as a guide to a specific diagnosis.

CYANOTIC HEART DISEASE WITH DECREASED PULMONARY BLOOD FLOW

First, let us consider the infant with reduced pulmonary blood flow and cyanosis. There are five major diagnoses to consider in this situation: 1) tricuspid atresia; 2) pulmonary atresia with intact ventricular septum (hypoplastic right heart syndrome); 3) critical pulmonic stenosis with intact ventricular septum; 4) tetralogy of Fallot; and 5) Ebstein's disease. All of these lesions have in common the presence of pulmonary hypoperfusion, but within this classification both anatomy and physiology may vary greatly. Differential diagnosis therefore becomes of great importance in planning medical and surgical management.

The ECG has been extremely helpful in the differential diagnosis of these defects. Left axis deviation and left ventricular hypertrophy is the characteristic finding in tricuspid atresia. Marked right axis deviation and right ventricular hypertrophy is the rule in tetralogy of Fallot and in pulmonary stenosis with intact ventricular septum.

In pulmonary atresia (hypoplastic right heart syndrome), the left ventricle is also dominant, but the axis tends to be "normal" in contrast to the left axis deviation seen in tricuspid atresia.

The ECG of Ebstein's anomaly is quite distinctive. The findings include: right bundle branch block, a prolonged PR interval, right atrial enlargement and usually decreased right ventricular forces.

CYANOTIC HEART DISEASE WITH INCREASED PULMONARY BLOOD FLOW

Under this classification there are four major defects to consider: 1) transposition of the great arteries; 2) total anomalous pulmonary venous drainage; 3) hypoplastic left heart syndrome; and 4) truncus arteriosus. Differential diagnosis of these four lesions is somewhat more difficult. The ECG characteristically shows right axis deviation and right ventricular hypertrophy in all.

Individual lesions are discussed in detail in Chapter 7, Cardiovascular Disorders.

PERSISTENT FETAL CIRCULATION SYNDROME

True right-to-left shunting may occur in babies without organic heart disease through fetal channels (patent foramen ovale, patent ductus arteriosus) secondary to increased pulmonary vascular resistance (9, 10, 15). This syndrome may be seen in association with hyperviscosity of the blood, neonatal hypoglycemia and atypical RDS, or it may be of the idiopathic variety.

Infants with persistent fetal circulation syndrome have certain characteristics in common: 1) they are likely to be of fullterm gestation; 2) cyanosis is striking, but the amount of respiratory distress is variable; 3) signs begin within the first 24 hours of life; 4) the classic history and the clinical and roentgenographic profile of RDS is absent; 5) mild to moderate cardiomegaly may be noted, but there are no murmurs or other signs of primary heart disease, nor is there evidence of frank congestive heart failure; 6) the ECG shows right ventricular predominance within normal limits for a newborn infant.

HYPERVISCOSITY

Cyanosis, respiratory distress and CNS symptoms have been reported in newborn infants with hyperviscosity of the blood (11). Intrauterine or early postnatal anoxemia may play an important role in the genesis of polycythemia by stimulating erythropoietin and thus increasing erythrocyte production. Chromosomal abnormalities and maternal, twin or placental transfusions are also associated with polycythemia in neonates.

ATYPICAL RESPIRATORY DISTRESS SYNDROME

A respiratory distress syndrome in term infants may result from early systemic hypoxemia, which also produces severe pulmonary vasoconstriction and markedly elevated pulmonary vascular resistance. Right-to-left shunting via the patent foramen ovale and ductus arteriosus results, but unlike classic RDS in premature babies, marked acidosis and hypercarbia are absent in the face of striking hypoxemia. Large true right-to-left shunts have been quantitatively documented both in experimental RDS and in clinical

RDS in man. A group of patients with atypical RDS has been reported by Roberton et al (13), who noted that most of the infants had a history of birth asphyxia.

Since shunting in this group of patients is not predominantly intrapulmonary, immediate improvement with administration of oxygen may not occur, and heart disease can easily be misdiagnosed in these cyanotic full-term infants. However, careful observation and evaluation of the clinical course will allow a correct diagnosis to be made in the great majority of patients. Cyanosis will gradually subside and the infant will improve if oxygenation and an adequate circulation can be maintained during the first few days of life. Transient tachypnea of the newborn infant may represent a mild variation of this syndrome.

HYPOGLYCEMIA

Infants with neonatal hypoglycemia may display cyanosis as a presenting sign prior to CNS manifestations or respiratory signs. Right-to-left shunting secondary to elevated pulmonary resistance is the most likely explanation for arterial oxygen desaturation in these infants, many of whom are offspring of diabetic mothers.

Central nervous system injury can produce both hypoglycemia and cyanosis (alveolar hypoventilation), but infants with symptomatic hypoglycemia have no other evidence of CNS abnormalities. Also of interest is that 12% of infants with transient hypoglycemia have temporary, but significant, polycythemia. Hypoglycemia may also coexist with congenital heart disease in the neonatal infant. Serial blood sugar determinations must be part of the evaluation of every cyanotic newborn infant. If the primary diagnosis of hypoglycemia is established, immediate administration of 50 per cent glucose is mandatory (see section Carbohydrate Metabolism, Ch. 12).

IDIOPATHIC

Symptomatic infants with cyanosis and respiratory distress may shunt right-to-left

through fetal circulatory pathways as a result of pulmonary vascular obstruction, in the absence of any known cause of pulmonary vasoconstriction. These are usually term infants with no history of birth asphyxia, nor findings of significant hypoglycemia or polycythemia. Blood gas and cardiac catheterization studies show only severe pulmonary artery hypertension with right-to-left shunting via the foramen ovale and ductus arteriosus. In one infant, postmortem examination revealed no anatomic abnormalities to explain the clinical course of severe cyanosis and cardiorespiratory collapse. Occasionally the pulmonary obstruction resolves during the first month of life, the infants surviving with no evidence of residual illness.

PALLOR

Pallor in the newborn infant immediately postpartum is an ominous sign, often reflecting a severe underlying abnormality. Differentiation between intrapartum blood loss or hemolysis and asphyxia as the cause of pallor is often difficult; however, since intact survival depends on prompt diagnosis and specific therapy, the distinction is vital.

The normal newborn infant has a ruddy appearance. Mild, transient cyanosis of the extremities (acrocyanosis) may occur in cold-induced peripheral vasoconstriction and is nonpathologic. Generalized postpartum cyanosis indicates intrauterine hypoxia. In very severe hypoxia associated with cardiovascular collapse, the infant may appear pallid rather than cyanotic, with only the mucous membranes and nail beds showing evidence of cyanosis. These infants are usually markedly obtunded with slow or absent respirations and moderate or severe bradycardia.

Successful resuscitation associated with restoration of a normal circulation will produce a normal appearing, ruddy infant, thereby confirming the diagnosis of intrauterine asphyxia and eliminating blood loss as the reason for the pallor.

Pallor may also be associated with a deficient number of circulating erythrocytes (anemia), reflecting either acute or chronic blood loss. Chronic anemia is most commonly due to intrauterine hemolysis secondary to Rh or ABO incompatibility, fetal bleeding into the maternal circulation and intertwin transfusion between monochorionic twins. Acute blood loss may be secondary to placenta previa or abruptio placentae, bleeding into the maternal circulation at the time of parturition, accidental cutting of the placenta during cesarean section, internal bleeding, rupture of a normal or abnormal umbilical cord and tearing of anomalously inserted placental blood vessels.

Diagnosis and treatment are discussed in the section Anemias, Chapter 8.

LETHARGY

Lethargy and unresponsiveness may be apparent in an infant from the moment of birth or may occur in one who was previously normal, and may be due to either prenatal or postnatal factors. Prenatal factors include intrauterine asphyxia, maternal analgesia and anesthesia, therapeutic agents (e.g., magnesium sulfate) and lithium carbonate administered to mother. Postnatal factors include sepsis and meningitis, hypothermia, hypoglycemia, CNS bleeding, polycythemia, hypocalcemia, bilirubin encephalopathy and aminoacidurias.

POSTNATAL FACTORS

The onset of lethargic behavior in a newborn infant whose activity had been previously normal may be a warning of the development of serious illness. Since signs of illness may be subtle in the neonate (especially in the premature infant), changes in activity of the infant must not be ignored. Being told by the mother or nurse that "the infant just isn't behaving right," or isn't interested in his feeding, should be the basis for a careful medical evaluation.

A variety of abnormal conditions may lead to the onset of lethargic behavior.

Lethargy may be the first presenting sign of sepsis or meningitis. The presence of unexplained lethargy is sufficient to warrant a diagnostic evaluation for sepsis, including lumbar puncture, chest x ray and blood culture, to preclude the presence of life-threatening infection. Even if the results of the diagnostic work-up are inconclusive, and pending final results from the laboratory, lethargy alone may justify the institution of antimicrobial therapy.

Hypothermia may be responsible for signs of lethargy. Although great care is taken in most newborn nurseries to keep both low-birth-weight and full-term infants warm, inadvertant cooling may occur, especially in transport from the delivery area to the nursery. If the axillary temperature is subnormal in a lethargic infant, it may mean that either the lethargy is secondary to accidental cooling or that both the lethargy and hypothermia are secondary to more serious illness. While preparations are being made for further diagnostic procedures, the infant should be slowly warmed.

Lethargy, either as an isolated finding or together with irritability and tremulousness, may be one of the first signs of hypoglycemia. Suspicion of hypoglycemia must be high in infants who are small for gestational age and infants of diabetic mothers. With adequate treatment, normal behavior should ensue.

Central nervous system bleeding may present with lethargic behavior. In the full-term infant, bleeding into the subdural space will produce a bulging fontanelle and separation of sutures in addition to other presenting signs. Subdural taps are indicated if there is even the slightest possibility of this diagnosis. Central nervous system bleeding in the premature infant is usually intraventricular; diagnostic and therapeutic measures in this condition should be aimed at the basic disorder, such as hypoxia or disseminated intravascular coagulation.

Since polycythemia may affect the CNS and lead to lethargic behavior and cyanosis, the hematocrit or hemoglobin concentration must be determined. A venous hematocrit of more than 65% or capillary hematocrit of over 70% will suggest this diagnosis.

Although hypocalcemia is usually associated with tremulousness and convulsions, lethargy may be present. It is advisable to determine serum calcium levels in lethargic infants if the diagnosis is not obvious.

Bilirubin encephalopathy may have lethargy as a presenting sign; although some permanent damage is likely to have occurred by the time this appears, exchange transfusion should still be carried out.

Various inborn errors of metabolism, such as galactosemia and maple syrup urine disease may also have lethargy as an early manifestation, and the medical and nursing staff must be constantly aware that any change in an infant's behavior warrants a prompt investigation.

JAUNDICE

Jaundice, an extremely common finding in the neonate, is usually clinically evident when the serum bilirubin concentration (primarily the unconjugated variety) exceeds 3 mg/100 ml. It may represent increased destruction of RBCs, a decreased capability to conjugate or excrete bilirubin or a combination of both.

Since unconjugated bilirubin is a potent CNS toxin capable of producing death or severe neurologic disability, the jaundiced infant must be promptly identified, an etiology established, and treatment begun, if necessary.

The appearance of jaundice within the first 24 to 48 hours of life is usually indicative of a hemolytic process most often due to a blood group incompatibility. Early onset of jaundice may also be observed in neonates with fetomaternal infection. Onset of jaundice after 48 hours of life is more often physiologic (a developmental delay in the infants ability to conjugate and excrete bilirubin). Its appearance at this time may also be a manifestation of postnatally acquired infection, G-6-PD deficiency and resorption of blood from a closed body space, e.g., cephalhematoma. It is uncommon for jaundice to appear after the first five to seven days of life. When this does occur,

such conditions as hypothyroidism, neonatal hepatitis, biliary atresia and metabolic disorders, such as galactosemia and α1-antitrypsin deficiency must be considered.

A complete discussion of diagnosis and treatment appears in the section Neonatal Jaundice, Chapter 8.

INAPPROPRIATE PASSAGE OF MECONIUM AND STOOL

Over 95% of normal full-term infants pass meconium by the end of the first day of life; nonpassage of meconium by the end of the second day may be considered pathologic (16). By the third day, the infant usually passes a transitional stool (a mixture of feces and meconium).

The number of stools an infant passes daily normally varies; a breast-fed infant may pass eight or ten stools or more per day. On the other hand, normal passage of stool may occur as infrequently as once every other day. An infant fed cow's milk formula (with a high casein and calcium content) tends to have harder and less frequent stools than a breast-fed infant.

CONSTIPATION AND OBSTIPATION

In intestinal obstruction, nonpassage of stool is usually accompanied by vomiting and abdominal distention. If the obstruction is relatively high or intermittent, small amounts of meconium may be passed (Fig. 22–2). In obstipation, especially if abdominal distention and vomiting are present, a plain x ray of the abdomen must be taken. In many cases, a definitive or presumptive diagnosis may be made on the basis of radiologic findings. If the x ray appears normal, a gentle examination of the rectum may be performed, either digitally or with a very soft lubricated rubber catheter. The passage of a meconium plug may be followed by normal defecation. Since the meconium plug syndrome may be associated with congenital megacolon (Hirschsprung's disease) (17), further observations and diagnostic studies are necessary in these infants. A sudden

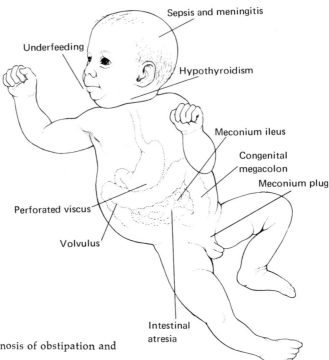

FIG. 22–2. Differential diagnosis of obstipation and constipation.

expulsion of gas and stool following rectal examination in newborn infants who are either constipated or have never passed stool is usually associated with congenital megacolon.

Premature infants of relatively low gestational age, especially those with RDS, sepsis or other debilitating illness, will often have decreased or absent peristaltic activity (paralytic ileus), resulting in a nonpassage of meconium.

In meconium ileus the obstipation is due to inspissated meconium. Family history, abdominal x ray and sweat test, all aid in making the diagnosis. The early establishment of this diagnosis is of the utmost importance since both surgical and nonsurgical treatment may be lifesaving (see section Meconium Ileus, Ch. 23).

Constipation may accompany congenital hypothyroidism, a rare but treatable disorder in newborn infants. If constipation is associated with any other signs of hypothyroidism (large tongue, hoarse cry, coarse features or umbilical hernia) thyroid function studies should be performed.

In hypertrophic pyloric stenosis, consti-

pation may accompany projectile vomiting.

Constipation may also accompany underfeeding, especially if the infant is being breast fed.

DIARRHEA

Although acute GI infection is the most frequent cause of diarrhea in the newborn infant, several other important etiologic factors must be considered (Fig. 22–3). A definition of diarrhea is often difficult in the neonatal period, as in later life. An infant may have many soft stools daily and yet show no disturbances in either water balance or acid-base homeostasis. On the other hand, two or three stools containing much fluid may cause serious metabolic disturbances.

Infants of heroin-addicted mothers who show signs of withdrawal often develop diarrheal stools. The etiology of this diarrhea (in the absence of a specific infectious etiology) is not known.

A side-effect occasionally seen in infants receiving phototherapy for hyperbilirubinemia is the frequent passage of watery

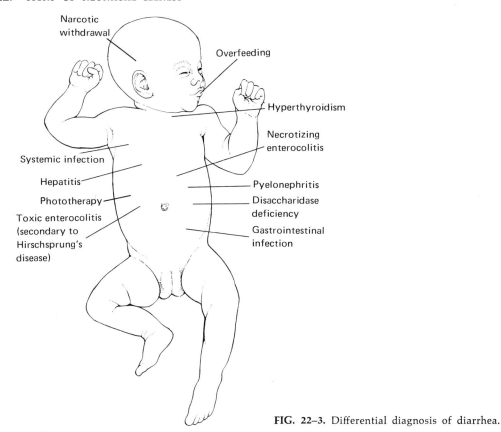

FIG. 22–3. Differential diagnosis of diarrhea.

stools. This may be due to the laxative action of breakdown products of bilirubin (secondary to photoxidation), which are excreted in the bile.

Diarrhea is occasionally seen in cases of congenital megacolon whose correct diagnosis has not yet been made. This diarrhea is the result of a toxic enterocolitis that probably has a noninfectious etiology. This entity is associated with a relatively poor prognosis and must be treated as a medical and surgical emergency.

Diarrhea, occasionally bloody, may be seen in necrotizing enterocolitis. This is a much less frequent sign than vomiting and abdominal distention.

In congenital hyperthyroidism, diarrhea may accompany other presenting manifestations. This rare syndrome is seen only in infants of untreated hyperthyroid mothers.

In both the congenital and acquired varieties of disaccharidase deficiencies, the diar-

rhea will be accompanied by a persistent acidic stool.

Infections other than those of the GI tract may be accompanied by diarrhea. Among these are pyelonephritis and hepatitis.

Management

Diarrhea in the newborn infant may have extremely serious consequences. The affected infant can easily develop a shock-like picture with a severe metabolic acidosis secondary to stool losses of water and bicarbonate. In some instances, the primary illness that is the underlying cause of the diarrhea, e.g., pyelonephritis, may jeopardize the well-being of the infant. If the diarrhea is infectious, a nursery-wide epidemic may start within hours, and appropriate precautions must be taken.

A specific etiology should be determined as quickly as possible. In addition to stool cultures, cultures of blood, urine and CSF should be obtained if there is any question of systemic infection. Our use of the fluorescent antibody technique to identify enteropathogenic *E. coli* has helped to abort several potential diarrheal epidemics. Frequent weighing of the patient and determination of acid-base balance are also of great importance in evaluating the infant with diarrhea, irrespective of the etiology, since dehydration and acidosis may develop rapidly. Prompt isolation of infants having infectious diarrhea together with the use of disposable gloves when handling infants will greatly aid in prevention of spread of the diarrhea.

VOMITING

Vomiting is frequently encountered among newborn infants (Fig. 22–4). It is associated with a wide range of illnesses and may be indicative of either primary GI or systemic illness, but it is also found in the absence of disease. It may be seen in infants who swallow significant amounts of maternal blood, amniotic fluid and debris. Vomiting following feedings is fairly common, especially in premature infants with limited gastric capacities who are overfed. It is essential that "pathologic" vomiting be differentiated from commonly encountered transient vomiting.

SURGICALLY RELATED

Early onset of persistent vomiting raises the question of possible intestinal obstruction. Time of onset and the content of the vomitus give clues as to the location of the obstruction. An early onset of vomiting mucus in the absence of abdominal distention is associated with a very high obstruction such as esophageal atresia. Vomitus that does not contain bile points to an obstruction proxi-

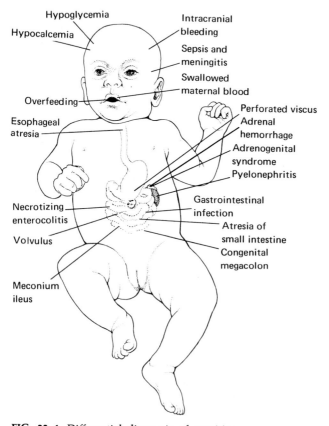

FIG. 22–4. Differential diagnosis of vomiting.

mal to the ampulla of Vater, while a more-distal obstruction would be likely with bilious vomiting. Significant abdominal distention is more likely to accompany the vomiting if the obstruction is relatively low. If constipation accompanies vomiting, a diagnosis of intestinal obstruction becomes increasingly likely. However, in the presence of a high or intermittent obstruction, such as an intussusception, small amounts of meconium may be passed. Fecal vomiting may occur with a low obstruction.

Hematemesis is unusual in a newborn infant with intestinal obstruction but is encountered occasionally with necrotizing enterocolitis. Hematemesis is most commonly seen when the fetus has swallowed maternal blood during delivery. Differentiation must be made from acute GI hemorrhage. This can be done by performing an alkali denaturation test to determine if the red blood cells are of maternal or fetal origin.

If vomiting occurs after an interval in which the infant has successfully retained oral feedings, several possibilities must be considered. Acute surgical emergencies, such as a perforated viscus or volvulus can present in this manner.

In meconium ileus, vomiting does not usually begin until the second day of life and is accompanied by abdominal distention. A positive family history of cystic fibrosis, palpation of doughy masses in the abdomen (inspissated meconium) and a positive sweat test all aid in confirming the diagnosis. Obstructive jaundice may also be seen. If intrauterine perforation has occurred, calcifications will be evident on an abdominal x ray, indicative of meconium peritonitis. Hirschsprung's disease must always be considered in the full-term infant with bilious vomiting, abdominal distention and constipation. A rectal examination will often be associated with the passage of gas and meconium, followed by a transient relief. An inspissated plug of meconium (meconium plug syndrome) may also produce the same clinical picture.

Vomiting and abdominal distention are primary presenting signs of necrotizing enterocolitis. This syndrome is usually seen in relatively immature, sick neonates after the first few days of life and may be associated with sepsis.

Hypertrophic pyloric stenosis is rarely seen as a cause of vomiting in the early neonatal period. The diagnosis can usually be confirmed by palpation of the pyloric tumor, nonbilious projectile vomiting and a hypochloremic, hypokalemic metabolic alkalosis. This diagnosis may sometimes be confused with congenital adrenal hyperplasia. In the latter condition, however, hyperkalemia is typical.

NONSURGICAL EMESIS

The differentiation between surgical and nonsurgical causes of vomiting in the neonate is often difficult. The GI tract of the newborn infant is sensitive to metabolic aberrations and functional ileus, and vomiting will be a common occurrence in many disorders.

Both intracranial bleeding and hypoxic encephalopathy lead to vomiting. In the full-term infant, a subdural hematoma may be an underlying cause; if suspected, subdural taps must be performed.

The onset of vomiting in an infant who has previously been well may also raise the suspicion of systemic bacterial infection, especially when accompanied by such other signs as lethargy or jaundice. A complete diagnostic evaluation, including blood cultures, lumbar puncture and urinalysis is indicated.

The presence of a flank mass, usually indicative of hydronephrosis, should raise a suspicion of pyelonephritis as the cause of the vomiting.

Vomiting may be the first sign of enteric infection; in addition to a stool culture, it is sometimes useful to perform fluorescent antibody studies to determine the presence of enteropathogenic E. coli.

Both hypoglycemia and hypocalcemia may on rare occasion present with vomiting. If vomiting is otherwise unexplained, blood glucose and calcium levels should be determined.

The adrenogenital syndrome may have

vomiting, occasionally projectile, as one of its earliest manifestations (see section Adrenal Cortex, Ch. 11). An elevated urinary 17-ketosteroid excretion together with hyperkalemia and clitoral hypertrophy in females will make the presumptive diagnosis. Since this is a potentially life-threatening but remediable cause of vomiting, it must always be kept in mind.

Other inborn errors of metabolism may cause vomiting in the late neonatal period. Galactosemia must be suspected if there is concurrent hepatomegaly, jaundice and cataracts. A galactose tolerance test will confirm the diagnosis here, as will decreased levels of galactose-1-phosphate-uridyl transferase in the erythrocytes. In hereditary fructose intolerance, vomiting may be an early sign, and elevated fructose levels in the blood and urine will make the presumptive diagnosis. The vomiting that occurs with glycogen storage disease is usually first noted after the neonatal period.

Vomiting may be an early sign of phenylketonuria, beginning during the first month of life. Routine screening of infants by the Guthrie test should detect all affected infants prior to the onset of clinical signs.

Chalasia (an abnormal relaxation of the musculature of the esophageal cardia) has regurgitation of feedings as the primary manifestation. The diagnosis can usually be made with a barium swallow and fluoroscopic examination.

Narrowing of the lower esophageal segment (cardiospasm or achalasia) may cause vomiting in the neonatal period. Here also, a barium swallow with use of fluoroscopy will confirm the diagnosis.

When the physician examines a newborn infant who is vomiting, he must decide if significant illness is present. If in doubt he must proceed with the appropriate diagnostic work-up. If operative intervention is entertained, an abdominal x ray must be taken and a surgical consultation obtained. During the period of observation, oral feedings should be discontinued and parenteral fluids started. Continued oral feeding of an infant who is vomiting may lead to aspiration pneumonia.

ABNORMAL TEMPERATURE

Abnormalities in the body temperature of a neonate (either hyperthermia or hypothermia) reflect either exposure to an inappropriate environmental temperature or the presence of serious illness.

In the premature infant, hypothermia is encountered much more frequently than fever. In most instances hypothermia is due to exposure of the infant to low environmental temperatures either in the delivery room, during transport to the nursery, or within the incubator. Hypothermia is more often a presenting sign of serious infection, such as sepsis and meningitis, than is fever. A subnormal body temperature may also be encountered in hypoxic premature infants, especially those with RDS. Fever in premature infants is usually caused by an overheated incubator. However, in some larger premature infants, this may be the first sign of serious infection.

Hypothermia is encountered much less frequently in full-term than in premature infants. It may be observed following severe cold stress in the delivery room. However, when noted in infants who have previously been well, sepsis and meningitis must be suspected and a full diagnostic evaluation undertaken.

A sudden rise in the infant's temperature must also raise suspicion of infection. However, an infant who is clothed and blanketed in the presence of very high nursery air temperatures may develop fever.

A full discussion of these problems appears in Chapter 13, Thermoregulation.

HEPATOSPLENOMEGALY

Enlargement of the liver and spleen may accompany a number of disease processes in the neonate. Normally, the liver edge may be palpable up to 2 cm below the right costal margin, while palpation of more than just the tip of the spleen may be considered abnormal.

Enlargement of both organs is commonly observed in isoimmunization secondary to both Rh and ABO blood group incompatibility. It may also be noted in other hemolytic anemias, such as congenital spherocytosis.

Hepatosplenomegaly is a frequent finding in perinatal infections. It is commonly seen in such prenatally acquired infections as rubella, toxoplasmosis, cytomegalovirus and congenital syphilis. Splenic enlargement may accompany bacterial sepsis, but its absence does not preclude this diagnosis. Hepatomegaly alone may be observed in both neonatal hepatitis and biliary atresia.

Hepatic enlargement may accompany right-sided congestive heart failure. It may also be noted in such disorders of carbohydrate metabolism as galactosemia and glycogen storage disease.

Bleeding into the liver and spleen may produce enlargement of these organs, as will metastasis from such neoplasms as neuroblastoma. Administration of excessive parenteral fluids may cause a circulatory overload and result in hepatosplenomegaly.

The clinician will often be faced with the problem of assessing a palpable liver and spleen in the neonate. If there is any doubt about the presence of illness, the physician must proceed with a diagnostic evaluation of the infant.

PETECHIAE, PURPURA AND ECHYMOSES

Bleeding into the skin is frequently observed in newborn infants. The trauma of delivery may normally produce scattered petechiae over the body, and a traumatic delivery (especially a breech) may result in echymoses over the presenting part. Echymoses may also be observed in the easily traumatized skin of premature infants.

Large numbers of petechiae and purpura are usually associated with a decreased number of circulating platelets (thrombocytopenia). This condition may be due to a variety of causes, such as isoimmunization, fetomaternal infection and disseminated intravascular coagulation. A full discussion of this subject appears in the section Thrombocytopenia, Chapter 8.

The clinician must recognize that the presence of purpura and petechiae in the neonate usually indicates a true medical emergency and that the underlying condition, if left undiagnosed and untreated, may result in bleeding into such vital organs as the brain, lungs, adrenal gland and liver.

ABNORMAL HEAD SIZE

The size and shape of the head of the newborn infant is primarily dependent on brain growth both during intrauterine life and early infancy. Occasionally, aberrations of skull development (premature closure of one or more sutures) may adversely affect the growth of a normally developing brain. Therefore, an infant whose head circumference is abnormally large or small, or who has a grossly misshapen head, is at a relatively high risk for abnormal neurologic development.

Inadequate fetal brain development, leading to microcephaly, may be due to several causes, including fetomaternal infection, fetal malnutrition and genetic abnormalities.

Abnormally large head size is usually due to an expansion of the brain secondary to accumulation of CSF under pressure (hydrocephalus). This is usually first noted following delivery, although it may begin in utero, especially when associated with such conditions as myelomeningocele and toxoplasmosis.

Hydranencephaly, a rare condition in which the cerebral cortex is paper thin and largely replaced by fluid, may be the cause of an enlarged head that is apparent either at delivery or during the neonatal period.

Frequently, the normal-sized head of a low-birth-weight infant who is small for gestational age may appear unusually large in relationship to the rest of the body. This condition should not be mistaken for hydrocephalus.

OCCIPITOFRONTAL MEASUREMENT

The assessment of neonatal head size is made by both inspection and measurement of head circumference at the greatest occipi-

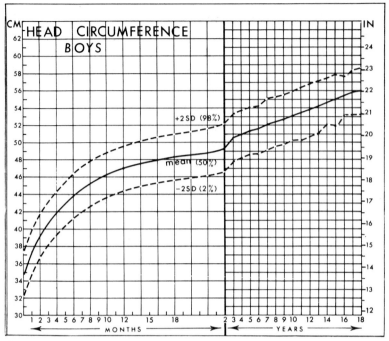

A

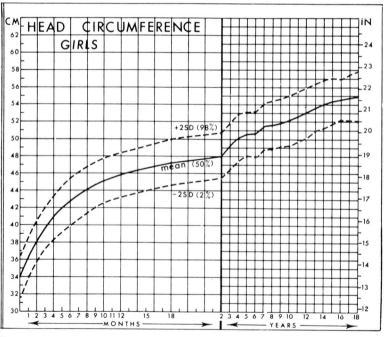

B

tofrontal diameter. This measurement reflects the volume of cranial contents (23). Although the diagnosis may occasionally be obvious on inspection alone, use of the tape measure and referral to a head growth graph is usually necessary.

With borderline abnormalities of head circumference, the infant's height and weight must be taken into consideration. For example, if all of these dimensions are at about the third percentile for gestational age, the infant may very well be normal. If, on the other hand, weight and length are at the 50th percentile or above; and the head circumference is at the 3rd percentile, true microcephaly must be considered.

The normal range of head circumference measurements for gestational ages of 26 to 42 weeks was determined on nearly 5000 newborn infants by Lubchenko et al (20) in 1966 (see section Intrauterine Growth Retardation, Ch. 4). Postnatal head growth has been assessed by a number of investigators and correlated in graphic form by Nellhaus (22) in 1968 (Fig. 22–5).

Measurement of head circumference must be a routine part of the physical examination of the newborn infant. In normal full-term infants, this measurement should be repeated at every follow-up well baby examination. In low-birth-weight infants, the head circumference should be determined at weekly intervals to assess abberations from expected growth. Although the rate of postnatal brain growth in premature infants does not necessarily reflect intrauterine growth rates, the Lubchenko intrauterine head growth curve can be used.

DIAGNOSIS AND MANAGEMENT

Although therapeutic possibilities are limited in the infant with abnormally slow intrauterine brain growth, every effort to establish an etiologic diagnosis must nonetheless be made.

FIG. 22–5. Postnatal head circumference from birth to 18 years. **A.** Head circumference, boys. **B.** Head circumference, girls. (Nellhaus G: Pediatrics 41:106, 1968)

If suspicion exists early in pregnancy that microcephaly is secondary to the encephalitis of fetomaternal infection, e.g., rubella, h. simplex, cytomegalovirus and toxoplasmosis, a complete diagnostic evaluation is required (see Ch. 20, Nonbacterial Infections).

Although little can be done to reverse the damage that has already occurred, future management of the infant may be guided by knowledge of the nature of the infection. Likewise, the family may be reassured about the limited possibility of reoccurrence after a subsequent pregnancy.

If small head size is secondary to a genetic disorder, chromosomal analysis is mandatory both for genetic counseling and for long-term management of the infant.

Decreased fetal brain growth resulting from severe intrauterine malnutrition may be at least partially amenable to treatment (19). These infants who are particularly prone to developing hypoglycemia, should have frequent blood sugar determinations performed. An adequate supply of calories must be provided since good postnatal nutrition may enhance brain development (and hence lead to "catch up" growth). Conversely, poor postnatal nutrition in infants who have had small head circumferences at birth leads to very severe retardation of brain development during the first year of life (23).

Prognosis

There is a clear correlation between microcephaly and mental retardation, especially if the microcephaly is pronounced. However, a small percentage of infants and children whose head circumferences are more than two standard deviations below the mean for their age will have normal mental development (18, 21). It is therefore imperative that all infants who have microcephalic head measurements receive careful serial neurologic and developmental evaluations.

An unusually large head circumference noted at birth, or a rapidly growing head, requires a full diagnostic work-up for hydrocephalus (see section Hydrocephalus, Ch. 23). Since a favorable prognosis is associated with early diagnosis and treatment, this condition alone would warrant frequent measurements of head circumference of all newborn infants.

ASCITES

Accumulation of fluid within the peritoneal cavity (ascites) is an unusual pathologic condition of the fetus and newborn infant that may be attributed to several etiologies (Fig. 22–6). It may occasionally be severe enough to cause dystocia. It must be distinguished from abdominal distension secondary to intestinal obstruction, perforated viscus or neoplasm. The diagnosis may be strongly suspected when abdominal distension is accompanied by either a fluid wave or shifting dullness on percussion and a diffuse haziness is apparent on abdominal x ray. Confirmation depends on removal of fluid by paracentesis.

The most common cause of neonatal ascites is lower urinary tract obstruction, usually due to posterior urethral valves (27, 28). Increasing hydrostatic pressure leads to

hydronephrosis, and there is transudation of urine from the kidney into the retroperitoneal space. The fluid then enters the peritoneal space through small tears in the posterior peritoneum. Rupture of the urinary collecting system resulting from the elevated hydrostatic pressure may also lead to ascites.

Intravenous pyelography will reveal the presence of hydronephrosis. Because of extravasation of dye from the kidneys, a faint perirenal halo will be apparent (24).

Treatment consists of removing ascitic fluid by paracentesis and decompressing the hydronephrotic kidneys, usually by bilateral nephrostomies. Definitive repair of the underlying lesion may be possible in some cases.

Urinary ascites has also been reported in an infant with a myelomeningocele and neurogenic bladder (25). The mechanism of ascites formation here is presumably the same as in obstructive uropathy.

In hydrops fetalis, secondary to hemolytic disease of the newborn, ascites may accompany the generalized edema. A pleural effusion may also be present. These findings are

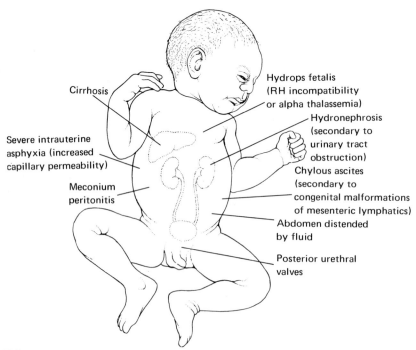

FIG. 22–6. Differential diagnosis of ascites.

presumably secondary to congestive heart failure caused by the severe anemia. Prevention and treatment are discussed in the section Bilirubin Metabolism, Chapter 8.

Ascites associated with generalized edema may also be seen following severe intrauterine asphyxia. This may be secondary to either congestive heart failure or increased capillary permeability.

Hepatic cirrhosis, usually secondary to such intrauterine infections as cytomegalovirus, toxoplasmosis or syphilis, may be associated with congenital ascites. Fetal tuberculosis with hepatic involvement and peritonitis may also be accompanied by ascites.

Ascites may be present in meconium peritonitis, which can be a complication of either meconium ileus or intestinal perforation. In this condition, the ascitic fluid is bile stained and usually sterile.

Chylous ascites, which may be seen in the neonatal period (26), is due to congenital malformation of mesenteric lymphatics. The ascitic fluid takes on the cloudy appearance only after milk feedings have been started. Treatment consists of low-fat diet and the judicious removal of ascitic fluid by paracentesis.

AMBIGUOUS GENITALIA

The discovery of ambiguous genitalia in a newborn infant presents a critical and very often perplexing problem to the physician. Although prompt diagnosis is a true medical emergency only in cases of the salt-losing variety of congenital adrenal hyperplasia, long delays in establishing the correct diagnosis may lead to adverse psychologic effects for both the family and patient.

The genetic sex of the infant is determined by the type of gonad present. Thus, an infant who possesses ovaries but has external genitalia resembling those of a male is a genotypic female and phenotypic male and is known as a female pseudohermaphrodite. The two most common causes are congenital adrenal hyperplasia (see section Adrenal Cortex, Ch. 11) and administration

of androgenic substances to the mother early in gestation. Maternal virilization, usually secondary to an androgen-producing neoplasm, can also lead to female pseudohermaphroditism. Female pseudohermaphroditism is also associated with GU anomalies, renal agenesis and esophageal atresia.

Male pseudohermaphroditism occurs when testes are present, but the external genitalia are either ambiguous or frankly female. Some examples of this are the syndrome of testicular feminization, "male" Turner's syndrome and the 3 β-hydroxysteroid form of congenital adrenal hyperplasia. Ambiguous genitalia may also be seen in genotypic males with certain congenital anomalies, among them the D trisomy syndrome.

True hermaphroditism, with the infant possessing both ovary and testis (or ovotestes), is extremely rare. The external genitalia here range from male with hypospadias to normal female.

Certain forms of sex chromosome mosaicism may also be associated with ambiguous genitalia. In the syndrome of mixed gonadal dysgenesis (XO/XY), there is one dysplastic gonad, representing the ovary, and a testis, which is usually undescended.

Embryologic development of the gonads and differential diagnosis and management of the infant with ambiguous genitalia is discussed in the section Disorders of Gonadal Development, Chapter 11.

CATARACTS

Cataracts are abnormal opacifications of the lens. Although not commonly detected in newborn infants, their occurrence is not rare. They may be difficult to detect (slit lamp examination is frequently necessary) and are often overlooked in a routine physical examination on a very young infant.

Cataracts may be hereditary (usually through an autosomal dominant mode of transmission) or acquired, either in utero or following delivery. In about one-half of all cases, other ocular abnormalities, such as microphthalmos, nystagmus, amblyopia, aniridia and dislocation of the lens, are seen. Congenital anomalies of other organ systems and mental retardation are often concomitant findings.

The most commonly seen inherited type is the zonular, or lamellar, cataract. The opacities are central and consist of lamellar areas surrounding relatively clear areas. Vision is usually normal or nearly so. Satellite and nuclear cataracts are less commonly seen, and as in the case of zonular cataracts, vision is usually not impaired.

Anterior and posterior polar cataracts are derived from the lens capsule. Although the former type does not interfere with vision, the latter often does.

Persistence of the primary vitreous, which normally disappears during the 11th week of gestation, may lead to a unilateral cataract and is often associated with microcephaly. This condition is nonhereditary.

Congenital cataracts occur in approximately one-fifth of cases of fetal rubella infection, and the opacities are usually bilateral (34). Two types of cataracts are associated with this syndrome. The entire lens may be involved, or the cataract may be centrally located, surrounded by a somewhat clearer peripheral zone (Fig. 22–7).

The rubella virus may be recovered for many months after delivery from the lenses of affected infants (36). It may also be recovered from the lens or anterior chamber of aborted fetuses and in infants of one to two years of age at postmortem examination.

Galactosemia, an inborn error of carbohydrate metabolism, may lead to cataract formation in about 70% of cases if left untreated (43). These cataracts, which are usually of the zonular or nuclear type, may be seen during the first few days of life. However, they may be small at this time and not recognized until later.

Although cataracts are seen in about 60% of cases of mongolism, they are rarely noted in the first weeks of life.

In Lowe's syndrome, which is characterized by mental retardation, hypotonia, renal rickets, aminoaciduria and glycosuria, there is about an 85% incidence of cataracts (31).

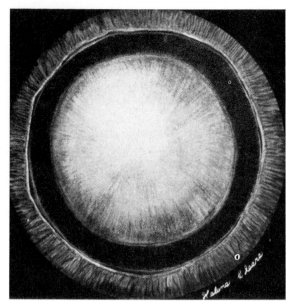

FIG. 22–7. Pearly white central rubella cataract. (Cordes FC. In Liebman SD and Gellis SS: The Pediatricians Ophthalmology, 1966)

In this sex-linked dominant condition, female carriers may also have lenticular opacities.

Other conditions that may be associated with congenital cataracts are craniosynostosis, Conradi's syndrome and the Hallermann-Streiff syndrome. A transient type of cataract, described in premature infants, is usually of little clinical significance (35). Treatment of congenital cataracts is usually conservative during the early months of life. Surgery is reserved for cases in which there is serious interference with visual acuity.

GLAUCOMA

Congenital glaucoma is rarely observed during the neonatal period; however, prompt diagnosis and treatment are vital if vision is to be preserved. Several clinical entities are associated with congenital glaucoma, a condition that is usually due to an abnormality of the tissues forming the angle of the anterior chamber of the eye. Primary developmental glaucoma has an autosomal recessive mode of inheritance and is usually bilateral.

About 50% of cases are apparent in the neonatal period. Glaucoma is an important ocular manifestation of congenital rubella (40) and, from a clinical point of view, resembles the hereditary variety. Other disorders that may be associated with congenital glaucoma are Lowe's syndrome, aniridia and retrolental fibroplasia.

The early signs of congenital glaucoma are excessive tearing, photophobia and blepharospasm. Later findings are corneal enlargement and clouding (which is secondary to edema). At birth, the cornea is normally 10 mm in diameter; this increases to 12 mm by adult life. A horizontal corneal diameter over 12.0 to 12.5 mm is highly suggestive of the diagnosis.

While intraocular pressure is usually normal at birth in congenital glaucoma, the pressure increases steadily. Digital palpation for measuring intraocular pressure is unreliable, and tonometry should be used. Other signs that may be useful in making the diagnosis are pupillary dilatation and the presence of a deep anterior chamber, which can be confirmed by gonioscopy. Funduscopy and slit lamp examination may also be of value.

The earlier the appearance of clinical signs, the poorer the prognosis. If mild corneal edema is present, the condition is usually reversible. With progression of the edema, irreversible loss of vision may ensue.

The treatment of congenital glaucoma is usually surgical since medical therapy alone is of little value. A goniotomy, or incision in the tissue of the anterior chamber, is generally the treatment of choice. Preoperative and postoperative use of pilocarpine or acetazolamide eye drops may be of ancillary value.

REFERENCES

RESPIRATORY DISTRESS

1. Avery ME: The Lung and its Disorders in the Newborn Infant, 2nd ed. Philadelphia, Saunders, 1968
2. Claireaux AE, Ferreira HP: Bilateral pulmonary agenesis. Arch Dis Child 33:364, 1958
3. France NE, Brown RJK: Congenital pulmonary lymphangiectasis: report of 11 examples with special references to cardiovascular findings. Arch Dis Child 46:528, 1971
4. Glass L, Rajegowda BK, Evans HE: Absence of the respiratory distress syndrome in premature infants of heroin addicted mothers. Lancet 2:685, 1971
5. Glass L, Rajegowda BK, Kahn EJ, Floyd MV: Effect of heroin withdrawal on respiratory rate and acid base status in the newborn. N Engl J Med 286:746, 1972
6. Swischuk LE: Transient respiratory distress of the newborn (TRDN). Am J Roentgenol Radium Ther Nucl Med 108:557, 1970
7. The Pediatric Clinics of North America: Respiratory Disorders in the Newborn. Philadelphia, Saunders, May, 1973

CYANOSIS

8. Gersony WM: Evaluating cyanosis in the newborn. Hosp Pract 4:43: 1969
9. Gersony WM: Persistence of the fetal circulation: a commentary. J Pediatr 82:1103, 1973
10. Gersony WM, Duc GV, Sinclair JC: "PFC" syndrome (persistence of the fetal circulation). Circulation 40:111, 1969
11. Gross GP, Hathaway WE, McGaughey HR: Hyperviscosity in the neonate. J Pediatr 82:1004, 1973
12. Lees MH: Cyanosis of the newborn infant. Recognition and clinical evaluation. J Pediatr 77:484, 1970
13. Roberton NR, Hallidie-Smith KA, Davis JA: Severe respiratory distress syndrome mimicking cyanotic heart disease in term babies. Lancet 2:1108, 1967
14. Shannon DC, Lusser M, Goldblatt A, Bunnell JB: The cyanotic infant—heart disease or lung disease. N Engl J Med 287:951, 1972
15. Siassi B, Goldberg SJ, Emmanouilides GC, Higashino SM, Lewis E: Persistent pulmonary vascular obstruction in newborn infants. J Pediatr 78:610, 1971

INAPPROPRIATE PASSAGE OF MECONIUM AND STOOL

16. Sherry SN, Kramer I: The time of passage of the first stool and the first urine by the newborn infant. J Pediatr 46:158, 1955
17. Van Leenwen G, Riley WC, Glenn L, Woodruff C: Meconium plug syndrome with aganglionosis. Pediatrics 40:665, 1967

ABNORMAL HEAD SIZE

18. Avery GB, Meneses L, Lodge A: The clinical significance of measurement microcephaly. Am J Dis Child 123:214, 1972
19. Chase HP, Dabiere CS, Welch NN, O'Brien D: Intrauterine undernutrition and brain development. Pediatrics 47:491, 1971

20. Lubchenko LO, Hansman C, Boyd E: Intra-uterine growth in length and head circumference as estimated from live births at gestational ages from 26 to 42 weeks. Pediatrics 37: 403, 1960

21. Martin HP: Microcephaly and mental retardation. Am J Dis Child 119:128, 1970

22. Nellhaus G: Head circumference from birth to eighteen years: practical composite international and interracial graphs. Pediatrics 41:106, 1968

23. Winick M, Rosso P: Head circumference and cellular growth of the brain in normal and marasmic children. J Pediatr 74:774, 1969

ASCITES

24. Dockray KT: The perirenal P sign. Am J Dis Child 119:179, 1970

25. Howat JM: Urinary ascites complicating spina bifida. Arch Dis Child 46:103, 1971

26. Kessel I: Chylous ascites in infancy. Arch Dis Child 27:79, 1952

27. Moncada R, Wany JJ, Love L, Bush I: Neonatal ascites associated with urinary outlet obstruction (urine ascites). Radiology 90:1165, 1968

28. North AF, Eldredge DM, Talpey WB: Abdominal distension at birth: due to ascites associated with obstructive uropathy. Am J Dis Child 111:613, 1966

AMBIGUOUS GENITALIA

29. Moloshok RE, Kerr JM: The infant with ambiguous genitalia. Pediatr Clin North Am 19:529, 1972

30. Schlegal RJ, Gardner LI: Ambiguous and abnormal genitalia in infants: differential diagnosis and clinical management. In: Endocrine and Genetic Diseases of Childhood. Edited by LI Gardner. Philadelphia, Saunders, 1969

CATARACTS

31. Abbassi V, Lowe CU, Calcagno PL: Oculocerebro-renal syndrome; a review. Am J Dis Child 115:145, 1968

32. Chandler PA: Congenital cataract. Pediatr Clin North Am 5:169, 1958

33. Cordes FC: Developmental and acquired cataracts of infancy and childhood. In: The Pediatrician's Ophthalmology. Edited by Liebman and Gellis. St Loius, Mosby, 1966

34. Gregg NM: Congenital cataract following german measles in the mother. Trans Ophthalmol Soc Aust 3:35, 1941

35. McCormick AQ: Transient cataracts in premature infants; a new clinical entity. Can J Ophthalmol 3:202, 1968

36. Menser MA, Harley JD, Hertzberg R, Dorman DC, Murphy AM: Persistence of virus in lens for three years after prenatal rubella. Lancet 2:387, 1967

37. Wilson WA, Donnell GN: Cataracts in galactosemia. Arch Ophthalmol 60:215, 1958

GLAUCOMA

38. Barkan O, Ferguson WJ: Congenital glaucoma. Pediatr Clin North Am 5:225, 1958

39. Chandler PA: Glaucoma in infancy and childhood. In: The Pediatrician's Ophthalomogy. Edited by Liebman and Gellis. St Louis, Mosby, 1966

40. Sears ML: Congenital glaucoma in neonatal rubella. Br J Ophthalmol 51:744, 1967

23

Surgical Problems

S. FRANK REDO

Surgery in the neonatal period should be performed in life-threatening crises only; elective procedures should be avoided. Surgical emergencies in newborn infants may involve thoracic or abdominal contents or the central nervous system, although the most commonly encountered problems are intraabdominal, and since there is very little room for error in the fragile infant, their successful management depends on careful attention to detail. The therapeutic aim should be to do as little as is necessary to save life. In some instances this may necessitate surgery in stages and several operations, but it is far better to proceed stepwise and ultimately achieve a viable infant than to attempt a single definitive procedure with a fatal outcome.

GENERAL PROCEDURES

PREOPERATIVE PROCEDURES

The basic tenets of preoperative care of the newborn infant are to establish a correct diagnosis utilizing the minimum number of procedures and to maintain normal homeostasis during this period (17).

From the point of view of diagnostic evaluation, the number and types of tests required to establish a diagnosis depend largely on the signs exhibited by the patient. If, for example, the problem is abdominal in nature, the presence or absence of a perforated viscus or intestinal obstruction must be established. Usually, plain films of the abdomen (flat and upright) will be adequate. Contrast studies should generally be limited to vigorous infants, but a barium enema is often vital in making the diagnosis of malrotation or megacolon, while a contrast study of the upper GI tract may be necessary for the diagnosis of esophageal atresia.

In the presence of unexplained dyspnea, a plain x ray of the chest may point to such surgical conditions as a pneumothorax or diaphragmatic hernia. In cardiac emergencies, special studies, including cardiac catheterization or angiography may be required. Serum electrolytes, blood gases and pH should be determined prior to surgery, especially in the presence of vomiting.

Since caloric deprivation usually accompanies a surgical condition, the infant must be managed in a strict thermoneutral environment. All procedures should be performed either inside of the incubator or under a radiant heater (see Ch. 13, Thermoregulation).

All fluid, acid-base and electrolyte disturbances should be corrected prior to surgery, and a normal blood glucose concentration must be maintained. The infant, of

---

The section Neurosurgical Problems (p. 508 ff) was prepared in association with Dr. Joseph H. Galicich.

course, must be adequately oxygenated, and any apparent or suspected infection must be treated.

Immediately prior to surgery, blood should be drawn for typing and cross-matching so that blood replacement can be provided at the time of surgery (10). In addition, a cutdown should be performed in order to insure an adequate route for IV instillation of fluids and blood during and immediately following surgery. A needle in a vein should not be relied on as a dependable IV route since during surgery these too often become dislodged or infiltrate. Consent for operation must be obtained from the parents, and the surgeon and neonatologist must carefully explain the situation to them.

OPERATIVE PRECAUTIONS

Temperature regulation is a major concern in newborn infants undergoing surgery (12, 15). Since the body cavity and viscera are usually exposed at operation, the surface area available for heat loss is markedly increased, and rapid cooling of the infant may ensue. It would be ideal if a warm environmental temperature were maintained over the operative field (14). If this is not possible, the dangers of heat loss may be minimized by placing the infant on either a heating mattress or an inverted instrument tray containing hot water bottles. Even with these precautions, however, it should be remembered that only that portion of the child in contact with the heat source will be heated. Usually this is only a small amount of the total body surface area.

As an additional aid, rubber gloves may be filled with warm water and applied to the groin or to both sides of the neck. Since large blood vessels traverse these areas, total body heating will be improved. Whenever heat in any form is applied to an infant, it is the responsibility of the person overseeing such application to make sure that the units being used are not so hot as to cause burns. Solutions in heating mattresses should not exceed body temperature, and similar precautions hold for hot water

bottles or gloves. During the surgical procedure there should be an indwelling thermometer of the type that can be connected to a constantly recording temperature gauge. In this way temperature changes can be monitored as the procedure progresses. Blood should be warmed before being used to replace any losses. Cold blood may lead to cardiac irregularities and fibrillation, especially if administered rapidly.

In thoracic procedures in which the pleural cavities are entered and in certain abdominal emergencies requiring maximum relaxation (such as in omphalocele repair) general endotracheal anesthesia may be mandatory, but most emergency procedures can be performed with local anesthesia. Xylocaine or procaine in 0.5% solution has been adequate in such extensive procedures as resection of intestinal segments as well as in less involved procedures, such as gastrostomy or colostomy. A minimal amount of agent should be employed. If care is taken not to exert pull or pressure on parietal peritoneum or mesenteries, the infant shows little discomfort and tolerates surgery well. It is important, however, despite the use of local anesthesia, that an anesthesiologist be in attendance throughout the procedure to properly monitor the child and to provide oxygen, stimulants or other medications as required.

Recent advances in monitoring equipment may enhance care of the infant during surgery (18). Blood pressures can now be measured accurately in newborn infants utilizing the Doppler principle, and telemetry permits the monitoring of cardiac rate and rhythm on an oscilloscope screen without the need for attaching wires from the infant to the monitoring device. Applying a stethoscope over the precordium and listening to heart sounds during surgery is a less-sophisticated means of monitoring the patient's cardiac status.

The unrecognized and uncorrected loss of even small amounts of blood may lead to a disastrous outcome when surgery is performed in the premature infant. Estimation of blood loss by the surgeon by visual means is wholly inadequate. In order to make as accurate an account of blood loss as is currently possible, all sponges used during the operation should be periodically discarded and weighed and the small amount of blood aspirated from the operative field should be suctioned into a small graduated cylinder, instead of the usual large discard bottle, for measurement. Based on sponge weights and aspiration losses, warmed blood should be administered to replace losses as accurately as possible.

POSTOPERATIVE MAINTENANCE

Attention must be paid to carefully maintaining homeostasis during the postoperative period. A strict thermoneutral environment must be maintained, especially when caloric intake is low. If the infant has had endotracheal intubation, a high environmental humidity should be maintained. In this case, care should be taken to avoid maceration and possible infection secondary to breaks in the skin.

Fluid, electrolyte and acid-base balance must be carefully maintained (8). During the postoperative periods, fluids and electrolytes are administered intravenously. Preparations containing potassium salts are not administered until the child has voided, after which solutions with potassium are begun. In addition to maintenance requirements, any abnormal fluid and electrolyte losses must be replaced with a satisfactory substitute. In general, if these abnormal losses are expected to persist over several days, it is better to have the fluid analyzed for electrolyte content and to replace it volume per volume with a solution prepared as nearly as possible having the same electrolyte constituents. If losses due to drainage are for short periods only, solutions containing approximately the same electrolyte concentration as the fluid lost may be employed, basing the evaluation of the types and amounts of electrolytes lost on readily obtainable average composition tables of fluids from various levels of the GI tract.

If the GI tract is expected to be nonfunctional for a prolonged period of time, total parenteral alimentation may be indicated.

Enteral feedings after an intraabdominal procedure should not be started until there is evidence of intestinal activity as manifested by: 1) lack of distension, 2) normal bowel sounds or 3) passage of stool or gas per rectum or per colostomy. In practice, the indwelling nasogastric tube is left in place until one or more of the above signs are manifest. Feedings are then usually withheld for an additional 6 to 12 hours after removal of the tube; then, following the criteria stated earlier, oral alimentation may begin. Paralytic ileus is not uncommon following intraabdominal surgery even in premature infants. Feeding such patients too soon may intensify the ileus and delay even longer the time to initiate oral alimentation.

AIRWAY AND THORAX

Breathing difficulties in the neonate and infant may be due to problems involving upper and lower air passages. Some of these problems become evident immediately after birth; others may not appear until later in infancy. Airway obstruction may be due to intrinsic or extrinsic factors.

CHOANAL ATRESIA

Choanal atresia is a congenital anomaly of unknown etiology, occurring in about 1:60,000 births (20, 22), in which there is no orifice through the posterior nares into the nasopharynx. The partition across the posterior nares may be membranous or bony. There may be small fenestrations, but these are usually not adequate to provide a satisfactory airway. When atresia is unilateral, the infant may not show signs of airway obstruction, and the condition may go unrecognized for years. However, when choanal atresia is bilateral the infant may manifest severe dyspnea because of reliance on nasal rather than on oral breathing. Indeed, it may take days or weeks for the infant to utilize his mouth for breathing as well as sucking. Therefore, the forms of dyspnea manifested can be related to the ability of the child to breathe by mouth. If the child cannot do so, dyspnea may be continuous with better aeration when the child cries and some air enters the tracheobronchial tree from the mouth. When an infant is able to mouth-breathe, dyspnea may be exhibited when he is sucking, since the mouth cannot be used for feeding and breathing at the same time. In these babies, dyspnea may not be apparent except at feeding time.

Choanal atresia should be considered in all instances of dyspnea in neonates. It can be readily demonstrated by attempting to pass a tube through the nose into the pharynx. If this cannot be done, choanal atresia probably exists. Definitive diagnosis can be made by instilling a small amount of water-soluble contrast agent into the posterior nares and obtaining a radiogram of the skull in the lateral position (Fig. 23–1).

Emergency treatment may be required to establish an airway (23). If the atresia is due

to a membranous partition, it can be punctured and polyethylene stents placed through the anterior and posterior nares without much difficulty. These should remain in place for several months. When a bony partition exists, treatment is more involved, and both the bony wall and soft tissue must be resected (21). Polyethylene stents are again used and left in place for several months. After removal of these stents, soft tissue or bone may grow and again decrease the size of the choanal opening. However, in such a situation, the infant no longer is dependent on nasal breathing and more definitive corrective surgery with more extensive choanal enlargement can usually be performed at this older age. Infants with choanal atresia who manifest dyspnea on sucking can be managed prior to surgical intervention by using gavage methods for feeding and, often, by inserting an oral airway.

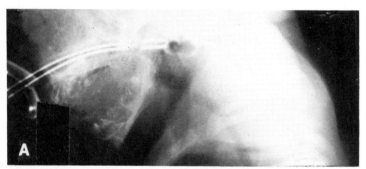

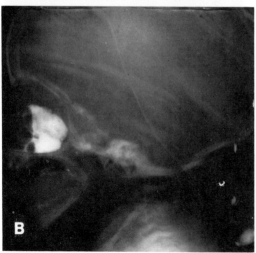

FIG. 23–1. Choanal atresia. Diagnosis is established by instilling a small amount of contrast agent into the posterior nares and obtaining a radiogram of the skull in the lateral position. **A.** Tube cannot be passed through nose into pharynx; **B.** water-soluble contrast material instilled into posterior nares does not enter pharynx.

EXTRINSIC LESIONS CAUSING TRACHEAL OBSTRUCTION

Respiratory obstruction may be caused by tracheal compression due to anomalous blood vessels, cystic hygroma and hemangioma in the neck, as well as by mediastinal cysts and tumors (29, 31). These latter problems will be discussed in their seperate sections below.

Vascular Anomalies

Vascular anomalies that may cause tracheal obstruction include double aortic arch, right aortic arch with a left ligamentum arteriosum, anomalous innominate artery, anomalous left common carotid artery and aberrant right subclavian artery (26, 30, 33). In many instances there may be esophageal compression as well, with some degree of dysphagia.

Clinical signs depend on the type of vascular anomaly and the degree to which tracheal and/or esophageal lumina are narrowed. Dyspnea may be present at birth or may appear within the first few weeks. The majority of infants have inspiratory stridor, although some may exhibit expiratory wheezing. This may persist during sleep and is more marked on crying. Cyanosis may be observed. Feeding is apt to accentuate stridor, increase dyspnea and cyanosis and precipitate coughing spells. All signs are aggravated by pulmonary infections, to which these infants are prone. In a classic case of double aortic arch, the child may assume an almost opisthotonic position with the head sharply extended. This position provides the maximum airway. Flexion of the head exaggerates the signs. Aberrant right subclavian arteries passing posterior to the esophagus and indenting it, rarely cause difficulty and usually require no treatment.

Diagnosis may be established by means of esophagram, tracheogram and angiocardiogram. Characteristically the esophagram and tracheogram will show narrowing or compression of the trachea, esophagus or both. Angiocardiography is helpful in precisely delineating the vascular anomaly.

Treatment consists in dividing the vascular elements that cause the ring, thus liberating and decompressing the trachea and esophagus. The particular technique to be employed obviously depends on the nature of the structures comprising the ring. The approach advocated by Gross (3) for dealing with these problems is a left anterolateral incision through the third intercostal space with division of the second, third and fourth costal cartilages. In the author's experience a left posterolateral incision has been equally effective and has been preferred.

Following the division of the ring it may be necessary with some of the anomalies to suture the aorta forward to the under surface of the sternum. At the conclusion of the operation a catheter is inserted into the left pleural space and placed on suction for from 24 to 48 hours, after which it may be removed.

HEMANGIOMA AND CYSTIC HYGROMA

Large cystic hygroma or hemangiomas in the neck (Figs. 23–2, 23–3) may cause tracheal and sometimes esophageal compression (25, 27, 28, 32, 34). In cystic hygroma, prompt excision with or without a temporary tracheostomy will alleviate the obstruction. In practice, the surgery is performed using an endotracheal tube, and in most instances tracheostomy is avoided. An occasional infant may require tracheostomy in the immediate postoperative period due to laryngeal edema, especially if there was difficulty in performing tracheal intubation. In these children the tracheostomy tube can usually be removed safely within two to three days and the stoma allowed to heal, which it does relatively rapidly. Hemangiomas causing tracheal or esophageal compression, or both, on the other hand, can rarely be removed in infancy. In these instances a tracheostomy must be constructed and usually must remain in place for one or more years until the hemangioma has resolved. These infants should not be irradiated because of the danger that this may cause laryngeal or tracheal stenosis as they grow. Within one or two years, most of these hemangiomas will spontaneously blanch and disappear or regress sufficiently so that they no longer compress the trachea or esophagus. Some cases require gastrostomy as well as tracheostomy if there is esophageal obstruction.

TRACHEOSTOMY

Many surgeons regard this procedure as hazardous and fraught with complications in the neonatal period. Our own experience, however, has led us not to hesitate about performing this operation when the indications for it exist. The prime indication, obviously, is upper airway obstruction for

FIG. 23–2. Large cystic hygroma of neck. **A.** External appearance. **B.** Exposure of mass at surgery.

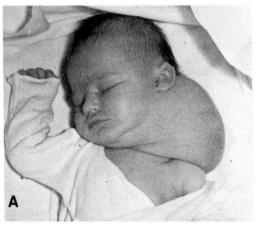

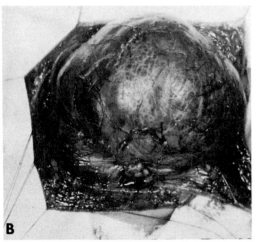

whatever reason. The technique, employed both in the surgical operating room and when it must be done as an emergency at the patient's crib, is simple and requires little advance preparation. Sterile tracheostomy sets, including tubes from #000 to #2 that are made especially short for pediatric use (36, 37), should be available. In most cases the child is intubated without anesthesia, and the tracheostomy is then performed under local or general anesthesia. After suitable sterile prepping and draping, a small collar incision is made just above the episternal notch; it is important to not make this too low or too high. Significant bleeding is rarely encountered. The incision is carried through the platysma and spread with a small self-retaining retractor. The strap muscles are separated in the midline, and the trachea is identified below the level of the thyroid gland. The indwelling endotracheal tube facilitates identification of the trachea, especially in cases where it may be displaced away from the midline. Although many authors suggest the excision of tracheal cartilage for placement of the tracheostomy tube, we have found it equally effective to simply grasp the trachea with a tracheal hook and make a cruciate incision extending one cartilaginous ring above and below the site of application of the hook. A tracheal dilator can then be inserted, after which the largest tube that will be accommodated by the trachea is inserted as the endotracheal tube is removed. The tracheostomy tube is inserted with its inner trochar. Immediately after insertion the trochar is removed and the inner tube inserted. The twill tape attached to the tube flange is then tied securely about the patient's neck, and the skin edges are loosely approximated with a few silk sutures. If it will be necessary to place the patient on a positive pressure respirator, a cuffed or tight fitting tracheostomy tube is employed.

Immediately after operation the patient is placed in a high humidity atmosphere. A special duty nurse is assigned to him exclusively and he is not left unattended for an instant. The inner tube is removed and cleaned every one to two hours as needed for the first three to four days and less-frequently thereafter. Suctioning through the tube is carried out for short periods at regular intervals and as required. The entire tracheostomy tube is replaced at weekly intervals (24, 35). Bacterial cultures of the tracheostomy tube and secretions should be taken at frequent intervals.

Complications that may occur during or following tracheostomy include pneumothorax, pneumomediastinum, subcutaneous emphysema, bleeding and blockage and dislodgement of tube. Pneumothorax and pneumomediastinum are usually due to entry into the pleura during the operation or too low placement of the tube. If the patient's neck is hyperextended at the time of the procedure and the tracheal opening is made low, on straightening the neck, the tracheal opening may be below the level of the episternal notch. In these cases subcutaneous emphysema of the neck, face and upper chest or pneumomediastinum, or both, may result. However, these usually require no treatment and will gradually subside as the air is absorbed. Pneumothorax may require aspiration if it is significant enough to cause respiratory distress. Bleeding is uncommon in our experience, but it may occur as a result of tears or lacerations of thyroid gland or blood vessels in the operative area. None of these complications should result from a carefully performed operation. Dislodgement or blockage of the tube, which may be due to poor nursing care in the immediate postoperative period, emphasize the importance of careful and frequent care. This includes suctioning the tracheostomy, cleaning or changing the inner tube, observing the patient's activities and checking the attachment of tube flange to neck by twill tape.

PULMONARY LESIONS

AGENESIS OF THE LUNG

Agenesis of the lung is an uncommon condition that may occur unilaterally or bilater-

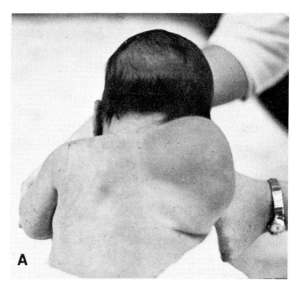

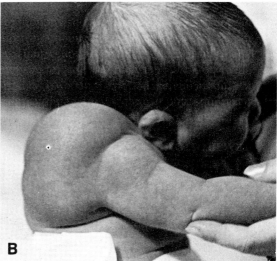

FIG. 23–3. Large cystic hygroma over right scapular region. **A.** Posterior view. **B.** Lateral view. There was no extension into chest.

ally (42, 56, 58). Bilateral pulmonary agenesis is extremely rare, fewer than ten cases having been reported. It may or may not be associated with absence of all or a portion of the trachea and with cardiac anomalies. Obviously, it is incompatible with life and there is currently no treatment for it.

Unilateral agenesis of the lung is also uncommon, but in 30 cases collected by Minetto (50), 17 involved the left side and 13 the right. Skeletal, cardiac and other anomalies are common in these infants.

Cyanosis, dyspnea, harsh breathing and other manifestations of respiratory distress occur. There is usually no associated chest wall deformity. The mediastinum is shifted, and breath sounds are absent on the affected side, which also elicits a dull percussion note. X rays reveal a homogeneous density, and the heart is located in the involved side. This may sometimes be interpreted as massive atelectasis. Bronchoscopy or bronchography may be required to make the diagnosis.

Although the majority of those with this problem die in infancy or early childhood, cases have been reported of patients 60 and 70 years of age. There is presently no surgical treatment, although the suggestion has been made that right-sided agenesis be treated surgically by plombage with the hope of preventing wide excursions of the mediastinal contents.

LUNG SEQUESTRATION

Sequestration of the lung and accessory lobes do not cause illness but may lead to misdiagnosis on x-ray examination. The sequestered lung appears as a smooth, soft tissue density between the dome of the diaphragm and the inferior surface of the lung, usually on the left side. The accessory lobe does not contain air and has no connection with the lung or tracheobronchial tree. Its blood is supplied directly from the aorta, as aortography clearly demonstrates (40, 57). Treatment is by surgical excision and is usually uncomplicated. However, the erroneous diagnosis of an accessory lobe as mediastinal tumor and its removal under that misconception with failure to recognize the aorta supplying its blood may lead to excessive bleeding.

CYSTIC DISEASE OF THE LUNG

Although uncommon in the neonate, cystic disease of the lung may be responsible for severe respiratory distress and constitute challenging diagnostic and therapeutic problems (38, 41, 51). The cysts may be single or multiple, unilateral or bilateral and filled with air, fluid or both; they are usually congenital. The lesions most frequently encountered are lobar emphysema, bronchogenic cyst, and cystic adenomatoid malformation of the lung.

LOBAR EMPHYSEMA

Abnormal distension of a pulmonary lobe can produce respiratory distress in otherwise normal newborns (45, 49, 53, 54). The disease is usually unilobular and is often confined to an upper or middle lobe, but it may be segmental, bilobular or bilateral or may involve an entire lung. Etiologic factors include mediastinal tumor, bronchial stenosis or some other form of partial bronchial obstruction or intrinsic alveolar disease which produces lobar hyperaeration. Progressive respiratory distress from birth to the second or third month of life may occur. There is usually cough, wheezing, dyspnea, tachypnea, tachycardia, expiratory stridor and intermittent cyanosis, often aggreveted by feeding. There may be retraction and bulging of the thorax, tracheal and cardiac shift, hyperresonant percussion tones and diminished breath sounds; chest roentgenograms in various views will establish the diagnosis (Fig. 23-4). Treatment by excision is specific and highly successful (Figs. 23-5, 23-6).

BRONCHOGENIC CYSTS

These may or may not have demonstrable communication with the tracheobronchial tree. They appear to be true congenital anomalies and have been described in 31-mm embryos, probably representing abnormal budding or diverticulum of the ventral component of the primitive foregut. Bronchogenic cysts are usually situated in the posterior part of the mediastinum at about the level of the carina and may occur on the right or left side. Although they have been classified on the basis of their location as paratracheal, carinal, hilar, paraesophageal and miscellaneous, the majority occur in the hilar area. Those in the carinal location are associated with highest mortality because of compression of both main stem bronchi, causing complete obstruction of the

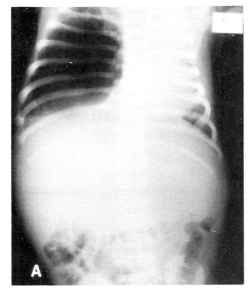

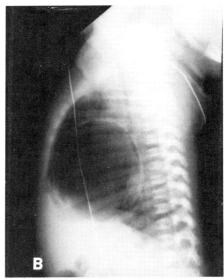

FIG. 23–4. Large emphysematous area occupying region of right middle lobe. **A.** Posteroanterior view showing mediastinum shifted to the left with compression of most of left lung. **B.** Lateral view with the emphysematous lesion well demonstrated.

airway. Roentgenogram of the chest is the most useful single examination in establishing diagnosis. If the cyst is not demonstrable in the posteroanterior view, it may be visible on the lateral or oblique projections or on tomograms of the lung fields. Associated signs that are helpful in making a diagnosis include deviation of the trachea or esophagus, or both; abnormal separation of the trachea and esophagus on the lateral or oblique views; and mediastinal shift. Areas of atelectasis or pneumonitis distal to the lesion; emphysema of the lung, indicating a ball valve type of obstruction; or compensatory emphysema of the uninvolved lobes or of the contralateral lung are all indirect evidence of bronchogenic cysts.

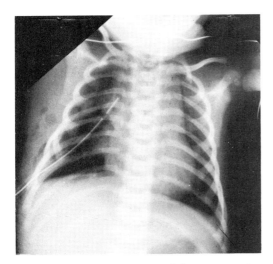

FIG. 23–5. Posteroanterior view following resection of right middle lobe. The mediastinum has moved back into near-normal position; left lung now well aerated; remaining right upper and lower lobes expanded.

FIG. 23–6. Resected right middle lobe with portion of area of emphysema opened.

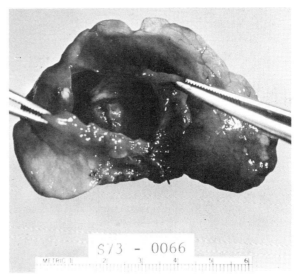

Occasionally, bronchoscopy or bronchography, or both, and angiocardiography may be required to establish the diagnosis unequivocally. Bronchoscopy and bronchography must be done cautiously and only when necessary to prevent further compromise of depressed respiratory function. Radiographically these cysts are usually sharply defined solitary round or oval shadows without calcification (55). Fluoroscopically, their attachment to the trachea or bronchus can be demonstrated by the motion of the lesion during swallowing.

The treatment of the mediastinal bronchogenic cyst is excision. It is clear from the collected experience that the presence of such a cyst is an urgent indication for surgical intervention (44, 46). These lesions must be properly diagnosed and treated to prevent progressive respiratory difficulty and to protect against the crippling effects of irreversible emphysema.

CYSTIC ADENOMATOID MALFORMATION OF THE LUNG

This is a rare lesion characterized by multiple cysts in one or more lobes of the lung, usually unilateral (39, 43, 47, 48). Pathogenesis is unknown, and there is no complete agreement among pathologists as to its classification. Some consider it hamartoma or congenital cystic disease of the lung. Five features of cystic adenomatoid malformation of the lung that differentiate it from congenital cystic disease of the lung have been described:

1. Absence of bronchial cartilage
2. Absence of bronchial tubular glands
3. Presence of tall columnar mucinous glands
4. Overproduction of terminal bronchiolar structures without alveolar differentiation, except in the subpleural areas and
5. Massive enlargement of the affected lobe that displaces other thoracic structures

Regardless of the nomenclature, this is a serious lesion that often increases in size rapidly with further compromise of already-restricted pulmonary function. Respiratory

distress and cyanosis occur immediately after birth. On physical examination, the chest may be barrel shaped, breath sounds may be poor or absent on the affected side with heart sounds shifted into the unaffected one. Diagnosis can be made by roentgenograms of the chest although in some instances, the film may suggest diaphragmatic hernia. On x ray the involved lung contains cystic and solid features with shift of the mediastinal structures to the opposite side and compression of the good lung (Figs. 23–7, 23–8). Because in our experience this has been a rapidly progressive

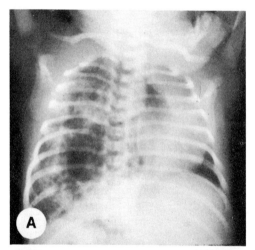

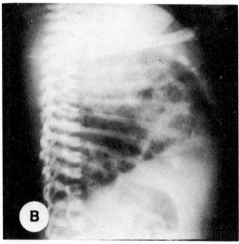

FIG. 23–7. Chest with large cystic and solid mass. **A.** Posteroanterior view of mass on right displacing mediastinum to left and compressed left lung. **B.** Lateral view demonstrates cystic areas better. The entire right lung appears involved.

process, surgical removal of the involved lobe or lung should be performed without delay. In most of the reported cases, resection can be limited to one or more lobes, without requiring removal of the entire lung. Surgery has been successful in more than 90% of the patients as compared to a uniformly fatal outcome when supportive measures alone were used (52). Postoperatively, the mediastinum returns to a more normal position, the good lung expands fully, and there is function of the remaining lung on the operated side (Fig. 23–9). Follow-up evaluation of our two patients two years after surgery reveals them to be in good health without respiratory problems and without evidence of recurrence or persistence of their disease.

PNEUMOMEDIASTINUM AND PNEUMOTHORAX

Pneumomediastinum and pneumothorax in the neonate are the result of a tear in an over-distended alveolus with subsequent interstitial emphysema. Air then migrates along the perivascular sheaths of the pulmonary blood vessels or peribronchial tissues to the mediastinum. If the process stops at this point, pneumomediastinum is apparent. However, if sufficient air accumulates, the mediastinal pleura may rupture, allowing air to enter one or both pleural spaces and producing pneumothorax (59, 63).

PNEUMOMEDIASTINUM

In most instances this is an asymptomatic condition that does not require surgical intervention (60, 66). Diagnosis can often be made on physical examination if there is a significant accumulation of air. Under these conditions, the sternum is thrust forward, there is a hyperresonant percussion note over it, and rarely a clicking noise may be heard synchronous with the heartbeat. Heart sounds may be distant. There may be cyanosis and, very unusually, signs of

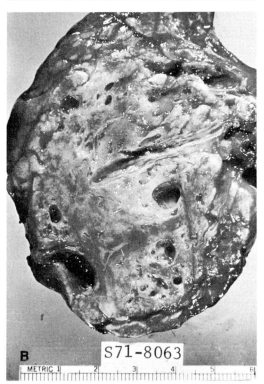

FIG. 23–8. Resected specimen (right lower and middle lobes). **A.** External view. **B.** Appearance after sectioning the tumor.

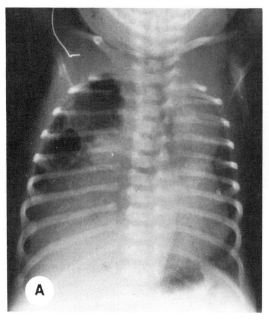

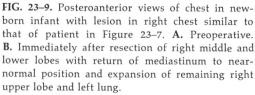

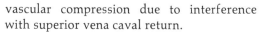

FIG. 23–9. Posteroanterior views of chest in newborn infant with lesion in right chest similar to that of patient in Figure 23–7. **A.** Preoperative. **B.** Immediately after resection of right middle and lower lobes with return of mediastinum to near-normal position and expansion of remaining right upper lobe and left lung.

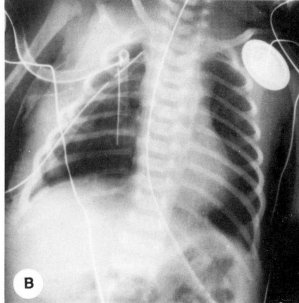

vascular compression due to interference with superior vena caval return.

Posteroanterior and lateral x rays of the chest will reveal a radiolucent area of variable degree behind the sternum and the characteristic "sail sign" produced by a collection of air outlining the thymus gland (Fig. 23–10). Treatment by retrosternal aspiration has been necessary in only one patient in our experience. The air usually will absorb spontaneously, but the condition may progress to a frank pneumothorax. Chernick and Avery (59) have demonstrated in animals that breathing 100% oxygen facilitates absorption of air from the chest. Although we have not used this technique for pneumomediastinum, it has been successfully used for the management of small pneumothoraces. This technique should be avoided in premature infants because of the danger of retrolental fibroplasia.

PNEUMOTHORAX

Asymptomatic pneumothorax occurs in about 1% of deliveries and symptomatic pneumothorax in 0.07% of live births (61, 62). In our own experience with 50 cases the left side was more often affected than the right, and bilateral involvement was not uncommon. Neonates with pneumothorax usually have associated complications, such as prematurity, hyaline membrane disease or aspiration. In many cases delivery is difficult, and because of the respiratory distress due to the associated complications mentioned, vigorous resuscitative efforts may be required (64). The combination of these factors probably leads to alveolar rupture and the progression to pneumomediastinum and pneumothorax.

The diagnosis should be suspected in any infant with respiratory distress. Classic signs on physical examination include diminished to absent breath sounds, hyperresonant percussion note and a shift of mediastinal structures to the unaffected side. Roentgenograms of the chest are usually diagnostic, but pneumothorax may be missed if the study is performed in the supine position. The diagnosis can be read-

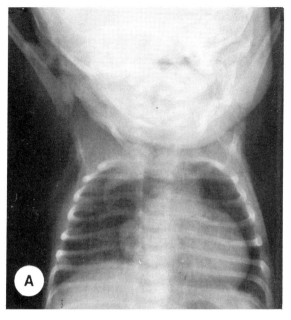

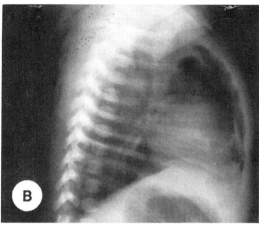

FIG. 23–10. Pneumomediastinum. **A.** Posteroanterior view of chest reveals characteristic "sail sign" produced by air outlining the thymus gland. **B.** Lateral view of chest shows radiolucent area behind sternum.

ily established by sitting posteroanterior x-ray views of the chest (Fig. 23–11).

Treatment depends on the extent of the pneumothorax (65). In infants with less than 25% involvement, the use of 100% oxygen breathing or simple observation is usually sufficient, and the air will resorb within a few days at most. Repeat physical examination of the chest at frequent intervals and x-ray studies as indicated by the findings should be performed to avoid the development of undetected tension pneumothorax.

If there is more than 25% involvement, initial treatment by simple aspiration with a post aspiration x ray may be performed. In some infants this may be all that is necessary, following which repeat examination in several hours should be done. If air has

FIG. 23–11. Sitting posteroanterior roentgenogram revealing significant pneumothorax on right with shift of mediastinum to the left.

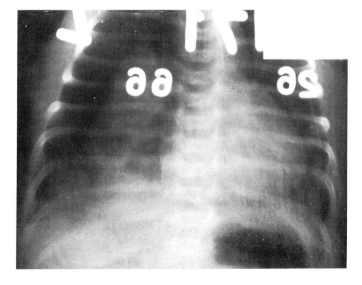

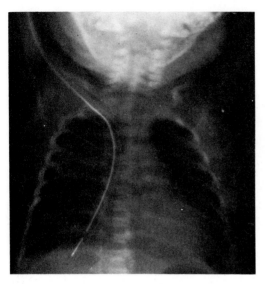

FIG. 23–12. Same patient as in Figure 23–11 immediately after insertion of chest tube. Right lung has partially reexpanded; pneumothorax is markedly decreased.

reaccumulated, obviously a persistent air leak exists. This is a definite indication for insertion of an intercostal catheter for chest drainage (Fig. 23–12). We prefer to connect this catheter to 8 to 10 cm of suction, although others simply attach it to an underwater seal. Small polyethylene tubes for drainage should be mentioned only to be condemned. They are rarely effective over a long period of time and may give a dangerous, false sense of security.

Our policy has been to leave the chest tube in place until bubbling stops in the collection bottle. The tube is then clamped and removed after 12 to 24 hours if there is no further accumulation of air. In patients with bilateral pneumothorax, chest tubes are inserted bilaterally. Usually such tubes are removed by withdrawing first one and then the other 12 to 24 hours later. If air leakage persists despite tube drainage, open thoracotomy may be necessary to identify the site of leakage and close it by suture. In our experience this has never become necessary. The outcome is largely dependent on the underlying cause of the air leakage. In those infants without serious underlying pulmo-

nary problems, e.g., respiratory distress syndrome (RDS), the prognosis is excellent and recovery without complications or sequelae is the rule. In contrast, simple control of pneumothorax is not effective in those patients with serious underlying pulmonary problems.

ESOPHAGUS

ESOPHAGEAL ATRESIA

Esophageal atresia is a condition in which the luminal continuity of the esophagus from the pharynx into the stomach is interrupted. In addition, there may be a fistulous communication between the esophagus and the trachea. Esophageal atresia is encountered in about 1:3000 to 1:5000 births, with a slightly increased incidence in males (70, 73). The disorder is due to a failure of complete separation of the primitive esophageal and tracheal tubes and probably occurs before the eighth week of gestation.

Because of the lack of luminal continuity of the esophagus these infants are unable to swallow amniotic fluid, and as a result polyhydramnios in the mother is an almost constant finding. The diagnosis can be suspected in newborn infants with an inordinate amount of oral secretions that require repeated aspiration. When feedings are offered, choking, coughing and cyanosis are apparent. Breathing may become labored, and there may be evidence of secretions within the tracheobronchial tree. The diagnosis can be made by attempting to pass a small catheter or feeding tube into the stomach. If the catheter stops abruptly 10 to 12 cm or less from the nares, the diagnosis is almost certain. In such situations, it has been our policy to withdraw the tube about 1 cm and tape it in place. The child is then taken to the radiology area and an x ray of the chest to include the abdomen is obtained. About ½ to 1 ml of water-soluble contrast material is introduced into the nasal tube. This will confirm the diagnosis and indicate the lower level of the blind upper esophageal segment. In addition the status of the lungs and heart can be evaluated on the chest film, and the presence or absence of air in the stomach can be noted in the abdominal portion (Fig. 23–13). It is important to use only a small amount of contrast material, since the overflow of substantial amounts into the tracheobronchial tree may lead to improper evaluation of possible tracheoesophageal fistulas and augment pulmonary problems already present (Fig. 23–14).

Esophageal atresias with and without tracheoesophageal fistula have been classified by many authors, often based on their own cases. However, the two most commonly used classifications are those of Vogt (81) and Gross (2). The Vogt classification lists three major variants: *Type I* is that in which there is a complete absence of esophagus; *Type II* consists of a blind upper and blind lower esophageal segment; *Type III* includes those cases of atresia in which there is also a tracheoesophageal fistula between (IIIa), upper esophageal segment and trachea, (IIIb), lower segment and trachea, or (IIIc), both upper and lower segments and the trachea. The Gross classification is more widely used, with designations extending from A to F. The A form of esophageal atresia consists of a blind upper and a blind lower esophageal segment without tracheoesophageal fistula. In the B, C and D forms there is an associated tracheoesophageal fistula: in the B type, from the upper esophageal segment; in the C from the lower segment; and, in D from both segments. The E variant is that situation in which there is no esophageal atresia but there is a tracheoesophageal fistula—this form is often referred to as the "H" fistula because of the "H" configuration provided by the vertical limbs of the esophagus and trachea and the horizontal limb of the fistula (90). The F type is included in their classification to complete congenital esophageal problems. In this condition there is stenosis or narrowing somewhere along the course of the esophagus without atresia and without a tracheoesophageal fistula. In our discussion we will use the classification

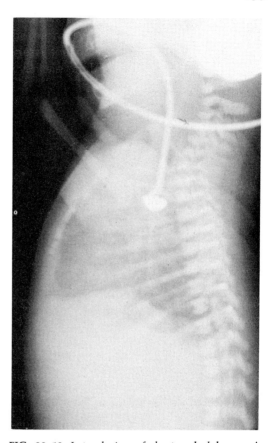

FIG. 23–13. Lateral view of chest and abdomen. A small amount of water-soluble contrast material has been instilled into the upper esophageal segment, outlining the blind pouch. Absence of stomach gas bubble reflects atresia of A type.

of Ladd and Gross rather than that of Vogt.

In a survey of 1058 patients with esophageal atresia conducted by the Surgical Section of the American Academy of Pediatrics covering the five-year period from 1958 to 1962 (72), the incidence of the various types of esophageal atresia was reported (in percent) as follows: Type A 7.7, B 0.8, C 86.5, D 0.7, E 4.2. In this series 52% of patients had some other anomaly in addition to the esophageal lesion. Congenital heart disease and gastrointestinal anomalies were found in about 20% of cases, while GU problems were present in about 10% of cases. The associated anomaly frequently affected survival. Management of the infant with esophageal atresia may be divided into two phases: 1) Presurgical and 2) Surgical.

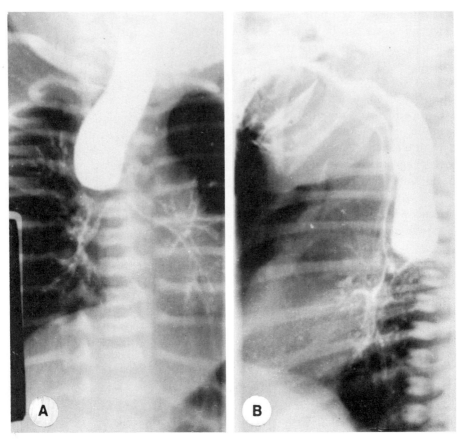

FIG. 23–14. Large quantity of contrast material given to infant by mouth with consequent overflow into trachea and bronchi produced an unintentional tracheobronchogram. **A.** Anteroposterior view. **B.** Lateral view of chest.

Presurgical

Treatment consists in decreasing the likelihood of aspiration from the upper pouch and regurgitation through the fistula. An indwelling nasoesophageal tube should be inserted into the upper pouch, the pouch emptied of secretions and the tube placed to constant suction using a negative pressure of about 5 mm Hg. It is vital that this tube be patent and functioning at all times. Recently a sump type of tube has been developed that functions in such a way as to keep the lumen clear at all times. To minimize the possibility of regurgitation through a tracheoesophageal fistula, the child should be placed in as near an upright position as possible (67). The child should be given IV fluids and should receive nothing by mouth; acid-base and electrolyte status must be carefully evaluated. Once these measures have been instituted, the patient can be evaluated regarding surgical treatment.

Surgical

Surgery for esophageal atresia should be considered an emergency, but the approach must be carefully planned (76). The operative procedure depends on the individual patient. Infants with esophageal atresia may be categorized as follows:

1. Mature or premature
2. Without pulmonary complications; with or without tracheoesophageal fistula; with or without associated anomalies
3. With pulmonary complications; with or without tracheoesophageal fistula; with or without associated anomalies

In general the premature infant is dealt with differently and will be discussed later. Treatment of the mature child will vary depending on the above factors.

Without Pulmonary Complications and Without Tracheoesophageal Fistula (Type A). In these infants a gastrostomy is performed under local anesthesia. An indwelling nasoesophageal tube is placed in the upper esophageal pouch and constant or intermittent suction is maintained. Feedings through the gastrostomy are begun 24 to 48 hours later. In the past, a cervical esophagostomy was then performed, and the child was followed until one or two years of age. Then a segment of the colon (usually ascending colon with or without the distal end of the ileum) would be interposed retrosternally between the cervical esophagus and the anterior wall of the stomach (68, 82). In general these children have done well postoperatively. However, it is reasonable to assume that reflux of gastric juice into the interposed colon may result in peptic colitis over the years. Because of this, several authors (74, 83) have advocated lengthening the upper esophageal segment—and the lower through the gastrostomy (78)—by introducing weighted bougies or catheters periodically. With this technique it has been possible to lengthen the esophageal segments sufficiently to perform a direct reconstruction of the esophagus (Fig. 23–15). Certainly this is theoretically a much better method than colonic interposition. However, the technique has not yet been widely used, nor have we had an opportunity to apply it.

With Tracheoesophageal Fistula (Type C). In these infants division and closure of the tracheoesophageal fistula with definitive reconstruction of the esophagus according to the technique of Haight (69) is the recommended treatment. A gastrostomy for feeding purposes and as a possible site for retrograde dilatations in the postoperative period is occasionally performed either just before or after the definitive correction.

Much has been written regarding the

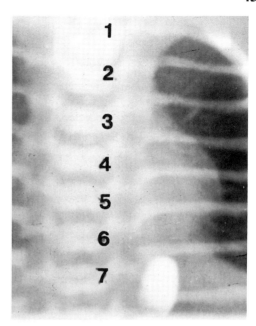

FIG. 23–15. Anteroposterior view of chest with contrast material in upper and lower esophageal segments indicating a gap equal to the distance across five vertebral bodies between the proximal and distal segments. Some authors have reported lengthening these segments by periodic bougienage to the extent that subsequent direct reconstruction of the esophagus is possible.

merits of retropleural versus transpleural correction of the atresia. Despite the theoretic advantages of a retropleural approach, should there be a leak at the anastomotic site, we have preferred a transpleural approach in which a broad pleural flap is elevated in such a manner as to expose the esophagus, essentially retropleurally. The incision is usually made through the fourth or fifth right intercostal space with the child in a full lateral position. The azygos vein is divided, the fistula identified, divided and then closed with 00000 silk sutures at the tracheal end. The lower pouch is then mobilized slightly to avoid compromising its blood supply. The muscularis of the lowermost portion of the upper pouch is then incised and a 2-mm cuff of it elevated from the submucosa. Then the lumen of the upper pouch is opened at its lowermost point, and the anastomosis is begun. All sutures of the posterior row are placed before tying them down with 00000 silk sutures on atraumatic needles in such a manner that the knots lie on the inside of the esophagus. Through-and-through bites are taken in the lower esophageal segment; the sutures pass through mucosa and submucosa alone of the upper esophageal segment. After all the sutures have been tied down, completing the posterior anastomotic line, the nasoesophageal tube, which is already in place, is passed down through the lumen of the esophagus into the stomach. This acts as a stent for the completion of the anastomosis and may be used as a feeding tube in patients without a gastrostomy. The anterior row of the anastomosis is now laid as was the posterior row. After the entire anastomosis has been completed, the muscularis cuff that was elevated from the upper esophageal segment is now sutured to the muscularis of the lower esophageal seg-

FIG. 23–16. Barium swallow with nasogastric tube in place, prior to removal, reveals adequate lumen throughout with only minimal indentation in region of anastomosis (arrow).

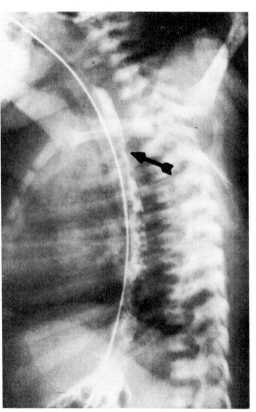

ment, sealing over the anastomosis. To avoid leaks, as few sutures as possible are used in constructing the anastomosis. Following the esophageal reconstruction, a soft catheter is inserted through the sixth or seventh intercostal space in the midaxillary line on the right and sutured both to the skin and, using a catgut suture, to the posterior chest wall so that its tip, into which additional holes have been cut, lies near but not on the area of the esophageal reconstruction. The large pleural flap is now allowed to fall back over the posterior mediastinal structures and the "retropleural" drainage catheter and is tacked down in several places. The lung is then reexpanded and a second catheter for pleural drainage is inserted into the pleural space through the sixth intercostal space anteriorly. Both tubes are attached to suction in the recovery room and are left in place for 10 days, after which the anterior tube (transpleural) is removed first and the retropleural catheter 24 hours later.

Postoperatively these infants are maintained in a high humidity environment for from five to seven days. A special duty nurse is assigned to the child for the same period in order to perform oropharyngeal suctioning as needed. These infants can usually swallow their saliva and pharyngeal secretions by the third to fourth postoperative day, but until that time the serious problem of possible aspiration exists and diligent nursing care is required. In infants with a gastrostomy, feedings may be given by this means at from 24 to 48 hours postoperatively. Those without a gastrostomy may be fed through the nasogastric tube at from one to two days after surgery. Prior to removal of the nasogastric tube (about ten days), an esophagram is obtained utilizing water-soluble contrast agent (Fig. 23–16). If the lumen of the esophagus appears adequate through the anastomotic site, the tube is removed. If there is significant narrowing, we prefer to do a gastrostomy and pass a heavy ligature through the gastrostomy and out the patient's nose so that retrograde dilatations may be performed. In our experience about one-quarter of the patients with primary repair of the esophagus have required dilatations for as long as two to three years. Retrograde dilatations are much safer than antegrade methods. Dilatations are usually performed weekly at the onset and then gradually at less frequent intervals up to from four to six weeks.

With Associated Anomalies. A significant number of infants with esophageal atresia may have other GI anomalies, in which case esophageal reconstruction may have to be delayed. Our policy in managing such patients depends on the location of the associated lesion.

Infants with esophageal and duodenal atresia are treated by gastrostomy and duodenojejunostomy and three to five days later undergo definitive esophageal surgery.

Infants with small bowel atresia are treated by gastrostomy and correction of the small bowel obstruction as the primary procedure followed in three to five days by esophageal reconstruction.

In infants with an imperforate anus and an externally draining fistula, the esophageal atresia is corrected first, and the external fistula dilated to permit emptying of the colon. (Management of the imperforate anus is delayed). In those without an externally draining fistula, a gastrostomy and colostomy are performed as the primary

procedure followed in one to two days by correction of the esophageal atresia. The imperforate anus is definitively treated at a later time.

With Pulmonary Complications. A gastrostomy is performed under local anesthesia and the pulmonary problem treated (Fig. 23–17). When the lungs have cleared sufficiently (one to two days, usually) proper treatment is instituted following the principles of management already discussed.

PREMATURE INFANTS

Following the successful division and closure of a tracheoesophageal fistula and primary reconstruction of the esophagus by Haight (69) in 1941, this became the standard technique for management of infants with esophageal atresia and tracheoesophageal fistula. This was a significant advance

FIG. **23–17.** Roentgenogram of one-day-old infant transferred to the New York Hospital. **A.** Right upper and middle lobe pneumonia with mediastinal shift. Stomach gas bubble indicates C type of esophageal atresia. **B.** Same infant 36 hours following insertion of nasoesophageal tube placed to aspiration and creation of gastrostomy. Pulmonary infiltrate markedly improved. Division and closure of tracheoesophageal fistula and reconstruction of esophagus was performed 24 hours later.

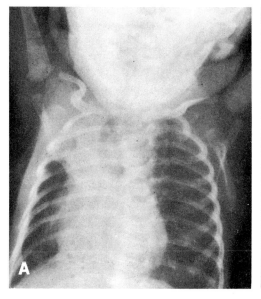
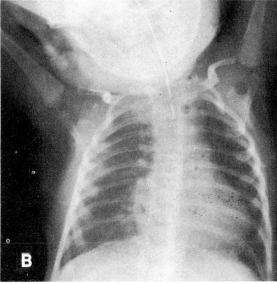

in therapy and preferred to the multiple stage procedures previously reported (77, 79), which were the first successful means of treatment. However, the mortality rate when primary repair was attempted in premature or critically ill neonates was extremely high. Holder, quoting from unpublished data of Gross and Wooley, indicated that in 62 patients treated by primary repair, infants weighing 3 to 5 lbs on admission had a 28% survival and those 5 to 7 lbs a 57% survival, while all patients over 7 lbs survived. On the basis of this experience, interest in a staged method of dealing with esophageal atresia and tracheoesophageal fistula in premature or critically ill neonates was reawakened. Holder et al (71) demonstrated that survival rate in these types of patients could be increased to almost 70%. The concept is a partial return to the initially successful methods of dealing with the problem. Having personally observed several of the patients cited by Holder et al, we were impressed with the technique and have adopted it. The smallest infant in our experience treated by the staged technique to be discussed weighed 1250 g. The child survived staged, complete correction only to develop Wilms' tumor at age 1 year, with death due to metastases at 18 months of age.

The Staged Technique (75)

This consists in 1) gastrostomy for decompression; 2) retropleural division and closure of the tracheoesophageal fistula, following which the gastrostomy is used for feeding; 3) restoration of esophageal continuity after the child reaches an adequate weight (usually 6 to 7 lbs).

Gastrostomy. This is performed under local anesthesia as soon as possible after the patient is admitted. A simple Stamm type of gastrostomy is made and the tube is placed to dependent drainage or low suction. This will decompress the stomach, correct any existing diaphragmatic elevation and improve pulmonary function. If pneumonia occurs, it should be treated before progressing to the next stage. The infant is placed in a 45° to 60° reverse Trendelenberg position to minimize the possibility of regurgitation through the fistula while awaiting the second stage. During this time, too, it is extremely important to provide for continuous aspiration of the upper esophageal segment by means of an indwelling nasoesophageal tube connected to low suction and to assign a special nurse to perform frequent suctioning of the oropharynx so as to prevent spillover of secretions into the tracheobronchial tree.

Division and Closure of Tracheoesophageal Fistula. This is usually performed under local anesthesia in a retropleural manner. Because of the thinness of the pleura, it is not unusual to make an opening into it during dissection. For this reason, an anesthesiologist is present to assist in respiration or to intubate the child if necessary in order to keep the lung of the operative side expanded. The child is placed in an almost full lateral position, and the posterior half of the fourth right rib is resected. The pleura is then reflected a short distance medially and extensively laterally and posteriorly to expose the azygos vein, which is then doubly ligated and divided. Following this the lower segment of esophagus and the tracheoesophageal fistula are identified. The fistula is freed up to its junction with the trachea and divided, and both ends are closed with 00000 sutures on atraumatic needles. The closed end of the distal esophagus is tacked up to the prevertebral fascia high in the chest to prevent it from retracting into the lower mediastinum. A drainage tube is placed into the retropleural space and attached to suction. This is usually left in place two to three days. We usually start feeding through the gastrostomy about 48 hours after closure of the fistula. The child is then fed until he weighs 6 to 7 lbs, at which time the third step is performed.

Definitive Reconstruction of the Esophagus. This is done under general anesthesia utilizing a transpleural approach. The technique is basically that of Haight, as already has been described. Postoperative management of the infant proceeds as discussed earlier. Some vigorous premature infants, close to 4 lbs in weight, may be treated by primary repair. In most premature infants, however, the staged method of management is superior to the primary technique in treating these problems. Although it may be desirable to accomplish complete repair at one operation, it is much wiser to stage the correction and end up with a survivor.

CHALASIA

Although this is not a condition requiring surgical intervention, it is worth considering because it may be confused with obstructive lesions of the esophagus or stomach.

Chalasia is manifested by vomiting after feedings, when the infant is in a horizontal position. This is thought to be due to a persistent relaxation of the lower end of the esophagus. No known etiologic factor has been demonstrable, but it has been assumed that chalasia is the result of a temporary neuromuscular imbalance. Effortless vomiting, which usually begins a few days after birth, can be avoided or minimized if the infant is held erect. The diagnosis can be established by fluoroscopic observation of the swallowing of barium. Relaxation of the cardioesophageal junction and retrograde filling of the esophagus are noted with increased intraabdominal pressure. The lack of projectile vomiting, prevention of vomiting by the erect position, lack of a pyloric tumor mass or demonstration of pyloric patency by barium examination of the stomach differentiate the problem from hypertrophic pyloric stenosis. Appropriate x-ray studies will rule out a hiatus hernia, with which it may be confused.

Treatment consists essentially in keeping the child propped up in a sitting position or erect, either continuously or at least for two to three hours after each feeding. The problem resolves spontaneously at from two to three months of age. Occasionally aspiration, airway involvement or pulmonary complications may develop with this syndrome.

DIAPHRAGMATIC HERNIA

Embryologically the diaphragm arises from the septum transversum. It is formed beneath the heart at about the eighth week of gestation and grows backward to meet and fuse with the dorsal mesentery of the foregut. On each side pleuroperitoneal folds form and extend posteriorly and laterally. Although these originally consist only of thin pleura and peritoneum, muscle fibers gradually grow in between these layers to complete the diaphragm, usually by the end of the ninth week of fetal life. The pleuroperitoneal canal closes first on the right and later on the left side. The posterior portion on either side is the last to close. Although the anterior portion is usually closed before the posterior, failure of fusion of the central and lateral portions may occur anteriorly. In addition to potential defects posterolaterally and anteriorly, several normal openings occur in the diaphragm through which the esophagus, aorta and inferior vena cava pass, and several lesser apertures also appear on either side through which the lesser and greater splanchnic nerves and on the left, the hemiazygos vein pass. With the exception of the esophageal hiatus, hernias through these apertures rarely if ever occur in infants or children. Thus, diaphragmatic hernias in infants and children are usually found in three locations (84, 91), including the: 1) posterolateral aspect (either side) foramen of Bochdalek (persistent pleuroperitoneal canal); 2) anterolateral–retrosternal aspect (either side) foramen of Morgagni; and 3) esophageal hiatus. The most common of these is the foramen of Bochdalek type, although hiatus hernias (esophageal) are currently being recognized and reported with greater frequency.

HERNIAS THROUGH
FORAMEN OF BOCHDALEK

These are about three to four times more common on the left than on the right. In only 5% to 10% of cases will there be a true hernia sac. The signs depend on the mass of abdominal viscera displaced into the pleural space as well as on the side involved. At or shortly after birth, respiratory distress is noted. This usually increases as the herniated abdominal viscera fill with gas, become distended and further compromise pulmonary ventilation. There is usually cyanosis, often of marked degree. On physical examination breath sounds are absent on the affected side, there is dullness to percussion, and heart sounds are displaced to the contralateral side. In some instances, particularly if the diagnosis has not been suspected and the condition treated within several hours, bowel sounds may be heard over the chest of the involved side. The abdomen is usually flat or scaphoid owing to the lack of viscera.

Diagnosis can be made readily by roentgenograms (87). In practice, we insert a radiopaque nasogastric tube prior to x-ray examination. Since the majority of Bochdalek hernias occur on the left, chest roentgenograms will show the stomach tube in the left chest and rule out congenital lung cysts or duplications that may sometimes give a similar x-ray picture. Hernias on the right may show a soft tissue density in the chest with an absent or smaller-than-normal liver shadow in the right upper abdomen. The stomach rarely extends into the right chest with such hernias, and the nasogastric tube in these instances may not be of diagnostic value. Mediastinal structures are displaced to the side opposite the hernia. Immediate surgical treatment is mandatory. However, while making arrangements, especially if the infant is to be transferred to another hospital for definitive care, a nasogastric tube should be inserted and attached to continuous suction and the patient placed with his affected side down. These two maneuvers tend to decompress the bowel and limit further distention of the herniated viscera, and they help ventilation by causing some mediastinal displacement away from the good (uppermost) side, thus allowing greater pulmonary expansion. In addition, the child should be placed in an incubator with oxygen to relieve the dyspnea and cyanosis. Prior to surgery pH, blood gases (arterial specimen) and electrolytes should be obtained. Since there is usually marked acidosis with accompanying hyperkalemia, immediate steps should be taken to begin correction. However, speed is essential and too much time cannot be used in these preliminary corrective measures. In most cases acidosis is due to the poor aeration, and prompt removal of the viscera from the chest will have an extremely beneficial effect. The operation may be performed using either a thoracic or abdominal approach; each has its advantages and disadvantages.

Thoracic Approach

The chest is usually entered through the seventh intercostal space on the affected side (88). The viscera are replaced into the abdomen and the edges of the defect in the diaphragm identified and approximated with heavy nonabsorbable sutures placed in horizontal mattress fashion. Following repair, the chest is closed in the usual way after a chest catheter has been inserted to drain the pleural space, usually through a separate stab wound at some distance from the main incision. Although this approach gives excellent exposure of the diaphragmatic defect, there may be great difficulty in reducing the herniated viscera back into the abdomen. Also, should there be associated malrotation of the bowel, this will probably not be recognized. For this reason we prefer to employ this technique only in children over one year of age or in those who have had a recurrence of a previously repaired diaphragmatic hernia.

Abdominal Approach

A paramedian incision is made on the affected side. On entry into the abdomen, a soft rubber catheter is inserted into the pleural space containing the herniated viscera in order to relieve negative pressure and facilitate reduction. We have followed Gross' recommendation (86) regarding the order in which the viscera should be removed from the chest: 1) right-sided hernia —small bowel first, then colon, and lastly, the liver; 2) left-sided hernia—stomach first, then small intestine, cecum, ascending and transverse colon, and finally splenic flexure and the spleen. After the viscera have been removed from the pleural space, the dome of the space is inspected for the presence or absence of a true hernia sac. If there is a sac, an opening is made at its apex to provide access to the true pleural space. The sac is then drawn down and the excess excised. The margins may then be included in the sutures used to approximate the rim of diaphragm. Although most hernias will be associated with an identifiable remnant of diaphragmatic muscle or tissue completely surrounding the defect, in some instances sutures may have to be placed directly into the structures of the chest wall posterolaterally. An imbricating type of repair with nonabsorbable sutures should be employed wherever possible, providing in essence a double-layer closure.

After the repair of the diaphragm has been completed, the bowel is inspected for malrotation. If it is present it is treated by the Ladd method. After the viscera have been replaced, the abdomen is closed in layers. Diaphragmatic hernia represents a situation in which the herniated abdominal viscera have had no domicile within the abdominal cavity. Indeed, this condition might be considered one of "intracorporeal omphalocele." Thus, there may not be enough space to accommodate the viscera. The usual dangers associated with omphalocele repair exist: 1) elevation of diaphragms with respiratory embarrassment or 2) inferior vena caval obstruction with cardiovascular embarrassment. It is primarily for this reason that we prefer the abdominal approach. If it is impossible to effect a complete layer closure of the abdominal wall, skin and subcutaneous tissue flaps may be created and simply approximated over the abdominal contents, as in the first stage of the delayed method for omphalocele repair (85, 90). The resultant ventral hernia can be corrected at a later time. Prior to completing the closure of the diaphragm, a catheter is introduced into the chest and brought out through a small stab wound. Regardless of

the operative approach, very little effort should be made by the anesthesiologist to attempt to expand the lung on the affected side. This lung rarely expands immediately and excessive pressure used in an attempt to accomplish this may lead to rupture of portions of the contralateral lung and development of pneumothorax on the unaffected side.

Postoperatively the chest tube is connected to underwater drainage with or without low suction. In our experience, the lung of the affected side has expanded as soon as three to four hours and as late as seven to eight days after repair of the hernia. Determinations of blood pH and gases should be obtained at frequent intervals, but despite early and proper treatment, acidosis may be impossible to correct in a significant number of cases, and they will succumb. In some cases, this may be due to continued poor aeration, either because of poor expansion of the lung on the affected side, pneumothorax or pulmonary involvement of the contralateral side or combinations of these factors. In others, there is a great likelihood that, despite the fact that there may be some lung expansion, alveolar hypoplasia will cause right to left shunts in the lung of the affected side that exaggerate the acidosis. It is apparent from experience that repair of the hernia alone is not the entire answer to the problems encountered in these infants. We have considered possible temporary banding of the pulmonary artery to the affected side in order to reduce the degree of right to left shunting of blood in the immediate postoperative period.

Diaphragmatic hernia may occasionally go undetected in the neonatal period and not be discovered for several months or years (Fig. 23–18). These children may present either with respiratory distress, with unusual chest findings on x ray or physical examination or with vomiting or poor physical development, or both, and signs of malnutrition. Once diagnosis of diaphragmatic hernia is established, surgical correction should be undertaken. As with any hernia, bowel in the hernia may become strangulated without warning. For this reason if no

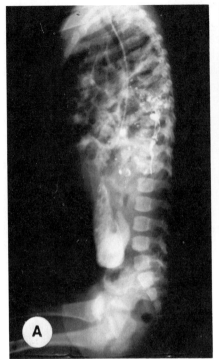
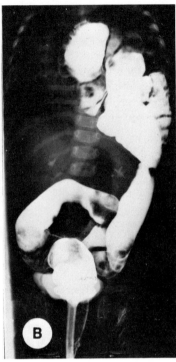

FIG. 23–18. Chest and abdomen of 14-month-old-girl demonstrating gas-filled loops of bowel in chest, some containing residual barium from a previous study. Although devoid of respiratory distress, the child had begun to vomit and showed signs of malnutrition. **A.** Lateral view. **B.** Barium enema reveals large portion of colon in left chest.

other, all diaphragmatic hernias of childhood (previously undetected or recurrent) should be operated on (Fig. 23–19). Postoperatively these infants are placed in an incubator or croupette with oxygen and a high-humidity atmosphere The patient's position is changed frequently. We have chosen to keep the child flat, turning him from side to side at a 30° angle about every 30 to 45 minutes. The child is maintained on IV feedings, receiving nothing by mouth, and constant nasogastric suction until there is evidence of intestinal activity.

HERNIAS THROUGH FORAMEN OF MORGAGNI

These are much less common than the Bochdalek variety in infants and children. There is a true sac that acts to confine the herniated bowel and thus limit pulmonary crowding. Signs of bowel obstruction may be more often encountered than cardiopulmonary embarrassment. Diagnosis is suggested by conventional anterioposterior and lateral x rays of the chest and proven by studies with radiopaque contrast materials. Repair may be accomplished either by transthoracic or abdominal approach. The diaphragmatic defect, of course, is anterior rather than posterolateral. The hernia sac must be excised or imbricated before the diaphragmatic opening is reapproximated. Postoperative management is essentially as previously discussed for management of hernias through the foramen of Bochdalek.

EVENTRATION OF THE DIAPHRAGM

This is characterized by an intact but thin, high diaphragm (89). The affected leaf of the diaphragm is stretched out and weak, having diminished muscular elements. The lung on the affected side is compressed, but the unaffected portion usually appears well

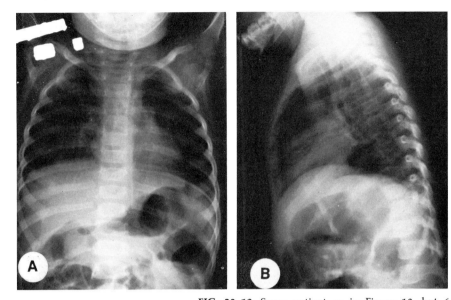

FIG. 23–19. Same patient as in Figure 18, but 6 months postoperative, demonstrating normal appearance of left diaphragm and chest. **A.** Anteroposterior view. **B.** Lateral views.

aerated and does not present the hazy appearance of the hypoplastic lung associated with true diaphragmatic hernia. Signs vary with the degree of elevation of the diaphragm and the amount of pulmonary compression and mediastinal shift. Diagnosis is readily made by chest roentgenograms, which reveal the leaf of the diaphragm on the affected side to be high in the pleural space, with abdominal organs below a definite arched structure separating the abdominal and pleural cavities (Fig. 23–20). Some have advocated the use of pneumoperitoneum to confirm the diagnosis when it cannot be otherwise established. Treatment is required only in those patients with severe signs due to lung compression. Operation is performed transthoracically. The thinned-out leaf of diaphragm is imbricated on itself and lowered, thus enabling the compressed lung to reexpand. There is usually sufficient tissue to effect a strong closure without the need for prosthetic materials for reinforcement. A chest tube is inserted for the first one to two postoperative days and attached to suction. General postoperative management is similar to that employed after the repair of diaphragmatic hernia, but the need for nasogastric suction and IV fluids does not persist as long.

FIG. 23–20. Anteroposterior view of chest and abdomen. Examination of the area reveals a definite arched structure on left, separating abdominal and pleural cavities. Mediastinum is shifted to right. Patient was asymptomatic.

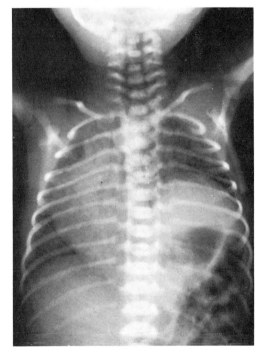

MEDIASTINAL TUMORS

The mediastinum is that portion of the thoracic cavity situated between the medial surfaces of the right and left pleura extending from the sternum anteriorly to the vertebral column posteriorly. Within it are contained all the thoracic viscera except the lungs. Conventionally the mediastinum is subdivided into four parts:

1. Superior: above the level of a line connecting the lower part of the fourth thoracic vertebra to the sternomanubrial junction
2. Anterior: bounded in front by the sternum, behind by the pericardium, above by the superior mediastinum and below by the diaphragm
3. Middle: the broadest part of the mediastinum, containing the pericardium and heart
4. Posterior: bounded in front by the pericardium, behind by the vertebral column, above by the superior mediastinum and below by the diaphragm

The structures usually contained within these various subdivisions are

1. Superior: aortic arch, innominate artery and thoracic portions of the left common carotid and left subclavian arteries, pulmonary arteries and veins, innominate and subclavian veins, superior vena cava, most of the thymus gland, vagus, cardiac, phrenic and left recurrent nerves, trachea, esophagus, thoracic duct, lymph nodes and lymphatic vessels
2. Anterior: portion of the thymus gland, loose areolar tissue, lymph nodes and lymphatic vessels
3. Middle: heart and pericardium, phrenic nerves, lymph nodes and lymphatic vessels
4. Posterior: thoracic part of descending aorta, azygos and hemiazygos veins, vagus and splanchnic nerves, sympathetic nerve trunks, esophagus, thoracic duct, lymph nodes and lymphatic vessels

Depending on the structures usually located in the various subdivisions of the mediastinum, certain tumors are more apt to occur in one section than another (96, 97). Thus, cystic hygroma, thymic tumors, and hemangioma are more common in the superior mediastinum, while lymphoma or lymphosarcoma, dermoids and teratoma are more common in the anterior mediastinum. Middle mediastinal tumors are apt to be lipomas or pericardial cysts, while those in the posterior mediastinum consist of enterogenous or bronchogenic cysts and tumors of neurogenic origin. In the infant or neonate, tumors of the mediastinum although uncommon are not rare. Signs are usually those associated with expanding, space-occupying lesions and may consist of apparent chest pain, respiratory distress, cough, dysphagia, hemoptysis, wheezing and weight loss.

Diagnosis may be made by roentgenograms of the chest, bronchography, bronchoscopy, esophagogram, esophagoscopy and occasionally by angiocardiography. Despite these modalities it may not be possible to establish the exact nature of the tumor preoperatively. Because of the possibility of malignancy and the danger of respiratory, cardiac, or esophageal embarrassment due to the location of the lesion, all mediastinal masses in infancy and childhood should be resected even though they may be asymptomatic when discovered.

ENTEROGENOUS CYSTS

These are located in the posterior mediastinum, but they may extend into either hemithorax as their size increases (99). They are usually muscle-walled tubular or spherical duplicated segments of the alimentary tract that may be partially or wholly detached from the parent viscus. Their mucosal lining is indicative of their site of origin, and the fluid they contain is similar to that which normally would be secreted by the parent tissue. Cervical or upper thoracic vertebral anomalies, such as hemivertebrae may be associated with these lesions (94). In addition, intraabdominal enterogenous cysts may occur. Although enteric cysts are often closely associated with the esophagus, dissection from this structure is not usually difficult. Because there is rarely a lumenal communication between the esophagus and these cysts, fluid produced by the epithelial lining accumulates, and the cysts may become very large. Those lined with gastric mucosa may lead to ulceration into the lung, bronchus or esophagus and may cause hemorrhage.

Treatment consists of resection through an appropriate thoracotomy incision. In rare cases the entire cyst may not be removable because of adherence to esophagus, bronchus or other vital structures, and it may be necessary to simply excise the mucosa of the cyst from the contiguous structure, leaving the wall. The usual regimen for patients who have had chest surgery is employed postoperatively. In general, results following the removal of such cysts are excellent.

TERATOMAS AND DERMOID CYSTS

These are common tumors second only to neuroblastoma in frequency (93). Located in the anterior mediastinum, they may reach large size and usually cause respiratory distress early in infancy.

Dermoid cysts consist of tumors of ectodermal origin. Grossly, they are characteristically thick-walled fibrous sacs lined by squamous epithelium and sometimes contain hair, teeth and various skin appendages.

Teratomas may be solid or cystic and are composed of tissue derived from all three embryonic germ layers. Some may be malignant, but their bizarre histologic pattern may make this aspect of the diagnosis difficult. The exact diagnosis of malignancy may depend on the ultimate course of the patient rather than on the histologic picture.

Diagnosis is often possible on routine chest roentgenograms if an anterior mediastinal mass with calcification or teeth, or both, is apparent. Early recognition and resection before either infection or malignant degeneration can occur are advocated.

TUMORS OF NEUROGENIC ORIGIN

Three tumors of neurogenic origin, all located in the posterior mediastinum, are encountered in neonates and infants (100).

These are distinguished histologically as 1) ganglioneuroma, 2) neurofibroma, benign lesions and 3) malignant neuroblastoma.

Ganglioneuroma

These arise from ganglia of the sympathetic chain and are the most common mediastinal tumor of neurogenic origin. The lesions tend to be large but are usually well encapsulated, so that most can be removed without difficulty. Symptoms generally do not develop until the tumor becomes large and a Horner's syndrome or tracheal deviation becomes apparent. Treatment by excision is usually possible and leads to excellent results.

Neurofibroma

These may arise from any of the nerves in the posterior mediastinum as isolated tumors or in conjunction with generalized neurofibromatosis of von Recklinghausen's disease. Signs and symptoms manifested by the patient depend on the size and location of the tumor. Some present as dumbbell-like masses extending from intervertebral foramina. Children with such lesions may have scoliosis. Treatment consists in removal of the tumor, or when this is impossible, resection of the bulk of the mass.

Neuroblastoma

This malignant neoplasm arises from a precursor of the ganglion cell of the sympathetic nervous system. Although most commonly encountered in the adrenal gland in infants, tumors arising in the mediastinum are not rare. Many cause no symptoms and are not detected until there is metastatic involvement. Chest roentgenograms reveal a well-circumscribed posterior mediastinal mass, often with evidence of calcification. There may be erosion of the neighboring ribs or vertebras.

Treatment consists of removal of the tumor. Because of spread to surrounding structures, it may be impossible to resect the entire tumor. When this is the case, as much of the mass should be excised as possible, since the prognosis may be improved following partial excision (98). These lesions are highly vascular and hemostasis may be difficult, particularly when complete removal is not possible. Infants undergoing surgery should have an adequate IV route (cut-down) and sufficient blood available for necessary replacement. Following surgery, radiation is employed to the tumor site (or residual tumor), and chemotherapeutic agents such as cyclophosphamide and vincristine alone or in combination are given. Obvious metastatic areas are also irradiated. In patients where complete removal is possible, vanilmandelic acid (VMA) determinations in the follow-up period after surgery may reveal metastatic activity in the absence of other findings. Except in those individuals with metastases to bone, the results after resection of mediastinal neuroblastomas followed by radiation and chemother-

apy are generally better than those obtainable with similar neoplasms in the abdomen.

CYSTIC HYGROMA AND HEMANGIOMA

Although these types of tumors may be present in the mediastinum alone, more often they extend into the mediastinum from a site of origin in the neck or axilla (92, 95). If signs are produced because of the size or location of such lesions, excision is the treatment of choice. In rare instances an irresectable hemangioma will lead to death due to compression of the distal trachea beyond the limit of palliation by tracheostomy.

ABDOMEN

INTESTINAL OBSTRUCTION

Intestinal obstruction in the neonate may occur at any level distal to the stomach and may be complete or incomplete (105, 109, 110). The complete form is usually due to atresia or volvulus, while the partial or in-

FIG. 23–21. Plain films of abdomen. **A.** Upper intestinal obstruction. Gas in stomach and loop of upper small intestine, calcific deposits in right half of abdomen and ground-glass appearance indicate intrauterine perforation with meconium peritonitis. **B.** Lower small intestinal obstruction. Many loops of bowel distended with gas.

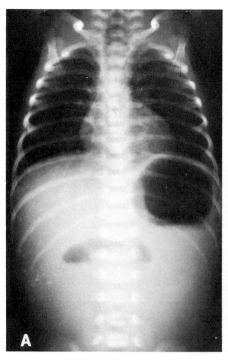
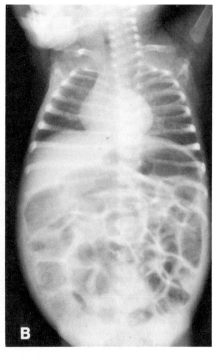

complete forms may be due to malrotation without volvulus, annular pancreas, stenosis, duplication or extrinsic pressure from an adjacent intraabdominal mass.

Signs of intestinal obstruction may vary in intensity or time of appearance depending on the level and degree of obstruction. In general, vomiting (usually of bile-stained fluid), distension, failure to pass meconium and irritability or lethargy suggest obstruction. The diagnosis may be confirmed by flat and upright roentgenograms of the abdomen (Figs. 23–21, 23–22) that reveal distended loops of intestine with air fluid levels. The degree of dilatation and number of loops will depend on the level of the obstruction and whether it is complete or incomplete. In infants judged capable of undergoing specialized radiographic studies, a barium enema may indicate the position of the bowel, establish the presence or absence of malrotation and provide information regarding the luminal size of the bowel. If this is very small, a so-called microcolon, it is

safe to assume that complete obstruction has existed from early in gestation and prevented the bowel from developing its normal caliber by precluding the flow of intestinal contents into it. In such situations the obstruction is probably due to intestinal atresia or to meconium ileus, which also results in microcolon. However, flat and upright roentgenograms of the abdomen are usually the only studies required since it is important merely to establish the diagnosis of obstruction. The exact cause of the obstruction can be readily determined at surgery, and appropriate steps can then be taken to correct the underlying cause. Contrast studies of the GI system by the oral route or from above by way of tubes are not

FIG. 23–22. Plain films of abdomen showing the so-called double-bubble sign indicative of duodenal obstruction. **A.** Gas does not pass beyond duodenum, which is highly suggestive of duodenal atresia but may be present in annular pancreas of malrotation. **B.** Small quantity of gas beyond duodenum (arrow), which presence rules out duodenal atresia.

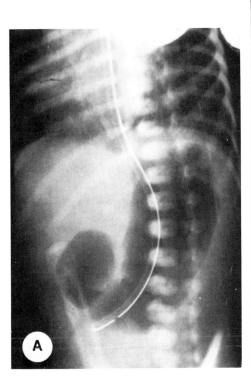

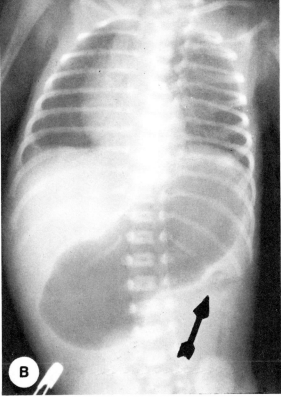

indicated since in the presence of obstruction the contrast material may be vomited and aspirated by the patient.

Intestinal obstruction in the neonate occurs most commonly in the ileum, next most commonly in the duodenum, less commonly in the jejunum and least in the colon (excluding imperforate anus). For a better understanding of intestinal obstruction the various causes will be considered separately.

Atresia

In this condition there is complete obstruction or lack of luminal continuity of the intestinal tract (106) occurring at one site (single) or involving several segments (multiple). There may be continuity of the bowel wall or portions of the bowel may be completely separated from proximal and distal segments (Fig. 23–23). Etiology may be failure of recanalization of the intestinal lumen after the period of occlusion by overgrowth of lining epithelial cells. However, it has

FIG. 23–23. Operative view of small bowel atresia, multiple with discontinuity. Above and to the left dilated proximal intestine ends blindly and is separated from more distal intestine (double arrow), which is much smaller in diameter. This in turn ends blindly and is separated from the next segment. Note the isolated portions with their own mesenteries (arrow).

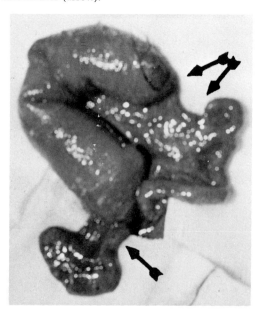

also more recently been postulated and experimentally demonstrated that atresia may be the end result of vascular accidents (impaired circulation) to segments of the intestine that cause necrosis with subsequent healing of the necrosed segment creating obstruction by scar tissue of the portion involved (107, 108).

Malrotation

During the 6th to 8th weeks of gestation, the midportion of the GI tract (duodenum to midtransverse colon), supplied by the superior mesenteric artery, grows at a much more rapid rate than does the abdominal cavity. As a result, this portion of the GI tract passes out into the umbilical stalk. From the 9th to 12th weeks, however, the size of the abdominal cavity increases, and the intestines return from the umbilical stalk to the abdominal cavity. Visualization of the manner of return is simplified if one imagines oneself facing the fetus. While the midgut is in the umbilical stalk, the duodenojejunal flexure is on the observer's left, the cecum on the right. As return to the abdominal cavity progresses in a counterclockwise direction (to the observer), the duodenojejunal flexure passes behind the superior mesenteric artery to end up in the left upper quadrant, while the cecum proceeds anterior to the superior mesenteric artery to reach the right lower quadrant. The failure of proper rotation in returning to the abdominal cavity leads to two potential dangers, neither of which are due to the failure of proper rotation per se; as a result of the abnormal mesenteric attachments associated with the malrotation, the cecum may end up in the epigastrium or in right upper quadrant (112–115). The mesenteric bands fixing the cecum and ascending colon now pass from these structures across the second and third portions of the duodenum, causing a variable degree of duodenal obstruction. In addition, the abnormal fixation of these mesenteries plus the abnormal attachment of the mesentery of the duodenojejunal flexure and small bowel may lead to a foreshortened or narrow mesenteric attachment of this portion of the gut, predisposing to the intestine rotating (clockwise) about the axis of the superior mesenteric artery. This causes volvulus of the midgut with possible vascular compromise of the bowel, dependent on the amount of vascular compression of the superior mesenteric artery, vein or both. Thus, in addition to a closed-loop type of obstruction of the midgut, vascular embarrassment to this segment of the intestinal tract may further complicate and increase the gravity of the situation. If obstruction is due to malrotation alone, the signs may be those of partial or incomplete obstruction. Should there be associated volvulus, the signs are usually those of complete obstruction.

Annular Pancreas

The pancreas is derived from a dorsal and ventral bud, the ventral ultimately swinging around the duodenum to fuse with the dorsal bud and form the entire pancreas. In some instances, rotation of the ventral bud is not complete, so that fusion with the dorsal bud results in a ring of pancreatic tissue that encircles the duodenum and causes incomplete or complete obstruction of the second portion of the duodenum (117–120).

Duplications

These are cystic, ovoid or tubular structures lined by mucosa of some portion of the alimentary tract and possessing a coat of smooth muscle. They are closely attached to a segment of the GI tract, usually along the mesenteric border or in the leaves of adjacent mesentery, and occur at all levels from the pharynx to the anus, but they are most common in relation to the ileum. The type of epithelial lining of a duplication need not be the same as that of the adjacent bowel to which it is closely adherent. Duplications may have communication with the adjacent portion of the GI tract proximally, distally or at both ends, or they may be closed segments without openings (Fig. 23–24). These structures usually contain fluid, the exact nature of which depends on whether there are communications with the lumen of the alimentary tract and on the type of mucosa that lines the duplication (121, 124, 125).

In addition to signs of intestinal obstruction, duplications may cause pain due to distention of the structure, bleeding secondary to slough of mucosa as a result of compression of mesenteric blood vessels or hemorrhage in those lined with gastric mucosa. Although several theories have been advanced to explain duplications, Bremer's (123) is the most widely accepted.

FIG. 23–24. Ileal duplication resected from three-day-old male. **A.** Unopened specimen. Appendix extends from base of cecum inferiorly to left. **B.** On cut section, lumen of duplication (arrow) communicates distally with normal ileum (upper mucosal-lined structure).

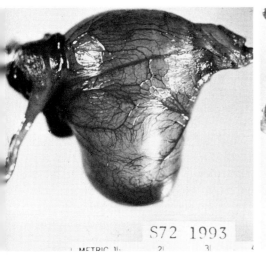

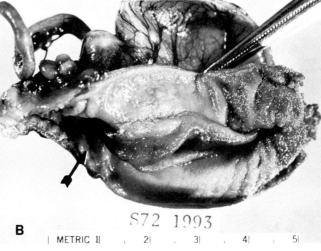

Bremer postulated that a few of the spherical and most of the tubular forms of duplications originate from an abnormal persistence of the vacuoles normally present during the "solid stage" of intestinal growth in the sixth or seventh week of gestation. "By the confluence of a chain of vacuoles a new channel is formed, parallel to the original lumen, and becomes separated from the latter by a union of the intestinal layers between the two. Since the duplication develops within the intestine, the outer wall of the duplicate portion always contains all of the tissue layers of the intestine."

Stenosis

In this condition there is narrowing of a portion of the intestinal tract (101, 106) at any level but most commonly in the duodenum. Stenosis usually manifests itself in partial or incomplete obstruction and depending upon the degree of narrowing may or may not be symptomatic in the neonatal period. Contrast studies of the small intestine may be necessary to establish the diagnosis.

SURGICAL TREATMENT OF INTESTINAL OBSTRUCTION

Intrinsic Duodenal Obstruction (Atresia; Stenosis)

These obstructions are surgically corrected by performing a bypass procedure, anastomosing jejunum to duodenum, proximal to the site of stenosis or atresia in a side-to-side fashion (103, 107, 108). In less than 5% of cases of duodenal atresia, the obstruction occurs proximal to the ampulla of Vater. In these instances, duodenojejunostomy may not be possible, and a gastrojejunostomy may be required.

Since these anastomoses rarely begin to function much before seven to ten days following surgery, a gastrostomy (102) is created at the original operation in order to provide for gastric decompression. The gastrostomy is usually placed to straight gravity drainage, although in some patients low

negative pressure may be applied to the tube. In addition to the gastrostomy tube, a second tube is usually inserted through the wall of the stomach above the gastrostomy site. This tube, which differs in size and color from the gastrostomy tube to prevent confusion, is threaded through the pylorus and proximal duodenum through the site of the duodenojejunostomy to lie well within the efferent limb of the anastomosis, extending several centimeters into the jejunum (Fig. 23–25). The proximal portion of this tube is brought out of the abdomen through a stab wound separate from the exit site of the gastrostomy tube and fixed securely to the skin. Two to three days following surgery, jejunostomy feedings (5 to 15 ml of glucose water or electrolyte solution) are begun through this tube. The quantity and quality of the feedings are gradually increased, and by the seventh day full formula can usually be given. In this way, the infant can be fed while the anastomosis is healing. At about the eighth to tenth day, thin barium is introduced through the gastrostomy tube to outline the duodenojejunostomy radiographically (Fig. 23–26). If this study reveals function at the anastomosis, the jejunostomy tube is withdrawn from the jejunum into the stomach, and at about the 14th postoperative day it is removed completely. Feedings by mouth can then be begun, and the gastrostomy tube is usually removed several days thereafter.

Extrinsic Duodenal Obstruction (Annular Pancreas; Malrotation)

The surgical treatment of annular pancreas is the same as that for duodenal stenosis or atresia, duodenojejunostomy, as has been described.

Management of the patient with malrotation depends in large part on whether there is associated volvulus and on whether the bowel involved in the volvulus is viable or not. A patient with malrotation and volvulus must have the volvulus corrected first. All of the small bowel must be brought out of the abdomen through the wound, and the volvulus must be reduced by counterclock-

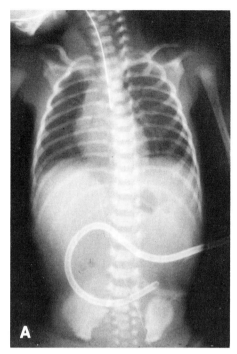
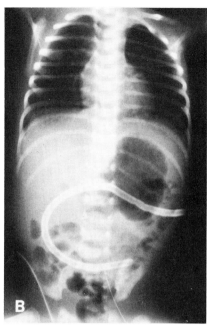

FIG. 23–25. Plain film of abdomen showing tube through duodenojejunostomy into efferent jejunum. **A.** Immediately postoperative (note the absence of gas in small intestine). **B.** Same patient seven days postoperative with gas widely distributed through bowel.

FIG. 23–26. Barium study through gastrostomy to demonstrate patency of duodenojejunostomy before removal of jejunostomy tube.

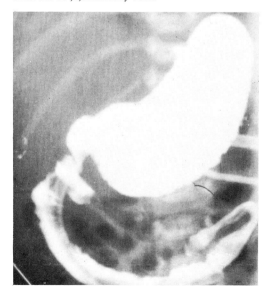

wise turning of the intestinal mass. If bowel appears compromised as a result of the volvulus, warm saline packs are applied, and the intestine is inspected for evidence of return to normal color and peristalsis. If there has been perforation or obvious gangrene of portions of the small bowel, these areas are resected and end-to-end anastomoses carried out to restore continuity.

In instances where the bowel is viable after reduction of a volvulus or where there has been extrinsic duodenal obstruction without volvulus, treatment consists in dividing the abnormal attachments or bands passing from the right upper quadrant across the second or third portions of duodenum to the malrotated cecum or ascending colon (111). These bands are usually avascular, and division of them is readily accomplished. Following complete division, the duodenum should fall into the right half of the abdomen almost vertically (the ligament of Treitz is also lysed as part of the operation). The entire small bowel lies in the right half of the abdomen, and the large bowel with cecum and appendix falls into the left half of the abdomen. Because of large raw-surface areas that result from division of the abnormal bands, appendectomy is not routinely performed, but parents are informed as to the new location of the appendix.

Gastrostomy is usually not performed in these cases, gastric decompression being accomplished by means of a nasogastric tube that can be removed usually after 36 to 48 hours. Feedings are begun 12 to 24 hours after tube removal, utilizing glucose water or electrolyte solution initially and progressing to formula within 24 to 36 hours.

Jejunum

Surgical management of jejunal obstruction is essentially resectional. Restoration of continuity may be accomplished by end-to-end, side-to-side or end-to-side anastomosis. In the typical obstruction due to atresia, the jejunum distal to the site of atresia will be small in calibre (microjejunum). In these circumstances, it may be better to employ a form of intestinal reconstruction that includes exteriorization of a portion of jejunum thus creating a jejunostomy. Two such procedures have been described: 1) Bishop-Koop (104) and 2) Santulli (108).

Bishop-Koop Exteriorization. After resection of the segment proximal to and including the area of atresia, the proximal (dilated) end of jejunum is anastomosed end-to-side to the distal microjejunum 6 cm distal to the original site of resection. The transected distal end is then brought out of the abdominal cavity through a separate stab wound, as a distal jejunostomy. A small catheter can then be threaded through this orifice into the distal jejunum. This catheter can be used for jejunostomy feedings and will promote more rapid development of a larger luminal area. As distal jejunum increases in calibre, intestinal contents will pass through the end-to-side anastomosis into the distal jejunum, and drainage from the jejunostomy will decrease gradually and in many instances cease entirely when the anastomosis is functioning maximally. This may take as long as ten days. Following

this, the distal jejunostomy tube may be removed. At about the third postoperative week the small exteriorized segment can be closed under local anesthesia, restoring jejunal continuity and eliminating the jejunostomy.

Santulli. This procedure is essentially the same as that just described with the fundamental difference being that the end-to-side anastomosis is constructed between the distal end of the jejunum and the proximal dilated segment. Thus the exteriorized segment is the proximal rather than the distal portion. A catheter can be threaded through this into the distal jejunum across the anastomosis for the purpose of instilling fluids or feedings into the distal segment to promote enlargement of the microjejunum. When external drainage has subsided and it is obvious that jejunal continuity across the anastomosis has occurred, the exteriorized segment may be resected as in the Bishop-Koop procedure.

When these operations are employed, it is important that the exteriorized segment is not so long that after excision of this segment and restoration of jejunal continuity, the patient is left with a "blind loop" that may lead to symptoms of the "blind loop syndrome" later.

An ancillary gastrostomy is created in all cases, including those treated by primary anastomoses (no exteriorization). This will serve to keep stomach and upper small bowel free of distension. The gastrostomy tube can usually be removed two weeks after surgery. Oral feedings may begin before this in most instances.

Ileum

Surgical treatment for ileal obstruction (treatment of meconium ileus will be described separately in the section dealing with that problem) is essentially resection of the involved segment, including the bulbous portion of ileum immediately adjacent to the site of obstruction, with restoration of continuity by end-to-end, side-to-side or end-to-side anastomosis. Exteriorization procedures such as Bishop-Koop or Santulli, which have been described above, may be employed.

The most widely used exteriorization procedure for ileal obstruction, however, is the Mikulicz procedure (2). This consists of suturing the antimesenteric borders of the distal and proximal segments of ileum, or ileum and ascending colon if the terminal ileum is included with the resected specimen, together with one or two rows of nonabsorbable sutures in continuous fashion. This approximation should extend 5 to 6 cm on each side of the intestinal segments following resection. Thus a double stoma is created and brought out of the abdomen through a separate stab wound. Both segments are fixed to the peritoneum with several sutures, and the main wound closed. Usually a single clamp grasping both stomata is left in place on the abdominal skin surface for 24 to 36 hours. After removing this, each stoma (proximal and distal) is identified and an appropriate spur-crushing clamp is inserted so that one blade of the clamp is through distal stoma and the other through proximal stoma. The clamp is then closed so that both blades impinge upon the approximated antimesenteric borders of the intestine, i.e., the contiguous wall or "spur." This clamp is progressively tightened. Within four to five days, the spur will be crushed and a single stoma created where previously there had been two. If the spur was of adequate length, after it has been crushed there will be spillage through the crushed area from proximal to distal segment. Initially, there will be drainage to the outside from the stoma. After several days, however, as distal "microintestine" increases in calibre and intestinal continuity becomes more normal, less spillage will drain to the outside. Usually three weeks after the initial procedure, the Mikulicz stump may be resected and closed under local anesthesia. Many surgeons have preferred this technique over direct primary anastomoses for ileal obstruction, believing it to be safer despite the fact that the infant must undergo two procedures instead of one.

Infants with multiple sites of atresia generally require individual resections and anastomoses at each site of atresia, but if these areas are relatively close and involve chiefly one segment of intestine, this entire segment with its multiple areas of atresia may be resected and only one anastomosis is required. Wherever possible, this is the preferred method of treatment. However, in most instances there are long segments of normal intestine between sites of atresia, and in such cases the removal of each involved segment with a separate anastomosis must be carried out in order to preserve as much small bowel length as possible.

Correction of Duplication

The surgical correction depends largely on the location and type of duplication (122). Where possible, resection with restoration of intestinal continuity by primary anastomosis is the procedure of choice. However, when cystic structures are encountered, e.g., stomach and duodenum, it may be possible to excise the duplication, including its mucosal lining, without incising the adjacent underlying mucosa of the parent organ. In some cases the contiguous mucosal septa may be excised, thus creating a single lumen where before there were two. In those cases where resection and primary anastomosis of the GI tract have been carried out, a gastrostomy is created for decompressive purposes.

Results of Treatment

In general, the high (duodenal) and low (ileal) obstructions are attended by higher survival rates than those in the jejunum or proximal ileum. Our survival rates have been 80% to 85% in cases of duodenal obstruction, 75% to 80% in ileal and 60% in patients with jejunal obstruction. With currently available methods for total parenteral alimentation, survival rates for obstruction at all levels should increase. Not only may fluid and electrolyte losses be adequately replaced but a high-caloric intake can be provided while normal intestinal function is being attained. Survival rates are lower in instances where multiple areas of atresia necessitate several anastomoses and cause the excision of so much small intestine that a very short small bowel results. In these infants, especially, IV hyperalimentation has provided the best chance for successful outcome.

Careful follow-up in regard to vitamin B_{12} and folic acid deficiency anemias with appropriate treatment is required for those infants in whom the terminal ileum including the ileocecal valve has been resected.

PERFORATED VISCUS

Any of the viscera within the abdominal cavity may perforate either prenatally or postnatally (127–129, 132). Etiologic factors may include an increase in intraluminal pressure, e.g., some instances of gastric perforation secondary to gavage feedings or of infants being bagged because of respiratory distress (133), but most perforations are due to vascular compromise or accident with subsequent necrosis of a portion of the wall of the viscus and later free perforation into the abdominal cavity (131). In neonates with prenatal perforation and spillage of meconium into the abdominal cavity, areas of calcification may be apparent on radiographic examination.

Although vomiting may be a presenting sign, in general the most apparent sign is abdominal distension, usually sudden in onset, with rapid decline in the baby's vital signs. Respiratory distress, tachycardia or bradycardia, pallor, lethargy or increased irritability, diarrhea or obstipation and acidosis occur. Changes in these infants occur rapidly, and prompt diagnosis and surgical intervention are required.

Diagnosis is established by flat and upright x-ray films of the abdomen (Fig. 23–27) that reveal free air within the peritoneal cavity. If the diaphragm is markedly elevated and interfering with respiration, it may be necessary to aspirate the free air by inserting a needle into the abdominal cavity. This is usually not a dangerous maneuver since the viscera are usually displaced posteriorly by the air when the infant is in the supine position.

Treatment

Surgical intervention is mandatory. Conservative methods of management are of no avail, and the precise identification of the perforated organ is usually not possible until exploration is done. If there has been a history of bagging or gavage feedings, the stomach should be suspected as the site of perforation. Small and large bowel perforation have no specific pathognomonic signs or x-ray appearance except in infants with necrotizing enterocolitis. The stomach is most commonly the perforated organ, next is the large bowel at the cecal or rectosigmoid level, and least common is the small bowel except in infants with unrecognized or untreated intestinal obstruction. Exploration is usually performed through a right paramedian or midline incision that may be extended caudad or cephalad as the situation demands. These incisions permit adequate exploration of all abdominal viscera including the region of the esophagogastric junction. At exploration, a systematic examination of all viscera must be performed. Beginning at the esophagogastric junction, the entire stomach surface, posterior as well as anterior, is carefully inspected. Though the quality of free fluid in the abdomen may often provide an indication of the level of perforation, a complete inspection must be carried out.

If the stomach is the site of perforation, surgical treatment will depend on the amount of stomach involved. In some instances, a near-total gastrectomy may be required (130). In other cases, the site of perforation may be small and closure after inserting a gastrostomy tube through the site of perforation may be adequate. Between these two extremes, partial gastrectomy may be required; often, infolding the site of perforation with sutures is sufficient. With all gastric perforations, the lesser sac must be entered and the posterior wall of the stomach carefully examined since often both anterior and posterior walls are in-

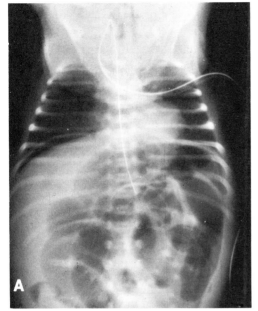

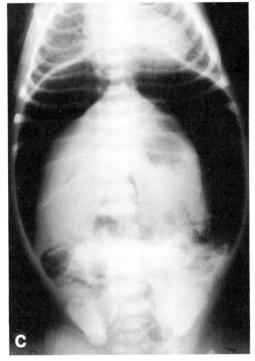

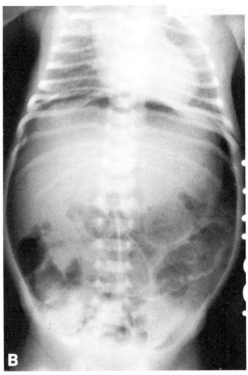

FIG. 23–27. Perforated viscus. **A.** Upright film of abdomen showing small crescent of air above right lobe of liver (suspect other than gastric perforation). **B.** Plain film of abdomen with more air apparent than in A. **C.** Upright film of patient in B demonstrates massive quantity of intraabdominal air and crowding of viscera into central mass (football sign), suggestive of large gastric perforation.

volved. Following adequate closure of the perforation, a gastrostomy is created. This is placed to low suction for 36 to 48 hours, then to dependent drainage for 12 hours after which, if bowel sounds have recurred, the child may be started on small amounts of oral feedings (usually glucose water or electrolyte solution) and gradually progressed to a normal diet.

If the stomach is not the site of perforation, the duodenum, small and large bowel are then carefully examined. It should be possible to locate any site of perforation, and an operation should not be considered adequate if no perforation is found. Small bowel perforation can be treated by resection of the involved segment with restoration of continuity by end-to-end anastomosis. Large bowel perforations may be treated similarly or in some instances by transverse closure of the involved site, if this is small. In some extremely ill patients, the site of large bowel perforation may be simply exteriorized in Mikulicz fashion, since this procedure can be carried out more quickly than a resection and reanastomosis. If there is a question about the integrity of the large bowel anastomosis where resectional surgery has been carried out, a proximal diverting colostomy may be indicated.

All infants with small or large bowel perforations require gastrostomy for decompression. Feedings are not begun until there is evidence of return of bowel activity. Ampicillin and kanamycin are given for five to seven days following surgery. The gastrostomy tube may be removed two weeks after surgery. In general, infants with gastric perforations have had the best survival rates—90% to 95%. Small bowel perforations not associated with lesions producing intestinal obstruction have had survival rates of 80%; while those with large bowel perforations have had a slightly less favorable outlook. Causes of death have included sepsis, secondary intestinal obstruction, pulmonary complications, prematurity and associated anomalies and, rarely, renal failure. The prompt recognition and treatment of perforated viscera should yield high salvage rates.

HIRSCHSPRUNG'S DISEASE

Described by Hirschsprung in 1888 (135), this condition was poorly understood and improperly treated until the monumental work of Swenson et al in the late 1940s (137, 138). They proved that the dilated portion of colon (megacolon) is not diseased, but simply the manifestation of a distal, functionally obstructive segment of colon that results from an absence or paucity of ganglion cells in the wall of the involved bowel.

Infants with aganglionosis present with signs suggestive of intestinal obstruction (140). The abdomen is markedly distended and passage of meconium is slight or absent. Digital rectal examination, insertion of rectal thermometer or catheter, or frank saline irrigation or enema is accompanied by passage of flatus and stool and decrease in the distension. The child may appear well for several hours or even for one to two days only to have a recurrence of distension and failure to pass stool. The severity and range of signs varies greatly, and many cases may not be identified in the neonatal period. In some instances, an initial diagnosis of meconium blockage syndrome may eventually prove to be Hirschsprung's disease.

Diagnosis is suspected by barium enema. Plain x-ray films of abdomen will reveal only marked distension, often of both large and small bowel (Fig. 23–28). Barium study may show redundant, large loops of colon or the colon may appear normal in size. The most important radiographic finding is that of retained barium in the colon 18 to 24 hours after the initial procedure (Fig.

FIG. 23–28. Lateral roentgenogram of abdomen revealing marked large and small bowel dilatation with gas in rectosigmoid colon.

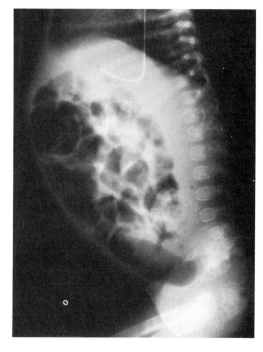

23–29), as this indicates poor evacuation (134, 136). With this finding, Hirschsprung's disease should be seriously considered. However, before undertaking surgery a rectal biopsy should be performed (139). This is usually done with the infant under general anesthesia and in a modified lithotomy position. The anus is dilated. The mucosa is incised several centimeters above the dentate line and is then dissected free of the underlying muscle wall of the rectum. A

FIG. 23–29. Hirschsprung's disease. **A.** Barium enema in lateral view demonstrating sharp cut-off area in rectum. **B** and **C.** Anteroposterior and lateral views 24 hours after barium enema showing retained barium and poor evacuation of colon.

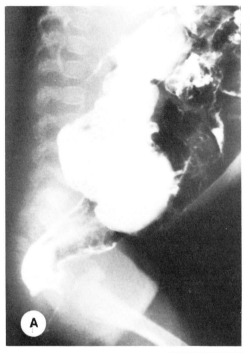

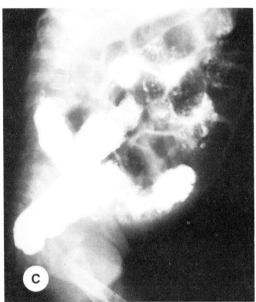

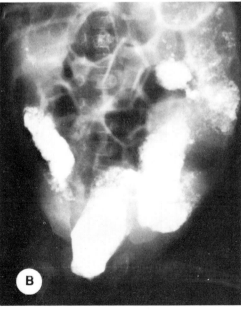

1-cm piece of the entire thickness of the muscle wall is then excised as the biopsy specimen. The muscle coat is then closed with absorbable suture material, after which the mucosa is reapproximated over the muscle-wall closure with absorbable suture material placed in continuous fashion. The specimen may be examined by frozen section technique or in the usual fashion (Fig. 25–30). Once aganglionosis has been established, further surgical treatment may be carried out.

Definitive treatment of Hirschsprung's Disease is not recommended for infants since the accepted forms of treatment are major operations that are best performed with a patient having a larger pelvis in which to work and better able to withstand a relatively long operation. The principle of management of Hirschsprung's Disease in the neonate entails simply decompressing the colon. Colostomy is the treatment of choice. Many surgeons prefer to perform this at the level of the sigmoid or descending colon; others have advocated a transverse colostomy. A sigmoid or descending colostomy if created can be removed at the time of the definitive procedure, thus saving the child an additional operation, namely, closure of the colostomy subsequent to definitive repair. A transverse colostomy may have the advantage of proximal diversion of the fecal stream while healing occurs at the site of the definitive correction and may outweigh the disadvantage of an additional operative procedure to subsequently close the colostomy. There is something to be said for each approach. Rather than establish a single definite policy, we suggest choosing where to perform the colostomy on the basis of the infant's colon as visualized on barium enema. If bowel is relatively short, sigmoid or descending colostomy is preferable since a transverse colostomy might limit the degree of mobilization of the colon possible at the time of definitive correction. If there is a large amount of colon with

FIG. 23–30. Photomicrograph showing **A.** ganglion cells in biopsy specimen of normal rectum (arrow). **B.** Presence of nerve fibers but absence of ganglia in myenteric plexus in rectal biopsy from patient with Hirschsprung's disease (arrow).

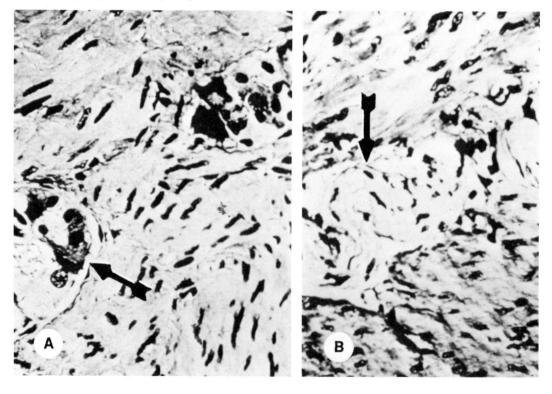

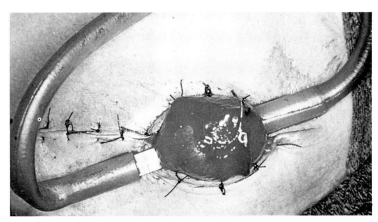

FIG. 23–31. Newly created transverse (loop) colostomy with glass rod beneath the exteriorized segment of colon. Decompressing catheter has not yet been placed.

redundant sigmoid (as is usually the case), transverse colostomy may be preferable.

In either event, the site selected for colostomy must be biopsied and frozen section examination of the wall done to establish the presence of ganglion cells at the proposed colostomy site. A colostomy must never be performed without confirmatory evidence of the presence of ganglion cells at the site chosen for its creation. The colostomy is made in loop fashion with a glass rod beneath the chosen loop (Fig. 23–31). At the time of fashioning the colostomy, a malecot catheter should be inserted into the proximal limb of the colostomy (through a small area of bowel inside a purse-string suture after the main wound has been closed and sealed off) so that a site for immediate decompression exists. After 24 to 48 hours, the colostomy is opened widely with cautery. The glass rod is removed after 12 to 14 days.

Complications

These infants do not usually require ancillary gastrostomy. A nasogastric tube is adequate for decompression and can be removed usually within one to two days. Although most colostomies are well tolerated, several problems may arise.

Skin excoriation about the colostomy site is especially likely in transverse colostomies made close to the hepatic flexure since stool may be less formed under these conditions than when colostomy is made in the distal

colon. Treatment is best accomplished by frequently changing the diaper or dressing over the colostomy site, using of a colostomy bag instead of a dressing, keeping the area dry by applying karaya powder and, probably most importantly, exposing the area as much as possible to the air under an ordinary light bulb (Fig. 25–32).

Superficial mucosal erosion or erosion of

FIG. 23–32. Abdomen of three-week-old infant revealing mild to moderate excoriation of skin surrounding transverse colostomy.

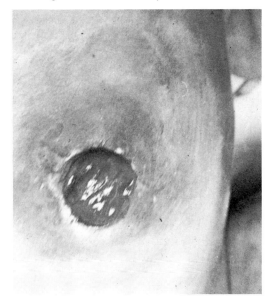

granulation tissue surrounding the colostomy bud may cause bleeding about the colostomy site. Careful handling of dressings in this area and the occasional use of silver nitrate to cauterize excess granulation tissue usually control this complication.

Stenosis of the colostomy may occur. Parents should be informed of the possibility of the stoma narrowing and instructed to dilate the opening on a weekly basis or more often as the situation demands. Rarely does a well-constructed colostomy become stenosed to the degree that colostomy revision is required.

Prolapse of colostomy may be an alarming complication to parents. A variable amount of proximal colon may prolapse. Small segment prolapse can usually be readily reduced by the parents. When moderate to severe degree of prolapse occurs, hospitalization may be required. Mild sedation and the use of cold 50% magnesium sulfate packs on the prolapse usually reduce it. If circulation of the colon begins to appear compromised, operative reduction and revision of the colostomy may be required.

Although these complications may be anticipated, most infants with a colostomy do well and except for mild skin excoriation tolerate the colostomy without incident until they have reached a size such that the definitive corrective procedure can be performed. Since definitive surgery is not carried out in the newborn period, discussion of the various techniques will not be discussed in this text.

NECROTIZING ENTEROCOLITIS

Although not exclusively a disease of premature infants, necrotizing enterocolitis occurs most frequently in this group. Since the early 1960s, this entity has become recognized as a frequent antecedent to GI perforation and an important cause of mortality in premature neonates. Conditions suggestive of necrotizing enterocolitis were reported as early as 1838 by Simpson (156), and in 1904 Maas (150) described pneumotosis intestinalis in a neonate. It was not until 1944, however, that the syndrome was first reported as a distinct clinical entity termed "malignant enteritis" by Willi (161) in Switzerland. The detailed clinical and pathological features were noted by Rossier et al (153) in the French literature in 1959 but did not become well known until the mid 1960s, when reports from the Babies' Hospital (143, 151, 159) in New York City as well as other centers (147, 157, 162) were published.

Signs are not usually manifested immediately after birth. Except for a history of minor apneic episodes the baby usually is doing well, eats normally and is free of bowel problems or abdominal distension. The onset of the disease is heralded by abrupt cessation of feeding, respiratory distress, and rapidly progressing abdominal distension. Vomiting has been noted in one-half of the reported cases. Stools may be scant, watery or blood-streaked, or there may be frank bloody diarrhea. Apneic spells and jaundice are common as the condition progresses. The disease is generally fulminant with rapid prostration and early death from intestinal perforation or sepsis. In one case encountered at the New York Hospital–Cornell Medical Center, however, the course was more protracted with signs presenting intermittently a month before perforation occurred. Blood counts and serum chemical determinations are nonspecific. Supine and upright films of the abdomen are the most useful diagnostic studies. Early, they may show generalized bowel distension, indistinguishable from mechanical obstruction or paralytic ileus. Later, the classic picture of gas within the wall of the intestine may be evident (152, 158), typically in the right lower quadrant (Fig. 23–33). Gas outlining the extrahepatic and intrahepatic branches of the portal vein (Fig. 23–34) may be noted as a late sign (155). Prognosis is grave under these circumstances, and only a few survivors have been reported (146). Free air in the peritoneal cavity indicates there has been GI perforation. Treatment of these infants is based largely on the findings at the time of diagnosis. Early in the disease medical management consisting of nasogastric suction, intravenous fluids and antibiotics (ampicil-

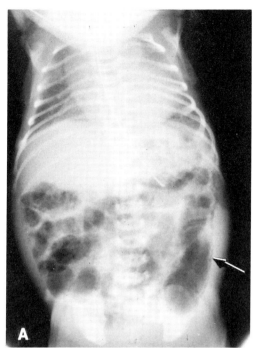 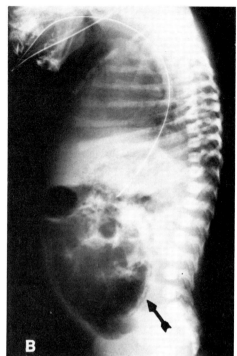

FIG. 23–33. Abdomen with gas within bowel wall (arrow). **A.** Anteroposterior view. **B.** Lateral view.

lin and kanamycin) as well as the usual supportive measures for infants of this size is employed. Surgical consultation is obtained, and pediatrician and surgeon both follow the patient carefully. Serial plain films of the abdomen are obtained. If the child's condition begins to deteriorate or there is progression as indicated by roentgenograms, early surgical exploration is required.

The exact indications for surgery are not well defined except in cases where there is pneumoperitoneum. However, waiting until free perforation occurs may be waiting too long.

From our experience, it appears that medical management carries with it a high mortality rate. Operation after free perforation has occurred similarly is associated with a grave prognosis. For these reasons, we feel that a more aggressive surgical approach is warranted and that these infants should undergo exploration if there is 1) generalized deterioration, 2) an increase in the amount or frequency of bloody diarrhea, 3) extension of intramural gas pattern prior to free perforation, or 4) gas present in the portal veins.

FIG. 23–34. Plain film of abdomen showing air in portal system (arrows).

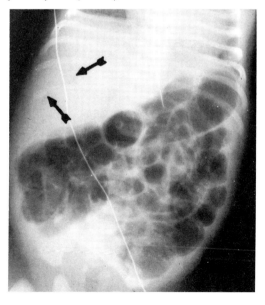

Surgery is performed through a mid-transverse, midline or long right paramedian incision. Necrotic bowel is excised, and depending on the level of involvement, GI continuity is restored either by the appropriate anastomosis, or if the terminal ileum or colon is involved, by an exteriorization type of operation such as a Mikulicz, Bishop-Koop, or Santulli procedure. If at surgery it is impossible to delineate the extent of bowel involved in the disease process, a simple loop ileostomy of the terminal ileum or an ileocolostomy of the Mikulicz type is performed. A gastrostomy is created and the child given optimal supportive management including antibiotics. Following successful surgery, feedings by mouth are instituted when it is apparent that normal intestinal activity and function have returned. The gastrostomy tube is removed several weeks after the infant has recovered

Results of management in infants with this disease vary widely among different institutions. The best results indicate an overall survival rate of as high as 67% with a survival rate of those undergoing surgery of 64%. In most of the published reports, survival rates for both medically or surgically treated cases does not exceed 50%. Follow-up of survivors indicates no residual difficulties except in the occasional infant who may develop stricture at the site of the previous disease or anastomosis.

The common pathologic feature is acute and frequently multiple mucosal ulcerations of the GI tract. Around these ulcers is a transitional area of intravascular congestion and thrombosis and mucosal coagulative necrosis with a scanty infiltrate of mononuclear cells. Eosinophilic infiltration may be present.

Pseudomembrane formation and gross and microscopic evidence of pneumatosis are characteristic. Perforations are frequent and often multiple. The involved area in the bowel may be limited or may involve nearly the entire bowel. The terminal ileum is reported to be the most common location, but over half the perforations described by Touloukian et al, (159) were in the colon or jejunum. Denes (145) describes only 2 of his 25 cases as involving the ileum alone. The majority of his cases were in the colon. Touloukian's group reported six cases in the stomach, and Hopkins' group (148) noted one in the duodenum and another with involvement of the stomach and esophagus.

While the etiology of this disease remains obscure, several theories have been advanced. In his original report, Willi suggested a bacterial origin but was unable to demonstrate the infecting organisms. However, the presence of enteric gram-negative bacteria cultured in these infants, particularly prior to the onset of signs in several series including the one reported by Asaph and Redo (142), suggests that these organisms may play a prominent role in the course of the disease, and there is now general agreement that the intestinal and portal vein gas is caused by these organisms. Schmid (154) hypothesized a viral origin, but he was unable to identify the organisms, and this theory has achieved little popularity. Agerty (141) suggested local factors such as volvulus or mucosal defect, but neither he nor subsequent authors have been able to observe these abnormalities. Stone et al (1958), however, have noted that multiple factors, including dehydration, ischemia, intestinal obstruction and hypoxia, can alter the mucosal barrier and result in bacterial invasion of the intestine. The small vessel thrombosis at the periphery of the ulcerations and other histologic similarities led Rossier (153) and later Herman (147) to postulate a Shwartzman phenomenon. They suggested that the bowel wall is sensitized by the somatic antigens of GI organisms and that subsequent bacteremia may then cause mucosal necrosis. Wilson and Woolley (162) have reported thrombocytopenia, which is characteristic of the Shwartzman reaction, in 9 of 16 cases of necrotizing enterocolitis. Attempts by my associates to reproduce the lesion in neonatal guinea pigs by sensitizing their bowel wall to suspensions of E. coli were unsuccessful, and it is unclear whether or not neonates are capable of developing Shwartzman reactions. Experimental evidence by Uhr (160) suggests that they may not be able to do so.

Blanc (144) demonstrates infected amniotic fluid in the GI tracts of infants born of mothers with amnionitis and suggests that this could cause gastroenteritis. Several subsequent series, including the one of Asaph and Redo (142), however, have failed to associate prolonged rupture of membranes or amionitis with the disease. Mizrahi et al (151) note the similarity of endotoxic shock in laboratory animals to that of clinical necrotizing enterocolitis and speculate that neonatal stress could cause splanchnic vascular ischemia with secondary ulceration and subsequent endotoxic shock. Touloukian et al (159) support this theory and suggest that the ischemia results in diminished mucin production, thus allowing proteolytic enzymes to attack the bowel wall normally protected by mucin. Mizrahi also notes that infants fed cow's milk, rather than being breast fed, have a lysozyme-deficient diet and an exceptionally gram-negative predominant GI flora, whereas a breast-fed baby's flora are mixed gram-negative and gram-positive. Citing Stetson's work Mizrahi also suggests that the susceptibility of animals to endotoxin may be directly related to the bacterial flora in the intestinal tract. Pitt et al (151a) have demonstrated that macrophages present in fresh breast milk protect hypoxic neonatal rats against necrotizing enterocolitis. Since it is likely that premature infants are generally not breast fed, this theory has some credence. However, a number of reported babies develop signs on the first day of life before any milk has been given, and thus it is unlikely that this is the cause of all the cases.

In 1969 Lloyd (149) advanced the interesting theory that the etiology may be related to selective circulatory ischemia, a phenomenon of asphyxial defense mechanism that shunts blood away from those areas of the body that are able to tolerate prolonged hypoxia to those areas that suffer irreversible damage if deprived of adequate circulation for relatively short periods of time. This phenomenon, known as the "diving reflex," is characteristic of diving mammals such as seals. He thinks there is evidence that this mechanism is operational in neonates in times of stress such as hypovolemia or hypoxia. Thus, the intense splanchnic vasoconstriction could lead to ischemic necrosis of the bowel.

It is this author's belief that necrotizing enterocolitis probably has a vascular-ischemic component as well as a bacterial factor. Which of these two is involved primarily is not clear from evidence presented to date.

MUCOVISCOIDOSIS (CYSTIC FIBROSIS OF THE PANCREAS) AND MECONIUM ILEUS

Cystic fibrosis is an inherited (autosomal recessive) disorder of the exocrine glands of many organ systems (164, 166). Pulmonary lesions dominate the clinical picture in childhood and ultimately lead to death of the individual.

Of surgical importance in the neonatal period is meconium ileus (172, 173, 180), which is due to lack of exocrine function of the pancreas. This occurs in about 5% to 10% of cases of neonatal cystic fibrosis and reflects failure of the meconium to undergo changes normally brought about by pancreatic secretions (168, 179). The meconium is thick, tenacious, and puttylike; it accumulates in the terminal ileum. Affected infants present with signs of intestinal obstruction. There may be a history of siblings with cystic fibrosis and possibly meconium ileus.

The diagnosis may be established by means of a sweat test (167, 170) that reveals elevated concentrations of sodium and chloride. Values of either ion greater than 60 mEq/l are diagnostic. However, during the first 48 hours of life, volumes of sweat may be insufficient to perform the analysis. Studies of nails and hair may also reveal elevated concentrations of these ions.

Meconium ileus may be diagnosed from flat and upright films of the abdomen that show distended loops of small bowel and often a "soap-bubble" appearance in the lower small bowel (Fig. 23–35). This soap-bubble appearance represents meconium admixed with intestinal gas (175). Contrast enema using radiopaque material shows a hypoplastic, microcolon since the abnormal meconium has not passed into the bowel. In

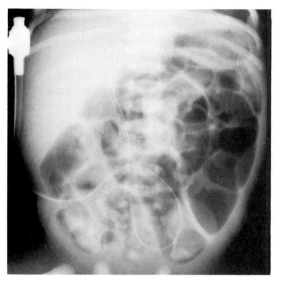

FIG. 23–35. Plain film of abdomen revealing dilated loops of bowel with suggestion of "soap bubble" appearance in right lower quadrant.

some instances, intrauterine perforation that may have occurred as a result of meconium ileus is revealed by calcific densities on abdominal roentgenograms (Fig. 23–36). Chest x rays should be obtained in these infants to evaluate the status of the lungs, which may not be involved at birth.

On physical examination, the abdomen is usually distended; loops of bowel with a doughy or rubbery consistency are often palpable. Rectal examination suggests a small anus and rectum. Tiny, dry, yellow-gray shreds suggesting meconium and mucus are occasionally passed after digital examination of the rectum, but true meconium does not appear at the anus. This helps differentiate meconium ileus from Hirschsprung's disease: infants with aganglionosis will pass gas and good amounts of meconium following rectal examination.

The pathologic picture at surgical exploration or postmortem examination is uniformly similar. The entire large bowel and distal 10 to 20 cm of ileum are small (microileum and microcolon). Within the narrow distal ileum are firm, rounded, yellow-gray pellets. Proximal to the hypoplastic segment, the ileum is markedly distended and bulbous, containing the bulk of the thick,

tenacious, abnormal meconium. More proximally the ileum continues enlarged for a variable distance, becoming more normal in calibre as the jejunum is approached. Microscopic examination of small bowel mucosa reveals abnormal glands, many of which are filled with thick, hyaline-staining secretions. Similar changes are evident in tracheobronchial glands, pancreas and liver. Bundles of fibrous tissue forming dense periacinal and interacinal bands are seen in the pancreas. In the neonate, the involvement of tracheobronchial glands and liver is often not striking. Ileal atresia may occur in patients who have had intrauterine perforation of this portion of the small intestine. If there is spillage of large amounts of meconium into the peritoneal cavity, subsequent calcification may lead to replacement of the small bowel by a stoney mass making treatment more difficult or impossible.

Meconium ileus may be treated surgically

FIG. 23–36. Anteroposterior view of abdomen showing calcific densities in right lower quadrant (arrow) and general ground-glass appearance suggesting intrauterine perforation with development of meconium peritonitis.

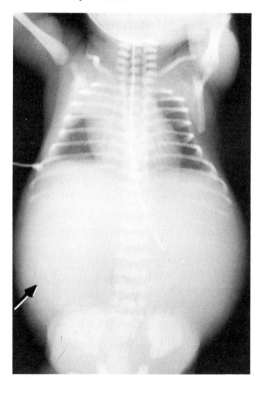

or nonsurgically. In the past, surgery has included ileostomy and evacuation of the thick meconium by mechanical, chemical or combinations of these means (163, 171). Hydrogen peroxide, saline and N-acetyl-cysteine have been employed to liquefy, soften or wash out the abnormal meconium, each with variable degrees of success (165, 174, 178). Most surgeons, however, preferred to excise the bulbous portion of dilated ileum that contained the bulk of the inspissated meconium and then carry out an exteriorization procedure similar to those of Mikulicz or Bishop-Koop (see section Intestinal Obstruction). Some performed end-to-end, end-to-side or side-to-side anastomoses to restore intestinal continuity.

A gastrostomy is performed for decompression. Where exteriorization has been performed, a small catheter is inserted into the distal stoma (Mikulicz) or the stoma of the exteriorized (distal) hypoplastic ileum (Bishop-Koop) through which pancreatic enzyme or fluids, or both, may be introduced to aid in the passage of mucus or accretions in the distal bowel and to promote development of a more normal luminal calibre. This catheter is usually removed in four to five days. Further management of the stoma resulting from these procedures has been discussed in the section Intestinal Obstruction.

In 1969 Noblett (176) reported a nonsurgical method of managing infants with uncomplicated meconium ileus (without evidence of perforation or peritonitis). This technique consists in using meglumine diatrozate (Gastrografin) as an enema. A catheter is inserted into the rectum, the infant's buttocks are strapped together, and under image-intensification fluoroscopy, warm enema solution is introduced by syringe through the catheter. The retrograde progress of this water-soluble contrast material is followed fluoroscopically until the entire colon is filled and the contrast agent flows back through the ileocecal valve into the distal hypoplastic ileum and then into the dilated bulbous portion filled with abnormal meconium. Contrast material is introduced until the more normal, more

proximal ileum is filled (Fig. 23–37). If this can be accomplished, the infant soon passes the instilled contrast material, meconium and gas, and distension is relieved. If it is impossible to achieve the desired retrograde passage of contrast material into the ileum, the procedure is halted and surgical correction is undertaken. Occasionally, although good passage of meconium may occur initially, the infant may continue to show signs of distension and may have no further passage of meconium per rectum. When this happens, a repeat enema may be carried out. In one infant in the author's experience, three separate enemas on four successive days were required to achieve ultimate nonsurgical correction of the meconium ileus. When this technique is used, a venous cutdown catheter should be in place and liberal fluids given during the procedure since Gastrografin is hyperosmolar and will draw

FIG. 23–37. Anteroposterior view of abdomen taken after completion of radiopaque medium enema (under image intensification fluoroscopy) showing that contrast has refluxed through the ileocecal valve and is well into proximal ileum. Treatment by this method is not considered to be successful unless significant reflux into the ileum is accomplished.

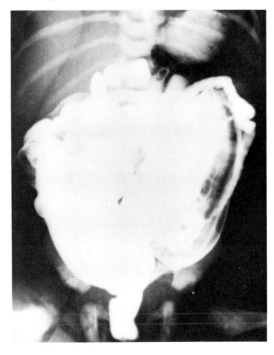

fluid from the intravascular compartment into the bowel. This not only dehydrates the child, but may also precipitate cardiovascular collapse. Careful medical management, with repeated assessment of fluid and electrolyte balance and vital signs, are required. Warming the Gastrografin is also vital since the relatively large volumes required could otherwise lead to a rapid fall in the infant's temperature with the possible untoward effects of hypothermia. Known perforation or gangrene are contraindications to this method.

In addition to the management of the problem of obstruction, whether by surgical or nonsurgical means, it is important to introduce pancreatic enzymes by mouth or through gastrostomy tube as soon as possible. From one-fourth to one-sixth teaspoonful of viokase is given twice daily to correct the pancreatic deficiency. It has been our practice to order kanamycin and ampicillin for seven to ten days following treatment. The results of treatment of the abdominal problems of meconium ileus by surgical means have led to survival rates of 70% to 75%. Nonsurgical treatment with the Gastrografin technique has led to over 90% survival in a small group of selected patients (169, 177, 181). All three infants so treated in the author's experience have survived the neonatal period. Genetic counseling is recommended for all parents with a child having mucoviscidosis.

ANORECTAL ANOMALIES

Congenital malformations of the anus and rectum occur in approximately 1:5000 live births and are slightly more common in males than females. The reader is referred to the excellent volume by Stephens and Smith (184) for a detailed discussion of the embryology and pathogenesis of the various anomalies and associated rectogenitourinary fistulous communications.

In order to appreciate the problems in diagnosis and management of anorectal anomalies, an understanding of the types encountered is essential. Many classifications have been described. That of Ladd and Gross (182) was once the most commonly used, but a classification outlined by Stephens (183) has come into greater use. Since Stephens' classification is slightly more complicated than that of Ladd and Gross (Fig. 23–38), for ease in visualizing the defect, the Ladd and Gross classification will be employed in this discussion.

The diagnosis of anorectal anomalies can usually be made by inspection of the perineum. If a small opening is visible at the anus through which a little meconium drains, a stenotic anus, or Type I anorectal malformation, exists. If there is no orifice at the anus but dark meconium is visible through the thin skin over the anal plate or if the area bulges when the child strains, there is a Type II anomaly, or anal membrane. In cases of Type III, with a low rectal pouch, there will be no anus. There may be an externally draining fistula to the perineum in the male or female (covered anus in Stephens' classification) or to the vagina (low) or fossa navicularis in the female (ectopic anus per Stephens). Type III anomalies with a high pouch will have no external fistulas in the male (anorectal agenesis of Stephens). Most Type III anomalies have rectourethral fistulas; a smaller number have rectovesical fistulas. In the female of this type (high pouch), high rectovaginal fistulas are common. The position of the genital tract between the urinary tract and the rectum generally precludes rectourinary tract fistulas in the female. Type IV anomalies (rectal agenesis of Stephens) present with what appears to be a normal anus externally. The anal canal and lowermost portion of rectum, however, are of variable length (usually short), and on rectal examination insertion of the entire extent of the examining finger may not be possible. Immediately after birth, the abdomen may appear unremarkable, but as gas enters the GI tract, distension occurs. If the condition goes undetected, there may be vomiting and signs of intestinal obstruction.

Diagnosis utilizing roentgen techniques are not necessary in the Type I or II anomalies, nor in the Type III with a perineal fistula in either sex or low vaginal or fossa navicularis fistula in the female since these are associated with a low pouch. In males

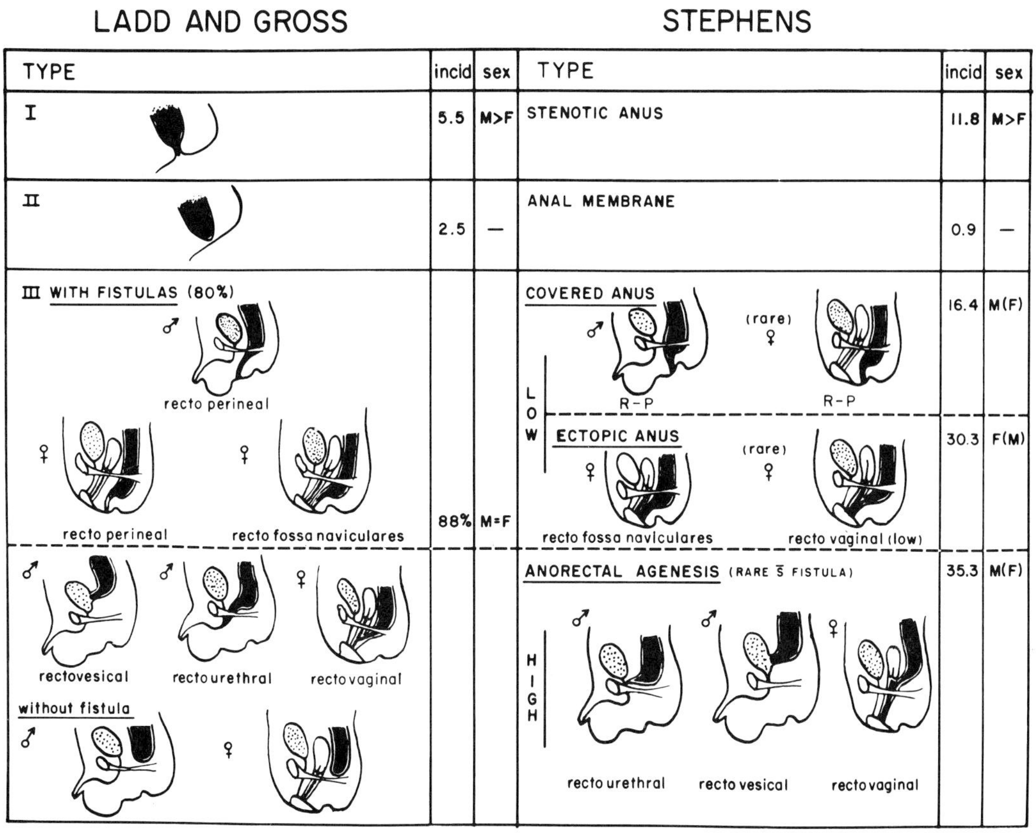

LADD AND GROSS — STEPHENS

TYPE		incid	sex	TYPE		incid	sex
I		5.5	M>F	STENOTIC ANUS		11.8	M>F
II		2.5	—	ANAL MEMBRANE		0.9	—
III WITH FISTULAS (80%) recto perineal (♂) recto perineal (♀) recto fossa naviculares (♀)	88%		M=F	COVERED ANUS (♂) (rare ♀) R-P / R-P	LOW	16.4	M(F)
rectovesical (♂) rectourethral (♂) rectovaginal (♀) without fistula (♂) (♀)				ECTOPIC ANUS recto fossa naviculares (♀) (rare ♀) recto vaginal (low)		30.3	F(M)
				ANORECTAL AGENESIS (RARE s̄ FISTULA) recto urethral (♂) recto vesical (♂) recto vaginal (♀)	HIGH	35.3	M(F)

FIG. 23–38. The more common types of anorectal anomalies according to the Ladd-Gross and Stephens classifications.

without an obvious externally draining fistula or in females with a high vaginal fistula, x-ray studies are helpful in establishing the diagnosis and type of anomaly. These should not be obtained until 18 to 24 hours after birth, so that gas in the colon will have time to reach the lowermost aspect of the rectal pouch. A radiopaque marker is placed over the perineum at the site where the anus should be (185). The infant is then placed in a head down position for several minutes, after which an abdominal roentgenogram is obtained in the lateral view. The upside down position is necessary to permit meconium to flow out of the distal portion of the rectal pouch and allow gas to reach that level. The distance between the radiopaque marker on the perineum and the limit of the gas-outlined rectal pouch indicates the level of the pouch. A low pouch is one located below the level demarcated by a line drawn between the upper border of the pubis and the coccyx, while a high pouch is one located above this level.

Treatment in the Type III anomalies will depend largely on whether the pouch is low or high. In males with Type III anomaly and a high pouch the presence of a rectourinary tract fistula may be established by noting meconium in the voided urine. The location of the fistula can be best demonstrated by means of a cystourethrogram. Since a high proportion of infants with anorectal anomalies have associated urinary tract anomalies, it is important than an IVP be performed early in order to identify urinary tract abnormalities, some of which may require surgical correction in the neonatal period.

Type I (Stenotic Anus)

This is best treated by frequent dilation, beginning in the immediate postnatal period. A small rubber catheter is used initially. As the anus becomes more patent, larger soft rubber catheters are employed. The mother can be instructed to do this daily, the physician checking the infant's progress at weekly, biweekly or monthly intervals as the dilatation progresses. Usually six to ten months of these dilations may be required before an adequate and persistent anus is achieved. The author has treated many neonates in this fashion with excellent results. Despite the length of time required to effect satisfactory dilation, surgery is not indicated in these patients.

Type II (Anal Membrane)

Surgical correction of this anomaly is relatively simple and in most instances may be performed under local anesthesia, although unless contraindicated, a light plane of general anesthesia may be preferable. An incision is made over the site of the anus into the rectal pouch, which usually lies immediately beneath the skin. Unless an injudicious procedure is carried out, there is no danger to the external anal sphincters, and the ultimate result should be excellent. Immediately on opening into the rectal pouch, meconium will be passed. This should be aspirated or removed by sponges after which the rim of the rectal pouch is sutured to the skin of the anal area using nonabsorbable sutures. The surgeon should insert his finger through the new anus to make sure that an adequate opening exists. The sutures are removed in 10 to 12 days, after which gentle dilations are begun. Dilations should be continued for three to six months to prevent cicatricial stenosis of the anus.

Type III With Rectoperineal, Rectovestibular or Rectovulvar Fistula (Covered or Ectopic Anus)

In the male, this type of anomaly may occur as a small subcutaneous tract from the perineum to the scrotal raphe or, as in the female, may be a small obvious opening in the perineum proper, usually just anterior to an area of pigmented skin or an anal dimple. Both varieties in the male and the rectoperineal variety in the female are treated by the so-called "cut-back" procedure. This is an uncomplicated technique usually performed under general anesthesia. In the male with a fistula extending to the scrotal raphe, a small probe is inserted into the tract and directed caudally. The tract is laid open in the midline with scissors. At the posterior aspect, the tract enters the anal pit that communicates with the rectal pouch. The incision is carried posteriorly until an adequate anal orifice is created. At the posterior margin of the incision, the opened rectal pouch is sutured to the skin with a few sutures of nonabsorbable material. In the classic picture of rectoperineal fistula (male or female) a curved clamp is inserted into the fistula and directed posteriorly. A scalpel is then used to incise the tissue overlying the slightly separated blades of the clamp. This is carried sufficiently posteriorly until an adequate orifice is obtained. The posterior portion of incised rectal pouch is sutured to the skin at the site of the anus with nonabsorbable sutures, as has been mentioned. Sutures are left in place for 10 to 12 days. After their removal, gentle dilations are carried out as described for the treatment of Type I and II anomalies.

Females with rectovulvar or rectovestibular fistulas are also treated by the cut-back procedure. Although some authors have employed anal transplant procedures, dissecting and mobilizing the lower rectal pouch and bringing this down through the external sphincter fibers, this more extensive operation probably is not warranted. The cut-back technique requires no dissection, and thus there is no danger of injuring the anal sphincter mechanism. Anal continence is the rule following cut-back, and the results utilizing this simple method are excellent.

Type III Without Externally Draining Fistula in Male, High or Small Rectovaginal Fistula in Female (High Pouch)

These types of anorectal anomalies have been associated with frequently poor results, chiefly due to anal incontinence following surgical correction. Failure to recognize the importance of the puborectalis muscle sling as a sphincter for the anus and the fact that definitive surgery was performed in neonatal period, when the pelvis is small and difficult to work in, caused many of these poor results. For either reason, the puborectalis sling may be damaged. If it is not identified and the colon is pulled through posterior rather than anterior to it, this important muscle will lose its sphincteric function. In addition, pelvic nerves may be injured during the dissection.

Because of these considerations, the author recommends treating infants with this type of anomaly by colostomy. This should be completely diverting in order to protect the urinary tract in the male from contamination by fecal spill-over from the proximal into the distal stoma and thence into a rectovesical or rectourethral fistula. (See section Intestinal Obstruction for discussion of creation, management and complications of colostomy.) The infant is followed and definitive correction of the anorectal agenesis, including division and closure of associated rectogenitourinary tract fistulas, is performed at approximately one year of life when the pelvis has increased in size. This facilitates surgery and provides the best chance for the child to gain an anus with good control.

In females with a low (or high) rectovaginal fistula that can be dilated to permit evacuation of colon contents, a colostomy is not necessary. If dilation of the fistula provides an adequate venting orifice, the definitive surgery may be delayed for several years. Understanding the importance of the puborectalis sling, delayed definitive correction and proper surgical management have led to markedly improved results in infants with this type of anorectal anomaly.

Type IV (Rectal Atresia)

The principles of management of this group are the same as those enumerated above, namely colostomy in infancy and definitive repair after one year of age. The various techniques for definitive correction of these types are well described in several excellent books of pediatric surgery. The treatment of anorectal anomalies is summarized in Table 23–1.

HERNIA AND HYDROCELE

Inguinal hernia and hydrocele may be considered minor congenital anomalies resulting from improper or incomplete closure of the processus vaginalis. In order to appreciate the possible variations, it is necessary to review the basic steps in the progression of the testes from their original location high on the posterior wall of the abdomen down through the inguinal canal into the scrotum.

The gubernaculum in some manner initiates the migration of the testis downward. At the same time, a bud of peritoneum begins to project through the fascial and muscle planes of the abdominal wall in the inguinal canal to reach the scrotum. The

TABLE 23–1. Treatment of Anorectal Anomalies

Type	Treatment or Intervention
I	(Nonsurgical), dilations
II	Incision of anal membrane followed by dilations
III	
1. With externally draining fistula	Cut-back procedure followed by dilations
2. Without externally draining fistula	Colostomy in neonatal period with definitive correction after age 1 year
VI	Colostomy in neonatal period with definitive correction after age 1 year

descending testicle is adjacent to this peritoneal outpouching (processus vaginalis). When both the testicle and processus have reached the scrotum, the testicle invaginates the bulbous distal portion of the processus vaginalis. The testicle is now enclosed in an envelope of the mesthothelial tissue of the processus. Following this, in the normal infant, the portion of the processus surrounding the testicle pinches off and forms the tunica vaginalis. The more proximal portion of the processus atrophies and disappears with complete closure at the abdominal side. The opening through which the testicle and its cord (vas deferens and blood vessels) pass out of the abdomen is known as the internal ring, the space through which it passes downward in the abdominal wall is

the inguinal canal, and the site at which it leaves the inguinal canal to pass downward into the scrotum is the external ring. The layers of the abdominal wall through which the testicle and cord pass provide three coverings for these structures, namely: 1) the external spermatic fascia from the external oblique muscle, 2) the cremaster fascia from the internal oblique muscle and 3) the internal spermatic fascia from the transversalis fascia.

The various anomalies of closure of the processus vaginalis lead to the different types of hernia or hydrocele encountered (Fig. 23–39). Of the various types of potential anomalies of closure of the processus vaginalis, inguinal hernia is the most common; hydrocele is next; and the combination separate hernia, cord and scrotal hydrocele is least common. Because the right testicle descends later than the left, hernias are more common on the right.

FIG. 23–39. The varieties of hernia and hydroceles associated with incomplete or anomalous closure of the original processus vaginalis. The upper panel shows steps in the normal investiture and disappearance of the processus vaginalis.

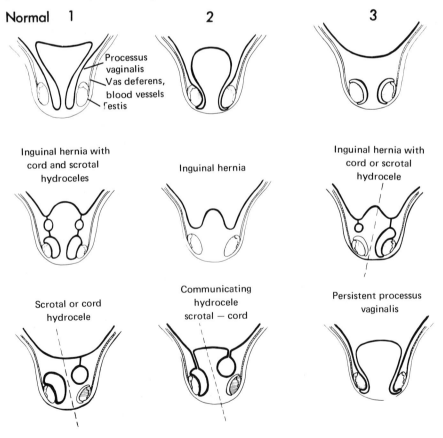

In the female, the same essential steps are repeated, and thus frank hernias and hydroceles occur. However, in the absence of a scrotum, hydroceles in the female are found only in the inguinal canal, i.e., hydroceles in the canal of Nuck.

Diagnosis of a hernia or hydrocele is made essentially by history, inspection and palpation. Unless the hernia has manifested itself at or shortly after birth, the mother is the first to become aware of an unusual bulge in the inguinal or pubic region, particularly when the child cries or strains. The bulge may disappear only to reappear at a later time when the child strains again. If a history suggestive of hernia is given by the mother, it may be necessary for the examining physician to elicit crying in the infant to demonstrate the defect. Palpation over the inguinal canal may lead to a sensation of two slippery surfaces gliding over each other, the so-called "silk glove" sign. Palpation through the scrotum and external ring, the usual method for detecting hernia in adults, is of no value in infants and should not be employed.

A hernia descending into the scrotum may be differentiated from a scrotal hydrocele in that it is possible in most cases to reduce the hernia, emptying the scrotum. A hydrocele of the cord may not be distinguishable from an incarcerated hernia. A scrotal hydrocele can be distinguished from a hernia since the cord structures above it can be felt and separated from the presenting mass. Transillumination of the mass is helpful but not diagnostic, since bowel herniating into the scrotum may also be transilluminated. If a mass in the scrotum transilluminates but cannot be reduced and is associated with thickening in the cord above the mass, an incarcerated complete hernia should be suspected. Flat and upright radiographs of the abdomen are helpful in such cases. If gas is demonstrable in the mass within the scrotum, the problem is that of an incarcerated hernia rather than a scrotal hydrocele. The diagnosis of communicating hydroceles is established if the fluid within the hydrocele can be evacuated by gentle pressure.

TREATMENT OF HERNIAS

Treatment of the varieties of defects depends on the specific pathology. Inguinal hernias should be treated surgically as soon as possible after the diagnosis is made since the possibility of incarceration or strangulation, or both, is great (186, 195). Surgery is performed under general anesthesia using an incision through the lowermost abdominal skin crease in order to produce the least disfiguring scar. The sac is dissected free of the cord structures up to its neck at the internal ring. The neck of the sac is then doubly transfixed with fine silk sutures and the excess sac excised. The integrity of the muscle layers of the inguinal canal is restored by utilizing a modified Ferguson type of hernia repair. Silk sutures are placed through the medial aspect of the aponeurosis of the external oblique muscle and the underlying internal oblique muscle and these are brought down to the shelving border of Poupart's ligament. As the level of the external ring is approached, the medial and lateral portions of the external oblique aponeurosis are merely reapproximated to provide a good exit site for the cord. Scarpa's fascia is closed with polyglycolic acid sutures. Subcutaneous tissues are brought together with similar suture material used in subcuticular fashion. Sterile plastic strips are placed across the wound to secure a fine skin closure. A small dry dressing is applied. The patient is usually discharged the following morning but may be allowed home several hours after surgery if the parents so desire and the patient's condition warrants.

It has been our policy to do bilateral procedures in all infants, even when only a unilateral hernia is demonstrable, unless there has been difficulty with anesthesia, the operation has taken more than 30 minutes or other problems exist that contraindicate prolonging the period of anesthesia and surgery. Whether bilateral exploration should be carried out when a hernia is demonstrable on one side only remains controversial (187, 189, 191, 193). In our experience, the finding of a hernia on the contralateral side is greater than 30%, and therefore we feel that bilateral exploration is indicated, with the reservations noted above.

Incarcerated Hernia

If an infant is admitted with a short history of incarceration and no clinical signs to suggest strangulated bowel, the child should be sedated and a gentle attempt made to reduce the hernia. This usually can be accomplished. The infant is observed, and surgery is carried out 24 to 48 hours later, permitting some of the edema to subside. This facilitates the operation and insures better closure and repair of the hernia.

Strangulated Hernia

This represents a true emergency since the bowel in the hernia may be undergoing necrosis. Surgery is carried out as previously described. However, care should be taken that the bowel not be reduced until the sac has been opened and the herniated viscera carefully inspected to evaluate their viability. If the herniated bowel becomes reduced due to relaxation caused by anesthesia or mishandling of the hernia sac, it may be necessary to make a separate incision in the right lower quadrant and examine the bowel for viability.

Usually a strangulated hernia is difficult to reduce since the internal ring is small. In such instances, the ring should be incised laterally in order to enlarge it and relieve the bowel of its strangulation. The bowel should not be returned into the abdominal cavity until the surgeon is satisfied that it is viable. This can best be determined by the return of peristalsis to the involved segment. The assumption of more nearly normal color or the presence of pulsations in the mesenteric vessels also help to establish its viability.

A question commonly asked by parents is whether surgery for hernia is necessary. In answer to this, it is generally accepted that an inguinal hernia does not disappear and therefore should be treated surgically. The one exception to this may be in premature infants. In these infants, the possibility of

closure of the processus after birth exists, and in this group a significant number of "hernias" may close spontaneously. Thus, these children may be observed at frequent intervals for several weeks to months following discharge from the hospital. If after a few months, the hernia is still present or larger, surgery should be recommended.

TREATMENT OF HYDROCELES

The treatment of hydroceles depends largely on the type observed. Scrotal hydroceles are not corrected during infancy, except in very unusual circumstances. Instead, the child is followed until at least the age of two years. If the hydrocele has not then disappeared, surgery is recommended. The surgical correction of a hydrocele consists in excising the hydrocele sac, leaving a 2 to 3-mm cuff of tunica surrounding the testicle proper. The operation is performed using the same incision and approach as for an inguinal hernia. In addition to excising the major portion of the hydrocele, the cord structures are inspected for an associated hernia, which if present is repaired.

Communicating hydroceles and hydroceles of the cord are treated as though they were inguinal hernias, that is, surgery is recommended as in the case of hernia. Hernia and hydrocele of canal of Nuck in the female are treated the same as hernia or cord hydroceles in the male (188, 190). The sac, in the female, is closely adherent to the round ligament from which it must be dissected. If this is not feasible, the round ligament may be divided with the sac. The ovary may present in an inguinal hernia in the female, thus making it in essence a sliding hernia with one portion of the sac consisting of the ovary and its blood supply. Surgical correction requires removing the hernia sac while preserving the ovary and its blood supply. This can be accomplished by opening the hernia sac opposite the side containing the ovary and then incising the sac on each side parallel to the ovary and its vessels. This flap is then tucked back into the abdominal cavity. A purse-string suture is then placed through the hernia sac and just through the outermost tissue of that segment of the wall of the sac containing the ovary and its vessels. The remainder of the repair is as has been described for male infants.

Postoperatively these infants are fed as soon as they have recovered from anesthesia. In general, they react as though no surgery had been performed. The plastic strips holding the skin edges together are removed after five to seven days. Until that time, we advise omitting immersion baths, preferring that the wound sites be kept dry. No other special instructions are required. The results of repair of inguinal hernia or hydrocele, or both, are excellent. Rarely there may be a recurrence. In general, these are not recurrences (hernia or hydrocele) but persistence of the defect due to the inadequate removal of the hydrocele or to a failure to resect the hernia sac at a high enough level. An adequate removal of hernia sac is indicated by retraction of the closed end of the sac beneath the internal oblique muscle after cutting the sutures closing the neck of the sac. The incidence of "recurrent" hernias should be less than 1% when the repair has been properly performed. Occasionally wound infection may occur and this is associated with the likelihood of a true recurrence of the hernia. Infection is usually due to poor technique in preparing the operative area. This type of surgery is clean in nature and wound infection should be rare.

A rare but serious complication of surgery for correction of hydrocele or hernia is atrophy of the testicle due to vascular injury to the blood vessels in the cord caused by poor surgical technique. Similarly, injuries to the vas deferens should not occur except when the operation has been carelessly performed.

UMBILICAL HERNIA

These are common in infants, rarely become incarcerated or strangulated and often resolve spontaneously within the first few years of life (194). It is not our policy to recommend surgery for umbilical hernia during the neonatal period.

OMPHALOCELE

This condition is a herniation of abdominal viscera into the umbilical stalk with normally located umbilical arteries and vein inserted into the sac. The extraabdominal viscera are covered only by peritoneum and the amniotic membrane. These coverings may be intact with viscera visible through them, or they may be ruptured with evisceration of abdominal contents. This defect in the abdominal wall may be explained by considering the embryology of the intestinal tract and the abdominal cavity (202). From the sixth to eighth week of gestation, the intestinal tract grows and elongates so rapidly that the developing abdominal cavity is too small to accommodate the viscera, and as a result these enter the umbilical stalk. From the eighth to tenth week of intrauterine life, the abdominal cavity enlarges and the intestines return to it. Failure of the abdominal cavity to enlarge sufficiently or, failure of the intestines to return to the abdominal cavity may lead to omphalocele. It is claimed that malrotation is a common concomitant of omphalocele, since the intestines never return to the abdominal cavity. However, the usual obstructive signs associated with malrotation are rarely encountered since it is not the malrotation per se but rather the abnormal posterior parietal peritoneal and mesenteric attachments that produce the symptoms attributed to malrotation.

Diagnosis is readily made by inspection. The thin membranous cover over the abdominal viscera can be clearly seen. If the membranes have ruptured, abdominal viscera will be seen extruding from the abdominal wall defect. Immediate surgical intervention is necessary, especially if the membranes are ruptured. While making preparations for operation, the omphalocele should be covered with warm, sterile saline packs. A cut-down should be performed and the child typed and cross-matched for blood replacement. Blood gases and serum electrolytes should also be determined and appropriate steps taken to correct metabolic aberrations that may be present.

The surgical procedure depends on the size of the omphalocele in relation to the size of the child, on whether membranes are intact or ruptured and on the presence of serious anomalies of other systems (201).

Correction and Repair

Primary Correction. This is usually employed in infants with an omphalocele small enough to be replaced into the abdominal cavity and the abdominal wall defect closed completely at one operation. In these cases, the umbilical vessels are suture-ligated proximally within the peritoneal cavity, and the distal segments are removed with or

without the amniotic membrane. The peritoneum is closed separately, and the abdominal wall is then reapproximated in layers. Obviously, these infants will lack an umbilicus after healing of the incision (Fig. 23–40).

Staged Correction. In infants with an omphalocele too large to replace into the abdomen, a primary repair is impossible. In these patients, skin and subcutaneous tissue flaps are elevated laterally and inferiorly from the infant's abdominal wall and then approximated in the midline. These babies are left after surgery with a large ventral hernia that can be repaired to restore the integrity of the abdominal wall at a later date. Very large omphaloceles may be man-

FIG. 23–40. Small omphalocele. **A.** Preoperative; **B.** following primary correction.

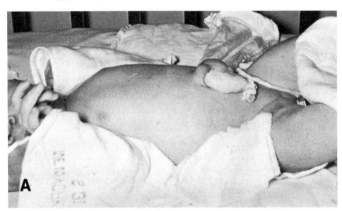

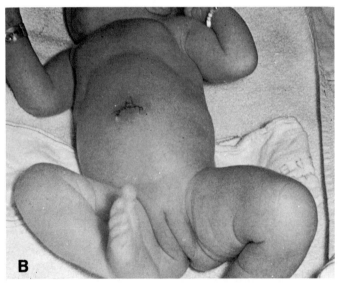

aged in this fashion. When large flaps are required, the skin near the central area of approximation may appear blue or pale, suggesting some degree of vascular embarrassment as a result of elevation of the flaps. Although there may be loss of some of this skin, local treatment consisting of the application of warm saline soaks is usually adequate to tide the infant over until the flap defects heal.

Correction Using Prosthetic Materials. Many surgeons have abandoned the use of skin and subcutaneous tissue flaps to cover large omphaloceles that cannot be repaired primarily. Instead, plastic bags consisting of Silastic reinforced with Dacron may be sutured around the margins of the omphalocele, placing the sutures through all layers of the abdominal wall at the rim of the omphalocele defect (196, 200, 205). Thus, the omphalocele becomes encased in a prosthetic pouch (Fig. 23–41). The upper end of the bag is sutured closed or a heavy ligature is applied. Antibiotic ointment or gauze pads soaked in antibiotic solution are placed over the bag. The apex of the bag may be compressed 24 to 48 hours after its application, replacing some of the viscera into the abdominal cavity. The portion of the plastic sac that has been compressed is tied. Progressing in this fashion, over a period of 7 to 14 days (depending on the size of the omphalocele), the contents of the omphalocele can be reduced into the abdominal cavity. The remaining portion of the plastic pouch can then be removed and the residual abdominal wall defect closed. In essence, this is a staged technique of omphalocele correction utilizing a prosthetic bag rather than skin and subcutaneous tissue flaps to accomplish the original covering of the omphalocele. The technique is well suited to the management of those infants with omphalocele with ruptured membranes. Unlike the traditional staged correction technique, complete repair can be accomplished in a shorter period of time, and the infant is not left with a ventral hernia that may exist for months or years until the second stage of the correction is completed.

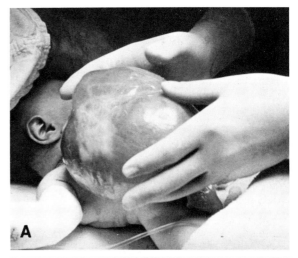

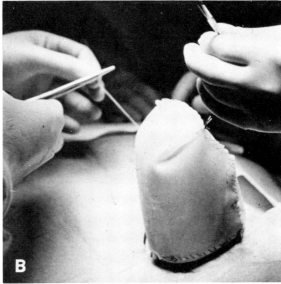

FIG. 23–41. Large omphalocele in small infant. **A.** Size of omphalocele in relation to child. **B.** Completion of encasement of the same omphalocele in prosthetic pouch.

Nonoperative Treatment. Although most omphaloceles can be treated successfully employing one of the methods described above, surgery is contraindicated for some infants in critical condition as a result of prematurity or serious anomalies of other systems. In such instances, the omphalocele can be managed using a 2% mercurochrome solution. This should be applied over the entire omphalocele sac hourly for two to three applications and then every 8 hours for the next 24 hours. This will lead

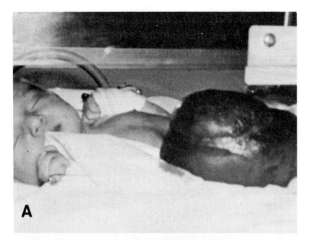

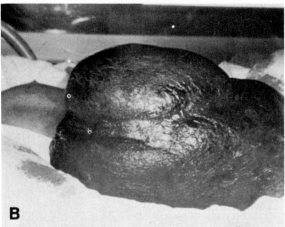

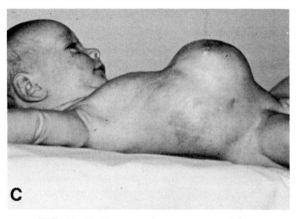

FIG. 23–42. Nonoperative treatment of larger omphalocele. **A.** Omphalocele after two applications of 2% mercurochrome. **B.** Close-up of omphalocele with beginning eschar. **C.** Appearance after complete epithelialization of omphalocele following treatment with 2% mercurochrome.

to the formation of a thick eschar over the omphalocele. Following this, epithelialization will progress from the skin at the margins of the omphalocele beneath the eschar, elevating the contiguous portion of the eschar (Fig. 23–42). The eschar should not be debrided, and care must be taken that the thick crust remains intact, but this is not a problem since after proper application of the mercurochrome solution, the resultant crust is tough and leathery. The time necessary for complete reepithelialization beneath the eschar depends largely on the size of the omphalocele (Fig. 23–43). Usually it takes from several weeks to months before this is completed. Once the defect has been epithelialized, the infant will resemble one who has had skin and subcutaneous tissue cover of the omphalocele as in the first stage of the staged technique for correction. The second stage or complete repair is per-

FIG. 23–43. Massive omphalocele. Because of associated serious cardiovascular anomalies, management with 2% mercurochrome was planned. Infant died immediately after birth before treatment could be started.

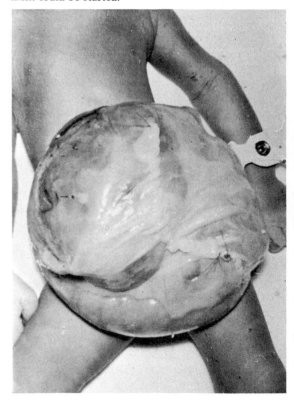

formed using the guidelines discussed in regard to the staged method of treatment.

A word of caution must be introduced in respect to the use of mercurochrome in these infants. If it is applied too liberally, the infant may develop signs of mercury poisoning. However, used judiciously the mercurochrome method of management has been satisfactory.

Results of Treatment

The ultimate outcome in these cases generally depends on the size of the omphalocele and the presence or absence of other congenital anomalies. Those with small omphaloceles who can have primary complete correction should have a universally good result unless there are other serious anomalies such as cardiac or GU defects. Those with large omphaloceles that, prior to use of plastic bag treatment, underwent the staged method of correction had a survival rate of about 70%, if there were no other serious anomalies. With the prosthetic bag, survival rates in infants without other serious anomalies has increased to 80%. Those treated initially with mercurochrome usually were very ill or had massive omphaloceles. In these, survival rates were about 60%.

The overall survival rate including all infants with omphalocele, prematures, those with other system anomalies and large omphaloceles in most series is about 60%. Mortality rates are much higher in infants with omphaloceles with ruptured membranes than in those with intact membranes (197, 204, 206).

GASTROSCHISIS

This is a congenital anomaly of the abdominal wall resembling an omphalocele with ruptured membranes (199, 203). However, it is a paraumbilical defect with prenatal evisceration of abdominal viscera. The umbilicus and umbilical cord are situated in normal position, and there are no covering membranes. Thus, it differs from an omphalocele and can be differentiated readily. The protruding viscera are edematous, and there is marked shortening and coiling of the small intestine and its mesentery.

Treatment is essentially that as described for omphalocele. In most instances, however, primary repair is not feasible, and either the staged method or the use of a plastic pouch may be necessary (198).

Results in our experience have been comparable to those for infants with omphalocele. With either defect, if the neonate can be treated successfully shortly after birth, the long-term follow up has generally revealed no subsequent GI problems.

APPENDICITIS

Appendicitis, while rare in the neonatal period (207), nonetheless poses a difficult diagnostic problem because of the nonspecificity of presenting signs. These include vomiting, fever, irritability, anorexia and occasionally diarrhea. The incidence of perforation is high, and significant morbidity and mortality is observed.

On physical examination, abdominal distension, tenderness and absence of bowel sounds are noted. The white blood count may be low, normal or elevated in this condition and is of little diagnostic value. The abdominal x ray reveals that ileus and free fluid are sometimes present. Definitive diagnosis is made only by laparotomy. Supportive medical treatment is the same as that for the infant with a perforated viscus or gangrenous bowel.

NEOPLASMS

Tumors encountered in the neonatal period include such minor lesions as epidermoid or dermoid cysts of the eyebrow and more serious ones such as retroperitoneal or sacrococcygeal teratoma, Wilms' tumor and neuroblastoma. These may be apparent on the surface (e.g., epidermoid or dermoid cyst of eyebrow and sacrococcygeal teratoma) or may be detected as an abdominal mass (e.g., retroperitoneal teratoma, Wilms' tumor and neuroblastoma).

SURFACE MASSES

Epidermoid or Dermoid Cyst of Eyebrow

This presents as a small, ovoid, relatively firm, slightly movable cystic mass usually near the lateral margin of and superior to the eyebrow. Diagnosis is made readily by physical examination. Treatment is surgical excision and can be easily accomplished. Operation, however, is not usually performed in the neonatal period but sometime after four to six months of age. An excellent result with no cosmetic deformity may be anticipated if the incision is placed properly at the time of excision.

ABDOMINAL MASSES

Retroperitoneal Teratomas

These are large tumors composed of tissue derived from all three primitive germ layers: 1) ectoderm, 2) endoderm and 3) mesoderm and usually consisting of solid and cystic elements (209, 210). In one series (208), histologic evidence of malignancy occurred in 6.8% of the cases. Most patients are found to have abdominal enlargement at birth or early in infancy. Flat films of the abdomen reveal a soft tissue density, often with calcification, filling a large segment of the cavity. Intravenous pyelograms demonstrate lateral displacement of ureters and some degree of hydronephrosis. Treatment consists of excision; this may be difficult because of adhesions between the tumor and major blood vessels or abdominal viscera. Therefore, complete removal may not be possible. The operative mortality recorded in Arnheim's series was 29% (208).

Sacrococcygeal Teratomas

These are relatively uncommon tumors that occur in about 1:40,000 births and present over the sacrococcygeal area as a rounded or lobulated mass, which may be cystic, solid or both (211–214). They vary in size from a few centimeters in diameter to an enormous bulk. The tumor may be attached to the coccyx by a stalk or may extend presacrally into the retroperitoneal region and be palpable on rectal examination. As in all teratomas, tissue is derived from all three primitive germ layers. Although some may undergo malignant degeneration, the majority are benign. Lateral and anteroposterior roentgenograms may reveal calcification, bone or teeth in the tumor as well as ventral displacement of the bowel if there is significant presacral and retroperitoneal extension. Intravenous pyelography may reveal ureteral displacement or obstruction with some hydronephrosis. Treatment is surgical. With the patient in a prone position and the legs abducted, a modified, inverted V-shaped incision is made over the mass. Skin and subcutaneous tissue flaps are developed. The sacrum is divided between the fourth and fifth segments, and presacral extension is dissected carefully from the peritoneum. The ventral aspect of the tumor is freed from the rectum by sharp dissection. After adequate hemostasis has been obtained, redundant skin is excised, and the wound is closed over one or more penrose drains. Postoperatively, the patient is maintained in the prone position until the sutures are removed. The drains are left in place for 48 hours or longer if indicated.

Since the operation is long and extensive, the usual precautions of having an IV cutdown in place and blood on call for replacement must be observed. In general, the results are good following surgery except when the tumor is initially malignant or a malignant recurrence develops. Operative mortality has been low in most series.

Wilms' Tumor (Nephroblastoma)

This is a rare neoplasm in the neonate that presents as an abdominal or flank mass. Urinalysis may reveal microscopic hematuria. Plain films of the abdomen reveal a soft tissue density displacing bowel. Intravenous pyelograms show compression, elongation and distortion of the pelvis or the calyces of the involved kidney. Unlike neuroblastoma there is no suggestion of calcification in the mass. The tumor may be confined by the capsule of the kidney, or it may extend through the capsule into any of the adjacent viscera or tissues, including the inferior vena cava. Metastases may result from lymphogenous or hematogenous spread. Secondary lung and liver involvement is not uncommon, but bone metastases are rare. Infants with hemihypertrophy are prone to develop Wilms' tumor on the affected or unaffected side and should be followed with periodic IVPs. Although bilateral Wilms' tumors are reported to occur in 5% of cases, none have been recorded in the neonatal period.

The treatment of Wilms' tumor is prompt surgical resection (220, 222, 223). A midline or bilateral transverse incision should be employed so that after removal of the involved kidney, the contralateral organ may be inspected, palpated and biopsied if necessary. The renal pedicle is usually dissected and ligated prior to mobilization of the kidney in order to minimize hematogenous spread of the tumor. In many instances, the bulk or extension of the tumor may make this impossible and it may be necessary to free up the kidney mass and local extensions before the renal pedicle can be safely ligated.

The author's regimen has been to limit preoperative abdominal palpation in children suspected of having Wilms' tumor, to give Actinomycin D immediately preoperatively and to institute radiotherapy as soon as the patient is released from the recovery room (217–219). In newborn infants, however, routine use of chemotherapy and radiotherapy is probably not warranted due to the less malignant behavior of this tumor in this age group. It has been recognized that nephroblastoma in the young infant has a better prognosis than in the older child (221). Some authors consider congenital nephroblastoma pathologically distinct from the true Wilms' tumor of childhood in that they are composed primarily of fibroblastic tissue and malignant epithelial elements are missing (215). Because of this, survival is excellent following nephrectomy alone. Thus, if the tumor, after complete surgical removal, reveals a predominantly mesoblastic structure on histologic examination, radiotherapy and chemotherapy are not required. In cases where the tumor has extended into adjacent structures, paraaortic lymph nodes, capsular blood vessels, lymphatics or renal vein, or when the tumor is poorly differentiated histologically, these additional modalities should be used.

From the recorded experience (no one institution has enough cases to provide valid statistics) the survival rate for children under one year of age is about 42% as compared with 18% for older children. Employing the rule of Collins (216), a newborn infant with congenital Wilms' tumor may be considered cured if he is free of disease at the time he is slightly over nine months of age.

Neuroblastoma

This is a malignant neoplasm arising from the adrenal medulla or ganglia of the sympathetic nervous system and occurring in any part of the body (224, 229). In the newborn infant, as in all age groups, the adrenal gland is the most frequent site of origin (almost 50%). Approximately 90% of neuroblastomas will be within the abdomen, 9% in the thorax and 1% in the cervical region. The tumor tends to be large and nodular and invades adjacent structures. Histologically it may be composed of undifferentiated small round cells, or these may be arranged in pseudorosettes. Unlike in older children, bony metastases are uncommon in the newborn infant, being reported (232) in 3.2% of cases. In the neonate, metastases to liver and subcutaneous tissues are far more common, the latter type being unique to this age group.

The actual incidence of neuroblastoma in the neonate may be very much higher than is clinically apparent. Wells (236) found four small in situ neuroblastomas in 3000 autopsies on fetuses and newborn infants. Others have reported similar findings (225, 231). Since the overall incidence of neuroblastoma in situ in newborn infants is about 60 times that of childhood neuroblastoma, the vast majority of these tumors must either undergo degeneration or be transformed into more mature, nonmalignant cell types.

Voûte et al. (235) have described such symptoms as sweating, pallor, headaches, palpitation and occasionally hypertension during the last weeks of pregnancy in mothers of fetuses with neuroblastomas. Measurements of urinary catecholamine levels in pregnant women with these symptoms may permit the diagnosis of fetal neuroblastoma. The placenta may be a metastatic site of neuroblastoma, but dissemination to the mother has not occurred.

Physical findings are obviously dependent on the location and extent of the disease. The intraabdominal type presents as a large mass that deep to palpation and may fill either side of the abdomen or flank or extend across the midline. The liver may be enlarged and hard. Subcutaneous nodules may be apparent over the trunk or extremities. The persistent blanching of these nodules that has been noted by Hawthorne (228) may be due to local vasoconstriction secondary to catecholamine release by tumor cells.

Plain roentgenograms of the abdomen show a posterior and laterally placed soft tissue mass with calcific specks. Intravenous pyelography reveals the kidney on the involved side to be displaced downward and laterally with compression of the renal pelvis if the tumor originates in the adrenal. Tumors arising from the sympathetic chain may produce lateral displacement of the kidney or ureter. Although bony metastases are not common in the neonatal period, a bone survey should be performed in all cases.

Diagnosis may be established from the physical and radiographic findings, however, bone marrow biopsy is done in all cases. Determinations of urinary catecholamine excretion, especially vanilmandelic acid (VMA), are important aids in diagnosis (234, 237, 238). The VMA test is extremely sensitive and may be used postoperatively as a prognostic sign. The VMA level should fall to normal within 10 to 100 days postoperatively. An increase in VMA excretion may be the first indication of metastasis or recurrence.

The ideal treatment is complete surgical removal. Where this becomes impossible because of local invasion of vital structures, as much of the tumor should be excised as is feasible; these are usually highly vascularized tumors, and there may be significant blood loss. If it appears that a direct attack on the tumor is not possible, a biopsy should be obtained to establish the diagnosis conclusively. In these latter two instances radiotherapy and chemotherapy are usually employed. Although concepts of chemotherapy undergo frequent change, in our institution, the present policy is to employ a combination of vincristine and cyclophosphamide with adriamycin or daunomycin. The first course of therapy extends over 7 to 10 days with subsequent repetition of the medications at 6 weeks, 3, 6, 9, 12 and 15 months. During the course of chemotherapy the blood count is followed closely including platelet determinations and the regimen altered should the white cell count fall below 1500/mm³ or platelets below 100,000/mm³. Side effects of these agents include alopecia, GI disturbances, ulceration of the mouth, muscular paralyses, depression of bone marrow and hematuria.

The prognosis of neuroblastoma in children is related to the extent of the disease at the time of its discovery. Staging for children with neuroblastoma has been proposed by Evans et al (226):

Stage I: Tumors confined to the organ or structure of origin

Stage II: Tumors extending in continuity beyond the organ or structure of origin but not crossing the midline. Regional lymph nodes on the homolateral side may be involved.

Stage III: Tumors extending in continuity beyond the midline. Regional lymph nodes may be involved bilaterally.

Stage IV: Remote disease involving skeleton, organs, soft tissues or distant lymph node groups (see IV-S)

Stage IV-S: Patients who would otherwise be Stage I or II, but who have remote disease confined only to one or more of the following sites: liver, skin or bone marrow (without radiographic evidence of bone metastases on complete skeletal survey) Because of the favorable prognosis in young infants with neuroblastoma some authors, including Thurman and Donaldson (233), question the validity of staging in this age group and exclude them from analysis.

The results of treatment of neuroblastoma in the neonatal period have been reviewed carefully by Schneider et al (230) in a collected series of 60 cases reported in the literature up to 1965. Twenty-nine had died, eight lost to follow-up and twenty-three were alive. This was a survival rate of 38.3% of all neonates with neuroblastoma, including stillborns, those untreated and those who died of other causes. Of 37 infants who had either biopsy alone or some therapy directed at the tumor, 23 survived, a survival rate of 62.2%. Ten of 31 neonates with metastases were long-term survivors (32.3%); 35% with liver metastases and 40% with subcutaneous metastases were alive and well. In general, the prognosis of neuroblastoma is better in the newborn infant than in the older child. Some of the tumors may mature to ganglioneuroma or there may be spontaneous disappearance of the neuroblastoma as reported by Gross (227). An aggressive attitude toward treatment is necessary in the neonate with this tumor even when it cannot be removed completely surgically or when there are metastases. Radiotherapy or chemotherapy should be employed with the hope that if the child can be maintained, the tumor may regress or mature to a more benign form.

MASSES OF GENITOURINARY ORIGIN

In addition to the neoplasms already discussed, any organ system can give rise to abdominal masses in the newborn infant (239–243). The most common are those of the GU tract.

Hydronephrosis

This usually is caused by ureteropelvic or ureterovesical obstruction due to stenosis, atresia, aberrant blood vessels or ureterocele. Palpation reveals a smooth, rounded mass. Intravenous pyelography may reveal nonfunction or delayed function with marked dilatation of the collecting system. Treatment consists of nephrectomy in cases of unilateral involvement and obvious lack of significant kidney parencyhma. In cases with bilateral disease, nephrostomy has been utilized in the neonate with definitive correction of the underlying defect at a subsequent time.

Multicystic Kidneys

Multicystic kidneys are common in the neonate; they may be bilateral but are more often unilateral (244, 248). There is usually atresia of the ureteropelvic junction and a deficiency of normal renal tissue on histologic examination. The mass is felt more anteriorly and tends to be lobulated in contrast to the smooth, rounded mass associated with hydronephrosis. There is usually only a thin shell of kidney tissue surrounding the cysts. Intravenous pyelography shows nonfunction on the affected side. Treatment is nephrectomy. This type of renal involvement differs from *polycystic kidney* (245–247), in which bilateral involvement is the rule. In the latter, the cysts are usually small and scattered throughout more normal renal tissue. Bilateral renal masses are palpable. Intravenous pyelograms reveal enlarged kidneys, a spongelike nephrogram effect, especially on delayed films, and poor delineation of the calyceal system. Retrograde pyelograms reveal elongated calyces. Unfortunately, there is no treatment available for these infants, who usually die in the neonatal period or shorly thereafter of renal failure.

MASSES OF GASTROINTESTINAL ORIGIN

These may arise from any segment of the GI tract and may be discovered as asymptomatic masses or may produce varying degrees of intestinal obstruction.

Mesenteric Cyst (Cystic Hygroma of the Mesentery)

These present as prominent, usually ballottable anterior masses that appear as soft tissue shadows displacing or crowding bowel on plain films of the abdomen. They may be unilocular or consist of small and large cysts with some elements of solid tissue. The cysts often contain chylous fluid and may contain serous or serosanguinous fluid. They may cause signs of partial intestinal obstruction or of acute distress if they should rupture. Mesenteric cysts are generally found in the small bowel mesentery, but they also occur in the mesentery of the large bowel and in the omentum. Treatment is surgical excision. If the cyst extends through only a short segment of the mesentery, resection with the adjacent bowel may be preferred. In other cases, especially if the lesion is extensive, the cyst may be dissected from the leaves of the mesentery, the surgeon being careful not to injure neighboring blood vessels; partial resection of the mass may be necessary if complete removal is not feasible.

Duplications

These have been discussed in the section Intestinal Obstruction.

Midgut Volvulus

This may arise in association with malrotation of the colon. The neonate usually presents with an abdominal mass and signs of intestinal obstruction. Plain films of the abdomen reveal a ground-glass density often with calcific deposits filling most of the abdomen. In those instances where the volvulus occurred early in gestation, most of the midgut will have undergone infarction and calcification. These infants have a poor prognosis since at surgery it will be necessary to resect all of the involved gut, leaving insufficient bowel for survival. Although IV hyperalimentation may aid in the immediate postoperative period, in most cases the remaining small intestine is insufficient to sustain life.

MASSES OF LIVER AND BILIARY TRACT ORIGIN

Hepatic Cysts

These may be large masses palpable in continuity with the liver edge or may be diagnosed with liver scan or sonographic techniques. Surgical excision is the treatment of choice, although simple drainage of the cyst with subsequent removal at a second operation may be necessary when the size of the cyst or general condition of the baby contraindicates a one-stage procedure.

Hepatic Tumors

These include hemangioma, lymphangioma, fibroma, adenoma, hamartoma, hemangioblastoma and hepatoma. Liver scan and sonography help to establish the location of such masses in the liver. Surgical excision is the procedure of choice if they are situated in an area that makes this feasible. Except in infants with an outright malignancy, the outlook following surgical removal is excellent.

Choledochal Cysts

These are rare cystic masses arising from the distal part of the common bile duct as a result of obstruction of the terminal portion of the duct. They may be large and may present as a mass in the right upper quadrant. There may be evidence of abdominal pain or discomfort and jaundice. Treatment consists of internal drainage, anastomosing the cyst to the duodenum or to the jejunum in Roux-Y fashion.

MASSES OF GENITAL TRACT ORIGIN IN THE FEMALE

Ovarian Cysts

These may occur in the neonatal period and because of their size may present as an abdominal mass, usually unilateral. The mass is often somewhat movable on palpation extending downward toward the pelvis. Plain films of the abdomen may reveal a ground-glass density. In rare instances calcific specks may be seen, suggesting a teratoma. The mass is generally asymptomatic, but should it undergo torsion with subsequent necrosis, infarction or both, the infant may be in acute distress. Treatment is surgical excision. At operation, the opposite ovary is inspected and palpated routinely. The prognosis following excision of this usually benign mass is excellent.

Hydrometrocolpos

This condition, secondary to an imperforate hymen, is most commonly encountered in older female children after the onset of menarche. However, in some neonates with imperforate hymen, the vagina may become markedly distended with secretions as a result of stimulation by maternal estrogens. In these cases, a lower midline mass may be noted on examination. If the hymen is imperforate and bulging, the diagnosis is established. Treatment consists of incision of the hymen and drainage of the retained vaginal secretions. It has been our practice to keep a small drain through the area of incision for ten days to two weeks to prevent resealing of the hymen. The prognosis is excellent. This condition must be suspected when there is a lower abdominal mass in a female neonate. If the abdominal mass is excised because this diagnosis has not been considered, the child will have had her uterus removed.

The prognosis for neonates with benign abdominal masses of the GI tract, hepatic or biliary tract or genital tract in the female, is excellent. Those babies with unilateral multicystic disease of the kidney similarly have a good outlook for the future since the contralateral kidney is usually normal. Infants with hydronephrosis usually can be managed by nephrostomy, salvaging the kidneys and performing definitive procedures after the child has grown. Prompt diagnosis, laparotomy and surgical excision of these masses should be carried out regardless of the size or gestational age of the baby.

GENITOURINARY TRACT PROBLEMS

Urinary tract disorders in the neonate are manifested by the presence of unilateral or bilateral abdominal mass or by anemia, acidemia and signs of infection. The problems usually encountered are those associated with obstructive uropathy (e.g., urethral valves, tight meatal stenosis, ureterovesical or ureteropelvic strictures and bladder neck obstruction), congenital multicystic or polycystic disease, agenesis or hypoplasia of the kidneys, nephroblastoma, deficiency of abdominal wall musculature (prune belly syndrome) and exstrophy of the bladder.

POSTERIOR URETHRAL VALVES

These are exaggerated mucosal folds that cause resistance to the flow of urine from the bladder and are found almost exclusively in males (249, 252, 254). Depending on the degree of obstruction, the infant may exhibit only mild trabeculation of the bladder or a severely damaged urinary tract that may be incompatible with life. In the neonatal period, the most common clinical findings are a suprapubic mass, failure to thrive and urinary tract infection. Diagnosis can be established by IVPs and cystourethrography, which usually reveal dilated posterior urethra, trabeculated and enlarged bladder and varying degrees of hydronephrosis and hydroureter. Most patients have decreased renal function. In a series of 28 cases (253), 8 became symptomatic during the first month of life and 16 during the first year of life. Since that report, 8 neonates have been encountered with urinary retention.

Successful treatment is based on prompt relief of the obstruction and drainage of urine. Waterhouse has achieved success in resecting the valves during the neonatal period by the transurethral route (255). If the infant is critically ill, if there is obstruction of the upper tract or if the ureters are severely dilated, nephrostomy and renal biopsy should be performed, with resection of the valves delayed for several weeks or months. However, most surgeons will only perform a nephrostomy during the neonatal period, postponing definitive surgery until the child is older. Following nephrostomy, good delineation of the urinary tracts can be obtained by pyelography through the nephrostomy tubes.

Serious secondary obstructive problems requiring further surgical procedures, such as straightening or resection of redundant portions of ureters with reimplantation into the bladder, may be observed in these infants (250).

Prognosis in these infants is largely dependent on the degree of urinary tract destruction related to secondary obstructive conditions. In those patients with minimal secondary change, resection of the obstructing valves will effect a cure. Those with secondary obstruction and reflux may require multiple surgical procedures, and the ultimate outcome will depend on the amount of functioning renal tissue that remains. In Waldbaum and Marshall's cases (253), one-third were cured by resection of the obstructing valves; one-third had good to fair renal function following resection of the valves, Y-V plasty of the bladder neck and reimplantation of ureters; the remaining one-third continued to have poor function despite nephrostomy drainage, and in some of these, renal transplantation may be necessary in order to sustain life. Obviously, the more extensive surgical procedures mentioned above are performed not in the neonatal period but are applicable to those patients who have been managed successfully into childhood.

URETEROPELVIC OBSTRUCTION

This problem with or without associated ureterovesical or bladder neck obstruction is encountered infrequently in the neonatal period. In a series of 192 patients operated on at the New York Hospital–Cornell Medical Center for ureteropelvic obstruction over the years 1950–1965, only 8 presented in the neonatal period. Six of these had primary ureteropelvic obstruction, while in the other two, there was also ureterovesical and

bladder neck obstruction. Five of the eight patients had bilateral involvement. In four cases, the condition was manifested by the presence of an abdominal mass.

Urinalysis may reveal pyuria, hematuria or casts, or it may be within normal limits. Diagnosis is established by IVP, which reveals hydronephrosis. Cystography may indicate reflux into one or both ureters.

Treatment includes nephrostomy initially, followed later by definitive correction of the obstruction, usually by the Y-V pyeloplasty. In those patients with ureterovesical and bladder neck obstruction in addition to the ureteropelvic obstruction, reconstructive procedures at the bladder neck or reimplantation of the ureters into the bladder may be required. Early recognition of the problem with appropriate staged management should yield a favorable prognosis.

CYSTIC DISEASE OF THE KIDNEYS

This has been discussed in the section Abdominal Masses.

CONGENITAL DEFICIENCY OF THE ABDOMINAL WALL MUSCULATURE (Prune Belly Syndrome)

This entity can be readily identified by physical examination (252–255). The deficiency in the musculature of the abdominal wall is manifested by a thin abdomen through which intestinal activity may be observed. The entire abdominal wall may be affected or the deficiency may be limited to one quadrant. The skin is redundant and wrinkled, thus giving rise to the descriptive sobriquet, prune belly. Serious obstructive urinary tract anomalies associated with this condition are responsible for its life-threatening nature. The muscular deficiency may impair respiration. Additional anomalies may include cryptorchism, GI tract deformities, thoracic cage defects such as pigeon breast or pectus excavatum and limb defects such as talipes, congenital dislocations and amputations.

The characteristic urinary tract findings are hydronephrosis; dysplastic or hypoplastic kidneys; severe dilatation and elongation of ureters; large, thick-walled bladder, often with a patent urachus; and a wide bladder outlet with a dilated prostatic urethra.

Diagnosis of the urinary tract anomalies is made best by cystography. Since reflux is usual, the status of the ureters and kidney pelves will be discernible in most cases. Intravenous pyelography may be of help, but since kidney function is often poor, delayed films several hours after initiating the study may be necessary to obtain any information.

Treatment depends on the degree of uropathy (260). In most instances, nephrostomy is done initially on each side. When maximal recovery of renal function has been achieved, straightening of the ureters and reimplantation into the bladder and cystostomy are performed.

Several weeks later pyeloureterography is done through the nephrostomy tubes, and these are removed at separate times if the situation warrants. The cystostomy tube is left in place for six or more months, and the patient is reevaluated at that time. Any evidence of bladder outlet obstruction is corrected by Y-V plasty before removal of the cystostomy tube. These patients must be followed closely and treated for any signs of urinary tract infection. Prognosis is dependent on the degree of urinary tract involvement. Some die shortly after birth because of extensive damage, hypoplasia or dysplasia of the kidneys. Those with salvageable urinary tracts, are greatly benefited by prompt diagnostic evaluation and corrective surgery.

EXSTROPHY OF THE BLADDER

This is a condition in which the entire bladder including the urethra down to the external meatus lies open and everted. The umbilicus is represented by fibrous tissue at the apex of the bladder. The skin and muscular wall of the central portion of the infraumbilical area is absent and replaced by the everted bladder. Ureteral orifices and trigone can be seen in the inferior aspect of the bladder folds. In the male, there is com-

plete epispadius with a short, upturned penis, the crura of which are widely apart on the ischiopubic rami. There may be unilateral or bilateral cryptorchism. In the female, the clitoris is bifid and the vaginal orifice can be seen below the ectopic bladder. This anomaly is three times more common in males than females with an estimated incidence of from 1:10,000 to 1:30,000 births.

Diagnosis is made by physical examination. At birth the upper urinary tract and kidneys are usually normal. However, exposure of the bladder mucosa and consequent edema may result in bacterial invasion, thickening squamous metaplasia and fibrosis. This in turn may lead to obstruction at the ureteral orifices causing hydroureter and hydronephrosis. Accompanying this anomaly, there is a wide separation of the rectus muscles below the umbilicus and a complete separation of the pubic bones (Fig. 23–44). The acetabula and femoral heads are rotated externally.

Definitive treatment (263, 265–267) of exstrophy of the bladder consists of: 1) urinary diversion by means of an ileal conduit together with closure of the defect of the abdominal wall or 2) functional reconstruction of the bladder, urethra and penis. In either case, it has been advocated that surgery be delayed until the infant is six or more months of age. However, many surgeons think that functional reconstruction of the bladder should be attempted in the neonatal period while the bladder is still soft and pliable and the surrounding skin free of infection and excoriation. The significant amount of blood lost when this is carried out has prompted some surgeons to propose simple turn-in or closure of the bladder and the abdominal wall defect with bilateral nephrostomy as a first step. Secondary procedures on the bladder and urethra may then be performed at a later date.

There are several techniques for achieving functional reconstruction of the bladder. Essentially, however, the operation consists of bilateral nephrostomy followed by separation of the bladder from the muscles of the abdominal wall and mobilization of

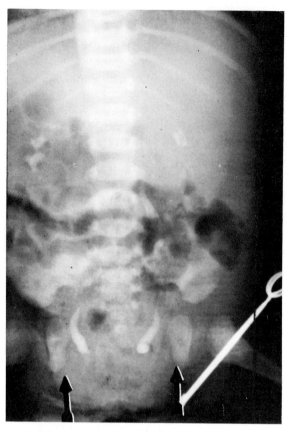

FIG. 23–44. Anteroposterior roentgenogram of abdomen showing complete separation of pubic bones (arrows) associated with exstrophy of the bladder in the neonate. Upper urinary tracts and kidneys are normal.

the urethra. The bladder is then inverted and the epispadius repaired. A cystostomy tube is placed in the bladder. The corpora of the penis are brought together about the reconstructed penile urethra, and the abdominal wall defect is then closed. Marshall and Muecke (263) advocate reimplantation of the ureters into the bladder during the reconstruction. A variation of this procedure includes the performance of bilateral iliac osteotomy a week prior to the bladder reconstruction to permit better apposition of the pubic bones (261, 264). The results of functional reconstruction have been poor largely because of the small size of the reconstructed bladder and poor urinary control following reconstruction. Although

some of these problems may be related to the fact that most patients did not undergo surgery in the neonatal period, Johnston (262) states that only 2 of 14 children in his series who had had reconstruction of the bladder as neonates achieved urinary control. Despite this, an attempt at functional closure is considered to be justified in most cases, especially in those where the bladder is large. If urinary control does not develop, an ileal conduit can be established for urinary diversion.

NEUROSURGICAL PROBLEMS*

The more common neonatal lesions of the nervous system and surrounding structures requiring neurosurgical evaluation and treatment result from birth trauma and maldevelopment (268). The spectrum of neurosurgical problems observed in the neonatal period is, however, much broader. Although not discussed in this section per se, it must be recognized that neurologic deficit in the neonate may also result from prenatal or postnatal infection, trauma, neoplastic and vascular disease. Accurate diagnosis and, in the case of neurosurgical disease, preoperative evaluation may therefore require tests such as isotopic brain scan, ventriculography, pneumoencephalography, myelography and cerebral angiography. In well-equipped and well-staffed pediatric neurosurgical centers, these neurodiagnostic techniques do not carry an appreciably higher risk in the neonate than in the older child and should not be withheld if the situation warrants. By the same token, neurosurgery should not be delayed solely on the basis of age.

TRAUMA

Trauma to the nervous system, spine and skull can result from seemingly normal delivery but more often follows a difficult one. Special attention must be paid to the neuro-

* Prepared in association with Dr. Joseph H. Galicich.

logic status of the infant following either premature delivery or dystocia, particularly breech delivery. Injury to the scalp, skull and peripheral nerves is usually apparent on the initial examination. Other trauma, especially that producing intracranial bleeding, however, may not result in obvious deficit for hours or even weeks following delivery.

Cephalhematoma and Skull Fracture

Injury to the scalp may result in hemorrhage beneath the galea or periosteum. Because of the laxity of the scalp in neonates, subgaleal hematomas may be extremely large. Blood loss into this space is occasionally great enough to require transfusion. Surgical treatment is not indicated unless the blood supply of the scalp appears to be jeopardized as a result of stretching by the underlying hematoma. In such cases the scalp is tense and shiny and shows poor capillary filling after blanching. Under these circumstances, needle aspiration may be attempted, but if a considerable clot is present, operative incision and evacuation of blood may be required to prevent scalp necrosis.

Subperiosteal hemorrhage is usually more localized and of lesser magnitude than subgaleal hemorrhage. It is, however, more often associated with and can mask an underlying fracture (269, 270). Subperiosteal hematoma can very often be diagnosed by the fact that it is firm and does not cross suture lines. Unless associated with a depressed fracture, treatment is rarely indicated. Skull fractures in the neonate are often depressed and have much the same appearance as dents in a ping-pong ball. They are the result of application of forceps or digital pressure during delivery. The depression will not resolve spontaneously and should be elevated surgically. The operation is relatively minor and consists of making a small incision over the fracture, drilling a small burr hole to one side of the depression and inserting an elevator beneath the skull to the center of the fracture. Surgery usually can be carried out on an elective basis at several days of age. Simple linear fractures of the skull require no treatment.

Spinal Cord and Peripheral Nerve Injury

Spinal cord injury at birth is usually the result of a difficult extraction of the head and shoulders in breech presentation. The most frequent site of injury to the spinal cord is in the region of the lower cervical and upper thoracic spine. Trauma to the spinal cord results from the stretching produced by angulation and forcible distraction of the vertebras. Injury to the spine itself is primarily ligamentous, and fractures and dislocation of the vertebral column are rarely demonstrable by x ray. Diagnosis should be suspected if there is lack of spontaneous movement or obvious weakness of the lower extremities. When paraplegia is present, the lower extremities are usually flaccid, but the reflex withdrawal of the feet and legs in response to pinprick on the sole and the persistence of deep tendon reflexes below the lesion may be misleading. Breathing is often primarily or solely diaphragmatic. A sensory or sweat level may be demonstrable. Myelography is valuable in determining the site of the lesion and often necessary before surgery. Emergent surgical exploration, i.e., laminectomy, should be carried out if there is clear evidence of progressive spinal cord dysfunction. Such progression is indicative of an expanding hemorrhage within the spinal canal. A complete block of the subarachnoid space demonstrated by myelography is also an indication for surgery. Unfortunately, most neonates with paraplegia resulting from trauma have sustained irreparable damage to the spinal cord.

The most common peripheral nerve injuries observed in the neonatal period are those of the brachial plexus and the facial nerve. The brachial plexus injury is usually associated with either shoulder dystocia or a breech delivery. Injury (Erb's palsy) is almost always unilateral. It most frequently involves the upper portion of the brachial plexus subserving the musculature of the shoulder and arm and is easily diagnosed. X rays should be taken to ascertain the presence or absence of frequently associated fractures of the clavicle and humerus.

Treatment consists of proper splinting of the affected extremity and physical therapy. Unless the nerve roots have been avulsed from the spinal cord, prognosis for spontaneous recovery is good. Surgical intervention is rarely indicated and should only be considered after adequate time has elapsed for recovery from a stretch injury. Injury to the facial nerve resulting from trauma of obstetric forceps also carries an excellent prognosis for recovery. Unless a laceration of the skin over the nerve is present, surgery is not indicated since the injury is a result of pressure and not disruption of the nerve. Protection of the eye on the involved side must, however, be carried out until the nerve recovers sufficiently to permit voluntary closure of the eyelids.

Subdural Hemorrhage

Subdural hemorrhage, the only form of intracranial bleeding in the neonatal period that is amenable to neurosurgical therapy is discussed in the section Intracranial Bleeding, in Chapter 9. This condition, which usually occurs in full-term infants following traumatic delivery, has become a rarity because of modern obstetric practices.

The diagnosis is suspected when lethargy, irritability and convulsions accompany a bulging fontanelle and separation of sutures of the cranial bones. The diagnosis is made by subdural taps. Echoencephalography and cerebral angiography may be valuable aids in localizing the extent of the clot.

CONGENITAL DEFECTS

Malformations of the nervous system and its surrounding structures, the meninges, skull and spine, account for more than one-half of all congenital defects. Some, such as anencephaly, are lethal. Others, such as minor degrees of spina bifida, are extremely common but produce no deficit and require no treatment. Within the diverse group of malformations that affect the nervous system directly or indirectly, there are anomalies that provide an actual or potential

communication to the surface of the body, produce compression of neural tissue, impede the circulation of cerebrospinal fluid (CSF), restrict growth of the brain, act as a source of intracranial bleeding or produce seizures. These all require surgical treatment. The more common malformations in this category include congenital forms of hydrocephalus, craniosynostosis, the overt forms of cranium and spina bifida, dermal sinus tracts, congenital tumors and vascular malformations. Only the more common malformations necessitating neurosurgical treatment in the neonatal period will be discussed. The reader is referred to neurosurgical texts for information regarding less-common anomalies.

INFANTILE HYDROCEPHALUS

Abnormal enlargement of the head in infancy is a common diagnostic problem of pediatric neurosurgery. The cranium of the young infant with normal sutures is a pliable and distensible structure. A change in the size and shape of the head at this age is therefore an accurate reflection of change in the volume and distribution of the intracranial contents (see section Abnormal Head Size, Ch. 22).

Hydrocephalus is the most frequent cause of abnormal head growth in the first three months of life, but other pathologic conditions, including subdural hematoma or effusion, brain tumor, true macroencephaly and lipid-storage disease, must first be ruled out. The term hydrocephalus, in modern usage, is synonymous with enlargement of the lateral or all cerebral ventricles. Occasionally, enlargement of the ventricles may be encountered in a child with a normal or small head secondary to atrophy of the brain, i.e., hydrocephalus ex vacuo. In this condition, intracranial pressure is normal. Hydrocephalus associated with increased intracranial pressure and head enlargement is caused by the obstruction of normal CSF pathways. One possible exception to this rule is the increased production of CSF by a choroid plexus papilloma. Cerebrospinal fluid is formed in all ventricles by the choroid plexus, flows out of the fourth ventricle into the subarachnoid space and re-enters the blood via the arachnoid villi that project into the major dural sinuses. Interference with this pathway at any point may produce an increase in CSF pressure, enlargement of the ventricles at the expense of the surrounding brain and, in the child, enlargement of the cranium.

In the infant, hydrocephalus is most often secondary to brain malformation including maldevelopment, i.e., "stenosis" of the aqueduct of Sylvius, the Chiari II malformation (Arnold-Chiari malformation) and the Dandy-Walker syndrome. In the Chiari II malformation, usually associated with myelomeningocele, the displacement of the medulla and cerebellar tonsils into the cervical spinal canal usually prevents normal egress of fluid from the fourth ventricle into the subarachnoid space. In the Dandy-Walker syndrome, there is a cystic expansion of the fourth ventricle that may be secondary to failure of development of the normal ventricular foramina of Lushka and Magendie. Aqueductal stenosis is by far the most common isolated congenital defect producing hydrocephalus. It is also present in many cases of myelominingocele in association with the Chiari II defect.

Other less frequent congenital causes of hydrocephalus include glial webs at the junction of the aqueduct and fourth ventricle, arachnoid cysts in the posterior fossa and aneurysm of the great vein of Galen. Vein of Galen aneurysms are the result of abnormal communication of the vein with one or more cerebral arteries. Enlargement of the vein resulting from the abnormally high intravascular pressure produces hydrocephalus by obstructing the underlying posterior third ventricle and the proximal portion of the aqueduct. Children with this abnormality frequently exhibit heart failure shortly after birth as a result of the arteriovenous shunt.

Hydrocephalus, even in the neonate, may be secondary to a neoplasm producing obstruction of the ventricles. The most common primary intracranial neoplasm of the neonate is the highly malignant medullo-blastoma. Benign and surgically curable tumors such as choroid plexus papilloma and cerebellar astrocytoma also occur. Other noncongenital causes of hydrocephalus in the neonatal period and early infancy include obliteration of the subarachnoid pathways by intrauterine or perinatal meningitis or subarachnoid bleeding.

Although enlargement of the head secondary to hydrocephalus may be apparent at or prior to birth, head circumference is often normal at birth even when there is CSF obstruction on a congenital basis. However, the anterior fontanelle in these children is frequently very large and palpation reveals increased tension.

The diagnosis of hydrocephalus in the infant is best confirmed by ventriculography. In this study, after tapping the subdural space bilaterally through the coronal suture to rule out subdural hematoma, a needle or catheter is inserted into the right lateral ventricle. Cerebrospinal fluid is removed and an equal quantity of air (approximately 30 ml) is injected. Radiologic examination of the entire ventricular system is then carried out by varying the position of the head, and the site of CSF block is determined. Ventriculography is also usually adequate for visualization of intracranial mass lesions that may be responsible for hydrocephalus but in some instances, e.g., when a vein of Galen aneurysm is suspected, angiography may be necessary for adequate diagnosis and treatment. Curable causes of hydrocephalus, e.g., choroid plexus papilloma, must be ruled out prior to other treatment. In the majority of infants with hydrocephalus, shunting of CSF from the ventricular system into the bloodstream, peritoneum or pleural space is necessary (273–275). The indication for shunting is a rapidly progressing hydrocephalus caused by a lesion that is not amenable to correction. Children in whom moderate enlargement of the ventricles has been documented and whose head circumference has been shown to have increased at a slow rate may be followed in the hopes that spontaneous resolution of the problem will ensue. Unfortunately, true arrest of hydrocephalus is infrequent (276).

The most common shunt utilized in the treatment of hydrocephalus is that from the right lateral ventricle into the right atrium of the heart, i.e., a ventriculoatrial shunt. In this procedure a small burr hole is placed in the right occipital region and the right internal jugular vein is exposed in the neck. Silastic catheters are then passed into the right lateral ventricle and, via the jugular vein, into the right atrium. A one-way valve is then interposed between the catheters. Ventriculoperitoneal shunts of similar design are frequently employed in the neonatal period. The most common cause of malfunction in either type of shunt is obstruction from inspissated protein, blood and ventricular debris (272, 277). Bloodstream infection and ventriculitis is another major complication of the ventriculoatrial shunt. Staphylococci are the most commonly encountered offending organisms. It has been demonstrated that preoperative and postoperative treatment with antibiotics can lower the rate of this complication. Both types of shunts need revision as the child grows. The prognosis for the child with hydrocephalus treated by a shunting procedure is dependent on several factors, including the degree of damage to the brain already present at the time of shunting, the presence of other malformations of the brain and the amount of success in keeping the shunt functional. Good results are now obtained in approximately 75% of these children, many of whom have reached their full intellectual potential (271, 278).

CRANIOSYNOSTOSIS

The cranial sutures normally remain patent until after completion of brain growth in the late teens. Closure of one or more cranial sutures early in life results in an abnormally shaped head and, if the coronal suture is involved bilaterally, in the restriction of brain growth and increased intracranial pressure. The cause of premature closure of the cranial sutures is unknown. It is rarely hereditary and most frequently occurs as an isolated abnormality. It may, however, be associated with premature closure of the facial bones (craniofacial dysostosis or Crouzon's disease) and polydactyly (Apert's syndrome). Isolated premature closure of the sagittal sutures, seen predominantly in males, occurs most often, followed by synostosis of the coronal sutures, which is more common in females. Closure of the metopic suture and various combinations of sutures including total craniosynostosis is less common. The coronal and lambdoid sutures may be involved on one or both sides.

The shape of the head in craniosynostosis depends on which sutures are involved and when they close. The skull normally enlarges by growth perpendicular to the sutures. When a suture closes prematurely normal growth is curtailed and compensatory abnormal growth occurs parallel to the suture. Premature closure of the sagittal suture therefore results in an elongated skull and of the coronal suture, in a wide and foreshortened skull. Because of the brain's rapid growth in the first two years of life, the distortion is greater the earlier the closure. Craniosynostosis is usually apparent shortly after the effects of molding of the head have subsided. Diagnosis is made by physical examination and confirmed by x ray. In addition to abnormal head shape, a ridge over the affected suture(s) is usually palpable, and in the case of coronal and sagittal synostosis, the anterior fontanelle is abnormally small.

Treatment is surgical (279, 280) and may be either therapeutic (to permit normal brain growth) or cosmetic. The operation consists of creating an artificial suture by the excision of a strip of skull, either at the site of the involved suture or parallel to it. The margins of the craniectomy are covered with plastic film to retard bony closure. The primary risk of surgery is blood loss and mortality should therefore be, and is, nil in pediatric neurosurgical centers. The operation must be carried out in bilateral coronal synostosis with or without accompanying synostosis of other sutures. Surgery should be carried out for both cosmetic and therapeutic purposes at an early age, usually at four to six weeks. In coronal and total synostosis it may be necessary to repeat the operation at intervals if the surgically created defects close.

SPINA BIFIDA AND CRANIUM BIFIDUM

A large proportion of the malformations that affect the central nervous system result from a defective closure of the neural tube, meninges, spine and skull. The common denominator in these lesions is a midline bony defect giving rise to the terms spina and cranium bifida. Such defects can occur anywhere in the dorsal midline along the neural axis but are most common in the lumbosacral and occipital regions. The spectrum of anomalies encountered is wide. In approximately 20% of the population there exists incomplete fusion of the two halves of the neural arch in one or more of the lower lumbar or upper sacral vertebras without defects in the skin or meninges. This bony defect termed spina bifida occulta is rarely symptomatic. Other more serious and surgically important defects in this category are dermal sinus tracts, meningoceles, myelomeningoceles and encephaloceles.

DERMAL SINUS TRACTS

Dermal sinus tracts are uncommon but important anomalies with which every pediatrician should be familiar. Embryologically, these tracts represent incomplete separation of neural from cutaneous ectoderm. They occur in the midline over the occiput or lumbar and upper sacral spine and open onto the surface of the skin. The opening is often extremely small but usually presents as a definite dimple with one or more hairs growing from it. In the occiput, the epidermis-lined tract often courses through a small midline skull defect through the meninges to the fourth ventricle. In the spinal variety they invariably course cephalad to the termination of the spinal cord, the conus medullaris. Within the subarachnoid space the tracts may expand into an epidermoid or dermoid tumor.

If untreated, these lesions often lead to serious damage of the nervous system either indirectly from meningitis and hydrocephalus or directly by compression of neural tissue. All newborn infants should be examined for the presence of the tell-tale cutaneous opening. Likewise, any child having had multiple bouts of meningitis or meningitis due to enteric or skin bacteria should be closely examined for a sinus tract even to the extent of shaving the occiput (286). Excision of the entire tract should be carried out as soon as is feasible after discovery. Since laminectomy or craniectomy may be required, the operation should be carried out by a neurosurgeon. Local excision of the opening on the skin is to be condemned.

MENINGOCELES

Meningoceles represent herniation of the dura and arachnoid through bony defects in the spine or skull. They usually present as fluid-filled sacs in the dorsal midline. As in the case of other closure defects, they are most common in the lumbosacral region and the occiput. Unlike myelomeningoceles, the sacs are often completely covered by skin at birth. They also rarely cause hydrocephalus or neurologic dysfunction. Communication with subarachnoid space at the neck of the sac is frequently quite small. Meningoceles can also occur in a ventral position projecting through a bony defect into the pelvis, chest and through the cribiform plate into the nasal cavities. The ventral lesions are rare but often misdiagnosed.

Surgical repair of meningoceles is carried out on an elective basis unless there is leakage of spinal fluid. Treatment is then essential to prevent meningitis. The operation consists of exposing the neck of the meningocele down to the normal level of the dura where it is amputated and a watertight closure of the dura accomplished. The sac is excised and the fascia and skin reapproximated. Ventral meningoceles are approached transdurally, and their communication with the subarachnoid space is obliterated by closure of the dural opening. The remaining sac is usually not removed.

MYELOMENINGOCELES

Myelomeningoceles are the most common of the closure defects. The incidence in various parts of the world ranges from less than

1:1000 to more than 5:1000 live births. In the United States the incidence is about 2.5:1000 live births. Although myelomeningocele is semantically distinguished from meningocele by the fact that the sac of the former contains neural tissue, the myelomeningocele does not represent a simple herniation of the spinal cord through a vertebral defect Rather, this anomaly invariably constitutes a serious defect in the development of the caudal as well as other portions of the CNS. In addition to the Chiari II malformation and aqueductal stenosis previously described, which is responsible for the almost constantly observed hydrocephalus, these patients are apt to have cerebral heterotopias, dysgenesis of the corpus collosum and abnormalities of the spinal cord proximal to the obvious lesion. Many have associated congenital anomalies of other systems, mainly GU and skeletal. All of these children have neurologic deficits, the extent of which depends on the level of the lesion. The child with the low-lying sacral meningocele may have only bladder and bowel dysfunction. Higher lesions produce paresis and sensory loss of varying degree in the lower extremities. Paraplegia is not uncommon.

Most myelomeningoceles occur in the low thoracic and lumbosacral region. They usually present as a large broad-based sac only partially covered by skin. The dorsum of the sac most often consists of a thin membrane, primarily arachnoid. At the cephalic end of the sac, the dysplastic cord can usually be observed, and frequently its dorsum is completely exposed. The bony defect consists of a wide spina bifida over three or more segments. Other anomalies of the spine, such as hemivertebrae, are frequent.

It has been adequately demonstrated that semiemergent surgical treatment of myelomeningoceles, i.e., within the first 24 hours after birth minimizes disability and length of hospitalization (281–285, 287). Many of the sacs rupture at birth or begin leaking shortly thereafter predisposing to meningitis. Damage to the exposed spinal cord from drying and infection also occurs if repair is delayed. The goal of treatment is to return the spinal cord and nerve roots to their proper level within the neural canal and to prevent further leakage of spinal fluid by closure of the dura, fascia and skin. Added technical advantages of early closure relate to the facts that the sac is smaller and more easily dissected from the contained neural tissue, the skin is more pliable and the cutaneous bacterial flora have not yet become established.

After repair of the myelomeningocele, the child is hospitalized for several weeks to insure proper healing of the wound and to observe the rate of head growth. The progression of hydrocephalus and its severity is roughly correlated with the size and level of the lesion. Some patients with small, low (usually sacral) myelomeningoceles may not develop clinically apparent hydrocephalus. Most patients, however, require shunting of CSF during the first weeks of life.

Prior to discharge from the hospital, the child should have x rays of the skull, entire spine and hips, IVP and urine cultures as well as urologic and orthopedic consultations. The long-term care of these individuals involves multiple disciplines and is best carried out in a combined clinic in which pediatrics, urology, orthopedics and neurosurgery are represented.

ENCEPHALOMENINGOCELES

Encephalomeningoceles are the cranial counterpart of the myelomeningocele. Most occur in the occipital region; they are frequently extremely large and often contain major portions of the occipital lobes or cerebellum. The ideal treatment of these lesions is to return the herniated portions of the brain into the cranium and repair the overlying dura and scalp. However, the brain within the sac is often infarcted or maldeveloped and, not infrequently, the skull is too small to allow return of the neural tissue. The amputation of nonfunctioning tissue is therefore carried out and the best possible closure made. As with myelomeningocele, these patients often develop hydrocephalus.

ORTHOPEDIC PROBLEMS

The common orthopedic problems encountered in the neonatal period are fractures related to birth trauma, congenital dislocation of the hip, talipes equinovarus (club foot), congenital amputations and deformities of the limbs, fingers or toes.

FRACTURES

Fractures associated with birth trauma are most common in the humerus and, in descending order of frequency, the clavicle and femur (288–290). Depressed fracture of the skull and epiphyseal injuries of the humerus or femur may occur but are infrequent.

Humerus

The humerus may be broken in a difficult delivery, especially in breech extractions. The fracture occurs usually just below the deltoid insertion at the junction of the upper and middle thirds of the bone; it is usually transverse and most often complete. There is marked deformity, obvious swelling and shortening of the arm. The upper fragment may be abducted with gross upward displacement of the lower fragment. If there is associated radial nerve injury, the arm hangs limp. The baby does not move the limb. Diagnosis can be confirmed by radiography. Treatment consists in inserting a pad between the chest wall and the upper arm and bandaging the arm to the chest with the elbow flexed so that the fingers are directed toward the opposite shoulder. Because of the radial paresis usually accompanying this injury, the wrist should be maintained in dorsiflexion. The simplest methods should be used for reduction and immobilization of these fractures since nature provides perfect restoration of a deformed bone regardless of the degree of displacement or angulation. The bandage is maintained for 10 to 14 days after which callus may be palpable. Fractures of this type heal well regardless of how treated. Recovery of nerve function is almost universally complete.

Clavicle

Fractures of this bone may occur as the result of injury in breech deliveries, in vertex deliveries where the clavicle of the anterior shoulder may be broken or spontaneously in the course of easy labor. The fracture occurs most often unilaterally, although it is occasionally bilateral. The site of injury is most commonly at the junction of the outer and middle thirds. There may be a complete fracture or one of the greenstick variety.

The related arm is not used by the baby and the Moro reflex is usually absent on the affected side. If suspected, the diagnosis can be confirmed by roentgenograms. If the injury is not noted, it may not be detected until a "lump" (callus) is felt by the mother a week or ten days later.

Treatment has consisted of bandaging the arm to the chest wall for 10 to 17 days; however, if left untreated, the end result is the same. The prognosis is excellent with no permanent deformity. The parents must be informed of the mass of callus that will develop and reassured that it will disappear as healing progresses.

Femur

These fractures occur most frequently in association with breech deliveries when the lower limb is brought down or when groin traction is applied. The break is usually transverse or oblique at about the midshaft. The upper fragment is abducted, flexed and externally rotated; the lower fragment is pulled upward and there is obvious shortening. The baby does not move the extremity. The thigh is swollen, and there is evidence of pain on motion of the limb. Diagnosis is confirmed by roentgenography. Treatment consists in traction suspension for 10 to 14 days. This can be accomplished by modification of Bryant's traction, in which both legs with skin traction applied are suspended from a frame. The feet are suspended by rubber bands from the bar of the frame, and the frame may be mounted on a board with a foam rubber pad to permit transportation and care of the child at home. However, it has been our practice to keep the child hospitalized and under medical observation until callus forms. This occurs rapidly; the break is usually solid within 10 to 12 days and well healed within three weeks. Moulding and remodelling takes place within a short time, the functional result is good, and the ultimate prognosis is excellent. The parents may be assured that the appearance of the limb will be normal and that there will be no delay in onset or impairment of walking.

CONGENITAL DISLOCATION OF THE HIP

This condition is one in which there is displacement of the head of the femur from the acetabulum. In a series reported by von Rosen (297) covering a period of almost eight years, 40 cases were encountered in about 24,000 births, an incidence of 1.7:1000. The etiology has been thought due to a shallow acetabulum and increased anteversion of the femoral neck (292), although some consider the defect due to excessive laxity of the joint capsule (295, 299). Diagnosis should be made in the neonatal period. In 1936, Ortalani (296) described a test in which with the child, supine and hips flexed to 90° and knees flexed and together, the hips are slowly abducted. If there is a dislocated hip, during abduction the head of the femur will slip back into the acetabulum causing a "click" as the head snaps over the wall of the socket. This test is not completely satisfactory in neonates since the dislocated head may slide smoothly over the low rim of the acetabulum without making a click. A technique described by Barlow (293) is very reliable in small infants up to six months of age. This test is done with the baby supine, its feet facing the examiner. With the child's hips flexed at a right angle and the knees fully flexed, the middle finger of each hand of the examiner is placed over the greater trochanter, and the thumb of each hand is applied to the innerside of the thigh opposite the lesser trochanter. The thighs are spread to midabduction and forward pressure is exerted behind the greater

trochanter by the middle finger of each hand in turn while the other hand holds the opposite femur and pelvis steady. The diagnosis of hip dislocation is made if the femoral head slips forward into the acetabulum.

Limited abduction at the hip is an unreliable test in the newborn infant since this sign is due to adaptive shortening of the abductors in cases of relatively long-standing dislocation. Abnormalities of skin creases of the buttocks or upper thighs, although not pathognomonic, should alert one to the need for further testing for dislocation of the hip.

The diagnosis can be confirmed by radiography. Using the technique described by von Rosen, an anteroposterior view is taken with the hips extended and the legs fully rotated inward and each abducted 45°. When the long axis of the femur on the normal side is projected upward and medially, it crosses the spine at the lumbosacral junction. On the side with the dislocated hip, a similar projection of the long axis of the femur crosses the lumbar spine at a higher level. Conventional x rays of the hip are of no value.

Treatment of congenital dislocation of the hip consists in placing the child in a von Rosen splint with the legs in the position of abduction and lateral rotation, the position in which the dislocated head of the femur is reduced. The von Rosen dorsal splint consists of two longitudinal bars made of thin malleable strips of aluminum covered by rubber and held together by a similar horizontal piece. The baby is placed supine into the splint with the legs abducted and externally rotated. Each longitudinal bar is then adjusted so that the upper end fits over the shoulder, the lower beneath the thigh maintaining the position of closed reduction. The horizontal piece is curved about the baby's lower thorax and upper abdomen to hold the child and keep the splint in place. The infant can be washed and otherwise attended to without removing the splint. Examination of the hip is performed weekly or biweekly. When the reduction seems stable, usually after six to eight weeks, the child may be removed from the splint for short periods to permit more thorough bathing and skin care. The splint is generally no longer required after the 12th to 14th week.

Results following this form of treatment in the newborn infant have been excellent (291, 294, 298). Splinting within the first week of life leads to a hip that is clinically normal before the child begins to walk and which will remain stable.

CONGENITAL TALIPES EQUINOVARUS (CLUBFOOT)

In this easily recognizable defect, the child's foot is inverted, abducted and plantar flexed. It is a congenital deformity of the tarsus. The equinus or plantar flexion component occurs at the ankle joint and the varus in the subtalar joint.

Although club foot may occur in association with arthrogryposis or malformations of the nervous system, such as spina bifida, it most often is encountered in children who are otherwise normal. There is no specific etiology but some cases are due to abnormal intrauterine position and increased mechanical pressure, leading to a foot molded into equinovarus position. Bone, ligament, and muscle abnormalities are commonly encountered in this deformity. Diagnosis is made by physical examination. The foot is turned inward and downward and appears clublike. The heel is elevated and small, the forefoot broad and twisted. On the dorsum of the foot, the talus is palpable. The lateral malleolus is prominent while the medial malleolus is buried on the inner aspect of the ankle. Muscles of the calf are underdeveloped or atrophic, and the foot is smaller than normal. In some infants, the foot may appear as a clubfoot but can be passively corrected. Such infants do not have clubfoot. The deformity may be due to weakness of the peronei that disappear in the first few weeks of infancy after which the foot will appear normal. This condition can be differentiated from true clubfoot in that it can be completely corrected passively and is not a fixed deformity.

Treatment of the true clubfoot in the neonatal period is by conservative means (300, 301). The general principle as practiced in our institution is to place the foot in close-fitting, molded plaster casts as soon after birth as possible. At the time of application, the foot is manipulated to correct, as much as possible, the adduction and varus deformities initially and the equinus anomaly thereafter. Plaster is changed, and the foot is manipulated weekly for the first two months, then every two weeks until correction has been achieved, which may take one to two years. When correction appears to be satisfactory by roentgenography and is stable, plaster may be discontinued, and a Denis-Browne bar or splint may be used intermittently or at night. Corrective shoes should be ordered when the child begins to walk.

The results of treatment are largely dependent on the severity of the clubfoot. In those infants with a relatively mild form, the results are uniformly good. In children with a severe form of clubfoot, about 50% will respond well to the conservative measures as outlined. The other 50% may require a variety of surgical procedures in childhood for correction or further improvement.

ANOMALIES OF THE EXTREMITIES

Although many infants with severe deformities of the extremities may be stillborn or die shortly after birth because of associated anomalies of a serious nature, a significant number of infants will nonetheless be encountered with abnormalities of the limbs. In the past decade, physicians and laymen alike suddenly became aware of significant defects in the limbs of children born of mothers who had used thalidomide during pregnancy (307). A broad spectrum of limb defects may occur, including congenital amputations of fingers, toes or portions of an extremity, due presumably to intrauterine destruction of the part, as well as to a variety of defects probably caused by primary inhibition of development of growth (302–306). With the exception of thalidomide no specific etiologic agent for these

TABLE 23–2. Types of Anomalies of the Extremities

Term	Description
Amelia	Absence of limbs
Hemimelia	Absence of portion (distal) of limb
Phocomelia	Reduction in size of proximal part of limb and retraction of distal part toward trunk
Acheira	Absence of hand
Apodia	Absence of foot
Adactylia	Absence of fingers
Aphalangia	Absence of phalanges
Polydactyly	Supernumerary fingers or toes
Syndactyly	Fusion of the webbing (skin) or bones of adjacent fingers or toes
Lobster claw	Deep clefts or split in hand or foot with associated syndactyly of adjacent fingers or toes
Brachydactyly	Abnormal shortness of fingers or toes
Macrodactyly	Hypertrophy of fingers or toes

defects has been identified. The terms applied to some of these anomalies are listed in Table 23–2.

Although these anomalies are obvious in the neonate, treatment is deferred until later in infancy or childhood. The specific treatment is based on the particular defect and may require multiple orthopedic and plastic procedures as well as the use of prosthetic devices in some cases. The reader is referred to orthopedic texts for further information.

NERVE INJURIES

The nerve injuries most commonly associated with birth trauma are those of the brachial plexus (308–311) that occur as a result of traction applied to the head while delivering the shoulder or by pulling to bring the arm down in a breech. Two types of paralyses may be observed: 1) Erb's palsy and 2) Klumpke's palsy.

Erb's Palsy

In this form, the fifth and sixth cervical roots are injured. The involved arm cannot be abducted from the shoulder or externally rotated; the forearm loses the power of supination. The child's arm is characteristically adducted and internally rotated with the forearm in pronation. There is no Moro reflex on the affected side. In general, power in the forearm and hand is preserved unless the lower part of the plexus is involved.

Klumpke's Palsy

This occurs less often and is due to injury of the seventh and eighth cervical and first thoracic roots. The child presents with a paralyzed hand. There may be meiosis and ptosis on the same side if the sympathetic fibers of T_1 are affected. Unless there has been a complete tear of the nerve fibers, these babies will recover completely within four to six months.

Treatment is nonoperative and consists in placing the child's arm in a suitable splint so that the paralyzed muscles are relaxed. Physiotherapy during this period is helpful.

REFERENCES

1. Brown JJM: Surgery of Childhood. Baltimore, Williams & Wilkins, 1963
2. Gross RE: The Surgery of Infancy and Childhood. Philadelphia, Saunders, 1953
3. Gross RE: An Atlas of Children's Surgery. Philadelphia, Saunders, 1970
4. Haller JA, Talbert JL: Surgical Emergencies in the Newborn. Philadelphia, Lea & Febiger, 1972
5. Holman CW, Muschenheim C: Bronchopulmonary Diseases and Related Disorders, Vol 1, part III. Hagerstown, Harper & Row, 1972
6. Levine MI, Mascia AV: Pulmonary Diseases and Anomalies of Infancy and Childhood. New York, Hoeber Med Div, Harper & Row, 1966
7. Mustard WT, Ravitch MM, Snyder WH Jr, Welch KJ, Benson CD: Pediatric Surgery, 2nd ed. Chicago, Year Book Med Pub, 1969
8. Paulsen EP: Postoperative fluid, electrolyte and caloric requirements in children. Am J Surg 107:390, 1964
9. Ravitch MM: Pediatric Surgery. In: Surgery Principles and Practice, 4th ed. Edited by JE Rhoads, JG Allen, HN Harkins, CA Moyer. Philadelphia, Lippincott, 1970
10. Rickham PP: Investigation of blood loss during operations on newborn infants. Arch Dis Child 29:304, 1954
11. Rickham PP, Johnston JH: Neonatal Surgery. New York, Appleton-Century-Crofts, 1969
12. Roe CF, Santulli TV, Blair CS: Heat loss in infants during general anesthesia and operations. J Pediatr Surg 1:266, 1966

13. Schaffer AJ, Avery ME: Diseases of the Newborn, 3rd ed. Philadelphia, Saunders, 1971

14. Shaw A, Franzel I, Bordiuk J: Prevention of neonatal hypothermia by a fiber optic "hot pipe" system: a new concept. J Pediatr Surg 6:354, 1971

15. Silverman WA, Sinclair JC, Scopes JW: Regulation of body temperature in pediatric surgery. J Pediatr Surg 1:321, 1966

16. Swenson O: Pediatric Surgery, 3rd ed. New York, Appleton-Century-Crofts, 1968

17. Swenson O: Neonatal physiology. In: Pediatric Surgery, 3rd ed. New York, Appleton-Century-Crofts, 1969

18. Talbert JL: Intraoperative and postoperative monitoring of infants. Surg Clin North Am 50:787, 1970

19. White RR: Atlas of Pediatric Surgery. New York, Blakiston Div, McGraw-Hill, 1965

AIRWAY AND THORAX

Choanal Atresia

20. Beinfield HH: Bilateral choanal atresia in the newborn. Arch Otolaryngol 73:659, 1961

21. Cherry J, Bordley JE: Surgical correction of choanal atresia. Ann Otol Rhinol Laryngol 75:911, 1966

22. Hobolth N, Buchmann G, Sandberg LE: Congenital choanal atresia. Acta Paediatr Scand 56:286, 1967

23. McGovern FH: Early management of choanal atresia. Laryngoscope 71:480, 1961

Larynx and Trachea

24. Aberdeen E: Tracheostomy and tracheostomy care in infants. Proc R Soc Med 58:900, 1965

25. Baker DC Jr, Pennington CL: Congenital hemangioma of the larynx. Laryngoscope 66:696, 1956

26. Blumenthal S, Ravitch MM: Seminar on aortic vascular rings and other anomalies of the aortic arch. Pediatrics 20:896, 1957

27. Campbell JS, Wiglesworth FW, Latorocca R, Wilde H: Congenital subglottic hemangiomas of the larynx and trachea in infants. Pediatrics 22:727, 1958

28. Ferguson CF, Flake CG: Subglottic hemangioma as a cause of respiratory obstruction in infants. Trans Am Bronchoesoph Assoc 41:27, 1961

29. Ferguson CF: Treatment of airway problems in the newborn. Ann Otol Rhinol Laryngol 76:762, 1967

30. Holinger PH, Johnston KC, Zoss AR: Tracheal and bronchial obstruction due to congenital cardiovascular anomalies. Ann Otol Rhinol Laryngol 57:808, 1948

31. Holinger PH, Johnston KC, Schiller F: Congenital anomalies of the larynx. Ann Otol Rhinol Laryngol 63:581, 1954

32. Littler ER: Asphyxia due to hemangioma in trachea. J Thorac Cardiovasc Sur 45:552, 1963

33. Neuhauser EBD: Roentgen diagnosis of double aortic arc and other anomalies of the great vessels. Am J Roentgenol Radium Ther Nucl Med 51:1, 1946

34. Redo SF, Williams JR, Bass R, Neumann K: Respiratory obstruction secondary to lymphangioma of the trachea. J Thorac Cardiovasc Surg 49:1026, 1965

35. Smythe P: The problems of detubating an infant with a tracheostomy. J Pediatr 65:446, 1964

36. Stool SE, Campbell JR, Johnson DG: Tracheostomy in children: the use of plastic tubes. J Pediatr Surg 3:402, 1968

37. Talbert JL, Haller JA Jr: Improved silastic tracheostomy tubes for infants and young children. J Pediatr Surg 3:408, 1968

Pulmonary Lesions

38. Albert HM, Potts WJ: Congenital lung cysts in infants. Pediatrics 12:283, 1953

39. Birdsell DC, Wentworth P, Reilly BJ, Donohue WL: Congenital cystic adenomatoid malformation of the lung: a report of eight cases. Can J Surg 9:350, 1956

40. Boyd G: Intralobar pulmonary sequestration. Dis Chest 24:162, 1953

41. Brunner S, Poulsen PT, Vesterdal J: Cysts of the lung in infants and children. Acta Paediatr Scand 49:39, 1960

42. Burger RA: Agenesis of the lung. Am J Dis Child 73:481, 1936

43. Craig JM, Kirkpatrick J, Neuhauser EBD: Congenital cystic adenomatoid malformation of the lung in infants. Am J Roentgenol Radium Ther Nucl Med 76:516, 1956

44. Eraklis AJ, Griscom NT, McGovern JB: Bronchogenic cysts of the mediastinum in infancy. N Engl J Med 281:1150, 1969

45. Hendren WH, McKee DM: Lobar emphysema of infancy. J Pediatr Surg 1:24, 1966

46. Herrman JW, Jewett TC Jr, Galletti G: Bronchogenic cysts in infants and children. J Thorac Surg 37:242, 1959

47. Hutchin P, Friedman PJ, Saltzstein SL: Congenital cystic adenomatoid malformation with anomalous blood supply. J Thorac Cardiovasc Surg 62:220, 1971

48. Kwittkin J, Reiner L: Congenital cystic adenomatoid malformation of the lung. Pediatrics 30:759, 1962

49. Leape LL, Longino LA: Infantile lobar emphysema. Pediatrics 34:246, 1964

50. Minetto E, Galli E, Boglione G: Agenesis, aplasia, ipoplasia polmonare. Minerva Med 49:4635, 1958

51. Moffat AD: Congenital cystic disease of the lungs and its classification. J Pathol 79:361, 1960

52. Moncrieff MW, Cameron AH, Astley R, Roberts KD, Abrams LD, Mann JR: Congenital cystic adenomatoid malformation of the lung. Thorax 24:476, 1969

53. Murray GF: Congenital lobar emphysema. Surg Gynecol Obstet 124:611, 1967

54. Raynor AC, Capp MP, Sealy WC: Lobar emphsema of infancy: diagnosis, treatment and etiologic aspects. Ann Thorac Surg 4:374, 1967

55. Robbins L: Roentgenologic appearance of bronchogenic cysts. Am J Roentgenol Radium Ther Nucl Med 50:321, 1943

56. Rosenberg DML: Pulmonary agenesis. Dis Chest 46:68, 1962

57. Talalak P: Pulmonary sequestration. Arch Dis Child 35:57, 1960

58. Wexels P: Agenesis of the lung. Thorax 6:171, 1951

Pneumomediastinum and Pneumothorax

59. Chernick V, Avery ME: Spontaneous alveolar rupture in newborn infants. Pediatrics 32:816, 1963

60. Hans SY, Rudolph AJ, Teng CT: Pneumomediastinum in infancy. J Pediatr 62:754, 1963

61. Krueger CS, Sherafat M, Reagan LB: Spontaneous pneumothorax in newborn infants. Surgery 64: 498, 1968

62. Logan WD Jr, Pausa SG, Crispin RH: Spontaneous pneumothorax in the newborn. Dis Chest 42: 611, 1962

63. Macklin CC: Transport of air along sheaths of pulmonic blood vessels from the alveoli to the mediastinum. Arch Intern Med 64:913, 1939

64. Oztalay AG, Beard AG: Tension pneumothorax: possible etiologic role of high intratracheal pressure. J Pediatr 63:530, 1963

65. Salyer JM, Camarata SJ: Considerations in the management of spontaneous pneumothorax in the newborn. Am Surg 35:27, 1969

66. Srougi MN: Pneumothorax and pneumomediastinum in the first three days of life. J Pediatr Surg 2:410, 1967

Esophageal Atresia

67. Castilla P, Irving IM, Rees GJ, Rickham PP: Posture in the management of esophageal atresia; variations on a theme by Dr. E. B. D. Neuhauser. J Pediatr Surg 6:709, 1971

68. Gross RE, Firestone FN: Colonic reconstruction of the esophagus in infants and children. Surgery 61:955, 1967

69. Haight C, Towsley HA: Congenital atresia of the esophagus with tracheoesophageal fistula. Extrapleural ligation of fistula and end-to-end anastomosis of esophageal segments. Surg Gynecol Obstet 76:672, 1943

70. Holden MP, Wooler GH: Tracheoesophageal fistula and esophageal atresia: results of 30 years' experience. Thorax 25:406, 1970

71. Holder TM, McDonald VG Jr, Wooley MM: The premature or critically ill infant with esophageal atresia: increased success with a staged procedure. J Thorac Cardiovasc Surg 44:344, 1962

72. Holder TM, Cloud DT, Lewis JE Jr, Pilling GP IV: Esophageal atresia and tracheoesophageal fistula. Pediatrics 34: 542, 1964

73. Holder TM, Ashcraft KW: Esophageal atresia and tracheoesophageal fistula. Ann Thorac Surg 9:445, 1970

74. Howard R, Meyers NA: Esophageal atresia: a technique for elongating the upper pouch. Surgery 58:725, 1965

75. Koop CE, Hamilton JP: Atresia of the esophagus: increased survival with staged procedures in the poor-risk infant. Ann Surg 162:389, 1965

76. Koop CE: Recent advances in the surgery of esophageal atresia. Prog Pediatr Surg 2:41, 1971

77. Ladd WE: The surgical treatment of esophageal atresia and tracheoesophageal fistula. N Engl J Med 230:625, 1944

78. Lafer DJ, Boley S: Primary repair in esophageal atresia with elongation of the lower segnemt. J Pediatr Surg 1:585, 1966

79. Levin NL: Congenital atresia of the esophagus with tracheoesophageal fistula: report of extrapleural ligation of fistulous communication and cervical esophagostomy. J Thorac Surg 10:648, 1941

80. Schneider KM, Becker J: The "H-type" tracheoesophageal fistual in infants and children. Surgery 51:677, 1962

81. Vogt EC: Congenital Esophageal Atresia. Am J Roentgenol 22:463, 1929

82. Waterston D: Colonic replacement of oesophagus (intrathoracic). Surg. Clin North Am 44:6, 1964

83. Young BG: Successful primary anastomosis in oesophageal atresia after reduction of a long gap between the blind ends, by bouginage of the upper pouch. Br J Surg 54:321, 1967

Diaphragm

84. Allen MS, Thomson SA: Congenital diaphragmatic hernia in children under one year of age: a 24-year review. J Pediatr Surg 1:157, 1966

85. Brown WT: Artificial abdomen in diaphragmatic hernia. Am Surg 36:737, 1970

86. Gross RE: Congenital hernia of the diaphragm. Am J Dis Child 71:579, 1964

87. Kirklin BR, Hodgson JR: Roentgenologic characteristics of diaphragmatic hernia. Am J Roentgenol Radium Ther Nucl Med 58:77, 1947

88. Koop CE, Johnson J: Transthoracic repair of diaphragmatic hernia in infants. Ann Surg 136:1007, 1952

89. Laxdal OE, McDougall HA, Mellin GW: Congenital eventration of the diaphragm. N Engl J Med 250:401, 1954

90. Meeker IA, Kincannon WN: The role of ven-

tral hernia in the correction of diaphragmatic defects in the newborn. Arch Dis Child 40:146, 1965

91. Snyder WH Jr, Greaney EM Jr: Congenital diaphragmatic hernia. Surgery 57:576, 1965

Mediastinal Tumors

92. Bergstrom VW: Hemangioma of the mediastinum causing death in a newborn. NY State J Med 45:1869, 1945

93. Ellis FH, Du Shane JW: Primary mediastinal cysts and neoplasms in infants and children. Am Rev Tuberc 74:940, 1956

94. Fallon M, Gordon ARG, Lendrum AC: Mediastinal cysts of foregut origin associated with vertebral abnormalities. Br J Surg 41:520, 1954

95. Gross RE, Hurwitt ES: Cervicomediastinal and mediastinal cystic hygroma. Surg Gynecol Obstet 87:599, 1948

96. Hope JW, Koop CE: Differential diagnosis of mediastinal masses. Pediatr Clin North Am 6:379, 1959

97. Hope JW, Borns PF, Koop CE: Radiologic diagnosis of mediastinal masses in infants and children. Radiol Clin North Am 1:17, 1963

98. Koop CE, Kieswetter WB, Horn RC Jr: Neuroblastoma in childhood: survival after major surgical insult to the tumor. Surgery 38:272, 1955

99. Mixter CG, Clifford SH: Congenital mediastinal cysts of gastrogenic and bronchiogenic origin. Ann Surg 90:714, 1929

100. Schweisguth O, Mathey J, Renault P, Benet JP: Intrathoracic neurogenic tumors in infants and children. Ann Surg 150:29, 1959

ABDOMEN

Atresia and Stenosis

101. Aitken J: Congenital intrinsic duodenal obstruction in infancy. J Pediatr Surg 1:546, 1966

102. Becker JM, Schneider KM: Tube gastrostomy in the treatment of upper intestinal obstruction in neonates. Surg Gynecol Obstet 116:123, 1963

103. Benson CD, Lloyd JR, Smith JD: Resection and primary anastomosis in the management of stenosis and atresia of the jejunum and ileum. Pediatrics 26:265, 1959

104. Bishop HC, Koop CE: Management of meconium ileus: resection, Roux-en-Y anastomosis and ileostomy irrigation with pancreatic enzymes. Ann Surg 145:410, 1957

105. Brown JJM: Small intestinal obstruction in the newborn. Ann R Coll Surg Engl 20:280, 1957

106. Fonkalsrud EW, de Lorimier AG, Hays DM: Congenital atresia and stenosis of the duodenum: a review compiled from the members of the surgical section of the American Academy of Pediatrics. Pediatrics 43:79, 1969

107. Nixon HH, Tawes R: Etiology and treatment of small intestinal atresia: analysis of a series of 127 jejunoileal atresias and comparison with 62 duodenal atresias. Surgery 69:41, 1971

108. Santulli TV, Blanc WA: Congenital atresia of the intestine: pathogenesis and treatment. Ann Surg 154.939, 1961

109. Santulli TV, Amoury RA: Congenital anomalies of the gastrointestinal tract. Pediatr Clin North Am 14:21, 1967

110. Zachary RB: Intestinal obstruction. Prog Pediatr Surg 2:57, 1971

Malrotation

111. Bill AH, Grauman D: Rationale and technique for stabilization of the mesentery in cases of nonrotation of the midgut. J Pediatr Surg 1:127, 1966

112. Estrada RL: Anomalies of Intestinal Rotation and Fixation. Springfield, Ill, Thomas 1958

113. Rees JR, Redo SF: Anomalies of intestinal rotation and fixation. Am J Surg 116:834, 1968

114. Snyder WH Jr, Chaffin L: Embryology and pathology of the intestinal tract: presentation of 48 cases of malrotation. Ann Surg 140:368, 1954

115. Soderland S: Anomalies of midgut rotation and fixation. Clinical aspects based on 62 cases in childhood. Acta Paediatr Scand [Suppl 135] 51:225, 1962

Annular Pancreas

116. Feuchtwanger MM, Weiss Y: Side-to-side duodenoduodenostomy for obstructing annular pancreas in the newborn. J Pediatr Surg 3:398, 1968

117. Gross RE, Chisholm JC: Annular pancreas producing duodenal obstruction. Ann Surg 119:759, 1944

118. Hope JW, Gibbon JF: Duodenal obstruction due to annular pancreas. Radiology 63:473, 1954

119. Jackson JM: Annular pancreas and duodenal obstruction in the neonate. Arch Surg 87:379, 1963

120. Kiesewetter WB, Koop CE: Annular pancreas in infancy. Surgery 36:145, 1954

Duplication

121. Basu R, Forshall I, Rickham PP: Duplications of the alimentary tract. Br J Surg 47:477, 1960

122. Bishop HC, Koop CE: Surgical management of duplications of the alimentary tract. Am J Surg 107:434, 1964

123. Bremer JL: Diverticula and duplications of the intestinal tract. Arch Path 38:132, 1944

124. Fisher HC: Duplications of the intestinal tract in infants. Arch Surg 61:957, 1950

125. Gross RE, Hilcomb GW, Farber S: Duplication of the alimentary tract, Pediatrics 9:449, 1952

Perforated Viscus

126. Agarty HA, Ziserman AJ, Schollenberger CL: A case of perforation of the ileum in a newborn infant. J Pediatr 22:237, 1943

127. Lloyd JR: The etiology of the gastrointestinal perforations in the newborn. J Pediatr Surg 4:77, 1969

128. Miller RE, Rhamy RK: Acute perforations in infants. Surg Gynecol Obstet 117:61, 1963

129. Parrish RA, Sherman RT, Wilson H: Gastroenteric perforations in newborns. Ann Surg 159:244, 1964

130. Rees JR, Redo SF: Neonatal gastric necrosis and perforation treated by gastrectomy and esophagogastric anastomosis. Surgery 64:472, 1968

131. Shaw A, Blanc WA, Santulli TV, Kaiser G: Spontaneous rupture of the stomach in the newborn: a clinical and experimental study. Surgery 58:561, 1965

132. Shaw A: Perforations of the gastrointestinal tract in newborns and infants. Hosp Pract 6:131, 1971

133. Walstad PM, Cocklin WS: Rupture of the stomach after therapeutic oxygen administration. N Engl J Med 264:1201, 1961

Hirschsprung's Disease

134. Berdon WE, Baker DH: The roentgenographic diagnosis of Hirschsprung's disease in infancy. Am J Roentgenol Radium Ther Nucl Med 93:432, 1965

135. Hirschsprung H: Stuhltiagheit Neugeborner in Folge von Dilatation und Hypertrophie des Colons. Jahrb Kinderheilk 27:1, 1888 (quoted in Pilling GP, Cresson SL: Pediatric Surgery, 2nd ed. Chicago, Year Book Med Pub, 1969

136. Hope JW, Borns PF, Berg PK: Roentgenologic manifestations of Hirschsprung's disease in infancy. Am J Roentgenol Radium Ther Nucl Med 95:217, 1965

137. Swenson O, Rheinhard HF, Diamond I: Hirschsprung's disease. N Engl J Med 241:903, 1949

138. Swenson O, Neuhauser EBD, Pickett LK: New concepts of the etiology, diagnosis, and treatment of congenital megacolon (Hirschsprung's disease). Pediatrics 4:201, 1949

139. Swenson O, Fisher JH, McMahon RE: Rectal biopsy as an aid in the diagnosis of Hirschsprung's disease. N Engl J Med 253:632, 1955

140. Swenson O: Congenital megacolon. Pediatr Clin North Am 11:187, 1967

Necrotizing Enterocolitis

141. Agerty HA, Ziserman AJ, Hollenberger CL: A case of perforation of the ileum in a new-

born infant with operation and recovery. J Pediatr 22:233, 1943

142. Asaph JW, Redo SF: Neonatal necrotizing enterocolitis–a report of eight cases. Med Bull USAREUR 28:320, 1971

143. Berdon WE, Grossman H, Baker DH, Mizrahi A, Barlow O, Blanc WA: Necrotizing enterocolitis in the premature infant. Radiology 83:879, 1964

144. Blanc WA: Amniotic infection syndrome. Pathogenesis, morphology, and significance in circumnatal mortality. Clin Obstet Gynecol 2:705, 1959

145. Denes J, Gergely K, Wohlmuth G, Leb J: Necrotizing enterocolitis of premature infants. Surgery 68:558, 1970

146. Goldstein WB, Gusmano JV, Gallagher JJ, Hemley S: Portal vein gas: a case report with survival. Am J Roentgenol Radium Ther Nucl Med 97:220, 1966

147. Hermann RE: Perforation of the colon from necrotizing colitis in the newborn: report of a survival and a new etiologic concept. Surgery 58:436, 1965

148. Hopkins GB, Gould VE, Stevenson JK, Oliver TK Jr: Necrotizing enterocolitis in premature infants. Am J Dis Child 120:229, 1970

149. Lloyd JR: The etiology of gastrointestinal perforations in the newborn. J Pediatr Surg 4:77, 1969

150. Maas H: Demonstration eines Preparates von Emphysema des grossen Netae. Berl Klin Wschr 41:401, 1904

151. Mizrahi A, Barlow O, Berdon W, Blanc WA, Silverman WA: Necrotizing enterocolitis in premature infants. J Pediatr 66:697, 1965

151a. Pitt J, Barlow B, Heird WC, Santulli TV: Macrophages and the protective action of breast milk in necrotizing enterocolitis (abstr). Pediatr Research 8:110, 1974

152. Rabinowitz JG, Wolf BS, Feller MR, Krasna I: Colonic changes following necrotizing enterocolitis in the newborn. Am J Roentgenol Radium Ther Nucl Med 103:359, 1968

153. Rossier A, Sarrut S, Delplanque J: L'enterocolité ulcero-necrotique du premature. La Semaine de Hopitaux. Ann Pediatr (Paris) 34:1428, 1959

154. Schmid O, Quaiser K: Ueber eine besondere Schwere Verlaufende Form von Enteritis beim Saeugling. Oest Z Kinderserzte 8:114, 1953

155. Sheiner NM, Palayew MJ, Sedlezky I: Gas in the portal vein: a report of two cases. Can Med Assoc J 95:611, 1966

156. Simpson JY: Peritonitis in the fetus in uterus. Edin Med Surg J 15:390, 1838

157. Stevenson JK, Graham CB, Oliver TK Jr, Goldenberg VE: Neonatal necrotizing enterocolitis: a report of twenty-one cases with fourteen survivors. Am J Surg 118:260, 1959

158. Stone HH, Allen WB, Smith RB III, Haynes CD: Infantile pneumatosis intestinalis. J Surg Res 8:301, 1968

159. Touloukian RJ, Berdon WE, Amoury RA, Santulli TV: Surgical experience with necrotizing enterocolitis in the infant.. J Pediatr Surg 2:389, 1967

160. Uhr JW: Effect of bacterial endotoxin in the newborn guinea pig. J Exp Med 115:685, 1962

161. Willi H von: Ueber eine Boesartige Enteritis bei Sauglingan der ersten Trimenons. Ann Paediatr 162:87, 1944

162. Wilson SE, Woolley MM: Primary necrotizing enterocolitis in infants. Arch Surg 99:563, 1969

Meconium Ileus (Mucoviscidosis)

163. Bishop HC, Koop CE: Management of meconium ileus: resection, Roux-en-Y anastamosis and ileostomy irrigation with pancreatic enzymes. Ann Surg 145:410, 1957

164. Bodian M (ed): Fibrocystic Disease of the Pancreas: A Congenital Disorder of Mucus-Production. New York, Grune & Stratton, 1953

165. Bowring AC, Kern IB, Jones RFC: The use of Tween 80 in meconium ileus. Australian Pediatric Association Thirteenth Annual Meeting, Canberra, April 1968 (quoted in Noblett HR: Treatment of uncomplicated meconium ileus by gastrografin enema: a preliminary report. J Pediatr Surg 4:190, 1969)

166. Di Sant'Agnese PA, Talamo RC: Pathogenesis and physiopathology of cystic fibrosis of the pancreas. N Engl J Med 277:1287, 1967

167. Elian E, Shwachman H, Hendren WH: Intestinal obstruction of the newborn infant: usefulness of the sweat electrolyte test in differential diagnosis. N Engl J Med 264:13, 1961

168. Farber SJ: The relation of pancreatic achylia to meconium ileus. J Pediatr 24:387, 1944

169. Frech RS, McAlister WH, Ternberg J, Strominger D: Meconium ileus relieved by 40 per cent water-soluble contrast enemas. Radiology 94:341, 1970

170. Gibson LE, Cooke RE: Test for concentration of electrolytes in sweat in cystic fibrosis of pancreas utilizing pilocarpine by iontophoresis. Pediatrics 23:545, 1959

171. Graham WP III, Halden A, Jaffe BF: Surgical treatment of patients with cystic fibrosis. Surg Gynecol Obstet 122:373, 1966

172. Holsclaw DS, Eckstein HB, Nixon HH: Meconium ileus: 20-year review of 109 cases. Am J Dis Child 109: 101, 1965

173. Macdonald JA, Trusler GA: Meconium ileus: an eleven year review at the Hospital for Sick Children, Toronto. Can Med Assoc J 83:881, 1960

174. Meeker IA Jr, Kincannon WN: Acetylcysteine used to liquefy inspissated meconium causing intestinal obstruction in the newborn. Surgery 56:419, 1964

175. Neuhauser EBD: Roentgen changes associated with pancreatic insufficiency in early life. Radiology 46:319, 1946

176. Noblett HR: Treatment of uncomplicated meconium ileus by gastrografin enema: a preliminary report. J Pediatr Surg 4:190, 1969

177. Rowe MI, Furst AJ, Altman DH, Poole C: The neonatal response to gastrografin enema. Pediatrics 48:29, 1971

178. Shaw A: Safety of n-acetylcysteine in treatment of meconium obstruction of the newborn. J Pediatr Surg 4:119, 1969

179. Shwachman H: The sweat test. Pediatrics 30:167, 1963

180. Shwachman H, Pryles CV, Gross RE: Meconium ileus. Am J Dis Child 91:223, 1956

181. Wagget J, Johnson DG, Borns P, Bishop HC: The nonoperative treatment of meconium ileus by gastrografin enema. J Pediatr 77:407, 1970

ANORECTAL ANOMALIES

182. Ladd WE, Gross RE: Congenital malformations of the anus and rectum: report of 162 cases. Am J Surg 23:167, 1934

183. Stephens FD: Imperforate anus. Med J Aust 2:803, 1959

184. Stephens FD, Smith DE: Ano-rectal Malformations in Children. Chicago, Year Book Med Pub, 1971

185. Wangensteen OH, Rice CO: Imperforate anus. Ann Surg 92:77, 1930

Hernia and Hydrocele

186. Clatworthy HW Jr, Thompson AG: Incarcerated and strangulated inguinal hernia in infants: a preventable risk. JAMA 154:123, 1954

187. Clausen EG, Jake RJ, Binkley FM: Contralateral inguinal exploration of unilateral hernia in infants and children. Surgery 44:735, 1958

188. Gans SL: Sliding inguinal hernia in female infants Arch Surg 79:109, 1959

189. Gilbert M, Clatworthy WA Jr: Bilateral operations for inguinal hernia and hydrocele in infancy and childhood. Am J Surg 97:255, 1959

190. Goldstein R, Potts WJ: Inguinal hernia in female infants and children. Ann Surg 148:819, 1958

191. Gunnlaughsson GH, Dawson B, Lynn HB: Treatment of inguinal hernia in infants and children: experience with contralateral exploration. Mayo Clin Proc 42:129, 1967

192. Kiesewetter WB: Hernias and hydroceles. Pediatr Clin North Am 6:1129, 1959

193. Kiesewetter WB, Parenzan L: When should hernia in the infant be treated bilaterally? JAMA 171:287, 1959

194. Kurbweg FT: Inguinal and umbilical hernias in infancy and childhood: contrast in management. South Med J 51:961, 1958

195. Rowe MI, Clatworthy HW: Incarcerated and strangulated hernias in children. A statistical

study of high risk factors. Arch Surg 101:136, 1970

Omphalocele and Gastroschisis

196. Allen RG, Wrenn EL Jr: Silon as a sac in the treatment of omphalocele and gastroschisis. J Pediatr Surg 4:3, 1969

197. Collins DL, Schumacher AE: Omphalocele ruptured before birth. Proc Paediatr Surg Cong (Melbourne) 1:21, 1970

198. Cordero L, Touloukian RJ, Pickett LK: Staged repair of gastroschisis with silastic sheeting. Surgery 65:676, 1969

199. Denes J, Leb J, Lukacs FV: Gastroschisis. Surgery 63:701, 1968

200. Ein SH, Fallis JC, Simpson JS: Silon sheeting in the staged repair of massive ventral hernias in children. Can J Surg 13:127, 1970

201. Firor HV: Omphalocele—an appraisal of therapeutic approaches. Surgery 69:208, 1971

202. Izant RJ, Brown F, Rothmann BF: Current embryology and treatment of gastroschisis and omphalocele. Arch Surg 95:49, 1966

203. Rangarathnam CS, Lal RB, Swenson O: Gastroschisis. Arch Surg 98:742, 1969

204. Rickham PP: Rupture of exomphalos and gastroschisis. Arch Dis Child 38:138, 1963

205. Shim WKT: Lateral plication of synthetic sack for large gastroschisis and omphalocele defects. J Pediatr Surg 6:143, 1971

206. Williams DK: Ruptured omphalocele of the newborn. Am Surg 35:793, 1971

Appendicitis

207. Meyer JF: Acute gangrenous appendicitis in a premature infant. J Pediatr 41:343, 1952

NEOPLASMS

Retroperitoneal Teratoma

208. Arnheim EE: Retroperitoneal teratomas in infancy and childhood. Pediatrics 8:309, 1951

209. Engel RP, Elkins RC, Fletcher BD: Retroperitoneal teratoma. Cancer 22:1068, 1968

210. Keramidas DC, Voyatzis NG: Retroperitoneal teratoma. J Pediatr Surg 7:434, 1972

Sacrococcygeal Teratoma

211. Donellan WA, Swenson O: Benign and malignant sacrococcygeal teratomas. Surgery 64:834, 1968

212. Emery JL: Teratomas. Pediatr Clin North Am 6:573, 1959

213. Gwinn JL, Dockerty MB, Kennedy RL: Presacral teratomas in infancy and childhood. Pediatrics 16:239, 1955

214. Walker JM, Foster RJP: Sacrococcygeal teratomas in the newborn. Arch Surg 61:1138, 1950

Wilms' Tumor

215. Bolande RP, Brough AJ, Iyant RJ Jr: Congenital mesoblastic nephroma of infancy. A report of eight cases and the relationship to Wilms' tumor. Pediatrics 40:272, 1967

216. Collins VP: Wilms' tumor: its behavior and prognosis. J La State Med Soc 107:474, 1955

217. D'Angio GJ: Clinical and biologic studies of actinomycin D and roentgen irradiation. Am J Roentgenol Radium Ther Nucl Med 87:106, 1962

218. Fernbach DJ, Martyn DT: Role of dactinomycin in the improved survival of children with Wilms' tumor. JAMA 195:1005, 1966

219. Johnson DG, Maceira F, Koop CE: Wilms' tumor treated with actinomycin D.: the relationship of age and extent of disease to survival. J Pediatr Surg 2:13, 1967

220. Koop CE: Current management of nephroblastoma and neuroblastoma. Am J Surg 107:497, 1964

221. Lattimer JK, Melicow MM, Uson AC: Nephroblastoma (Wilms' tumor): prognosis more favorable in infants under one year of age. JAMA 171:2163, 1959

222. Ledlie EM, Mynors LS, Draper GJ, Gorbach FD: Natural history and treatment of Wilms' tumors: an analysis of 335 cases occurring in England and Wales. Br Med J 4:195, 1970

223. Louw JH: The management of Wilms' tumor. S Afr Med J 45:1065, 1971

Neuroblastoma

224. Bill AH, Koop CE (eds): Conference on the biology of neuroblastoma (Sept. 15, 16, 1967). J Pediatr Surg 3: Suppl, 1968

225. Bolande RP: Benignity of neonatal tumors and concept of cancer repression in early life. Am J Dis Child 122:12, 1971

226. Evans AE, D'Angio GJ, Randolph J: A proposed staging for children with neuroblastoma. Cancer 27:374, 1971

227. Gross RE, Farber S, Martin LW: Neuroblastoma sympatheticum: a study and report of 217 cases. Pediatrics 23:1179, 1959

228. Hawthorne HC Jr: Blanching subcutaneous nodules in neonatal neuroblastoma. J Pediatr 77:297, 1970

229. Koop CE: The neuroblastoma. Prog Pediatr Surg 4:1, 1972

230. Schneider KE, Becker JM, Krasna IH: Neonatal neuroblastoma. Pediatrics 36:359, 1965

231. Shanklin DR, Sotelo-Avila C: In situ tumors in fetuses, newborns and young infants. Biol Neonate 14:316, 1969

232. Sutow W: Prognosis of neuroblastoma in childhood. J Dis Child 96:269, 1958

233. Thurman WG, Donaldson MH: Neoplasia of Childhood. Chicago, Year Book Med Pub, 1967, p 176

234. Von Studnitz W, Kaser H, Sjoerdsma A:

Spectrum of catecholamine biochemistry in patients with neuroblastoma. N Engl J Med 269:232, 1963

235. Voûte PA Jr, Wadman SK, Putten WJ van: Congenital neuroblastoma. Symptoms in the mother during pregnancy. Clin Pediatr 9:206, 1970

236. Wells HG: Occurrence and significance of congenital malignant neoplasms. Arch Path 30:535, 1940

237. Williams CM, Greer M: Homovanillic acid and vanilmandelic acid in diagnosis of neuroblastoma. JAMA 183:836, 1963

238. Young RB, Steiker DD, Bongiovanni AM, Koop CE, Eberlein WR: Urinary vanilmandelic acid (VMA) excretion in children: use of a simple semiquantitative test. J Pediatr 62:844, 1963

Abdominal Masses

239. Benson CD, Reiners CR: Asymptomatic masses in infants and children. Arch Surg 76:688, 1959

240. Boles ET Jr: Tumors of the abdomen in children. Pediatr Clin North Am 9:467, 1962

241. Hendren WH: Abdominal masses in newborn infants. Am J Surg 107:502, 1964

242. Longino LA, Martin LW: Abdominal masses in the newborn infant. Pediatrics 21:596, 1958

243. Wedge JJ, Grosfeld JL, Smith JP: Abdominal masses in the newborn: 63 cases. J Urol 106:770, 1971

Cystic Kidney Disease

244. Goodyear WE, Beard DE: Unilateral multicystic kidney in infancy. Am J Dis Child 76:203, 1948

245. Gwinn JL, Landing BH: Cystic diseases of the kidneys in infants and children. Radiol Clin North Am 6:191, 1968

246. Hoeffel JC, Jacottin G, Bourgeois JM: Classification of renal cysts in children. Aust Paediatr J 6:123, 1970

247. Johnston JH: Renal cystic disease in childhood. Prog. Pediatr Surg 2:99, 1971

248. Spence HM: Congenital unilateral multicystic kidney: an entity to be distinguished from polycystic disease and other cystic disorders. J Urol 74:693, 1955

GENITOURINARY TRACT

Obstructive Uropathies

249. Ellis DG, Fonkalsrud EW, Smith PJ: Congenital posterior urethral valves. J Urol 95:549, 1966

250. Hendren WH: A new approach to infants with severe obstructive uropathy: early complete reconstruction. J Pediatr Surg 5:184, 1970

251. Hendren WH: Recent advances in the management of low urinary obstruction in the newborn. Prog Pediatr Surg 2:115, 1971

252. Nesbit RM, Labardini MM: Urethral valves in the male child. J Urol 96:218, 1966

253. Waldbaum RS, Marshall VF: Posterior urethral valves: evaluation and surgical management. J Urol 103:807, 1970

254. Waterhouse K, Hamm FC: The importance of urethral valves as a cause of vesical neck obstruction in children. Trans Am Assoc Genitourin Surg 53:138, 1961

255. Waterhouse K: Personal communication, 1973

Prune Belly Syndrome (Abdominal Musculature Deficiency)

256. Bruton OC: Agenesis is abdominal musculature associated with genitourinary and gastrointestinal tract anomalies. J Urol 66:607, 1951

257. Eagle JF Jr, Barrett GS: Congenital deficiency of abdominal musculature with associated genitourinary abnormalities: a syndrome; report of 9 cases. Pediatrics 6:721, 1950

258. Gellis SS, Feringold M: Congenital absence of abdominal muscles (prune belly). Am J Dis Child 109:571, 1965

259. McGovern JH, Marshall VF: Congenital deficiency of abdominal musculature and obstructive uropathy. Surg Gynecol Obstet 108:289, 1959

260. Waldbaum RS, Marshall VF: The prune belly syndrome: a diagnostic therapeutic plan. J Urol 103:668, 1970

Bladder Exstrophy

261. Caskie JD, Borski AA: One-stage plastic repair of exstrophy of bladder combined with bilateral osteotomy of the ilia. J Bone Joint Surg 45A:161, 1963

262. Johnston JH: Exstrophy of the bladder. Prog Pediatr Surg 2:171, 1971

263. Marshall VF, Muecke EC: Functional closure of typical exstrophy of the bladder. J Urol 104:205, 1970

264. Shultz WG: Plastic repair of exstrophy of the bladder combined with bilateral osteotomy of the ilia. J Urol 79:453, 1958

265. Swenson O, Moussatos GH, Fisher JH: Results of repair of exstrophy of the bladder. Surg Clin North Am 43:151, 1963

266. Symposium on treatment of complete exstrophy of the urinary bladder. Ann Chir Infant 6:359, 1971

267. Williams DI, Savage J: Reconstruction of the exstrophied bladder. Br J Surg 53:168, 1966

NEUROSURGICAL PROBLEMS

General

268. Matson DD: Neurosurgery of Infancy and Childhood. Springfield, Ill, CC Thomas, 1969

Trauma

269. Cleveland D: Skull fracture and craniocerebral injuries. In: Fractures in Children. Edited by WP Blount. Baltimore, Williams & Wilkins, 1954

270. Kendall N, Woloshin H: Cephalhematoma associated with fracture of skull. J Pediatr 41: 125, 1952

Hydrocephalus

271. Carney A, George DB, Simpson DA: Long-term results in the treatment of hydrocephalus. Proc Paediatr Surg Cong (Melbourne) 1:65, 1970 (cited in J Pediatr Surg 6:515, 1971)

272. Hemmer R: Complications of ventriculo-atrial shunts and their prevention. Z Kinder Chir 5:1, 1967

273. Murtagh F, Lehman R: Peritoneal shunts in the management of hydrocephalus. JAMA 202: 1010, 1967

274. Overton MC III, Snodgrass SR: Ventriculo-venous shunts for infantile hydrocephalus: a review of five years' experience with this method. J Neurosurg 23:517, 1965

275. Pudenz RH: The ventriculo-atrial shunt. J Neurosurg 25:602, 1966

276. Schick RW, Matson DD: What is arrested hydrocephalus? J Pediatr 58:791, 1961

277. Tsingoglou S, Forrest DM: Complications from Holter ventriculo-atrial shunts. Br J Surg 58:372, 1971

278. Yashon D: Prognosis of infantile hydrocephalus: past and present. J Neurosurg 20: 105, 1963

Craniosynostosis

279. McLaurin RL, Matson DD: Importance of early surgical treatment of craniosynostosis: review of 36 cases treated during the first 6 months of life. Pediatrics 10:637, 1952

280. Mount LA: Premature closure of sutures of cranial vault. A plea for early recognition and early operation. NY State J Med 47:270, 1947

Spina Bifida and Cranium Bifidum

281. Bunch WH, Cass AS, Bensman AS, Long DM: Modern Management of Myelomeningocele. St Louis, Warren H. Green, 1972

282. Lipschitz R, Beck JM, Froman C: An assessment of the treatment of encephalomeningocoeles. S Afr Med J 43:609, 1969

283. Rickham PP, Mawdsley T: The effect of early operation on the survival of spina bifida cystica. Dev Med Child Neurol (Suppl) 11:20, 1966

284. Sharrard WJW, Zachary RB, Lorber J, Bruce AM: A controlled trial of immediate and delayed closure of spina bifida cystica. Arch Dis Child 38:18, 1963

285. Symposium on Myelomeningocele. American Academy of Orthopedic Surgeons (Hartford, Conn., Nov. 1970). St Louis, Mosby, 1972

286. Walker AE, Bucy PC: Congenital dermal sinuses: a source of spinal meningeal infection and subdural abscesses. Brain 57:401, 1934

287. Zachary RB: Recent advances in the management of myelomeningoceles. Prog Pediatr Surg 2:155, 1971

ORTHOPEDIC PROBLEMS

Fracture

288. Altman DH, Smith RL: Unrecognized trauma in infants and children. J Bone Joint Surg 42A:407, 1960

289. Ferguson AB Jr: Orthopedic Surgery in Infancy and Childhood, ed 3. Baltimore, Williams & Wilkins, 1968

290. Truesdell ED: Birth Fractures and Epiphyseal Dislocations. New York, Paul B Hoeber, Inc, 1917

Congenital Dislocation of Hip

291. Andren L, von Rosen S: The diagnosis of dislocation of the hip in newborns and the primary results of immediate treatment. Acta Radiol 49:89, 1958

292. Badgley CE: Correlation of clinical and anatomical parts leading to a conception of the etiology of congenital hip dislocation. J Bone Joint Surg 31A:341, 1949

293. Barlow TG: Early diagnosis and treatment of congenital dislocation of the hip. J Bone Joint Surg 44B:292, 1962

294. Bost FC, Hagey H, Schottstaedt ER, Larsen LJ: The results of treatment of congenital dislocation of the hip in infancy. J Bone Joint Surg 30A:454, 1948

295. Carter C, Wilkinson J: Persistent joint laxity and congenital dislocation of the hip. J Bone Joint Surg 46B:40, 1964

296. Ortolani M: Un segno poco noto e sua importanza per la diagnosi precoce di prelussazione congenita dell'anca. Pediatria (Napoli) 45:129, 1937

297. von Rosen S: Diagnosis and treatment of congenital dislocation of the hip joint in the newborn. J Bone Joint Surg 44B:284, 1962

298. von Rosen S: Further experience with congenital dislocation of the hip in the newborn. J Bone Joint Surg 50B:538, 1968

299. Wynne-Davies R: Acetabular dysplasia and familial joint laxity: two etiological factors in congenital dislocation of the hip: review of 589 patients and their families. J Bone Joint Surg 52B:704, 1970

Congenital Talipes Equinovarus (ClubFoot)

300. Ferguson AB Jr: Orthopedic Surgery in Infancy and childhood, ed 3. Baltimore, Williams & Wilkins, 1968

301. Salter RB: Congenital malformations of the lower extremities. In: Pediatric Surgery, 2nd ed. Edited by WT Mustard, MM Ravitch, WH Snyder Jr, KJ Welch, CD Benson. Chicago: Year Book Med Pub, 1969

Anomalies of Extremities

302. Conway H, Bowe J: Congenital deformities of the hands. Plast Reconstr Surg 18:286, 1956

303. Frantz CH, O'Rahilly R: Congenital skeletal limb deficiencies. J Bone Joint Surg 43A:1202, 1961

304. Kanavel AB: Congenital malformations of the hand. Arch Surg 25:1, 1932

305. Patterson TJS: Classification of the congenitally deformed hand. Br J Plast Surg 17:142, 1964

306. Patterson TJS: Congenital anomalies of the hand and upper extremity. In: Plastic Surgery: a concise guide to clinical practice. Edited by WC Grabb, JW Smith. Boston, Little, Brown, 1968

307. Smithells RW: Thalidomide and malformations in Liverpool. Lancet 1:1270, 1962

Nerve Injuries

308. Bonney GLW: Prognosis in traction lesions of the brachial plexus. J Bone Joint Surg 41B:4, 1959

309. Craig WS, Clark JMP: Peripheral nerve palsies in the newly born. J Obstet Gynaecol Br Commonw 65:229, 1958

310. Wolman B: Erb's palsy. Arch Dis Child 23:129, 1948

311. Wickstrom J: Birth injuries of the brachial plexus: treatment of defects in the shoulder. Clin Orthop 23:187, 1962

24

Special
Problems
of
Neonatal
Radiology

WALTER E. BERDON

There are two major problems in the radiographic examination of neonates. The first is technical: obtaining radiographs of diagnostic quality on small patients, frequently utilizing portable equipment. The second is to determine if abnormalities are indeed present; this requires a knowledge of the "range of normal," an area still not precisely defined. Thus mistakes continue; normal findings are called abnormal, and abnormalities are overlooked as normal findings.

This chapter will emphasize important helpful technical points and stress important areas. For a complete review the reader can find recent references in the bibliography. The latter is limited to only a few references, but they, in turn, contain comprehensive reviews of the recent literature.

CHEST

Applying the above criteria to problems of interpreting neonatal films, the chest is certainly the most difficult. Not only is it hard to know what observed densities represent in films of critically ill infants, but technically this represents the area where the equipment usually has to be brought to the patient. Most films are still taken with portable equipment; even so, it is possible with care to obtain adequate films in noncrying infants taken without *motion* (the single most important technical point) in frontal and lateral views. With collimation to screen off the gonadal areas, it is nevertheless important to include examination of the neck and upper abdomen, since apparent chest disease may relate to both upper airway problems and intraabdominal catastrophies.

LUNG FLUID

Fetal lungs are partially fluid filled; with parturition, this fluid must be displaced and replaced by air. Most of this exchange is probably caused by compression of the tracheobronchial tree and chest during vaginal delivery, the rest being resorbed by veins and lymphatics. Films taken in the first hours of life give the greatest problem of interpretation since they frequently show a pattern that looks like pulmonary edema, with marked vascular congestion, fluid in the fissures and what looks like mild cardiomegaly (Fig. 24–1). Some of these infants are ill, and others have tachypnea, while many seem clinically normal. These patients and their x-ray films create controversy about transient tachypnea, "wet" lung syndrome and atypical respiratory distress syndrome (RDS). We believe that these problems are resolved by the infant's clinical course rather than the interpretation of any specific pattern on one single film.

Respiratory Distress Syndrome (RDS)

Contrasted with this nonspecific vascular engorgement pattern is the clear-cut x ray of a typical patient with RDS. Fine granular densities extend symmetrically through both lung fields, and an air bronchogram pattern extends out into the lung fields (Fig. 24–2). Overinflation of the thorax is *not* usually a feature of this disease. With the utilization of continuous distending airway pressure, complications of treatment have begun to appear on chest radiographs. These include the fine bubbles of interstitial pulmonary emphysema on the first and second day (Fig. 24–3) and the later-appearing, larger bubbly areas of so-called bronchopulmonary dysplasia, representing true emphysema, side by side with areas of atelectasis.

Interstitial Emphysema and Free Air

Interstitial pulmonary emphysema is a warning that the patient may be in the process of developing tension pneumothorax, pneumomediastinum, pneumopericardium and even pneumoperitoneum, in the form of a chronic, ongoing air leak. When tension pneumothorax develops in such infants diaphragmatic inversion rather than lung collapse occurs (Fig. 24–4). This reflects the decreased compliance of the lung that prevents complete collapse.

The more chronic emphysematous changes of bronchopulmonary dysplasia are probably the end result of a variety of problems, including oxygen therapy, and in the Babies Hospital have been observed much more frequently than the idiopathic bubbly lungs described by Mikity and Wilson. Any discussion of these raises the question of magnification chest films (Fig. 24–2) since

this would seem the ideal way to carefully examine the fine bubbles and other features. Unfortunately, in the past, magnification equipment has been available only within main x-ray departments. Currently (1975) portable equipment with a 0.3-mm focus spot is being devised so that magnification films can be taken in any nursery, as long as the infant can be placed half-way between the x-ray tube and the x-ray film, with an air gap below the patient equal to the air gap between the tube and the patient. We believe that good quality conventional films will give adequate information to plan treatment on these babies without using magnification, the latter being reserved for specialized centers and for teaching purposes.

/ The combination of pulmonary interstitial emphysema and tension pneumothorax has emerged as a problem in the treatment of RDS. This is distinguished from the more benign form of pneumomediastinum seen in full-term babies who have aspirated meconium and have over-distended lungs with flat diaphragms and large thoracic cages. Presumably, their pneumonediastinum arises from areas of interstitial pulmonary emphysema, but the latter can only be appreciated if there is diffuse disease surrounding the bubbles. In the typical case of meconium aspiration it is not possible to see where the air is leaking from in the lungs. Pneumomediastinum in these cases is best seen on lateral views as a large, retrosternal translucent area (Fig. 24–5). Subcutaneous emphysema is uncommon in this age group.

Occasionally, the occurrence of pneumothorax and pneumomediastinum is a sign that the infants have a form of Potter's syndrome, due either to renal agenesis or to severe urologic obstructive malformations associated with oligohydramnios. For this reason, intravenous pyelograms (IVPs) and cystograms should be considered in newborn infants with severe signs of air block.

Placement of Tubes and Catheters

One important aspect of chest films in critically ill neonates concerns the placement of endotracheal tubes and umbilical catheters; both clinician and radiologist should look at

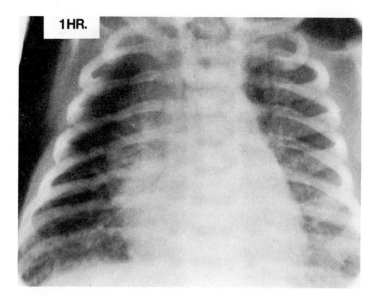

FIG. 24–1. One-hour-old infant with no significant respiratory distress. The "vascular engorgement" resembling pulmonary edema may represent areas of unabsorbed fetal lung fluid and/or areas of incomplete expansion of alveoli or both. (Courtesy of Dr. L. S. James)

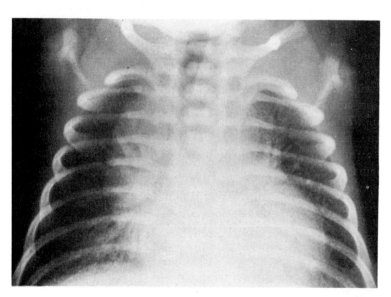

FIG. 24–2. Newborn infant with typical "respiratory distress syndrome" (i.e., hyaline membrane disease). Fine granular densities and air bronchogram pattern are typical. Original film 14x14 in. by magnification technique with 0.31-mm focal spot. (Courtesy of Dr. R. Ablow)

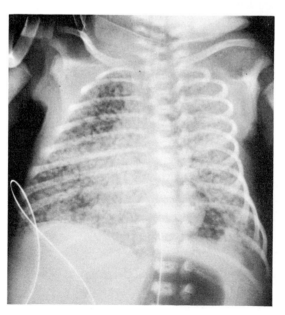

FIG. 24–3. Thirty-six-hour-old infant treated with continuous lung distending pressures who developed pulmonary interstitial emphysema complicating respiratory distress syndrome. Small lucent areas in perivascular spaces and lymphatics represent interstitial air.

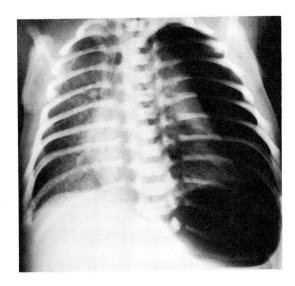

FIG. 24–4. Infant with respiratory distress syndrome. Diaphragmatic inversion is evidence of left tension pneumothorax since lung is so stiff it does not readily collapse.

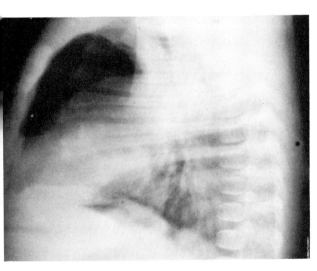

FIG. 24–5. Pneumomediastinum seen as retrosternal air space in infant with meconium aspiration syndrome. Aspiration of air was not required.

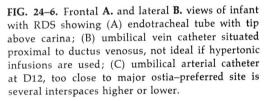

FIG. 24–6. Frontal **A.** and lateral **B.** views of infant with RDS showing (A) endotracheal tube with tip above carina; (B) umbilical vein catheter situated proximal to ductus venosus, not ideal if hypertonic infusions are used; (C) umbilical arterial catheter at D12, too close to major ostia–preferred site is several interspaces higher or lower.

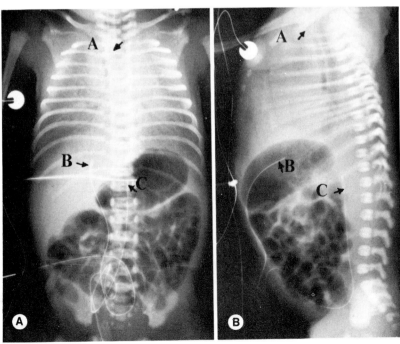

films in two projections and the tip of each tube should be identified for proper placement (Fig. 24–6).

STRUCTURAL ANOMALIES ASSOCIATED WITH RESPIRATORY DISTRESS

Heart Disease

The only comment on heart disease to be made is that the most severe anomalies, such as hypoplastic left heart syndrome, may have surprisingly few radiographic findings. The largest hearts in newborn infants can be seen in patients *without* intrinsic heart disease, as in cardiac dilatation secondary to large extracardiac shunts (e.g., CNS and liver–Figs. 24–7A, 24–7B) or in cases of fetal hypoxia. The thymus can also widen the apparent cardiac size and may lead to a false diagnosis or cardiomegaly.

FIG. 24–7. Huge heart in infant with heart failure secondary to arteriovenous shunting through hepatic hemangioma. Umbilical aortogram shows arteriovenous shunts in liver.

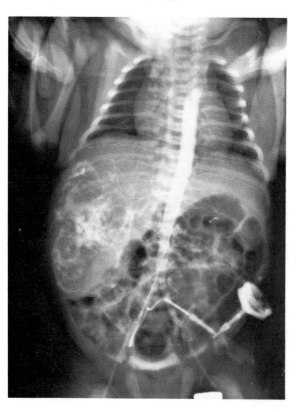

Surgical Causes

Surgical causes of respiratory distress, especially esophageal atresia as well as diaphragmatic hernia, are the *main* reason for taking chest films in the neonate. Diaphragmatic hernia usually occurs on the left side with the liver and small bowel loops herniated into the left hemithorax. In the sickest infants, the bowel loops may not be air-filled (Fig. 24–8A). Injection of air through a nasogastric tube is a useful technique in such patients. Hopefully, this will identify bowel loops in the chest (Fig. 24–8B). If an umbilical venous catheter has been passed, urographic contrast material can be injected and branches of the portal venous system in the chest outlined, again making the diagnosis quite easy.

Bony Structures

Examination of the chest should include inspection of bony structures. This will identify the baby with a constrictively small thorax whose asphyxial state represents the thoracic dystrophy of Jeune. Other bony causes of respiratory distress include multiple rib fractures in osteogenesis imperfecta.

GENITOURINARY

THE INTRAVENOUS PYELOGRAM (IVP)

The major technical differences between older children and neonates in the examination of the urinary tract relates to the rapidly changing glomerular and tubular function in the latter group. It has proven necessary to increase the IVP dose of contrast medium to almost 3 ml/kg in *well-hydrated* neonates in order to obtain adequate urograms. This experience led to the realization that such doses are safe and also emphasized the importance of keeping the patient well hydrated. Such urograms may require a 30- to 60-minute period to obtain adequate concentration in the kidneys. Renal outlines are difficult to see in neonates because of the

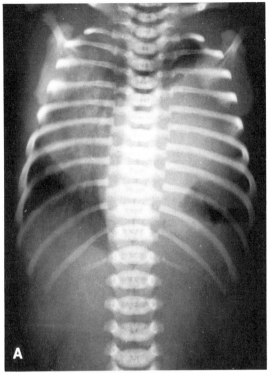

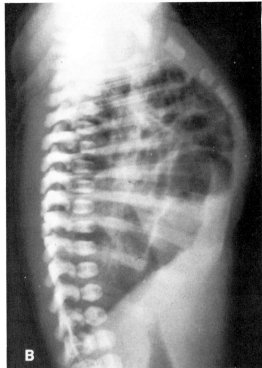

FIG. 24–8. **A.** Left-sided diaphragmatic hernia–herniated small bowel not filled with air in this depressed infant. Note gasless abdomen and mediastinal shift to right. If in doubt, diagnosis can be confirmed by putting air through nasogastric tube. **B.** Typical lateral view of scaphoid abdomen and loops of bowel in chest in infant with left-sided diaphragmatic hernia.

absence of perirenal fat. All overlying bowel gas is resolved in the obtaining of one or two laminographic sections at 3 or 4-cm levels, which will blur out bowel gas and show calyceal anatomy quite well.

The newborn infant handles the contrast agent in several ways. In one group there may be good visualization of the kidneys after the injection of from 5 to 10 ml of contrast medium; no special techniques are needed in such patients although the prone position is valuable in displacing obscuring bowel gas. A second group may fail to concentrate even 10 ml of contrast material, yet this group may prove to have normal IVPs when the study is repeated at one to two weeks of age. For this reason screening IVPs in patients with other anomalies but without GU signs are best deferred to at least one week of age in order to avoid repetition of the study. Why 3 ml/kg should fail to outline renal structures is not clear. Such a dose in an adult would reach 200 ml (as opposed to the usual 30 to 60 ml in use as a standard IVP dose for adults).

A third group deserves comment. Such infants may have a history of slightly enlarged kidneys or of passing urine loaded with casts. Their IVPs show bladder opacification, and normal calyces can be seen (Fig. 24–9). The picture is dominated by a progressive stasis of contrast material in the tubules. This can be diffuse (Fig. 24–9) or spotty (Fig. 24–10) in content, slightly simulating polycystic kidneys. However, the patients do not have renal impairment on a follow-up study, and the kidneys are normal on serial IVPs; the main diagnostic challenge is to avoid labeling such patients as having "sponge kidneys" or obstructed kidneys. Speculation on the mechanism has included tubular stasis of urates, urinary glycoprotein or impaired renal circulation.

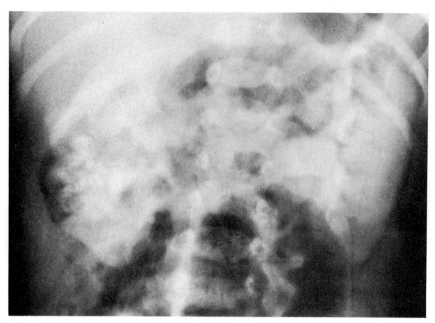

FIG. 24–9. Nephrogram of newborn infant showing symmetric bilateral "stasis." Kidneys are normal in size and excretion adequate of contrast occurred with filling of bladder. This should not be confused with renal tubular necrosis or polycystic kidney disease.

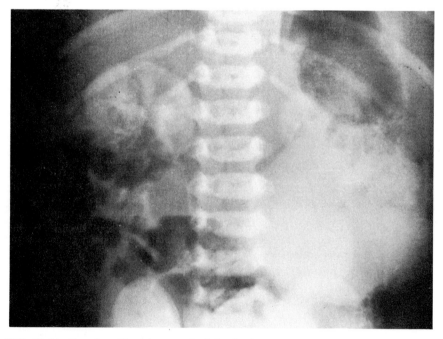

FIG. 24–10. One-day-old infant with left flank mass. Right stasis nephrogram (spotty distribution) with left ureteropelvic junction obstruction. Right kidney totally normal on repeat IVP next day.

Mild cases may pass unnoticed unless delayed films happen to be obtained. Our own cases have not gone on to renal papillary or tubular or cortical necrosis, although others claim this has occurred.

The neonatal stasis nephrogram can be considered as a radiographically abnormal but pathologically nonserious finding in most cases—hydration and time usually "open up the kidneys." One should not resort to unnecessary and potentially dangerous studies such as retrograde pyelograms or aortograms; we have seen lethal complications of such studies in this group of patients.

ABDOMINAL MASSES

The finding of an abdominal mass in a newborn infant should lead to obtaining an IVP as the basic screening examination because most such masses relate to the urinary tract in the form of either a hydronephrotic kidney (Fig. 26–10) or a multicystic kidney. The former shows function in the form of parenchymal rims and calyceal crescents, usually with final visualization of the hydronephrotic renal pelvis (the most common site of obstruction being at the ureteropelvic junction). Multicystic kidney merely shows a bunching of bubbly lucencies on the early films as a reflection of the "total body opacification" phenomenon. There is no function in the usual case.

Renal Tumors

Emergency surgery need no longer be mandatory for newborn retroperitoneal masses for fear of missing a Wilms' tumor since it has become apparent that newborn renal tumors are usually benign hamartomas. Radiographic techniques start with urograms, but umbilical angiography can be used to outline the vascular supply to such masses (Fig. 24–11). It should be emphasized that in interpreting angiograms "neovascularity" is a sign only of the vascular nature of the mass and not of whether it is benign or malignant.

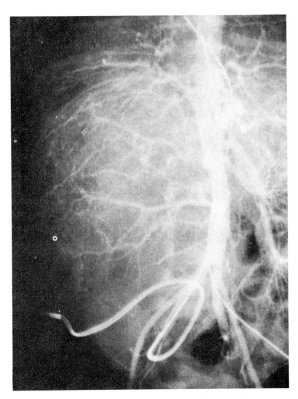

FIG. 24–11. Right flank mass in newborn infant. Umbilical aortogram shows two renal arteries supplying tumor circulation. (IVP had shown distorted calyces in upper pole of mass.) Pathology was benign hamartoma, not a Wilms' tumor.

Another mass involving the GU system is adrenal hemorrhage, which can be unilateral or bilateral. This may present with jaundice due to breakdown of blood pigments within the hematoma. A typical case shows flattening of the top of the kidney and displacement of the kidney laterally and inferiorly. Total body films show a large lucent suprarenal mass (Figs. 24–12A, 24–12B). Within a few days the mass changes size and shape and calcifications begin to appear. Ultrasonography may be of help in showing the mass to be essentially echo free. In the usual case, surgery can be avoided because of radiographic and clinical findings compatible with adrenal hemorrhage. The problem case may require exploration and biopsy in order to exclude a neuroblastoma.

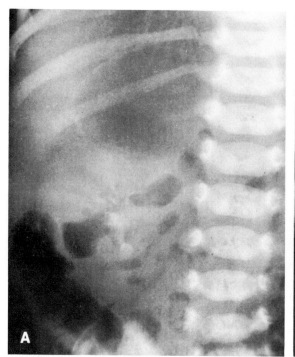 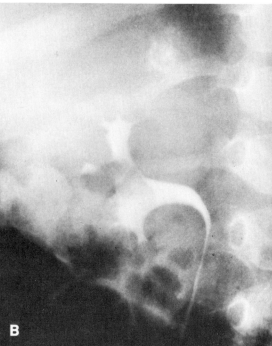

FIG. 24–12. A. Right flank mass in eight-day-old infant. Right kidney flattened and displaced slightly down and laterally. Suprarenal mass has faint calcific rim and "lucent" center due to avascularity. B-mode ultrasonogram was echo free, indicative of cystic nature. Diagnosis made of adrenal hemorrhage; no operation. **B.** Same patient one year later. Mass gone with small calcified area in adrenal; adrenal function normal.

LOWER GENITOURINARY (GU) TRACT

Posterior Urethral Valves

Lower urinary tract obstruction in the newborn infant is a significant problem. The most frequent diagnosis in the male is posterior urethral valves (Figs. 24–13A, 24–13B). Such patients may have typical findings of a large bladder and tubular masses in the flanks representing dilated ureters. Cases in which the urinary tract is ruptured and there is both retroperitoneal and intra-abdominal urine create a much more difficult diagnostic problem. Any newborn male with ascites should be evaluated in terms of posterior urethral valves being the most likely diagnosis. Voiding cystourethrography is the key diagnostic procedure (Fig. 24–13A), and

we believe it should precede the IVP (Fig. 24–13B) in such patients, as it immediately reveals whether valves are present and whether there is massive reflux.

Ureterocele

Ectopic ureterocele usually presents with similar abdominal findings with masses in the flank representing dilated ureters. This condition is more common in females. Characteristic findings are of large lucent masses within the bladder representing the terminal portion of the massively dilated ureters. An IVP may show displacement of the lower poles of one or both kidneys by the hydronephrotic upper poles, the latter leading to the ureterocele. Well-performed cystograms and IVPs should permit this diagnosis to be made with certainty.

"Prune Belly" Syndrome

The prune belly syndrome (undescended testes, hydroureters and abnormal kidneys and defective abdominal wall musculature) shows a spectrum of renal abnormalities

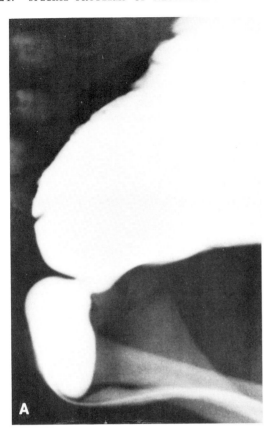

FIG. 24–13. **A.** Lateral voiding cystogram in male newborn infant with bladder felt up to umbilicus; typical ballooned posterior urethra secondary to obstructing valves; valves per se not visualized. Note tiny caliber of urethra just below dilated segment. Reflux not present to ureters. **B.** IVP shows rims and crescents of hydronephrosis on one-minute film. Delayed film shows dilated ureters down to bladder.

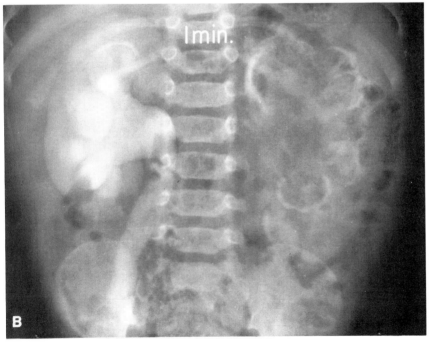

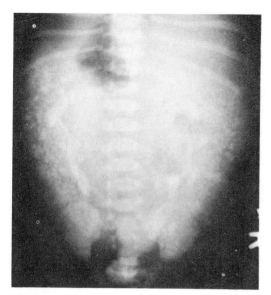

FIG. 24–14. Polycystic kidneys. Streaky nephrogram is seen in huge kidneys. Patient lived despite azotemia and hypertension.

ranging from nonfunction and Potter's syndrome to hydronephrosis to normal function. Clinical diagnosis is evident in most cases.

Renal Polycystic Disease

Bilateral polycystic kidneys are rare. They present as bilateral flank masses and are visualized on urograms if there are sufficient functioning nephrons. A streaky nephrographic pattern develops (Fig. 24–14) and cystic dilated tubules finally fill and may trap contrast material for as long as a week. The most severely involved patients present with Potter's syndrome, hypoplastic lungs, pneumothorax and pneumomediastinum; less severely involved patients may survive for months or even years.

Renal Vascular Insults

The newborn infant may have vascular insults to the kidneys as well as to the adrenals. This can include renal vein thrombosis, which may be suspected when a mass rapidly develops and is associated with hematuria and a nonfunctioning kidney. Contrast material injected into a leg vein will show clots

extending into the vena cava. Umbilical angiography is available to study the renal arterial supply to the kidneys. Renal cortical and tubular necrosis usually presents with nonfunctioning kidneys and if the patient survives papillary necrosis and even cortical calcification may develop.

GASTROINTESTINAL (GI)

INTESTINAL OBSTRUCTION

Immediate problems in neonates with gastrointestinal tract disorders usually re-

FIG. 24–15. Esophageal atresia. The wrong way to outline the proximal pouch: the infant was fed by bottle and aspirated huge amounts of contrast that was well handled. (Barium has proven safer than water soluble agents in this area). Gasless abdomen shows absence of fistula between tracheo-bronchial tree and distal esophagus.

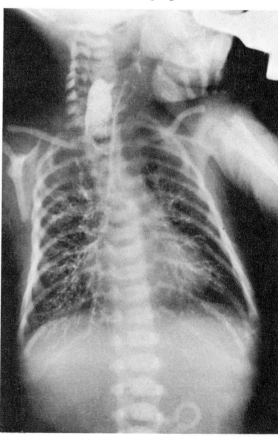

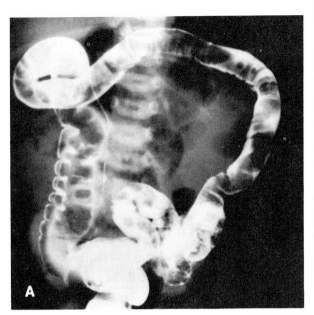

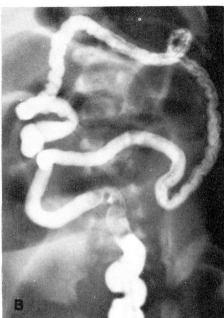

FIG. 24–16. A. Aganglionosis of entire colon in infant with dilated small bowel loops. Note that colon is not tiny as in usual organic distal small bowel obstruction. B. Distal small bowel obstruction due to inspissated meconium in meconium ileus of fibrocystic disease. Note the "microcolon." C. Lethal colitis in unrecognized Hirschsprung's disease of the usual low sigmoid transition. Note that colitis (ulcers, edematous mucosa) is in "normal" (i.e., ganglionic) bowel while aganglionic rectum is spared.

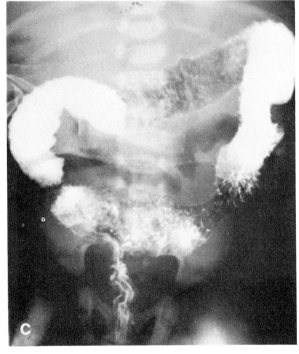

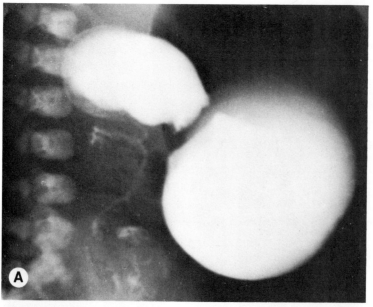

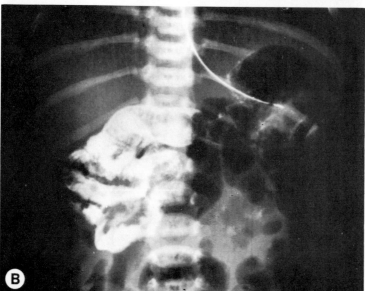

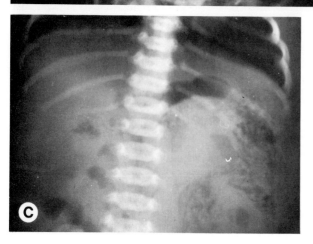

FIG. 24–17. **A.** Malrotation and volvulus–almost total lumen obstruction of duodenum. Note the spiral course of unfixed duodenojejunal junction that is diagnostic of malrotation. **B.** Malrotation and volvulus–partial lumen obstruction of duodenum with edematous jejunal loops due to venous engorgement. **C.** Gangrene of small bowel due to unrecognized malrotation. Bubbles of gas through upper abdomen represents gas in wall of infarcted bowel.

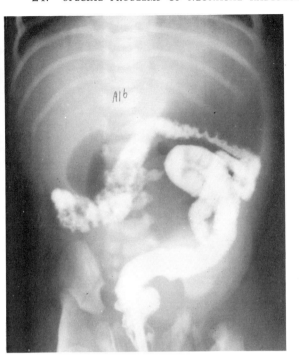

FIG. 24–18. Barium enema showing malrotation in infant with total duodenal obstruction. The upper GI series obviously cannot be used to check for malrotation when there is total duodenal obstruction.

prefer the latter route since it allows us to control the study more carefully. All fluoroscopy should be performed with an image intensifier; 70-mm spot film recording has proved ideal for us as applied in this situation.

Obstruction is assessed by size and number of the distended loops. The more numerous the loops, the lower the obstruction. Colonic examination is utilized to distinguish those patients with intrinsic colon disease (such as Hirschsprung's disease) where at least part of the colon will be dilated from those infants whose obstruction is above the colon in the lower small bowel. In the latter situation, colon size will range from almost normal in the case of total Hirschsprung's disease (Fig. 24–16A) to the microcolon in fibrocystic disease (Fig. 24–16B). Unrecognized Hirschsprung's disease can lead to a lethal colitis (Fig. 24–16C).

MALROTATION AND MALFIXATION

The only true GI surgical emergency in the newborn infant is malrotation with midgut volvulus, and for that reason this anomaly will be discussed in some detail.

Malrotation is a poor term, a better term being malfixation. These babies have a small bowel literally "hanging around" the superior mesenteric artery without adequate fixation at the ligament of Treitz or in the right lower quadrant. If volvulus occurs, not only is there luminal duodenal obstruction with bilious vomiting (Fig. 24–17A), there is also vascular obstruction (Fig. 24–17B), and unless the diagnosis is readily made the midgut may become gangrenous (Fig. 24–17C). For that reason, any infant who vomits bile should have abdominal films taken to see if there is any evidence of midintestinal obstruction. Even if the films appear normal, bilious vomiting is an indication for performing a contrast study. Identification of the malrotation and malfixation can be done either by barium enema or by upper GI series. The enema studies are utilized not only to exclude microcolon and Hirschsprung's disease in the infant who is vomiting bile, but to ascertain that

late to *total* obstructions in the form of atretic segments. The higher the obstruction, the more likely a maternal history of hydramnios. Obstructions located in the stomach, duodenum and proximal small bowel usually do not require positive contrast studies since air is an excellent contrast agent. Esophageal obstruction, on the other hand, can be studied with carefully performed contrast studies of the proximal pouch to see if there is a proximal pouch fistula and to ascertain the level of the pouch (Fig. 24–15).

As a general point of technique, no infant should be studied with contrast material unless fluoroscopy is available. Barium contrast agents should be used rather than water-soluble agents in investigation of the upper gastrointestinal tract since the aspiration of water-soluble material by vomiting or through an H fistula can rapidly produce pulmonary edema. The barium can be given by bottle or through a nasogastric tube; we

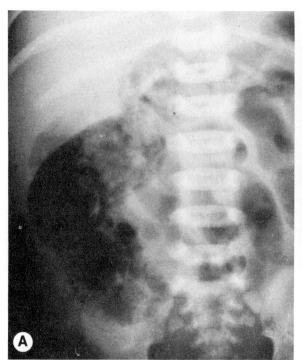

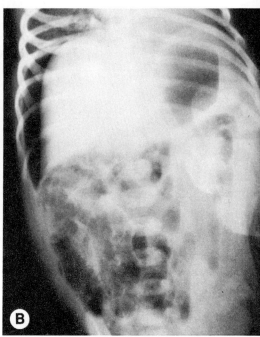

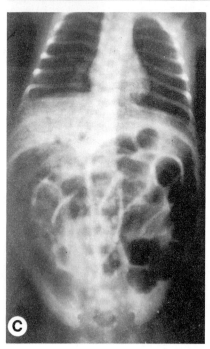

FIG. 24–19. A. Necrotizing enterocolitis–distal loops in right lower abdomen with intramural air. **B.** Necrotizing enterocolitis–free air seen in right flank on left lateral decubitus film. Note the intramural air in right lower quadrant loops. (Courtesy of Dr. A. Shaw) **C.** Necrotizing enterocolitis. Note the air in intrahepatic radicles of portal vein. Perforated ileum was found at necropsy.

the cecum is in its normal position in the right lower quadrant (Fig. 24–18). The detection of a cecum high on the right side or in the midline in an infant vomiting bile suggests malrotation as the basic problem.

We have increasingly utilized the upper GI series to evaluate malrotation and malfixation. Partial duodenal obstruction should be looked for (Fig. 24–17B). The single most important finding is the identification of the duodenojejunal junction. Normally this is on the left, about the same level as the duodenal bulb; a lower than normal duodenojejunal junction with a jejunum that passes downward and to the right (Figs. 24–17A, 24–17B) is diagnostic of malfixation and should lead to emergency surgical consultation in order to evaluate the possibility of malrotation and volvulus. Some of the sickest infants have the most benign plain films and for that reason contrast studies are mandatory in the infant who vomits bile.

NECROTIZING ENTEROCOLITIS

The final area of newborn GI pathology that deserves detailed discussion is necrotizing enterocolitis. Whether this represents a breakdown in immunologic defenses of the premature infant's bowel with bacteria entering the wall, or whether this is an ischemic disease is not clear. Such infants present with abdominal distension, blood-streaked stools and bile emesis; their radiographs show small bowel distension, bubbles and strips of intramural gas and occasionally perforation (Fig. 24–19A, 24–19B) or air extending through the venous drainage of the small bowel into the portal radicals of the liver. This is a highly lethal clinical situation. Interestingly, many

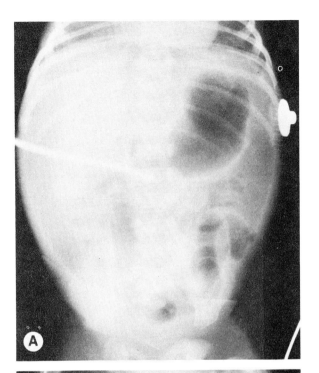

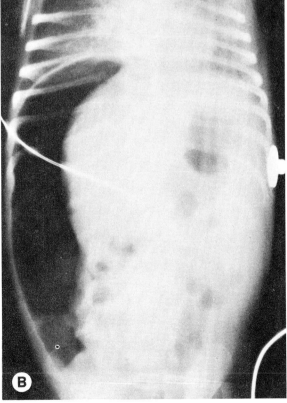

FIG. 24–20. Ileal perforation. **A.** Supine film shows free air as bulging flanks, vague lucency over abdomen with curved white line of falciform ligament slightly to right of midline over liver area. **B.** Left lateral decubitus position shows free air rising to right flank. This 850-gm premature survived following surgery.

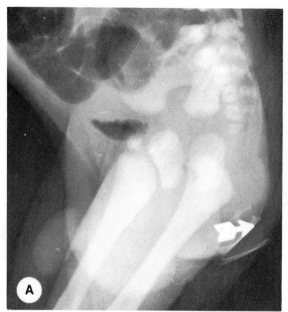
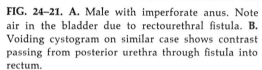
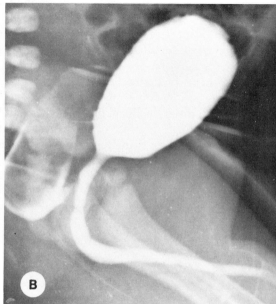

FIG. 24–21. A. Male with imperforate anus. Note air in the bladder due to rectourethral fistula. **B.** Voiding cystogram on similar case shows contrast passing from posterior urethra through fistula into rectum.

of our cases have their abdominal findings detected on chest films taken for apneic episodes, which emphasizes the point made previously that at least the upper abdomen be included on chest radiographs.

Massive perforation is readily diagnosed when free air is observed under the diaphragm. If, however, the infant is examined in the supine position, the physician should be aware of the findings of free air in this projection. This includes outlining the falciform ligament by air on either side of it (Fig. 24–20A). The "football" sign refers to the stitching of the football represented by the falciform ligament and the bulging flanks creating the football shape. We have preferred using decubitus films with the infant lying on the left side, the right side elevated and the x-ray beam horizontal (Fig. 24–20B). This will allow free air to be seen in the right flank, and at the same time, the liver can be studied to see if there is air within the branches consistent with necrotizing enterocolitis and to see if there are

dilated loops, air/fluid levels or intramural air.

ANORECTAL MALFORMATIONS

Anal and rectal malformations are basically a clinical, rather than radiographic diagnosis. The radiologist's main role is to look for associated spinal anomalies, perform a neonatal urologic evaluation because of the high index of associated malformations and occasionally to pin-point the site of the fistula between the rectum and the urinary tract (as soon as air is seen in the bladder in the male—Fig. 24–21A, 24–21B). There are too many technical factors to make films of the inverted infant particularly helpful in assessing the level of the rectal atresia.

REFERENCES

1. Berdon WE, Baker DH: Pediatric x-ray diagnosis, 6th ed. Section 10. The Neonate and Young Infant. Chicago, Year Book Med Pub, 1972

2. Swischuk LE: Radiology of the Newborn and Young Infant. Baltimore, Williams & Wilkins, 1973

3. Wesenberg RL: The Newborn Chest. Hagerstown, Harper & Row, 1973

25

Medicolegal Aspects

DAN J. TENNENHOUSE

BASIC PRINCIPLES

CRIMINAL AND CIVIL LAW

The law is arbitrarily divided into two traditional categories: criminal and civil. Criminal law deals with acts that harm society as a whole. A district attorney, representing the people, prosecutes the defendant and asks for punishment by fine or imprisonment. He must produce sufficient evidence to prove the defendant guilty beyond reasonable doubt. The existence of an injured party is immaterial. Civil law deals with acts that harm individuals. A private attorney, representing a plaintiff, prosecutes the defendant and asks for either money damages or a court order to prevent the defendant from causing irreparable harm. To prove the defendant liable he must produce a preponderance of evidence to that effect, i.e., more than half of the evidence must support liability. The existence of a living individual who has been or will be injured by the defendant's conduct is essential.

CRIMINAL LAW

Criminal indictments rarely arise out of the practice of medicine. Although the technical requirements for crimes such as assault and battery, defamation or false imprisonment are sometimes present in medical practice, they are not generally brought to the attention of the criminal courts unless there are also elements of malice and substantial injury.

Certain types of medical negligence can result in a felony conviction, however. If serious injury or death results from a physician's criminal negligence, the physician can be convicted of battery or manslaughter. Criminal negligence requires a reckless disregard for the patient's safety, such that serious injury or death is a natural and likely consequence. For example, presume that a newborn infant presents with fever, irritability and a high-pitched cry. Failure to further evaluate this condition may be negligence, but while death or serious injury is possible, it is not inevitable. Now presume that lumbar puncture reveals purulent cerebrospinal fluid. Failure to treat at this point may be *criminal* negligence because the addition of information making death or serious injury probable, instead of possible, can change simple negligence to criminal negligence. Thus, failure to evaluate a child who has sustained head trauma may be negligence, but failure to evaluate a child known to have a unilateral dilated pupil following head trauma may be *criminal* negligence.

The attention of the criminal courts may

also be drawn to the physician who deliberately misrepresents expensive treatment that he knows to be unnecessary as being necessary. This is fraud, and such treatment is battery, or manslaughter if death results. If the misrepresentation is for financial gain, an additional crime akin to grand larceny may also be present.

Criminal prosecution is possible for any violation of a criminal statute regulating the practice of medicine. Though usually based on a violation of drug and narcotic control laws, such prosecutions may also result from violations of state criminal statutes requiring, for example:

1. Reporting of reportable diseases to a public health agency
2. Administering prophylaxis for ophthalmia neonatorum
3. Testing newborn infants for phenylketonuria and other inborn errors of metabolism
4. Testing pregnant patients for Rh factor and syphilis

CIVIL LAW

Tort

Tort means a "civil wrong" and applies to certain acts that cause harm to persons or property. There are three broad categories: 1) intentional torts, 2) negligent torts and 3) liability without fault.

Intentional Torts. The defendant in this case caused harm by an intentional act, which means there was an intent to commit the act, but not necessarily an intent to cause harm. Treating a patient without consent may be an intentional tort called battery, which is similar to the crime of battery discussed above. A battery is considered sufficient "harm" to warrant damages in a civil lawsuit even if no physical injury has resulted, since the plaintiff's bodily privacy has been violated.

False imprisonment means restraint of a person against his will and is an intentional tort that may occur with restraint of a patient. Such restraint may be physical, by

drugs or by threat of physical force. When restraints are necessary to protect the patient from harm, the physician probably has a legal privilege, which is generally based on a statute, and he would not be liable for false imprisonment.

Improper release of medical information may be an intentional tort. If a physician releases *untrue* information regarding a patient to third persons, it may be defamation. A defamation in writing is libel; a defamation that is spoken is slander. His belief that the information was true is immaterial. If a physician releases *true* information regarding a patient to third persons without the patient's consent, it may be invasion of privacy.

As in the criminal law, intentional torts without substantial elements of malice and serious injury rarely result in successful civil lawsuits against physicians.

Negligent Torts. The defendant in this instance caused harm by a negligent act. Professional negligence, or "malpractice," is a negligent tort. The negligent manufacture or use of medical equipment or drugs may also injure patients, and involve both physicians and manufacturers in negligence lawsuits. Defamation and invasion of privacy can be negligent torts if a physician negligently releases improper medical information. Automobile and industrial accident litigation that involves the physician as an expert witness is also in the negligent tort category.

Liability Without Fault. The defendant in this case is liable for reasons of social utility. Defective drugs or medical products may permit a lawsuit against the manufacturer even when negligence cannot be proved. The manufacturer, although innocent of negligence, is considered to be in a better position to pay for an injury caused by his defective product than is the equally innocent victim. Also, if recurrences are preventable, the manufacturer should be given the incentive to develop safeguards. Therefore, society is better served by finding "strict liability" of the manufacturer.

For similar reasons a hospital may be

liable for the negligence of its employees, including salaried physicians, and a private practitioner may be liable for the negligent acts of his employees or of other physicians. It is well established in the law that a physician is liable for the negligence of his office nurse or any other employee. A physician is also liable for the torts of other physicians if an "agency" relationship existed between them at the time of the tort. In partnership practice every partner is liable for the torts of every other partner within the scope of the practice. However, even without a partnership, "agency" may be construed if the patient reasonably believed that an agency relationship existed between the physicians at the time of treatment. In any given case, agency may be found if the negligent physician

1. Consulted or worked closely with the defendant physician
2. Was in training, and under the defendant's supervision
3. Substituted for the defendant
4. Received the patient as a referral from the defendant
5. Administered anesthesia for the defendant surgeon
6. Shared an office with the defendant
7. Billed the patient on the defendant's stationary (1)

The courts sometimes rely on tenuous theories in order to find a solvent defendant.

Contract

The physician who agrees to "cure" his patient or to achieve some specific goal with treatment may be making a contract. The physician can then be sued for breach of contract, despite the best medical care, if he fails to achieve that goal. Careful explanation that no medical treatment is guaranteed can prevent breach of contract lawsuits.

Insurance

Recent cases suggest that the physician has a duty to complete a patient's insurance forms when these are reasonably related to his medical care. If failure to do so results in an economic loss to the patient, the physician may be liable.

Medical testimony may also be valuable in probate, child custody, commitment and other civil proceedings. When the custody of an infant is contested, objective medical opinion may be the most reliable basis for the court's decision.

MEDICAL NEGLIGENCE

Three elements essential to a lawsuit for medical negligence are: negligence, damages and causation.

NEGLIGENCE

Medical negligence is failure to apply the ordinary or accepted skill and learning that are applied in similar circumstances by others with the same level of training. The law does not require above-average care. Negligence can also be defined as failure by a physican to exercise proper diligence and his best judgment in a particular medical situation, exposing the patient to an unreasonable risk of harm. Any competent, well-respected physician may occasionally be negligent in his usual practice of medicine.

A pediatrician must use at least the same degree of care commonly used by other pediatricians. If a newborn infant develops mild clinical jaundice in the first 24 hours, with hepatosplenomegaly, a pediatrician should consider a possible diagnosis of erythroblastosis fetalis and follow the patient with hemoglobin and Coombs' tests. A nonspecialist, inexperienced with neonates, could confuse this clinical picture with physiologic neonatal jaundice and fail to order the appropriate tests. If a jury believes the testimony of medical expert witnesses that no more could be expected of a nonspecialist in this situation, failure to make an early diagnosis would be within the nonspecialist's standard of care and would not be negligent. A pediatrician, or anyone holding himself out to be a pediatrician, would be found negligent in the same circumstances. A specialist in family practice would probably be held to a standard of care somewhere between the two, depending on his training and experience. If the nonspecialist was aware of progressive jaundice, but rather than confusing it with another clinical entity, was simply unconcerned and did nothing, there may be breach of the standard of care requiring referral to a specialist.

Reasonable errors of professional judgment are not negligence. Suppose the serum bilirubin level of a Coombs positive infant was 12 mg/100 ml within 24 hours of birth. Failure to order an exchange transfusion at that time is a reasonable medical judgment, and as such it probably would not give rise to liability irrespective of the consequences. However, a bilirubin level of 20 mg/100 ml may be beyond the range at which a decision not to transfuse is considered reasonable.

When a physician is sued for negligence, a reasonable error of judgment may be his strongest defense. Testimony should show that, in hindsight, the physician used his best medical judgment under the circumstances, and an untoward result can occur despite good medical practice.

DAMAGES

Damages are the money given by juries to compensate patients for certain injuries, whether past or future, which result from negligence. They may include the actual costs of medical and other supportive care, lost income (including predictable losses for as much as an entire lifetime), and pain, suffering, loss of comfort or companionship, etc.

Punitive damages may be awarded if the defendant's harmful act was intentional. But intent alone will not generally sustain punitive damages without a substantial element of malice. Proof of malice is difficult, particularly as to physicians, and punitive damages are rarely seen in health care litigation. Since the civil law takes on the character of criminal law in dealing with intentional torts, the jury is permitted to award the plaintiff any amount of punitive damages necessary to sufficiently punish the defendant for his conduct.

If a patient dies, a wrongful death lawsuit may compensate the loss suffered by the family as a consequence of a patient's death. If an infant dies shortly after birth as a result of medical negligence, the damages available to the family in a wrongful death lawsuit are likely to be small. Costs of medical care have not been substantially affected. Anticipated income that is lost to the family by the infant's death is so remote and speculative that it will probably be excluded from consideration by the jury. Emotional injury for the loss of a baby to whom there was little opportunity to become emotionally attached may be the major basis for damages.

The compensation might, however, be very large in those instances where the infant does not die but suffers severe brain damage. Not being a wrongful death case, the infant as well as both parents may recover damages for all injuries, including emotional distress and anticipated costs of medical and supportive care for a lifetime.

CAUSATION

Legal causation is a complex concept that requires the negligent act to be either the actual cause of the injury or a substantial contributing factor to the injury. For example, since anaphylaxis is not dose dependent, the appearance of that condition following the administration of a negligently excessive dose of medication does not give rise to liability. The negligent act was not an *actual* cause of the injury. If however, a drug administered without proper indication caused unforeseeable anaphylaxis, the requirement of *actual* causation would be satisfied. The administration of a nonindicated drug is negligent because the benefits do not warrant the risks, and the physician will be responsible for any untoward reaction that results.

Causation also applies to indirect injuries that ultimately result from forces set in motion by the negligent act. Presume that negligent failure to control toxemia of pregnancy resulted in premature delivery. Presume also that the premature infant was given excessive oxygen in his incubator by a different physician and developed retrolental fibroplasia. The physician who failed to control the toxemia is then liable for the retrolental fibroplasia despite the presence of an intervening negligent act.

Since some indirect injuries are so far removed from the negligent act that an injustice would result if liability for them were permitted, legal limitations on causation exclude certain categories of remote indirect injuries. Presume that in the preceding example, the excessive oxygen was administered by a disgruntled intern trying to punish the hospital for making his life unbearable. This is an example of an intentional tort, and as such it would supercede the prior negligent act and terminate the legal causation.

DEFENSES

A medical negligence lawsuit may be defended by showing that either negligence, causation or damages is absent. However, if all are present, additional defenses may still be available. These include contributory negligence, statutes of limitations and the Good Samaritan statute.

Contributary Negligence

If the plaintiff's own carelessness contributed to his injury, contributory negligence exists. Since newborn infants cannot be considered to be capable of negligence, contributory negligence does not apply to them. Parental negligence, however, is a defense to the injuries claimed by the parents. For example, presume that a physician negligently prescribes a fetotoxic drug to a pregnant patient and that the patient negligently takes an overdose of it. Despite the physician's negligence, if fetal injury results, the mother's lawsuit against the physician for her own emotional distress and increased medical costs can be completely barred. The lawsuit on behalf of the child is not affected by contributory negligence.

In some states the doctrine of "comparative negligence" has replaced contributory negligence. This permits the verdict against the physician to be decreased, but not barred, by the patient's contribution to her own injury. Even in states with contributory negligence, comparative negligence may sometimes be secretly applied by juries despite instructions to the contrary. As a result, the defense of contributory negligence is not always totally effective.

Statutes of Limitation

Every state has its own statutes limiting the time period in which lawsuits can be initiated. These periods vary greatly. Limitation periods may also vary with factors such as

1. The type of defendant (e.g., physician, hospital, government entity)
2. The type of action (e.g., negligence, battery, breach of contract)
3. The type of injury (e.g., wrongful death, birth injury)
4. Point of time when the statute went into effect (e.g., commission of the negligent act, discovery by the patient of negligence, termination of treatment)

Generally, statutory time limitations for initiating lawsuits on behalf of children are postponed until the child reaches the age of majority, although little evidence would remain to support a lawsuit after many years. There are, however, exceptions to this general rule. For example, in California special statutes create a six-year limitation period for injuries arising prior to or during birth and a one-year limitation period for claims by children against public hospitals. Also, if the physician was aware of his own negligence, but failed to so inform the patient or family, the limitation period may be postponed indefinitely.

Good Samaritan Statute

All states have statutes protecting physicians from malpractice claims based on emergency treatment rendered at the scene of an accident or outside the usual scope of practice. These statutes are seldom considered since claims rarely, if ever, arise from such situations.

ECONOMIC REALITIES OF LITIGATION

PROBABILITY OF LITIGATION

Contingency Fee

The contingency fee system is a contract arrangement between lawyer and client, whereby the lawyer advances the cost of litigation out of his own pocket, then takes for his fee a percentage of any judgment awarded to his client. Lawyer's fees may be in the range of from 30% to 35% for cases settled before trial and from 35% to 50% for cases that go to trial. If judgment is for the defendant, the lawyer loses the litigation costs and receives no fee.

Litigation is expensive. Lawsuits for medical negligence often cost thousands of dollars to prosecute, with large sums required to purchase medical expertise. Therefore, the lawyer takes a considerable risk initiating any litigation that lacks reasonable chance of success. Unless the patient is severely injured, the average lawyer will not prosecute a claim for medical malpractice. However, some attorneys occasionally accept poor cases after obtaining a retainer fee from the client.

In many states the judge may have the discretionary power to alter certain aspects of the contingency fee arrangement if the client is a minor. This may include decreasing the attorney's fee and placing money judgments in trust for the child to be administered by a court-appointed trustee.

Although the contingency fee system tends to discourage frivolous lawsuits, recent trends in jury verdicts suggest that cases involving serious injuries have good potential for a plaintiff's verdict irrespective of weak evidence of medical negligence. Thus, the brain-damaged infant evokes such jury sympathy that weak evidence of obstetric negligence is greatly magnified. This phenomenon may induce speculation by a few lawyers who will prosecute any case having a large potential for damages however preposterous the theory of negligence.

Extrinsic Influences

The outcome of litigation may be influenced by certain extrinsic factors unrelated to the merit of the case. Lawsuit is less likely with

1. Little sympathy for the plaintiff (e.g., injuries resolved without sequelae—damages are based primarily on past discomfort)
2. Prejudice against the plaintiff (e.g., plaintiff has a contributing history of alcoholism or venereal infection)
3. Little credibility of the plaintiff (e.g., the plaintiff has a psychiatric history or a demeanor suggesting untruth or poor memory of events)
4. No malice by the defendant (e.g., the physician has written no malicious or unprofessional comments into the medical records)
5. Credibility of the defendant (e.g., the physician projects a confident and respectable image)
6. The physician not being employed by a "target defendant" organization (e.g., the physician is in private practice rather than employed by a hospital or medical group with a reputation in the community for poor quality care)
7. Prejudice in favor of the defendant (e.g., the physician is well known and liked in the community from which the jury is drawn)
8. The physician being an effective witness (e.g., the physician has a reputation for being familiar with the medical records and is adequately counseled by the defense attorney at the time of deposition or trial)
9. A trial location unfavorable to the plaintiff (e.g., juries drawn largely from a rural or conservative population, who tend to believe that money damages awarded to a plaintiff constitutes an unearned windfall)

SETTLEMENT

One function of the defense lawyer is to determine the likelihood of a successful defense. Where the physician firmly believes that "truth" is in his favor, the defense lawyer realistically understands that "truth" is not before the jury. Only the evidence is before the jury, and if it supports the plaintiff, any favorable settlement out of court is a victory. Therefore, the defense lawyer objectively weighs the risk of facing a jury against the cost of settlement, and the physician should respect that judgment.

Since a primary purpose of the civil law is to promote social utility, the modern legal system is often more concerned with providing sustenance for the patient unable to work due to an injury sustained during medical care, than it is with determining who was "right" and what is "fair." Medical malpractice litigation could thus be viewed as a type of accident insurance for the patient, paid for by increased medical fees covering the cost of increased malpractice insurance premiums. To view such litigation as stamping the physician with guilt is to invite unnecessary grief when the inevitable finally happens. Juries cannot award damages without first finding negligence, and they are loath to send the patient away penniless when they believe that the insurer must pay; the physician's only loss is to his pride. Even though the doctor believes himself blameless, he should accept the economic reality of litigation and cooperate fully with his defense lawyer's efforts to make a favorable settlement.

LEGAL REPRESENTATION

Generally, a physician defendant in a civil lawsuit is well represented by the lawyer retained by the malpractice insurer. There are three situations, however, in which the physician should consider seeking independent counsel.

The quality of legal representation being inversely proportional to the lawyer's caseload, a lawyer with too many case assignments will be unable to devote sufficient time to preparation of the physician's defense. Unfortunately, some large defense lawfirms increase their profit margins by maximizing each lawyer's caseload. As a result, a defense lawyer may be assigned many more cases than the opposing plaintiff lawyer.

The overburdened lawyer may dangerously delay obtaining all medical records relating to the plaintiff's condition; he may also delay seeking medical consultation and expert witnesses or fail to adequately prepare witnesses and defendants for deposition and trial. If this is apparent, a physician defendant who is seriously concerned about the effect on his reputation of losing a lawsuit should consider obtaining independent counsel.

A lawyer who represents the insurer of both the physician and the hospital may be unable to represent the best interests of all defendants in a lawsuit. For example, in a negligence lawsuit against a physician and a hospital, the physician may be expected to suppress his knowledge of a negligent act by a hospital nurse which may prove the case against the hospital. Although such evidence could permit the physician to escape liability, a lawyer representing the insurer may be willing to risk an unfavorable verdict against the physician on the chance that lack of clear evidence of negligence will result in a favorable verdict for all defendants. No other verdict would benefit the insurer since damages will be as large whether against one or all defendants.

If the amount of damages sought in a lawsuit exceeds the physician's malpractice insurance policy limits, the physician should consider seeking independent counsel. The insurer, acting in its own best interest, could take an action that exposes the physician to a verdict in excess of his policy limits.

AVOIDING LITIGATION

THE USE OF EVIDENCE

In a jury trial, the jury must determine the facts, and the judge must decide how the law should apply to those facts. The jury's determination of fact is based on evidence including the testimony of witnesses and tangible materials such as medical records, and a lawyer's decision to sue is based largely on the anticipated effect of that evidence on a jury.

Medical Records

The outcome of a trial often depends on the credibility of witnesses. If the physician and the patient have different recollections of an event, the patient's version is likely to be believed. However, a written record supporting the physician's recollection can swing the balance of credibility in his favor. Sometimes a single relevant statement in the chart can win or prevent a lawsuit.

Medical records should be complete but limited to factual information and opinions intended to assist other physicians in the care of the patient. Illegible, altered or missing records and statements that criticize other medical personnel or indicate hostility toward the patient may create an inference of wrongdoing by the physician and invite lawsuit. Statements in the records denying fault or explaining away a bad medical result may suggest a "guilty conscience" and also invite lawsuit.

Consultants

Medical negligence lawsuits generally require proof that the defendant made an unreasonable decision. Since proving a decision was unreasonable is very difficult if that decision was supported by consultation, the appropriate use of consultants is an excellent safeguard against lawsuit. Many hospitals have bylaws requiring the use of consultants in certain situations. Violation of those bylaws may create an inference of negligence by the physician.

Physician–Patient Relationship

An excellent physician–patient relationship is the most important single deterrant of medical lawsuits. A substantial percentage of lawsuits arise because patients with no actual knowledge of medical negligence seek legal assistance for vindictive reasons.

In perinatal practice this hazard is relatively great. The demands and expectations that parents place on physicians are frequently unreasonable, and this leads to angry parents. If one single factor is responsible for more litigation than any other, it is inadequate explanation of what parents should expect from medical care. Physicians who must deal with parents can minimize such problems by reserving more time for discussion and explanation, thereby precluding the ignorance that breeds anger. This is an investment of time and money, but it can pay dividends in community reputation as well as in reducing the danger of lawsuit.

PERINATAL MEDICOLEGAL HAZARDS

PRENATAL

CONTRACEPTIVE FAILURE

"Wrongful life" lawsuits are not uncommon following the failure of contraception. These lawsuits arise often because the physician failed to advise the patient that no method of birth control, short of hysterectomy, is 100% reliable. If unexpected pregnancy occurs, the patient presumes that physician error was responsible.

Wrongful life lawsuits tend to be of doubtful merit. Although the costs of bearing and rearing a child and the emotional strain of caring for an additional child are ample bases for damages in many states, parents seeking such damages can expect little jury sympathy. The claim that the child is not worth the cost will receive a cold reception in the courtroom. Such lawsuits probably have their greatest merit when the parent is indigent and will suffer great economic hardship because of the additional child.

The physician should not rely on the defense argument that abortion is available for patients with unwanted pregnancies. For emotional reasons, patients who use contraceptives are often unwilling to submit to abortion, and juries readily accept such attitudes unless the patient has sought abortion in the past.

Temporary and Permanent Contraception

The patient may allege physician negligence for improper choice of a birth control method or for insufficient instruction in its use. Occasionally, a patient requests treatment for menstrual irregularity believing that the drug prescribed will also provide contraception. If pregnancy occurs, she may insist that her primary reason for seeing the physician was contraception.

Surgical sterilization failures are just rare enough to create an inference of physician negligence when they occur. Resulting lawsuits, though common, usually end favorably for the physician. But if the physician tells the patient that surgery will produce sterility, failure to achieve that goal may be breach of a contract. A breach of contract theory is advantageous to the patient because physician negligence need not be proved. In many states, however, the physician must make an express warranty (a statement that sterilization is guaranteed) before he can be found liable for breach of contract.

ABORTION

If the physician intentionally and carefully performed an abortion with the patient's consent, no civil liability would result. Nevertheless, a criminal indictment could ensue if the abortion violated a criminal statute of that state. All such criminal statutes set forth exceptions under which the abortion can be performed legally, but these exceptions have traditionally been narrow. For example, to be legal in many states abortion must be performed

1. By a licensed physician
2. With approval of a committee or specific number of physicians

3. With consent of spouse, or parent if a minor
4. For the purpose of saving the life of the mother, following rape or if the child would be born defective

State statutes may, however, be reviewed by the federal courts and ruled unconstitutional. The court must find the statute overbroad and infringing on the freedom of individuals, without sufficient benefit to the state's own interests to warrant such infringement. This happened in two 1973 landmark decisions: *Roe* v. *Wade* and *Doe* v. *Bolton* (5, 14), where the United States Supreme Court limited the permissible scope of state abortion statutes. Now, no state statute may prevent abortion

1. In the first trimester if, in the physician's judgment, it is medically indicated. This is almost no limitation at all.
2. In the second trimester unless such restriction on abortion is reasonably related to the mother's health. A reasonable relation to health may still be construed very broadly.
3. In the third trimester if the abortion is necessary to preserve the mother's life or health. This limitation is essentially unchanged from the older laws.

Statutes may still require that only licensed MDs perform abortions. The power of a state to require spousal consent or parental consent for abortion in a pregnant minor was not settled in these decisions but see the section Lack of Consent: Battery, infra.

If the physician treats a patient who is probably the victim of an illegal abortion, there may be a statute requiring him to report the circumstances to a local law enforcement agency. Violation of this statute may result not only in criminal liability, but also in civil liability if the physician's inaction exposes the patient to further harm.

Unsuccessful attempted abortion may result in the birth of a deformed child. A lawsuit on behalf of the child is likely and has good potential for a large verdict against the physician.

Occasionally, an abortion procedure may fall within the scope of a state's murder-manslaughter statute. Such statutes can only apply if the fetus fits the legal definition of a *person* protected by the statutes.

Under the old common law rule, a fetus does not become a *person* until it lives separate from the mother (i.e., with live delivery), although a particular state may vary this by statute. The *Roe v. Wade* and *Doe v. Bolton* decisions, supra, appear to create an additional requirement of viability, such that state criminal statutes cannot directly protect the life of a fetus that cannot survive separate from its mother. It should be kept in mind, however, that this entire area of law is rapidly changing and that legal definitions of *fetus* and *person* are often unclear and in need of much judicial interpretation.

Thus, an abortion procedure which requires the delivery of a viable fetus, followed by some deliberate act to terminate its life, could technically violate a murder-manslaughter statute in many states. An abortion procedure which causes death-in-utero of a viable fetus could expose the physician to a murder-manslaughter indictment only in a state with statutes differing from the old common law rule. The question of viability may be decided by a jury.

Convictions for murder and manslaughter in abortion cases will probably remain exceedingly rare. Perhaps the most important single factor in successful criminal prosecution is local public opinion strongly adverse to abortion.

MISDIAGNOSIS OF PREGNANCY OR GESTATION

Accidental abortion during dilatation and curettage of an undiagnosed pregnancy is a possible basis for lawsuit. Insufficient damage, however, decreases the probability of lawsuit unless the patient has no living children, an infertility problem, and fails to become pregnant again by the time of trial.

The use of teratogenic or fetotoxic drugs or biologicals during early undiagnosed pregnancy can result in a lawsuit with large potential damages. If a patient might be pregnant, the physician could have a duty to test for pregnancy before prescribing such drugs. The physician certainly has a duty to rule out probable pregnancy by history before exposing the patient (see Fetotoxic and Teratogenic Drugs, infra).

Misdiagnosis of pregnancy as a tumor, with irradiation of the uterus, has also produced deformed infants and resulted in lawsuits.

Misdiagnosis of gestation period with early induction of labor unnecessarily exposes the infant to the complications of prematurity. Complete reliance upon the patient's menstrual history for computing the estimated date of delivery is dangerous practice, especially if induction of labor is contemplated. Furthermore, the availability of tests for fetal maturity may create a duty to test every fetus for maturity before undertaking routine induction or repeat elective cesarean section.

MATERNAL DISEASE

Toxemia of pregnancy, uncontrolled diabetes mellitus and other serious complications of pregnancy may result in a lawsuit if diagnosis or adequate treatment is delayed. The physician thus has a duty to maintain a high index of suspicion and to recheck the patient at frequent intervals to reduce the possibility of fetal injury. Failure of the patient to return regularly for follow-up appointments can provide the physician with a contributory negligence defense, but as such a defense may require proof that the patient understood the importance of keeping the appointments, the physician should be certain that he has advised the patient of the importance of regular follow-up care and that this advice is clearly reflected in the records.

The physician who treats a pregnant patient also treats a delicate and vulnerable fetus for which a jury may find the highest duty of care. The inadequate treatment of seemingly minor maternal respiratory infection or anemia may be linked to fetal anoxia, and vaginitis may be linked to amnionitis. Therefore, minor maternal disorders with any potential for fetal injury deserve extra attention.

Rubella, accidental drug exposure and other teratogenic events during pregnancy create a dilemma for the physician. If he knows or should know that the fetus may be deformed, he probably has a duty to advise the patient that abortion should be considered. Failure to advise the patient of this option, resulting in the birth of a deformed child, may permit the parents to sue for the actual and emotional costs of rearing a deformed child. The courts would not, however, permit the *child* to sue the physician for failing to recommend its own abortion.

As new tests become available for the diagnosis of congenital defects, the physician may have a duty to utilize them whenever indicated. Amniocentesis and x ray of fetal bone structure may have application in this area.

FETOTOXIC AND TERATOGENIC DRUGS

Numerous drugs have been implicated in fetal injury, and resulting lawsuits are common. The physician has a duty to be aware of the drug's potential hazards to a fetus (as described in the manufacturer's literature) and to make a reasonable effort to diagnose the pregnancy.

A reasonable effort to diagnose pregnancy probably requires an adequate history and a pregnancy test, if indicated. However, the precise indications for a pregnancy test may be a central issue varying with the circumstances and expert testimony in each case. There is no duty to perform a pregnancy test too early in gestation for reasonable accuracy of the test.

Occasionally the pharmaceutical manufacturer is named as a defendant in the lawsuit. The manufacturer may attempt to escape liability by blaming the injury on physician error. Therefore, the physician will also be a primary defendant in the lawsuit. The manufacturer may be at a disadvantage, however, due to the common bias against large profit-oriented corporations. Manufacturers have been found liable for drug advertising overpromotion, mislabeling, failure to provide adequate warning literature and failure to properly test a drug before marketing it.

Excessive smoking or the abuse of drugs such as aspirin, antacids, alcohol or antihistamines by the patient may increase the risk of fetal injury. The physician should advise the patient of this risk and carefully note in his records evidence of the patient's failure to follow medical advice.

STATUS OF THE FETUS AS A PERSON

A child may have the right to sue the physician who negligently caused his prenatal injury. A general rule of law, however, requires that the fetus have the status of a legal "person" at the time of injury since only a person has the protection of the law. Person status has usually been interpreted by the courts to mean a viable fetus, i.e., one capable of living independent of the mother. Thus, a child may have no right to sue for injuries sustained at six months' gestation, whereas the same injury sustained a month later may permit lawsuit. Determination of viability depends on expert medical testimony. A few states have adopted more liberal rules and permitted lawsuits for previable injuries. Further changes in the law may eventually permit a child to sue for injuries from a chromosomal defect sustained by a parent prior to the child's conception. This rule does not affect the parents' right to sue for their own economic and emotional injury resulting from the child's injury.

If the prenatal injury is fatal, a wrongful death lawsuit may be available to the family or to the child's estate. Most states require that the child be born alive, but about 20 states have now adopted the rule that wrongful death lawsuits are permitted for stillborn infants if the injury occurred when the fetus was viable.

Lawsuits for death of a fetus or newborn infant rarely result in large verdicts.

PRENATAL LABORATORY TESTING

The availability of anti-Rh immunoglobulin and its potential for substantially decreasing the probability of hemolytic disease may create a duty to evaluate and treat pregnant patients at an early stage for potential Rh incompatibility. Testing of pregnant patients for Rh factor is now required by statute in some states. Lawsuits for failure to do so may be common in the future.

Now that rubella vaccine is widely available, rubella susceptibility should probably be determined in every patient being treated for infertility. The courts may eventually find that physicians have a duty to treat rubella susceptibility in any patient likely to become pregnant, including unmarried but sexually active patients.

The physician has a duty to advise the patient that pregnancy is contraindicated for a period of time following rubella vaccination. This should be carefully noted in the medical records.

The duty to order routine prenatal tests such as serology, hemoglobin and urinalysis is so well established that failure to do so would be almost indefensible in the courtroom.

INTRAPARTUM HAZARDS

ABANDONMENT AND DELAYED HOSPITALIZATION

Abandonment is a type of medical negligence in which the patient is left unattended and without sufficient opportunity to find another physician of her choice and as a result sustains a medical injury. This may occur in numerous ways.

The physician may agree to deliver the patient but fail to explain that another qualified physician will take his place in the event that he is required elsewhere at the time of delivery. Then if another physician must stand in for him and the patient can prove that she was harmed by the substitution, a lawsuit may be based on negligent abandonment and possibly on breach of contract. Such a lawsuit has little merit, however, because a reasonable patient would be aware of such a possibility; damages would usually be small, and the physi-

cian could probably prove that he had little choice of action. Although these constitute no legal defense, jury sympathy would tend to favor the physician.

If the attending physician chose an unqualified or incompetent substitute, a lawsuit having strong merit could be based on negligent abandonment, as the physician retains the primary responsibility for his patient when he delegates duties to others. Particular caution is required when responsibility is delegated to students, interns and residents.

While in active labor, the patient may insist on being delivered at home. If the physician refuses, a lawsuit based on negligent abandonment and breach of contract will probably have no merit unless the physician had earlier agreed to deliver the patient at home or no practical means was available to transport the patient to the hospital.

While in active labor, the patient may insist on "natural childbirth" or some other specific form of medical care that conflicts with the physician's best judgment. If the physician ignores the patient's request and proceeds with his own preferred treatment, he may be sued for battery. If the physician refuses to carry out the delivery, he may be sued for negligent abandonment. If the physician follows the patient's demands and knowingly gives negligent care, he may still be sued for the negligence. That the patient asked for negligent care does not excuse the physician for giving it. How then, does the physician escape this dilemma?

If the patient demands a specific mode of treatment that clearly involves negligent medical practice, the physician should refuse. If the patient refuses to consent to some aspect of needed medical care, such as a blood transfusion or a spinal anesthetic, and has a full understanding of the danger involved, failure to give that aspect of care will not be abandonment or negligent practice. The physician should still provide all other care to the best of his ability in order to offer the patient the best chance for a favorable outcome despite the deficit. Unless the patient is temporarily psychotic, the physician probably has no privilege to commit a battery and should conform to the patient's refusal. The circumstances should be carefully documented in the medical records. Whenever the patient refuses to cooperate with the physician and understands the danger, a contributory negligence theory may protect the physician. If the physician's actions are *reasonable* under the circumstances, a lawsuit will have little merit.

If the patient is unable to pay for medical services, the physician may refuse to perform the delivery. If the patient then has insufficient time to find another physician prior to delivery, there is negligent abandonment with jury sympathy strongly in the patient's favor, and a successful lawsuit against the physician is likely to result.

A hospital may refuse to admit a patient in active labor on technical grounds (e.g., no Blue Cross card), but if she is delivered outside the hospital with resulting injury to the infant, the hospital may face a lawsuit for negligence with jury sympathy strongly in the patient's favor.

Abandonment may also result from examination by a nurse. A patient in active labor was refused admission to the hospital because the nurse who examined her decided she was not in active labor and sent her home. An incorrect decision could result in a meritorious lawsuit primarily because the patient was not examined by a physician. The attending physician may be negligent in delegating to a nurse his duty to examine the patient. The hospital, too, may have a duty to provide every patient who may be in labor with examination by a physician and may also be liable for a negligent policy of permitting nurses to make such decisions. The jury may refuse to accept an allegation that a physician would have made the same decision as did the nurse in a specific case.

FETAL ANOXIA

Perhaps the most common single basis for lawsuits in perinatology is fetal anoxia during labor and delivery. Brain injury in a neonate may produce large verdicts as jury

sympathy favors the infant. The defense that such injury may result from natural causes will probably not be accepted if there is any basis for physician negligence.

With the induction of labor, a special duty of care probably arises due to the increased danger to the fetus. This duty can usually be satisfied with more frequent monitoring and more careful evaluation for the complications of induction.

The frequency with which fetal heart rate and progress of labor is monitored deserves special comment. Insufficient monitoring is a strong basis for a negligence lawsuit. The issues are easily understood by jurors, who may have high expectations for the care of patients in labor. Also, a hospital that fails to hire sufficient qualified nursing staff may appear to be placing economic considerations above those of patient welfare. This could anger a jury.

Unavailability of proper surgical facilities, equipment or personnel for emergency cesarean section have been the bases for lawsuits against hospitals. Any hospital that maintains a delivery suite has a duty also to maintain a continuous capability for emergency cesarean section.

Routine drug orders may create an inference of negligence since they tend to violate the principle that drugs should be tailored to the specific patient and used in the smallest sufficient dosage. When fetal anoxia occurs, unnecessarily large drug dosages are often implicated. Therefore, routine drug orders should be formulated in such a way as to encourage the modification of dosages. Requiring the physician at least to fill in the dosages of the more dangerous drugs when routine orders are stamped in the patient's chart would help minimize this problem.

Delayed diagnosis of uterine inertia, cephalopelvic disproportion or other complications of labor may be linked to fetal injury, and used as the basis for a negligence lawsuit. Unless the physician's care was obviously reckless, proof of medical negligence in such cases is generally difficult. The physician need only provide care consistent with the accepted practice of other respected practitioners. If, for example, a long trial of labor is considered accepted practice at a large medical center, or in a respected obstetric text, it would probably be found by a jury to fall within the standard of care.

Another complication that has resulted in negligence lawsuits is prolapse of the umbilical cord. The artificial rupture of membranes occurring prematurely and causing prolapse of the cord and fetal injury may strongly infer physician negligence. Delay in treatment of a known cord prolapse has also resulted in lawsuits against physicians and nurses.

General anesthesia used for delivery with inadequate indications is a strong basis for negligence since fetal anoxia may be presumed due to depressive effects of the anesthetic. Neurologic deficits discovered subsequently will be blamed on the anesthetic.

PHYSICAL INJURY

Traumatic injuries to a newborn infant during delivery usually result from the misapplication of forceps or from excessive traction. Laymen expect physicians to use extraordinary care in the handling of neonates and therefore see traumatic injuries during delivery as suggesting physician negligence. Furthermore, when neurologic injuries are involved, they are apt to be severe, as with intracranial hemorrhage, brachial plexus injury and even spinal cord transection, and may result in large verdicts.

The application of forceps should be viewed as a delicate and hazardous surgical procedure demanding the greatest care. Injuries from the application of foreceps by physicians who do not use forceps regularly are particularly difficult to defend.

POSTPARTUM HAZARDS

INITIAL RESPONSIBILITY FOR CARE

Rarely is a pediatrician present in the delivery room during an uncomplicated delivery. Therefore, the obstetrician must be responsible for both neonate and mother if they require simultaneous attention. Such

potentially hazardous circumstances can be avoided if another physician trained in neonatal resuscitation is immediately available to every delivery. Although a well-trained nurse can greatly reduce this hazard, neonatal injury could result in lawsuit primarily because no other physician was available. If the jury believes that the unavailability of another physician was a negligent policy that substantially reduced the chance of successful resuscitation, a verdict for the plaintiff must be found.

When the division of medical responsibility for a patient is not clearly defined, all physicians involved may be jointly liable. For example, if two physicians receive copies of an abnormal laboratory report, and each believes that the other will provide the medical follow-up, both may be liable for every aspect of the patient's care. Lack of communication among physicians is an important basis for negligence in litigation, especially if no single physician assumes primary responsibility for the patient's total care.

The problem of division of medical responsibility in perinatology is particularly complex since care of the child as a separate entity should begin early in pregnancy, and care of the mother during pregnancy unavoidably affects fetal well-being.

ROUTINE POSTPARTUM PROCEDURES

Confusion as to the identity of a newborn infant occasionally results in lawsuit based on negligent hospital identification procedures or on nursing negligence. Damages require proof of emotional harm to the parents, which is due partly to permanent uncertainty as to the child's true identity. Sometimes unauthorized circumcision adds to the potential damages. These lawsuits usually result in small verdicts because of the lack of substantial injury.

Failure to carry out routine procedures such as prophylaxis for ophthalmia neonatorum or PKU testing, can result in severe neonatal injury and lawsuit. Although such procedures are usually performed by nursing staff, the ultimate legal responsibility may rest with the physician.

In many states, certain of these procedures are required by statute, and since statutes establish the standard of care, violation of a statute is negligence per se and no further proof is required that an accepted standard of medical care has been violated. The jury can be instructed that the physician was negligent *as a matter of law*, and the jurors need decide only the amount of damages to be awarded. Thus, the physician should see to it that routine nursing procedures are being reliably carried out.

INCUBATOR HAZARDS

Malfunction and Misuse

Defective equipment or careless use of equipment by newborn nursery staff may result in neonatal exposure to dangerous temperatures or oxygen concentrations. Lawsuits for incubator injuries may be directed against

1. The incubator manufacturer for an equipment defect
2. The hospital for negligent maintenance of the equipment
3. The hospital, physicians and nursing staff for negligent use of equipment known to be defective

Much as pathologists must actively conduct quality control evaluation of clinical laboratory testing procedures, the physicians may have a duty to investigate the quality and use of the incubators. The extent of this duty is naturally limited to whatever a jury believes to be reasonable, but considering the magnitude of potential harm to be averted by a small investment of the physician's time, definite routine procedures for incubator quality control appear to be essential.

If the hospital is sued for negligent choice of inferior equipment or for inadequate maintenance of equipment, the hospital may also appear to have placed economic considerations above those of patient welfare.

Retrolental Fibroplasia

As with all disorders commonly considered to be iatrogenic, retrolental fibroplasia has been a frequent source of perinatal lawsuits. When it results from physician error or equipment malfunction, a lawsuit with strong merit can be anticipated. Jury sympathy for a blind infant may amplify the least evidence of negligence, and lead to a large plaintiff verdict.

RESPIRATORY DISTRESS SYNDROME (RDS)

Since serious sequelae of RDS are common despite the best medical care, lawsuits based on improper treatment may be difficult to prosecute. If RDS results from prematurity, however, and the prematurity is linked to physician negligence, the patient may have a stronger case.

JAUNDICE

Lawsuit is likely following kernicterus since the damages are large and the possible sources of negligence many. Negligence could be based on:

1. Failure to take appropriate prophylactic measures during pregnancy
2. Failure to distinguish erythroblastosis fetalis from physiologic jaundice of the newborn
3. Failure to adequately monitor neonatal bilirubin levels in erythroblastosis fetalis
4. Unreasonable delay in initiating exchange transfusion

THE NEONATE AS OUTPATIENT

INFECTION

Infection in the young infant is a frightening experience for parents, who may irrationally blame themselves for the illness and be frustrated by the physician's relatively calm reaction. If a serious complication arises, the parents may blame the physician for insufficient treatment. This sets the stage for lawsuit.

A frequent theory of negligence used in these cases is delayed diagnosis; therefore, a febrile infant that is not hospitalized should be watched with extreme caution. Infections that commonly result in lawsuit include

1. Tetanus, often seen when delivery occurs outside of a hospital
2. Meningitis
3. Tracheobronchial infections, especially those with a potential for airway obstruction such as epiglotitis
4. Conjunctivitis
5. Bacterial enteritis with dehydration
6. Staphylococcal disease, especially with such complications as pneumonia or osteomyelitis

Occasionally a hospital infection results from poor isolation techniques or failure to discover and treat carriers on the hospital staff. Although the highest standard of care applies in the prevention of such infections in infants, some evidence of deviation from good medical practice is still necessary to prove negligence. Therefore, the mere presence of a hospital infection in an infant will not generally establish liability.

DEHYDRATION

The infant with vomiting, diarrhea, fever and poor oral intake may be sent home only at considerable risk. Critical electrolyte difficulties with possible brain damage or death may be only a few hours away. Reliance on parental judgment in such cases is a difficult defense in the courtroom since the parents' lack of medical training and inability to make objective decisions under the circumstances will be quickly pointed out. Any history of poor parental judgment is additional evidence that the physician was negligent in trusting them.

DRUGS

Occasionally immunization produces a serious adverse reaction with permanent sequellae. If a lawsuit results, it will probably be directed at both the physician and the pharmaceutical manufacturer. The physician cannot be found liable unless there is evidence of physician error. However, the pharmaceutical manufacturer may attempt to avoid liability by alleging that injury resulted because the physician gave the immunization improperly or in the presence of a contraindication. The physician's defense must be based on proper use of the biological according to the manufacturer's directions. These lawsuits usually end favorably for the physician.

One frequent complication of intramuscular injection in infants is peripheral nerve injury. Because the gluteal muscle mass is small, the danger of sciatic nerve injury increases unless special care is used. Injections into the upper arm of an infant may produce radial nerve injury. Lawsuits based on negligent injection often have strong merit and moderately large potential damages.

If the parents are to administer oral medication to an infant, the physician must carefully explain the drug's use and possible side effects. Parents may be slow to recognize signs of an adverse reaction or overdose in an infant, and toxic drug levels can accumulate rapidly. Parental negligence is a difficult defense for the physician since parents will claim that the physician spent little time explaining use of the drug. Jurors drawing on their own experience with physicians may well believe the parents' testimony. The physician's best defense is a careful explanation to the parents with adequate documentation in the medical records.

CONGENITAL AND MECHANICAL PROBLEMS

The delayed diagnosis of congenital orthopedic problems, such as dislocation of the hip, metatarsus varus, tibial torsion and torticollis, which may benefit from early treatment, may result in a lawsuit years later when the deformity becomes obvious to the parents and an orthopedist advises them of a diminished prognosis.

Potentially life-threatening GI problems such as pyloric stenosis, megacolon, intussusception, volvulus and incarcerated hernia may present with little more than vomiting and abdominal distension in an infant (7). Therefore, delayed diagnosis of serious organic disease can occur despite the best medical care. Nevertheless, an unreasonable delay, where findings suggested organic disease long before proper diagnostic studies were carried out, can result in a meritorious lawsuit.

CHILD ABUSE

Child abuse is a crime for which one or both parents can be prosecuted and for which the custody of the child can be taken from the parents by court order. Most states have laws requiring that child abuse be reported to local law enforcement agencies. Therefore, the physician may have a legal duty to report this diagnosis whenever it should reasonably have been made. However, child abuse is rarely reported since physicians tend to fear legal complications and realize that the child's only hope for medical care rests on parental confidence in the physician. The average district attorney's office has a poor record of convictions in such cases, and the chance that custody will actually be taken from the parent is rather small.

The physician who fails to report a clear case of child abuse may face a civil lawsuit. For example, suppose the infant's parents are separated, the mother has custody, and she abuses the child producing permanent injury. If the physician knew or should have known of abuse and failed to report it, thereby failing to protect the infant from the injury, he may be sued by both the father and the infant for damages arising from the injury. Furthermore, the physician may be negligent as a matter of law (i.e., irrespective of any finding by a jury) if a statute exists requiring physicians to report child abuse.

OTHER THEORIES OF LIABILITY IN PERINATOLOGY

LACK OF CONSENT: BATTERY

Without consent, any "touching" of a patient is battery. Touching includes physical examination, ordering injection or any other act producing physical contact. A physician may be liable for injury resulting from a battery irrespective of the quality of medical care given. Requiring no proof of medical negligence, battery theory as used in lawsuits may compensate the patient for unavoidable complications of properly indicated procedures.

A patient above the legal age of majority may give or withdraw consent at any time. Consent may be verbal or in writing. If the patient is an infant, however, the power to consent resides in the legal guardian, usually a parent.

In an emergency, where the patient's legal guardian cannot be reached by telephone or other reasonable means, a mature relative or anyone with a written authorization to secure medical treatment for the infant may give consent. If no authorized person is available, consent is implied, and the physician may proceed with the treatment.

Occasionally, a parent or legal guardian refuses consent, and the infant faces serious injury or death as a result. A court may order the necessary medical procedure pursuant to a statute for that purpose or, in the absence of such a statute, may appoint a new legal guardian to give consent. Judicial consent has upheld cases for blood transfusion, amputation, immunization and other necessary care. The proper channel through which to obtain judicial consent is generally the hospital's administrator or legal counsel.

Generally, only the parents have power to consent to medical care of a minor. There are, however, several important exceptions to this:

1. Statutes may permit pregnant minors to consent to any pregnancy-related medical care. This has been interpreted to include abortion in some states.
2. Statutes may "emancipate" certain minors by giving them the power of consent. Such statutes may affect married, financially independent and other minors.
3. Some courts now tend to find the power of consent in any minor with sufficient "maturity" to comprehend the significance or appreciate the hazards of the medical care to which she consents.

In about nine states, statutes deny un-emancipated minors the right to obtain abortions without parental consent. In 1973 a federal court in Florida found the Florida statute unconstitutional (3), and this finding may apply to all such statutes unless reversed by the United States Supreme Court.

The physician who is asked to treat a pregnant minor without parental consent faces a dilemma. If he refuses to treat her, she may fail to find proper medical care or injure herself in desperation; if he treats her, the parents may initiate a vindictive lawsuit, especially if complications arose from the treatment. The physician's defense may depend on difficult legal concepts applied to the particular circumstances of the case. Therefore, he would be well advised to discuss the laws of his own state with an attorney before undertaking to treat pregnant minors without parental consent.

LACK OF INFORMED CONSENT: NEGLIGENCE

The physician's duty to obtain consent before undertaking treatment has always been clear. The degree of explanation to the patient necessary to obtain consent, however, has never been well defined. Often in the past the physician made the decisions, the patient remained uninformed, and consent was an empty formality. However, the current wave of "consumerism" is influencing the attitudes of modern courts and creating dissatisfaction with the traditional method of obtaining consent. The patient, as consumer, now claims the right to make the final decision, and the courts support that claim. In the past several years, state supreme courts have shown a trend to establish legally imposed standards for informed consent, and this trend will probably result in relatively uniform law throughout the country in the next few years. These legal standards set forth a minimum amount of information that must be available to the patient for an informed consent. The physician has a duty to provide that information, and breach of this duty is negligence.

Requirements for an Informed Consent (2)

The courts will probably require an adequate explanation in lay terms of the nature of, alternatives to and risks of the contemplated medical procedure. The patient must understand, for example, which parts of the body will be affected and how they will be affected, what subjective impressions should be expected, what follow-up care will be necessary, and what sequellae or impairments should be anticipated. The patient must also understand what reasonable alternatives there are to the procedure. For example, an informed consent for contraceptives may require understanding of the problems inherent in every alternative method of contraception, as well as the dangers of having no contraception at all.

The most difficult concept in informed consent for the physician to grasp, or for the courts to clearly define, is the principle that distinguishes those risks of a procedure which must be disclosed to the patient for an informed consent. Inconsequential or extremely rare complications are clearly not among the risks that must be disclosed. Relatively uncommon complications probably need not be disclosed unless they are very serious. Therefore, the frequency and severity of a complication are the factors that determine the need for disclosure. The purpose of explaining the risks is to assist the patient in making his decision. If the knowledge of any complication is material to the consent decision, that complication should be disclosed as a risk. In the courtroom, a jury that must base its decision on the importance of the undisclosed risk to the patient's decision will decide if consent was given with sufficient understanding.

If a procedure is clearly mandatory, and there are no reasonable alternatives, no decision is necessary. Thus, informed consent is not required. But the more elective the procedure, the more necessary is an explanation of the risks, alternatives and dangers inherent in those alternatives. Elective experimental procedures require the greatest care in obtaining an informed consent.

Legal Effect of Informed Consent

For negligence based on lack of informed consent, the plaintiff must prove that

1. A risk, material to his decision of consent, was not disclosed by the physician
2. If he had known of this risk, he would have refused to consent
3. The procedure resulted in injury

The strict legal theory of lack of informed consent even appears to permit recovery by the plaintiff for complications that were disclosed. For example, if surgery is necessary, and the surgeon discloses the risk of hemorrhage but not infection, the patient's consent is not informed. If the patient can prove that he would have refused to consent if he had known of the infection risk, then he can recover damages for *any* injury sustained as a result of the surgery. Therefore, if hemorrhage occurs, the patient can recover damages for resulting injury despite his prior knowledge of the risk of hemorrhage.

Negligent lack of informed consent allows the patient monetary recovery for unavoidable complications of medical procedures. It also allows lawsuits to be based more on the relative credibility of the witnesses than on medical standards of care, and this may in turn reduce the attorney's need to rely on expert medical testimony and permit the case to be evaluated by a jury when the attorney is otherwise unable to prove medical negligence.

Unless the physician's conduct was outrageous, lack of informed consent is usually a weak malpractice theory. Reasonable patients do not ordinarily refuse consent to treatment recommended by physicians having superior medical knowledge and judgment, and most plaintiffs cannot convince a jury that the procedure would have been refused had the risk been disclosed.

When Informed Consent May Be Unnecessary

If the physician determines that the patient is not sufficiently stable to objectively weigh the risks and reach a proper decision, he may have a privilege to withhold information. The physician, however, must prove that this opinion was justified. Such proof may be based on the concurring opinion of a psychiatrist or of the patient's family. Careful documentation is essential.

The patient may spontaneously request that the physician make the decisions and not disclose the risks. This waiver of rights also requires careful documentation.

Proof of Informed Consent

The nature of the information disclosed to the patient prior to obtaining consent is probably best documented in the physician's office records or progress notes. Form letters containing this information and signed by the patient are of limited value. Since the signature does not prove that the patient read and understood the material, form letters should be supplemented by hand written notes in the medical records. Tangible evidence should show that special care was taken to satisfy the unique needs of each individual patient.

The physician's note need not be lengthy and should not contain an exhaustive list of alternatives and risks of the procedure. It should be general, covering alternatives and risks categorically. It may also be good practice to mention that the patient appeared to understand.

LIABILITY OF THE NURSE

Standards of Care

The nurse, like the physician, can be liable for breach of a professional standard of care. If the nurse is employed, her employer is also liable for her negligence and may be the primary defendant in a lawsuit. Nursing standards of care are generally based on the skill and knowledge of nurses with similar training and experience. For example, if testimony by experts shows that experienced obstetric nurses should recognize a complete prolapse of the cord and hold the fetal head off the cord until a physician arrives, less care by an experienced obstetric nurse may be negligent. Although a less experienced nurse might not be negligent in the same circumstances, the supervising nurse who assigned the duty, the hospital that failed to provide sufficient qualified personnel, or the physician who unreasonably relied on the observations of an unqualified nurse may be found negligent instead.

If the physician errs, a nurse may have a duty to call attention to the error. For example, an experienced nurse should recognize a dangerous deviation in the physician's order for a frequently used medication and inquire further before carrying out the order. Failure to do so could result in a lawsuit against both physician and nurse.

Oral Orders

Hospital policies regarding oral orders are usually clear, but have no legal effect other than to create an inference of negligence if a policy was violated. Generally, oral orders can authorize treatment by nursing or other paramedical staff. Exceptions may arise if a statute requires that certain orders, particularly those pertaining to narcotic drugs, be in writing. Whenever practical, orders should be written to prevent communication mishaps between physician and nurse. If oral orders are necessary, they should subsequently be reduced to writing. Proving the existence and precise wording of such orders several years later in a courtroom may otherwise be extremely difficult.

Emergencies

If no physician is immediately available in an emergency, nurses may provide all emergency care, including care that a physician would have otherwise given. Experienced obstetric nurses who must, for example, occasionally perform precipitous deliveries and resuscitate infants, are held to nursing standards of care and will not be liable for certain errors that physicians would not have made. Nevertheless, lawsuits may be directed at negligent hospital policies or medical decisions that permitted the medical emergency to occur with no physician present.

Alerting Physician

The nurse has a duty to call a physician when her observation of the patient indicates an urgent need for medical attention. In the absence of specific orders as to when the physician should be called, the nurse must rely on her own discretion and will be held to a standard of care commensurate with her training and experience. If a nurse is not trained to recognize a particular urgent problem, failure of the physician to write an appropriate order may be negligent. Therefore, the physician must be familiar with the training and experience of the nurses on whom he relies.

Occasionally, a physician may refuse or fail to respond to a nurse's urgent call for assistance. The nurse may then have a duty to call other physicians until she finds one who will come immediately. The period of time a nurse should wait for one physician before calling another varies with the circumstances, but it must appear reasonable if the nurse is to avoid liability.

THE DEFORMED NEWBORN INFANT

The law affecting the survival of severely deformed infants is in its formative stages. Great changes in this law may be anticipated in the near future; therefore, the concepts presented here must be based on both well-established legal principles and on prophesy. When a situation that may determine the life or death of a deformed infant arises, consultation with an attorney conversant with applicable current laws of the jurisdiction is mandatory.

From the standpoint of civil litigation, few cases involving severe and unavoidable congenital deformities have sufficient damages or jury appeal to offer substantial danger of lawsuit. Criminal prosecutors, however, tend to follow political rather than economic motives, and the indictment of physicians may provide that morbid sensationalism which readily attracts the news media. Although the jury system gives the physician excellent protection against conviction, the indictment alone may destroy a good medical reputation.

If the physician and the parents agree to provide necessary supportive care or affirmative intervention to preserve the life of a deformed newborn, no legal problems need be anticipated. The courts will not permit the child to sue for a decision that permitted his own survival. However, if the physician fails to properly disclose the extent of the deformities to the parents, thereby improperly obtaining their consent to preserve life, a lack of informed consent exists. It is very doubtful, however, that any court would entertain a lawsuit in such a case, since the basic premise of such a lawsuit would run contrary to the public policy to preserve life. The parents would first have to convince the court that they had the right to terminate their child's life: a highly improbable prospect.

If the physician recommends no supportive care or affirmative intervention despite medical indications, and the parents agree, civil lawsuit by the parents is very unlikely. The strongest basis on which the parents could have a meritorious lawsuit would probably be lack of informed consent due to the physician's failure to disclose the extent of the deformities. A jury may find that the parents would have requested proper care for the child if they had not been misled by the physician. If the child survives, with injuries aggravated by the lack of care, the lawsuit could be brought by the child as well as by the parents, and large damages are possible.

Criminal action against the physician is unlikely in cases involving failure to affirmatively intervene to save the infant's life. Failure to provide supportive care, however, may be a crime since the criminal law may impose a duty on the physician by virtue of his relationship with the helpless patient to preserve life. The extent of this duty is unclear. Basic nourishment, environmental needs and nursing care are probably required, however. If failure to provide supportive care is found to be a crime, ratifica-

tion by the parents offers no defense for the physician. A criminal act cannot be excused by the consent of anyone, including the victim.

Affirmative intervention to terminate the life of a deformed infant may result in a murder indictment against the physician. From the practical standpoint, conviction is unlikely unless the physician admits, for whatever reason, that he committed an act with intent to take a life. A jury would hesitate to convict a physician for the murder of a severely deformed newborn infant if there were any reasonable basis to find otherwise. But, nonviability of a newborn infant does not excuse the crime of murder.

If the physician refuses to treat a severely deformed infant and the parents have insufficient opportunity to obtain medical care elsewhere, a lawsuit for abandonment may result. Jury sympathy, however, would probably favor the physician.

If abandonment causes the death of a newborn infant, a criminal indictment for manslaughter is also possible.

If the physician wants to treat a deformed infant but the parents refuse consent, a court order must be obtained before treatment can be carried out. Following treatment pursuant to a court order, lawsuit against the physician for battery would be without legal basis.

If the parents refuse consent, and the physician elects not to seek a court order, thereby permitting the child to go untreated, criminal action against the parents is possible. The duty of the physician in such a case is unclear. If the courts find that the physician has a duty to seek a court order, then failure to do so may expose him to civil lawsuit by the child or to criminal prosecution if the child dies.

PERINATAL RESEARCH

Perinatal researchers should be especially familiar with two crimes. If the research terminates life a murder-manslaughter theory based on homicide may be possible. If the research involves physical or chemical contact with the fetus or neonate, a battery theory based on lack of consent may be possible.

Homicide can be committed only by terminating a life having the legal status of a person. The criminal law has traditionally defined a person as one living without reliance on maternal circulation. Thus, live birth is necessary before homicide is possible.

Without specific legislation, the criminal courts will probably continue to define the termination of life in utero as abortion and the termination of life in a spontaneously delivered neonate as homicide. But what of research that terminates life in a fetus removed from the uterus early in gestation and sustained by mechanical means? In *Roe v. Wade* and *Doe v. Bolton* described in the section Abortion, supra, the Supreme Court denied to the states the power to substantially protect the life of a fetus in the first two trimesters and thereby suggested that a previable fetus has little, if any, legal status as a person. It appears, therefore, that research which terminates the life of a previable fetus in utero with consent of the mother will probably not violate abortion laws. It is also probable that research which terminates the life of a previable fetus outside the uterus will not be homicide, although this matter may soon be better clarified in the courts.

Research on the fetus or neonate that does not produce injury may be battery despite parental consent. The courts may find that the parents' power to consent for a child is not absolute. It is likely that the courts will permit the parents to consent to experimental procedures that have direct benefit to the child or are totally innocuous, as with the simple drawing of blood samples. But the courts may determine that parents cannot consent to an experimental procedure that is of no direct benefit to the child and has a significant risk of harm.

Researchers may be able to avoid battery situations by framing their experimental protocols in terms of a medical benefit to the child. Research often produces test results that could serve as useful baseline studies if included in a patient's permanent records. Nevertheless, if the risk of harm outweighs the direct medical benefit to the child, future courts may find that the parents were without power to consent.

Another unsettled matter is the power of parents to consent to an organ transplant between sibling children. Subsequent civil lawsuit by the donor child based on a battery theory could be allowed by some courts. That the plaintiff would receive little sympathy from a jury is small consolation to the physicians involved. Without carefully worded legislation or favorable court decisions permitting such transplants, they probably carry a legal risk for the physician who performs them.

From the practical standpoint, researchers who act in good faith, without malice or substantial economic gain and for the benefit of medical science have little to fear from courts or juries. Occasionally, an attorney who seeks the benefits of publicity engendered by controversial court actions, will bring a frivolous lawsuit against researchers. These lawsuits have little chance of success. Unfortunately, our present legal system offers no effective means of controlling this problem.

Recent changes have taken place in the federal government with regard to fetal research. Most of these changes primarily involve political and ethical considerations and are, therefore, beyond the scope of this chapter. New federal statutes may regulate and even ban some aspects of fetal research since the federal legislature has broad discretion in such matters. Every researcher has a duty to be familiar with and comply with relevant statutes or possibly face prosecution for a federal crime. The increase in federal regulation of medical research will probably continue, consistent with the trend in other areas.

LEGAL TRENDS

The liability of physicians for negligence is generally based on the breach of a standard of care recognized by the medical profession. In recent years, however, the courts have shown a growing tendency to attack the practices of whole industries and professions when they conflict with the interests of the consumer. New trends in the law of informed consent are an example of court-created standards of medical care, but the most extreme example of such standards appears to be a 1974 decision by the supreme court of the state of Washington. *Helling* v. *Carey* (10) involved injury to a 32-year-old woman from undetected glaucoma. Medical experts agreed that patients under 40 are not routinely tested for glaucoma because the condition is too rare. The court, however, decided unanimously that glaucoma is so harmful and tonometry so simple and safe, that ophthalmologists must henceforth test all patients for glaucoma irrespective of age. The defendants were found liable for negligence, but this decision is probably an anomaly, and there is no indication that other states will necessarily follow it.

The implications of this type of decision could be extremely serious. If every harmless diagnostic procedure is required for every patient, irrespective of the rarity of the disorder it can detect, the resulting cost of medical care and shortage of physicians would render our present system of health care delivery unworkable.

Furthermore, three of the judges in *Helling* v. *Carey* recommended in a concurring opinion that strict liability rather than negligence be applied. Following this view, physicians would be liable for every poor medical result, and negligence would be immaterial. Such legal thinking has created the modern law of strict liability for defective products and could give rise to strict liability for defective services, including medical care that unavoidably results in injury. This is similar to the concept of no-fault medical insurance.

But certain features distinguish medical services from products. Injury from defective products is relatively rare, due often to undiscovered negligence, and easily paid for by the manufacturer. Untoward medical results, however, are common; they are usually unavoidable despite the best medical care, and they must be paid for ultimately by higher costs of medical care. Malpractice

insurers will not absorb the large losses certain to result, and a physician whose practice has an inherently high frequency of serious complications, such as an obstetrician or neonatologist, could soon find himself uninsurable.

Current legal trends seem to require that the hospital assume greater responsibility for the patient. Not only must a modern hospital provide competent personnel and safe equipment, it may have a duty to restrict the privileges of its medical staff. Common practice among hospitals now permits general and family practitioners to deliver and treat newborn infants within the hospital. Only when serious complications arise may the hospital have a duty to require consultation with a specialist. Future legal developments may require consultation in every case and eventually limit perinatal care in hospitals to specialists alone.

Hospitals probably have a duty in most states to maintain peer review and other committees for the purpose of detecting and preventing dangerous policies and habitual negligence of the medical staff. Breach of this duty may expose the hospital to lawsuit for the negligence of any physician on its staff whose dangerous practices were otherwise preventable (4). This concept may expand until hospitals require physicians to conform their entire manner of practice to rigid hospital standards in order to retain staff privileges.

Allied Health Professions

Nurse practitioners, physician's assistants, clinical pharmacists, and other allied health professionals are currently seeking greater responsibility in primary patient care. Legislation for their licensure is being drafted in some states, and training programs are expanding. However, the scope of training and responsibility in these fields is vague. Until the legislatures and courts have clarified the precise roles of allied health professionals, the physician may be forced to bear full legal responsibility for their medical decisions. The physician still retains primary responsibility for the patient and is the only member of the health care team presumed to be familiar with all aspects of the patient's problem.

The law will be slow to tolerate full delegation of any of the physician's obligations. Statutes purporting to establish the scope and responsibilities of allied health practice are not entirely reliable until interpreted by the courts. Future lawsuits against physicians may be based on inappropriate delegation of duties and failure to adequately supervise allied health professionals irrespective of legislation that appears to permit such practices.

CONCLUSION

Despite the many legal hazards discussed in this chapter, most physicians in clinical practice will rarely be confronted with legal problems. A conscientious practitioner who sets aside adequate time to communicate with his patients has little to fear from the law. If, however, a lawsuit does occur, its purpose is to compensate an injured patient. Proof of fault is a requirement of our legal system, and a lawsuit should be viewed neither as a personal attack on the integrity of the physician, nor as evidence of incompetent medical practice.

REFERENCES

1. Abbuhl RW: The Legal Responsibility of One Treating Physician for the Negligence of Another. J Legal Med 1 (4):19, 1973

2. Cobbs v. Grant, 8 Cal 3d 229, 104 Cal Rep 505, 502 P 2d 1 (1972)

3. Coe v. Gerstein, Case No. 72-1842-Cic-JE (D.C., Fla., Aug 14, 1973)

4. Darling v. Charleston Comm. Mem. Hosp., 33 Ill 2d 326, 211 NE 2d 253 (1965)

5. Doe v. Bolton, 93 S. Ct. 739 (1973)

6. Greenhill JP: Obstetrics. Philadelphia, Saunders, 1965

7. Haller JA: Pediatric Surgery. In: Principles of Surgery. Edited by S Schwartz. New York, McGraw-Hill, 1969

8. Harney DM: Medical Malpractice. Indianapolis, Allen Smith, 1973

9. Hayt E, Hayt LR, Groeschel AH: Law of Hospital, Physician and Patient. Berwyn, Ill, Physician's Record Co, 1972

10. Helling v. Carey, 519 P 2d 981 (Wash., 1974)

11. Jury Verdicts Weekly, Vol 14–18 incl. Santa Rosa, California, E. N. Raymond and Associates, 1970–1974 incl

12. Perkins RM: Criminal Law. Mineola, New York, Foundation Press, 1969

13. Prosser WL: The Law of Torts. St. Paul, West Publishing Co, 1971

14. Roe v. Wade, 93 S. Ct. 705 (1973)

15. Schaffer AJ, Avery ME: Diseases of the Newborn. Philadelphia, Saunders, 1971

16. The Citation, Vol 22–28 incl. Chicago, American Medical Association, 1971–1974 incl

Appendix A

ADDENDUM 1

PREVENTION OF PREMATURE DELIVERY
(See p. 67)

The effect of progestational agents in the prevention of premature delivery was studied by Johnson et al (1). In a controlled prospective investigation, 250 mg 17 α-hydroxyprogesterone caproate was administered intramuscularly at weekly intervals to 18 high-risk gravidas and a placebo administered to 22 matched controls. Premature delivery was not observed in the treated patients, but it occurred in 41% of those who were not treated. While the results of this study are promising, further investigations are necessary before this mode of therapy can receive widespread clinical application.

REFERENCE

1. Johnson JWC, Austin KL, Jones GS, Davis GH, King TM: Efficacy of 17 α-hydroxyprogesterone caproate in the prevention of premature labor. N Engl J Med 293:675, 1975

ADDENDUM 2

PERINATAL DIAGNOSIS OF THYROID DISORDERS
(See p. 244)

Further information of potential value in the antenatal diagnosis of thyroid disorders became available late in 1975.

Sack et al (2) measured thyroxine (T_4), free thyroxine (FT_4) and triiodothyronine (T_3) concentrations in amniotic fluid and found a progressive increase in T_4 levels with advancing gestational age. At term, amniotic fluid T_4 concentrations are much lower than either maternal or fetal serum levels. In contrast, amniotic fluid FT_4 levels are significantly higher than those found in maternal or fetal serum. T_4 and FT_4 concentrations in maternal or fetal serums do not correlate with levels in amniotic fluid of euthyroid fetuses. T_3 was undetectable in amniotic fluid.

Chopra et al (1) have found that an inactive thyroid hormone (3, 3', 5'-triiodothyronine or reverse T_3) is found in high concentrations in amniotic fluid, especially prior to the 30th week of gestation. Measurements of this hormone in amniotic fluid (especially when there is a history of fetal hypothyroidism in a previous pregnancy) may lead to diagnosis and treatment of hypothyroidism relatively early in pregnancy.

Since the placenta is relatively impermeable to thyroid hormones, treatment of the hypothyroid fetus would probably involve direct injection of the therapeutic agent into either the amniotic fluid or fetus. This has been carried out experimentally but has not yet been applied clinically.

REFERENCES

1. Chopra IJ, Crandall BF: Thyroid hormones and thyrotropin in amniotic fluid. N Engl J Med 293:740, 1975
2. Sack J, Fisher DA, Hobel CJ, Lam R: Thyroxine in human amniotic fluid. J Pediatr 87:364, 1975

ADDENDUM 3

HYPOGLYCEMIA AND HYPERAMINOACIDEMIA
(See p. 254)

It has been observed that serum concentrations of amino acids involved in gluconeogenesis (alanine, glycine, proline and valine) are significantly elevated in undergrown hypoglycemic infants (1,2). It is therefore likely that impaired hepatic gluconeogenesis is yet another factor responsible for hypoglycemia in these infants.

REFERENCES

1. Haymond MW, Karl IE, Pagliara AS: Increased gluconeogenic substrates in the small for gestational age infant. N Engl J Med 291:322, 1974
2. Mestyan J, Soltesz G, Schultz K, Horvath M: Hyperaminoacidemia due to the accumulation of gluconeogenic amino acid precursors in hypoglycemic small-for-gestational age infants. J Pediatr 87:409, 1975

ADDENDUM 4

NASOJEJUNAL FEEDING
(See p. 273)

At the end of 1975, nasojejunal (NJ) alimentation had achieved widespread successful use. Because of this, a description of the current technique for NJ feedings in our neonatal center is included.

A 15-inch radiopaque catheter (inner tube) is inserted into the lumen of a 15-inch No. 8 French feeding tube (outer tube), so that the end of the inner tube is about 1 inch distal to that of the outer tube. The two tubes are taped together securely.

The distance from the glabella to the heel of the infant is measured, and this distance is marked on the outer tube with a small piece of tape. After emptying gastric contents with a nasogastric feeding tube, the infant is attached to cardiac and respiratory monitors, and the NJ tube is inserted into the stomach through a nostril.

The infant is then positioned on his right side, and the tube is further advanced until the tape reaches the level of the nostril. During this procedure, the infant is carefully observed for signs of gagging, cyanosis, apnea, bradycardia and abdominal distension. The tube is then taped in place, and the infant is kept on his right side for about 24 hours. When alkaline, bile-colored fluid is aspirated, the end of the tube has passed into the jejunum. Anteroposterior and lateral abdominal x rays verify the position of the tube.

When the position of the tube has been ascertained, the inner radiopaque catheter is removed, and formula (0.67 calories/ml) is continuously delivered (using an infusion pump) at the rate of 80 to 100 ml/kg body weight/24 hr. Volumes are increased by 20 to 30 ml/kg/day until a volume of 180 to 200 ml/kg/day is reached. Formula must not remain at room temperature for more than 4 hours.

Loose stools and abdominal distension may occasionally be observed. Serious, life-threatening complications, such as necrotizing enterocolitis, small bowel perforation, and sepsis, have been reported.

All infants receiving NJ feedings must be very carefully observed, and the physician must be immediately notified if any changes in the clinical condition occur.

ADDENDUM 5

E. COLI K_1 ANTIGEN
(See p. 356)

Although there are over 1000 recognized *E. coli* capsular antigens, organisms having the K_1 antigen are responsible for the majority of cases of neonatal *E. coli* meningitis.[1] Organisms containing this antigen (which is morphologically and physicochemically similar to that seen in *N. meningitidis, H. influenzae, S. pneumoniae,* and *K. pneumoniae*) are transmitted to the infant by either the nursing staff or mother and are found in 20%–40% of rectal swabs obtained from a random population (including neonates). It is thought that host immune factors are responsible for the high degree of pathogenicity of the K_1 antigen for the neonate.

REFERENCE

1. Sarff LD, McCracken GH Jr, Schiffer MS, Glode MP, Robbins JB, Orskov I, Orskov F: Epidemiology of *Escherichia coli* K_1 in healthy and diseased newborns. Lancet 1:1100, 1975

Index

A

Abandonment, and litigation, 556–557
Abdomen, neonatal physical examination of, 332
Abdominal distension, and neonatal infection, 344
Abdominal pregnancy, ultrasound diagnosis of, 32
Abdominal masses, x rays of, 534, 535, 536
Abdominal surgery, 468–482
ABO incompatibility, 173–174
  diagnosis of, 181
  and hepatosplenomegaly, 432–433
Abortion(s)
  and litigation, 553–554,
  in history taking, 322
  and rubella, 70
Acetazolamide eye drops, 439
Achalasia, 432
Achondroplasia, 203, 204
Achromobacter, and meningitis, 356
Acid-base balance. See also Acid-base disturbance; Acid-base metabolism
  maintenance of, 41
  and meningitis therapy, 358
  in neonatal heroin withdrawal, 310
  in premature infants, 66
  and respiratory distress syndrome, 98
Acid-base disturbances
  combined acidosis, 223–224
  diagnostic terms for, 224
  late metabolic acidosis, 224–225
  metabolic acidosis, 224
  respiratory acidosis, 224
  respiratory alkalosis, 224
  and vomiting, 224
Acid-base metabolism, 220, 221–225
  disturbances of. See Acid-base disturbances
  and fetal physiology, 221
  in neonatal period, 221, 223–225
Acid citrate dextrose, and exchange transfusion in neonatal jaundice, 183

Acid elution (Kleihauer) technique, 162
Acidemia, and pulmonary atresia with intact ventricular septum, 139
Acidosis. See also Combined acidosis; Metabolic acidosis; Respiratory acidosis
  and congestive heart failure, 122
  and fetal oxygenation, 45
  and intravenous fluid therapy, 214–215
Acne, neonatal, 83
Adenocarcinoma of vagina, 400
Adenoviruses, and infectious diarrhea, 362
Adenylic kinase, and fetal malnutrition, 76
Adipose tissue, development of, 266
Admission, to normal nursery, 316
Adrenal cortex
  clinical aspects, 233–239
  congenital hyperplasia of, 235–239, 437
  fetal development and function of, 232–233
  and fluid and electrolyte balance, 213
  hemorrhage, 234–235, 421
  hypoplasia, 239
  normal neonatal, 233
Adrenocortical-pituitary axis, fetal, 233
Adrenogenital syndrome. See also Congenital adrenal hyperplasia
  and polycythemia, 163
  and vomiting, 431–432
Afferent limb, and perinatal immunology, 349
Aganglionosis, of colon, 539
Age
  gestational. See Gestational age
  maternal. See Maternal age
Agenesis of lung, surgery for, 447–448
Aircraft, for neonatal transport, 5, 7
Air Shields Negative Pressure Respirator, 107
Airway canalization, 89–90

Airway obstruction, surgery for, 443–447
Albinism, 265
Albumin
  and bilirubin metabolism, 169, 176–177
  -binding tests, 182
  and neonatal jaundice therapy, 188
Alcohol ingestion, in obstetric history, 323
Aldactone. See Spironolactone
Aldrich's syndrome, 168
Alkali infusion
  and metabolic acidosis, 76
  and resuscitation, 53
Allied health professions, and litigation, 567–568
Allopuranol, and Lesch-Nyhan syndrome, 265
Alpha-1-antitrypsin
  deficiency, neonatal jaundice and, 174
  respiratory distress syndrome and, 99
Alveoli
  at birth, 114
  and pulmonary surfactant, 93
Ambient temperature, and survival, 285–286
Ambiguous genitalia, 240, 437
  diagnostic criteria, 241–242
  management, 242
Ames Dextrostix, 256
Amino acid metabolism
  and maple sugar urine disease, 264–265
  and methymalonic acidemia, 265
  and neonatal seizures, 197
  and protein metabolism, 260–261
Aminoglycosides, 410–411
Aminopterin, congenital anomalies and, 402
Ammonia metabolism, 265–266
Amniocentesis, 36–37
  and genetic counseling, 303
  interpretation of, 178–179
  and Rh incompatibility, 177, 178, 179
Amnion mounts, and amniotic infection syndrome, 343
Amnionitis, maternal, and neonatal gastroenteritis, 484–485

R

Race
  and glucose-6-phosphate
    dehydrogenase deficiency,
    181
  in history taking, 322
  and Mongolian spots, 81
  in neonatal history, 324
  and perinatal morbidity and
    mortality, 20
  and preeclampsia, 21
  and prematurity, 64
  and Rh incompatibility, 173
  and sole crease development,
    73–74
Radiant heaters, 12, 283–284
  and assisted ventilation, 107–
    108
  and lumbar puncture, 357–358
  in neonatal resuscitation, 52
  and prematurity, 67
  for transport vehicles, 5
Radiant heat loss, and heat dis-
    sipation, 279
Radiation therapy
  and arteriovenous fistulae,
    123
  and hemangiomas, 88
Radioactive iodine uptake,
    maternal, 401
Radiology. See Neonatal
    radiology
Rales, in neonatal chest
    examination, 330
RBCs. See Red blood cells
RDS. See Respiratory distress
    syndrome
Reciprocal translocation, in-
    heritance of, 295
Recoil and ability, and evalua-
    tion of muscle tone, 338
Record-keeping, 18
Recovery area for post-cardiac
    surgery patients, 149
Rectal atresia, 491
Red blood cells
  and bilirubin metabolism, 169
  fetal formation of, 155–156
  increased hemolysis of. See
    Hemolytic disease of new-
    born
  and malaria diagnosis, 395
  and neonatal jaundice, 174
Reflexes, and evaluation of
    muscle tone, 338–339
Regional transport, and inten-
    sive care, 4–10
Renal anomalies, 329
Renal development
  embryonic, 207, 208
  and polycystic disease, 208–
    209
  and renal dysplasia, 208
Renal dysplasia, 208
Renal polycystic disease, x rays
    of, 538

Renal tumors, x rays of, 535, 536
Renal vascular insults, x rays of,
    538
Renal vein, and pulmonary dis-
    tress, 421
Renal vein thrombosis, and
    infectious diarrhea, 360
Resection of lobe, 449
Reserpine, effects on neonates,
    406
Respirations, neonatal, 90, 91,
    92
  in perinatal asphyxia, 49–50
  and physical examination, 325
  and pulmonary sufactant, 93
  and respiratory distress syn-
    drome, 94–95
  stabilization of, 92
Respirators, 5, 106–107
Respiratory acidosis, 224. See
    also Acid base disorders
  and assisted ventilation, 106
Respiratory alkalosis, 224. See
    also Acid base disorders
Respiratory collapse, and
    pulmonary hemorrhage,
    102
Respiratory depression, 308
Respiratory distress. See also
    Respiratory distress syn-
    drome
  and acquired pulmonary dis-
    ease, 420–421
  bony causes of, 532
  and congenital anomalies of
    respiratory tract, 419–420
  differential diagnosis of
    tachypnea and, 418–421
  and Group B streptococci, 377
  metabolic acidosis, and, 419
  narcotic withdrawal and, 418–
    419
  in neonatal physical exami-
    nation, 325
  nonpulmonary causes of, 421
  and polycythemia, 163
  prolonged, 100–102
  surgical causes, 532–533
  in total anomalous pulmonary
    venous connection, 136
  and transposition of great
    arteries, 132
Respiratory distress syndrome
    (RDS), 66, 92–100, 333,
    420
  antenatal diagnosis of, 96, 97
  and assisted ventilation, 104
  atypical, and cyanosis, 424–
    425
  chest x rays and, 529, 530, 531
  clinical manifestations of, 94–
    95
  and continuous distending
    airway pressure, 105–106
  differential diagnosis of, 95–96
  differentiation from total
    anomalous pulmonary
    venous connection, 137

Respiratory distress syndrome
    (*continued*)
  etiology of, 92–94
  follow-up of infants with, 100
  and intracranial bleeding, 201
  and litigation, 559
  and metabolic acidosis, 48
  in neonatal chest examination,
    330
  in neonatal lung examination,
    331
  and neonatal narcotic with-
    drawal, 309
  and neonatal oxygenation,
    46–48
  and patent ductus arteriosus,
    128
  pathologic factors, 99–100
  and physician-parent relation-
    ship, 319
  postnatal diagnosis of, 97–98
  prevention and treatment of,
    98–99
Respiratory failure, causes of,
    104
Respiratory monitors, 13, 14
Respiratory patterns, in neonatal
    chest examination, 330
Respiratory rate, in neonatal
    physical examination,
    326, 330
Respiratory tract, congenital
    anomalies of, 419–420
Respiratory virus infections, 392
Resuscitation
  and alkali infusion, 53
  and cardiac massage, 53
  in delivery room, 325
  equipment for, 50–51
  and pallor, 425
  and umbilical blood vessel
    catheterization, 54–55
Reticulocyte counts, neonatal,
    157
Retina. See also Retrolental
    fibroplasia
  in neonatal examination, 329
  and overoxygenation, 40
Retinitis, and toxoplasmosis,
    387
Retrolental fibroplasia
  active stages of, 59, 60
  cicatricial stages of, 60
  clinical considerations, 60–61
  and embryology, 59
  and glaucoma, 439
  historical background, 58–59
  and litigation, 559
  pathophysiology, 59–60
  prediction of, 67
Retroperitoneal teratomas, 500
Rh antibodies, 172–173
  immunization against, 177
Rh incompatibility, 172–173.
    See also Hemolytic dis-
    ease
  with ABO incompatibility, 174
  and amniocentesis, 37